MRI of the Upper Extremity

Bethany U. Casagranda
Editor

MRI of the Upper Extremity

Elbow, Wrist, and Hand

Springer

Editor
Bethany U. Casagranda
Department of Radiology
Imaging Institute, Allegheny Health Network
Pittsburgh, PA
USA

ISBN 978-3-030-81611-7 ISBN 978-3-030-81612-4 (eBook)
https://doi.org/10.1007/978-3-030-81612-4

This Springer imprint is published by the registered company Springer Nature Switzerland AG
The registered company address is: Gewerbestrasse 11, 6330 Cham, Switzerland

Acknowledgement

To the authors,

I would like to extend my deepest gratitude to every author of this female-dominant project who displayed their talents on the pages of this book. Some of you are my idols, my mentors, my colleagues and my former trainees. All of you are strong, brilliant and remarkable. Continue to contribute to this world as much as you do our beloved field and the world certainly will be a brighter place.

~BUC

To my daughters, Isabella and Eva Helene

I hope my work and service in this life pave a deliberate path in your life. A path where your voice will be easily heard, your place will be visibly present and your talents will be enthusiastically encouraged. The world needs all you have to offer. So when an opportunity arises to better the lives of a few or of many...

Give it all you've got!

~mom

To my husband, Dennis

I am thankful for the encouragement and patience it took to get our household through this project and all the daily endeavours we tackle as a family. Your direct contribution to this book is also appreciated. Any author would be grateful for such an excellent (and affordable) hand model. Much love and gratitude.

~BUC

Introduction

The upper extremity begins proximally at the shoulder and extends distally through the hand. *Shoulder is excluded from this text because it is discussed in a dedicated Springer book entitled MRI: Shoulder.* This text covers the biomechanical importance, anatomy, traumatic pathology and non-traumatic pathology of the remaining upper extremity joints.

Joint Structure

Joints can be classified by their structure and function. The basis for classifying the joint structure involves defining the material composing the joint and the presence or absence of a cavity. Structural classification of joints includes fibrous, cartilaginous and synovial joints. Fibrous joints, such as the cranial sutures, are bound by connective tissue and have no "joint space" or cavity. Therefore, fibrous joints are strong but produce very little movement. Cartilaginous joints include the articulations of the spine and pelvis and are either lined or connected to hyaline or fibrocartilage. Cartilaginous joints allow slightly more movement when compared to fibrous joints. Lastly, synovial joints are the only joints to structurally have a cavity or space between bones. This cavity is lined with synovium and occupied by synovial fluid. Synovial joints, supported by several static and dynamic stabilizers, allow for the greatest amount of joint movement allowing one to achieve daily acts of living [1]. All joints of the upper extremity are synovial joints allowing varying degrees of motion. However, the benefit of motion brings an increased vulnerability to injury.

Joint Function

Functional classification of the joint is determined by the motion produced when under force. The six types of synovial joints include pivot or rotary, hinge, saddle, plane, ball-and-socket and condyloid [2]. The upper extremity impressively comprises all of these joint types allowing gross and fine motor movement.

The shoulder joint is a ball-and-socket joint, although it is more correctly described as a ball-and-saucer joint. In contrast to the hip, the other ball-and-socket joint of the body, the socket is much shallower. This allows for less restriction of movement at the joint but compromises stability in the process. The elbow joint commonly referred to as a hinge joint which partially true but does not explain the ability to pronate and supinate the forearm. The articulation of the radial head and the radial notch on the ulna allows for this motion. This creates what is called a "pivot" joint, allowing the movement of one bone on another. The radiocarpal joint can be classified as an ellipsoidal or condyloid joint. Despite the intercarpal articulations being synovial joints, unlike their counterparts, they do not allow much movement. The interphalangeal joints of the hand are basic hinge joints [3]

Importance of the Upper Extremity

Many of our activities of daily living require proper function of the upper extremity including personal hygiene, dressing and feeding. More complex tasks categorized as instrumental activities of daily living also utilize the function of the upper extremity such as transportation, shopping, and meal preparation and overall household management. All of these tasks can be made incredibly difficult if pain or injury has rendered our upper extremity ineffective or if the patient has difficulty ambulating. Arm swing is an important component of human gait [4]. Despite being bipedal, literature shows how effective arm swing can help create core balance, improve breathing and decrease metabolic energy expenditure necessary to ambulate [5, 6]. Proper use of the upper extremity allows us to interact with the world. Therefore, the recognition of injury to its many parts carries great importance.

References

1. Classification of Joints | Boundless Anatomy and Physiologycourses.lumenlearning.com › boundless-ap › chapter.
2. The six types of synovial joints: examples & definition. *Study.com*, 20 Dec 2015, https://study.com/academy/lesson/the-six-types-of-synovial-joints-examples-definition.html. Chapter 14 / Lesson 1 Dominic Corsini
3. Forro SD, Munjal A, Lowe JB. Anatomy, shoulder and upper limb, arm structure and function. StatPearls Last Update: 10 Aug 2020.
4. Massé J. Advance Physical Therapy. The importance of arm swing during walking and running. 19 Dec 2016.
5. Meyns P, Bruijn SM, Duysens J. The how and why of arm swing during human walking. Gait Posture. 2013;38(4):555–62. PMID: 23489950.
6. Umberger BR. Effects of suppressing arm swing on kinematics, kinetics, and energetics of human walking. J Biomech. 2008;41:2575–80. S0021-9290(08)00271-6.

Contents

1 **Elbow: Importance and Biomechanics** 1
Bethany U. Casagranda

2 **Elbow: Anatomy and MRI Optimization** 5
Eira S. Roth and Lulu He

3 **Elbow Pathology: Traumatic** 37
Lindsay Stratchko, Lauren Ladd, and Donna G. Blankenbaker

4 **Elbow Pathology: Nontraumatic** 85
Sara M. Bahouth and Connie Chang

5 **Wrist: Importance and Biomechanics** 109
Bethany U. Casagranda

6 **Wrist: Anatomy and MRI Optimization** 113
Asako Yamamoto, Brady K. Huang, and Christine B. Chung

7 **Wrist Pathology – Traumatic** 133
Teresa T. Martin-Carreras and Jenny T. Bencardino

8 **Wrist Pathology: Non-traumatic** 151
Amanda M. Crawford, Maryam Soltanolkotabi, and Nancy Major

9 **Hand: Importance and Biomechanics** 183
Bethany U. Casagranda

10 **Hand – Anatomy and MRI Optimization** 189
Tetyana Gorbachova, Angela Atinga, and Linda Probyn

11 **Hand Pathology: Traumatic** 213
Erin F. Alaia

12 **Thumb Pathology – Traumatic** 229
Sarah I. Kamel and Suzanne S. Long

13 **Hand Pathology: Nontraumatic** 247
James Korf and M. K. Jesse

Index 275

Contributors

Erin F. Alaia Department of Radiology, Musculoskeletal Division, NYU Langone Health/NYU Langone Orthopedic Hospital, New York, NY, USA

Angela Atinga Department of Medical Imaging, University of Toronto, Sunnybrook Health Sciences Centre, Toronto, ON, Canada

Sara M. Bahouth Division of Musculoskeletal Imaging and Intervention, Massachusetts General Hospital, Boston, MA, USA

Jenny T. Bencardino Department of Radiology, Division of Musculoskeletal Imaging, Hospital of the University of Pennsylvania, Philadelphia, PA, USA

Donna G. Blankenbaker University of Wisconsin School of Medicine and Public Health, Madison, WI, USA

Bethany U. Casagranda Department of Radiology, Imaging Institute, Allegheny Health Network, Pittsburgh, PA, USA

Connie Chang Division of Musculoskeletal Imaging and Intervention, Massachusetts General Hospital, Boston, MA, USA

Christine B. Chung Department of Radiology, University of California San Diego, La Jolla, CA, USA

Department of Radiology, VA San Diego Healthcare System and University of California San Diego, La Jolla, CA, USA

Amanda M. Crawford Department of Radiology, University of Utah, Salt Lake City, UT, USA

Tetyana Gorbachova Department of Radiology, Einstein Healthcare Network, Sidney Kimmel Medical College at Thomas Jefferson University, Philadelphia, PA, USA

Lulu He Department of Radiology, Imaging Institute, Allegheny Health Network, Pittsburgh, PA, USA

Brady K. Huang Department of Radiology, University of California San Diego, La Jolla, CA, USA

M. K. Jesse University of Colorado, Department of Radiology, Musculoskeletal Radiology and Intervention, Aurora, CO, USA

Sarah I. Kamel Department of Musculoskeletal Radiology, Thomas Jefferson University Hospital, Philadelphia, PA, USA

James Korf University of Colorado, Department of Radiology, Musculoskeletal Radiology and Intervention, Aurora, CO, USA

Lauren Ladd Indiana University School of Medicine, Indianapolis, IN, USA

Suzanne S. Long Department of Musculoskeletal Radiology, Thomas Jefferson University Hospital, Philadelphia, PA, USA

Nancy Major Department of Radiology, University of Colorado, Aurora, CO, USA

Teresa T. Martin-Carreras Department of Radiology, Division of Musculoskeletal Imaging and Intervention, University of Wisconsin Hospital and Clinics, Madison, WI, USA

Linda Probyn Department of Medical Imaging, University of Toronto, Sunnybrook Health Sciences Centre, Toronto, ON, Canada

Eira S. Roth Department of Radiology, Virtual Radiologic, Eden Prairie, MN, USA

Maryam Soltanolkotabi Department of Radiology, University of Utah, Salt Lake City, UT, USA

Lindsay Stratchko University of Wisconsin School of Medicine and Public Health, Madison, WI, USA

Asako Yamamoto Department of Radiology, University of California San Diego, La Jolla, CA, USA

Elbow: Importance and Biomechanics

1

Bethany U. Casagranda

Elbow

> The moral arc of the universe bends at the elbow of justice. —Civil Rights Leader: Martin Luther King, Jr.

Importance and Biomechanics of the Elbow

The elbow joint serves as the important midpoint between the shoulder and the hand. Its concerted efforts with other joints of the upper extremity facilitate an arc of hand placement in space. This allows for lengthening and shortening of the upper extremity as necessary to grasp objects and navigate through the environment. It is comprised of several osseous and soft tissue structures that confer stability to the joint and contribute to its kinematics [1, 2].

Specifically, the elbow is comprised of three joints enveloped by a synovial capsule: ulnohumeral joint, radiocapitellar joint, and proximal radioulnar joint (PRUJ). Boney articulations of the joints and immediately adjacent ligaments act as static (passive) stabilizers. Dynamic (active) stabilizers refer to the surrounding musculature. Scientific literature has produced an abundance of research regarding the biomechanics and stabilizing structures of the elbow. These works have identified the key primary and secondary stabilizers along with description of how injuries to these stabilizers affect the elbow's function [3, 4].

Three primary static constraints include the ulnohumeral joint, the anterior bundle of ulnar collateral ligament (UCL), and the lateral collateral ligament (LCL) complex. The LCL complex is defined as the radial collateral ligament, lateral ulnar collateral ligament, and annular ligament. Stability relies on the ulnohumeral joint, the anterior bundle of UCL, and the LCL complex being intact. Secondary stabilizers include the radiocapitellar joint, common flexor tendon, common extensor tendon, and joint capsule. Dynamic stabilizers are comprised of muscles that cross the elbow articulations. The lines of pull from contraction of these muscles create balanced forces within the joint and produce motion [4, 5]. All of these components come together to form the "ring" concept of elbow stability (Fig. 1.1) [1].

Primary motion of the elbow at the level of the ulnohumeral joint is flexion/extension with the center of rotation involving 2–3 mm of area at the trochlea as described originally by Fischer in 1909 (Fig. 1.2). This hinge joint produces an axis of rotation revolving around an imaginary line between the inferior medial epicondyle and the center of the lateral epicondyle [4, 6]. The coronoid process acts as a buttress in prevention of posterior dislocation.

B. U. Casagranda (✉)
Department of Radiology, Imaging Institute, Allegheny Health Network, Pittsburgh, PA, USA
e-mail: bethany.casagranda@ahn.org

B. U. Casagranda (ed.), *MRI of the Upper Extremity*, https://doi.org/10.1007/978-3-030-81612-4_1

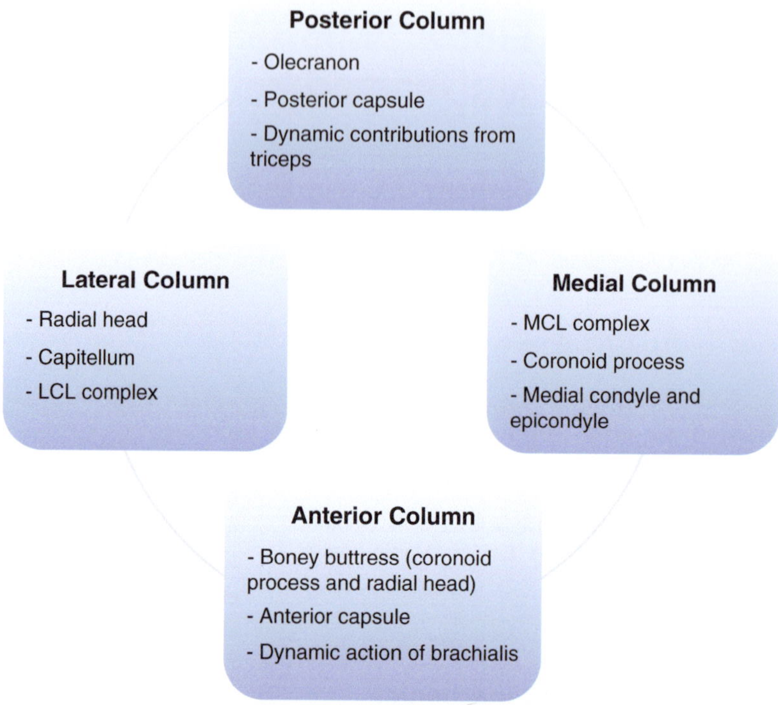

Fig. 1.1 "Ring" concept of elbow stability. (Copyright credit [1])

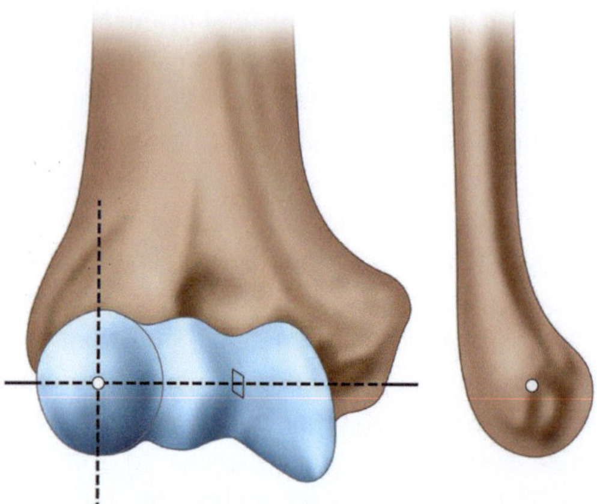

Fig. 1.2 Axis of rotation for flexion/extension of the elbow

The coronoid fossa houses the coronoid process in the setting of deep elbow flexion [7]. Normal elbow range of motion is from 0° to 150 and is limited by the previously described static and dynamic stabilizers. Specific factors limiting extension include the relationship of the olecranon with the olecranon fossa, the tension of the anterior bundle of the UCL, and the common flexor muscle group. Factors limiting flexion include the relationship of the coronoid process with the coronoid fossa, the radial head against the radial notch, the capsular tension, and the triceps muscle [4, 6].

Primary motion of the elbow at the level of the PRUJ is supination/pronation. This pivot joint produces an axis of rotation revolving around an imaginary line between the proximal radial head and the convex articular surface of the adjacent ulna known as the radial notch. Forearm rotation averages 75° pronation and 85° supination. Pronation and supination motions are restricted mostly by the passive stretch of antagonistic muscles as well as the quadrate ligament [4, 6].

With the arm extended in anatomic position, the humerus does not perfectly align with the bone of the forearm. This deviation from a straight line toward the thumb is referred to as the "carrying angle" (CA) of the elbow (Fig. 1.3). The purpose of the CA is to allow the arms to swing passed the hips unimpeded during normal gait. Recent studies have found the CA tends to

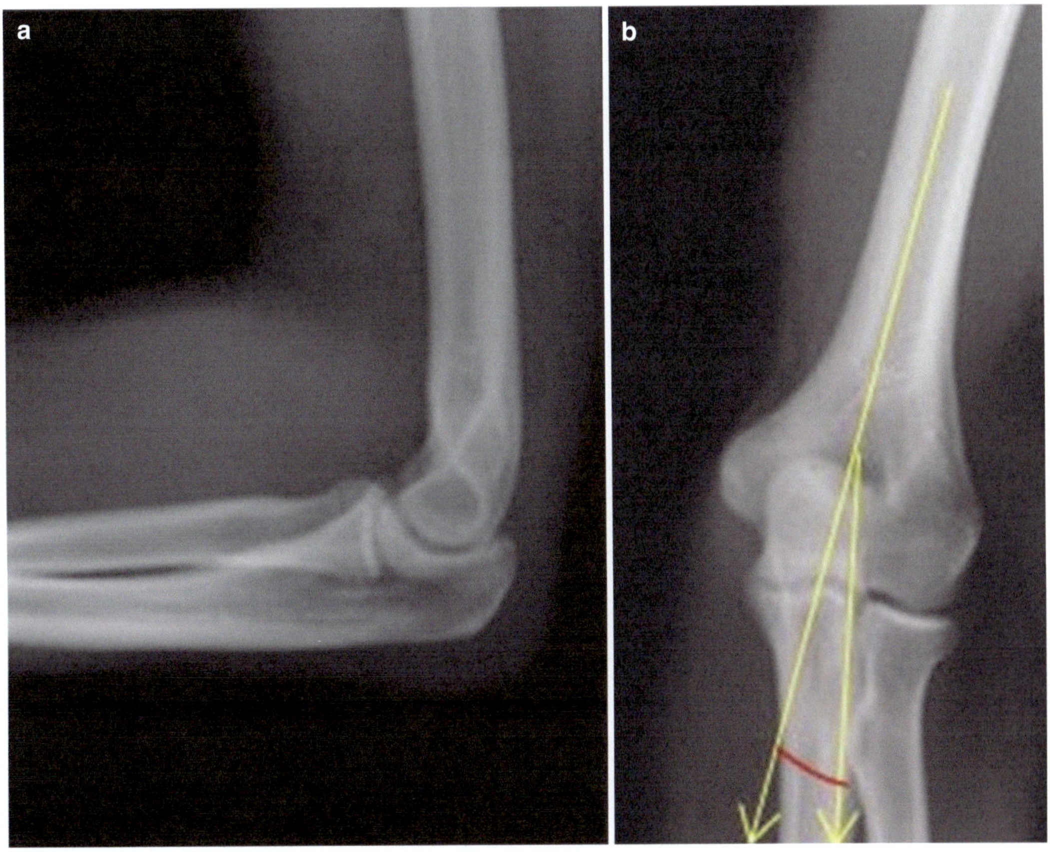

Fig. 1.3 Carrying angle. Lateral (**a**) and anteroposterior (**b**) radiographs of the elbow. AP radiograph annotated with carrying angle measurement

Table 1.1 Normal carrying angle measurements

Average carrying angle measurements	Degrees of variability
All: 12.88°	±5.92°
Men: 10.97°	±4.27°
Women: 15.07°	±4.95°

be larger in women than men with the difference being attributed to most women having smaller shoulders and wider hips than most men (Table 1.1). Regardless of gender, the CA is larger in the dominant hand when compared to the nondominant hand lending to the theory that increased forces on the joint increase the CA. Variability in CA has been found when comparing differences in stage of development, race, and age [8–10].

References

1. Aquilina AL, Grazette AJ. Clinical anatomy and assessment of the elbow. Open Orthop J. 2017;11:1347–52. https://doi.org/10.2174/1874325001711011347. PMID: 29290874; PMCID: PMC5721323.
2. Dimon T. The body of motion: its evolution and design. Berkeley: North Atlantic Books; 2011. p. 39–42.
3. Bryce CD, Armstrong AD. Anatomy and biomechanics of the elbow. Orthop Clin North Am. 2008;39(2):141–54, v. https://doi.org/10.1016/j.ocl.2007.12.001. PMID: 18374805.
4. Fornalski S, Gupta R, Lee TQ. Anatomy and biomechanics of the elbow joint. Tech Hand Up Extrem Surg. 2003;7(4):168–78. https://doi.org/10.1097/00130911-200312000-00008. PMID: 16518218.
5. O'Driscoll SW, Jupiter JB, King GJ, Hotchkiss RN, Morrey BF. The unstable elbow. Instr Course Lect. 2001;50:89–102. PMID: 11372363.
6. Morrey BF, editor. The elbow and its disorders. Philadelphia: WB Saunders; 2000.

7. Savoie FH. Orthobullets. Elbow anatomy & biomechanics. American Shoulder and Elbow Surgeons Updated: 2019 Dec 24. Available from: https://www.orthobullets.com/shoulder-and-elbow/3078/elbow-anatomy-and-biomechanics.
8. Steel FL, Tomlinson JD. The carrying angle in man. J Anat. 1958;92(2):315–7. PMID: 13525245; PMCID: PMC1249704.
9. Paraskevas G, Papadopoulos A, Papaziogas B, Spanidou S, Argiriadou H, Gigis J. Study of the carrying angle of the human elbow joint in full extension: a morphometric analysis. Surg Radiol Anat. 2004;26(1):19–23. https://doi.org/10.1007/s00276-003-0185-z. Epub 2003 Nov 26. PMID: 14648036.
10. Tükenmez M, Demirel H, Perçin S, Tezeren G. Measurement of the carrying angle of the elbow in 2,000 children at ages six and fourteen years. Acta Orthop Traumatol Turc. 2004;38(4):274–6. Turkish. PMID: 15618770.

2 Elbow: Anatomy and MRI Optimization

Eira S. Roth and Lulu He

The elbow is a unique and dynamic joint that provides a transition from the anatomic arm to the anatomic forearm. It is the second most commonly injured joint in the upper extremity, accounting for up to 20% of sports-related injuries, and merits particular attention by radiologists [1]. The elbow is comprised of three osseous articulations [2, 3]: the articulation made between the distal humerus and ulna, between the distal humerus and radius, and between the proximal ulna and the proximal radius. These are termed the ulnohumeral (also referred to as ulnotrochlear joint), radiocapitellar, and radioulnar joints, respectively (Fig. 2.1) [3].

The ulnohumeral and radiocapitellar joints create a synovial hinge joint, permitting arm flexion and extension [2–7]. The ulnohumeral joint serves as the primary osseous stabilizer of the elbow particularly when the arm is moved through the extremes of arm flexion and extension, such as when the elbow experiences greater than 120 degrees of flexion or less than 20 degrees of flexion [7, 8]. The radioulnar joint is formed by the abutment of the radial head with the radial notch of the ulna and functions as a pivot joint, thereby permitting forearm pronation and supination [7, 9].

When evaluating osseous anatomy, it is important to understand which components are considered principle stabilizers, since injury or instrumentation to these structures may predispose to joint instability. For instance, the olecranon process of the proximal ulna serves as a primary stabilizer in the prevention of anteroposterior displacement as the trochlear notch, also called the semilunar notch because of its crescent shape, encircles the trochlea by almost 180° (Fig. 2.2) [4, 8]. The coronoid process of the proximal ulna located anteriorly also serves to prevent posterior ulnohumeral dislocation [10, 11].

For the purposes of an anatomic review, elbow anatomy will be divided into four principle compartments. This approach is advocated when using ultrasound to evaluate the elbow, wherein the elbow anatomy is split into anterior, posterior, medial, and lateral compartments (Fig. 2.3) [12]. This organization can be applied to any modality but is particularly useful in approaching elbow MR imaging. The following sections review conventional elbow anatomy of each compartment as well as common anomalous anatomy including variations in origins, insertions, morphologies, or courses of the ligaments, tendons, and muscles. The most commonly encountered accessory muscles are also discussed.

E. S. Roth (✉)
Department of Radiology, Virtual Radiologic, Eden Prairie, MN, USA
e-mail: Eira.Roth@vrad.com

L. He
Department of Radiology, Imaging Institute, Allegheny Health Network, Pittsburgh, PA, USA
e-mail: Lulu.He@AHN.org

B. U. Casagranda (ed.), *MRI of the Upper Extremity*, https://doi.org/10.1007/978-3-030-81612-4_2

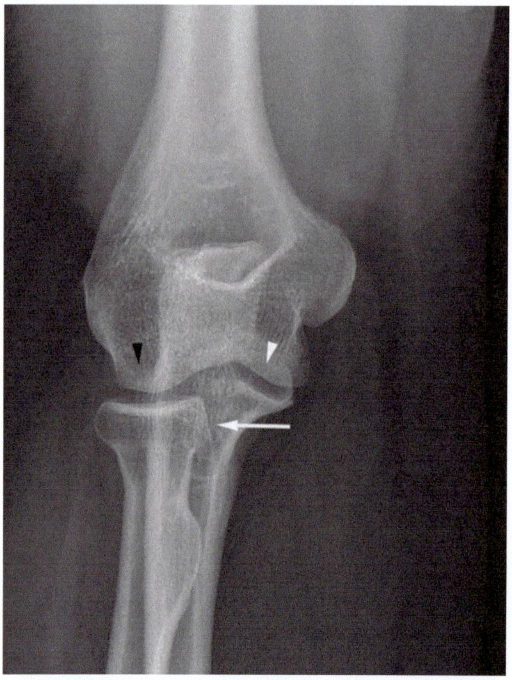

Fig. 2.1 AP radiograph of the elbow demonstrating the radiocapitellar joint (black arrowhead), ulnohumeral joint (white arrowhead), and radioulnar joint (white arrow)

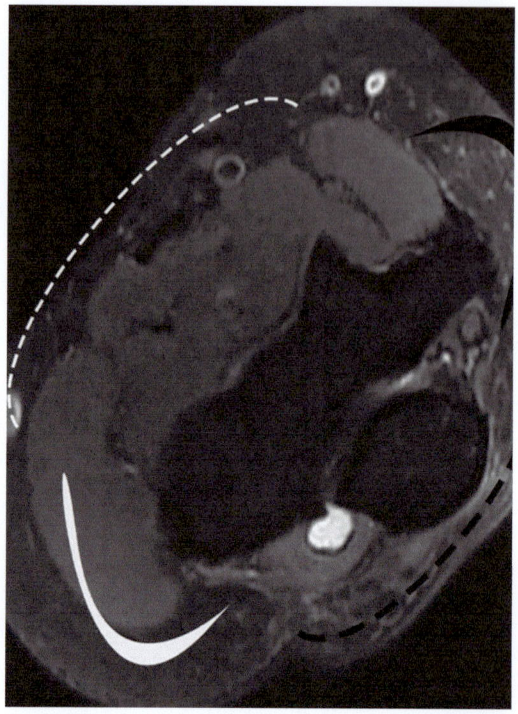

Fig. 2.3 AX PDFS image of the elbow showing the anterior compartment (white dashed arc), posterior compartment (black dashed arc), medial compartment (solid black arc), and lateral compartment (solid white arc)

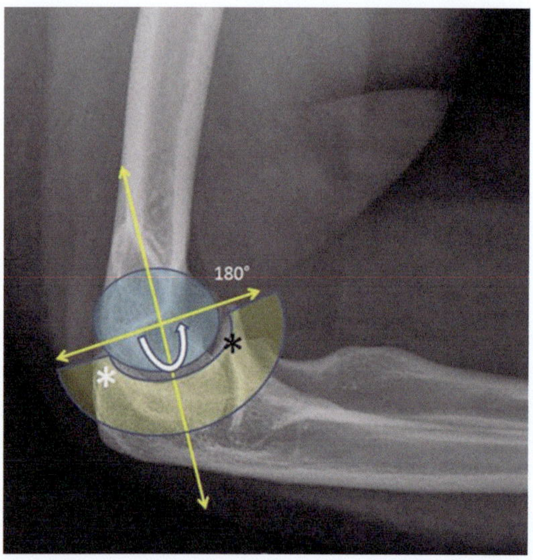

Fig. 2.2 Osseous stabilizers. Lateral radiograph of the elbow flexed 90° shows the trochlear notch of the ulna encircling the trochlea approximately 180°. The ulnohumeral joint is stabilized by the olecranon process posteriorly (white *) and the coronoid process anteriorly (black *)

The Anterior Compartment

Anterior Compartment Muscles

The anterior compartment consists of the ligaments, muscles, and tendons that reside deep and adjacent to the cubital fossa. The cubital fossa is also referred to as the antecubital fossa and is the visible skin and soft tissue depression that forms the anterior transition from the distal arm to the proximal forearm. Anatomically, the superior border is considered "an imaginary line" connecting the humeral epicondyles. The supinator and brachialis muscles form the inferior boundary, while the pronator teres is the medial margin, and the brachioradialis is the lateral margin, with the overlying skin as the "roof" (Fig. 2.4a) [5]. Deep to the cubital fossa, the anterior compartment contains three "B" muscle flexors and their distal

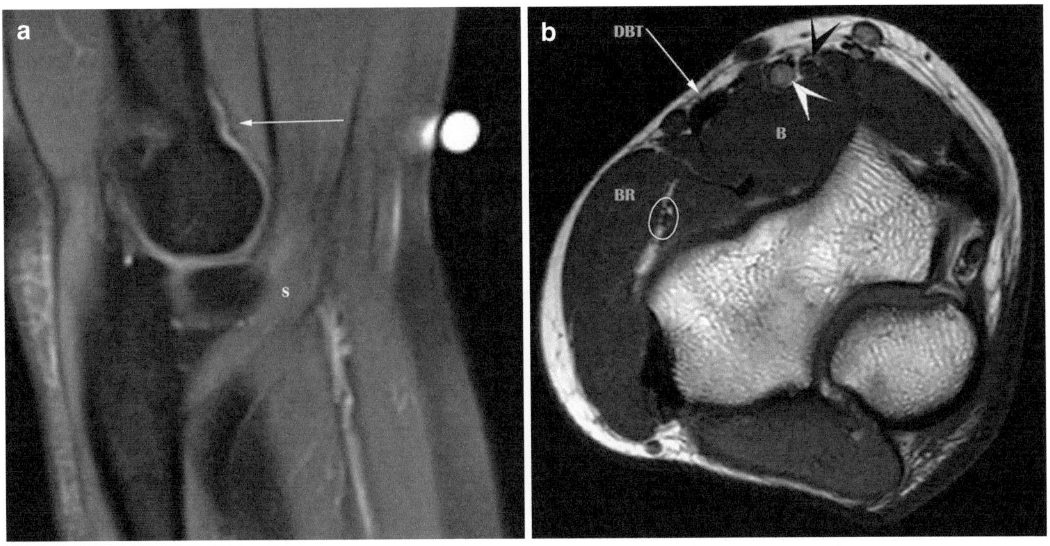

Fig. 2.4 (**a**) SAG TIFS POST with skin marker overlying the antecubital fossa, which extends from the humeral epicondyles superiorly (white arrow) to the supinator (S) and brachialis (not annotated) muscles inferiorly. (**b**) AX T1 shows the contents of the antecubital fossa and anterior compartment. These include the distal biceps and its tendon (DBT), the brachialis (B) and brachioradialis (BR) muscles, the median nerve (black arrowhead), the brachial artery (white arrowhead), and the branches of the radial nerve (circle)

tendons (Fig. 2.4b). They include the biceps brachii, brachialis, and brachioradialis. These, along with the median nerve, radial nerve, and brachial artery, are the principle anatomic structures evaluated when reviewing an elbow MRI. During ultrasound evaluation, anatomic inspection should also include a search for the anterior elbow fat pad and anterior synovial recess [1].

The Biceps Brachii

The first "B" anterior compartment muscle is the biceps brachii. The biceps originates proximally at the level of the shoulder as two separate heads. The long or lateral head originates from the supraglenoid tubercle. The short or medial head arises from the coracoid process of the scapula [4]. Distally, the biceps muscle belly provides dynamic reinforcement of the anterior elbow joint capsule, which is typically collapsed against the distal anterior humerus [8]. The conventional belief regarding the biceps is that both muscular heads merge, forming a single distal biceps tendon (DBT) that then descends obliquely to insert on the radial tuberosity of the proximal radius (Fig. 2.5a, b) [13]. Unlike other arm flexors, the biceps muscle is relatively short, with a long exposed distal tendon that measures an average of 7 cm long [1]. Furthermore, the tendon lacks a protective vascular sheath and instead relies on an extra-synovial paratenon similar to the Achilles tendon of the ankle [1]. The relatively exposed design of the distal tendon makes the DBT more vulnerable to injury.

The biceps is innervated by motor branches of the musculocutaneous nerve (C5–C7) and receives its blood supply from the muscular branches of the brachial artery. The biceps brachii participates in both elbow flexion and forearm supination [14]. When the arm is held in the neutral position, meaning that the palm of the hand is facing the ipsilateral thigh, the biceps primarily assists with forearm supination, permitting the palm to be rotated to face anteriorly. The biceps flexes the arm at the elbow when the forearm is held in the neutral and supinated positions. The combined actions of arm flexion and forearm supination create a proper biceps curl technique which necessitates rotation of the forearm from the neutral position followed by forward elbow flexion. This technique allows engagement of both biceps brachii components when performed properly.

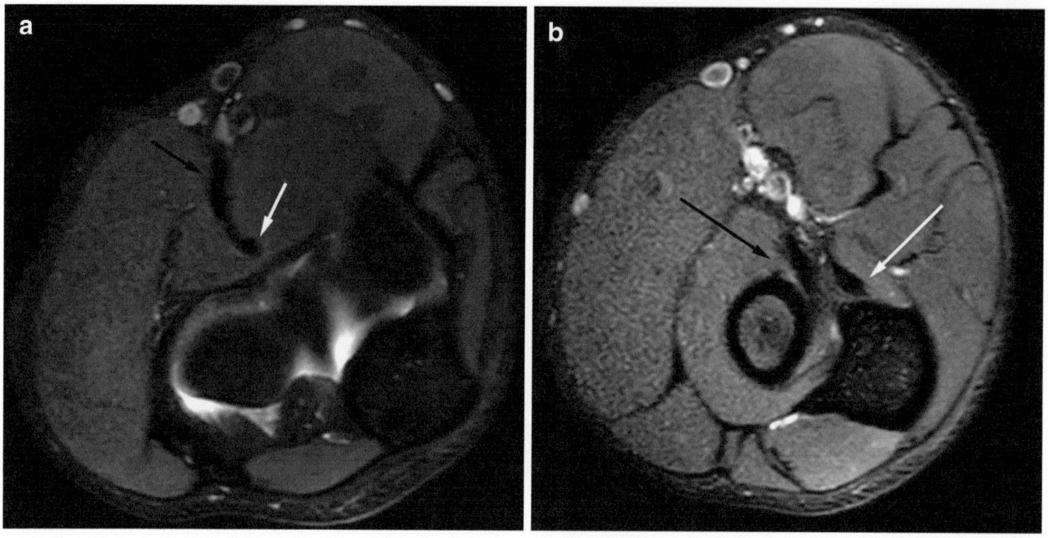

Fig. 2.5 (**a**) AX PDFS illustrating the superficial course of the biceps brachii (black arrow) relative to the brachialis tendon (white arrow). (**b**) AX PDFS – The DBT inserts on the radial tuberosity (black arrow), while the brachialis inserts on the coronoid process (white arrow) and ulnar tuberosity (not shown)

A common biceps variant is a bifurcated DBT believed to arise secondary from failed fusion between the two proximal biceps myotendinous components (Fig. 2.6). In this setting, both tendons insert normally upon the radial tuberosity [13]. Preservation of the normal distal attachment site is significant, as it can be useful in distinguishing an anatomic variant from a distal biceps tendon tear. However, more recent musculoskeletal ultrasound literature and anatomic literature postulate that the normal "single" distal tendon seen on MRI and CT may actually in itself represent two persistent tendons that insert so closely together that it is difficult to discern one from the other on modalities other than high-frequency ultrasound or gross anatomic dissection [1]. This raises the possibility that what we have been classifying as "normal" versus "variant" may in fact represent a spectrum of varying degrees of fusion. The important point is that regardless of whether the DBT is recognizable as a single tendon or two tendons, the tendons should be continuous throughout their course and continue to insert on the radial tuberosity [1, 5, 13]. Tendon discontinuity, failed connectivity with the radial tuberosity, and adjacent fluid are features suspicious for a tendon tear rather than anatomic variation.

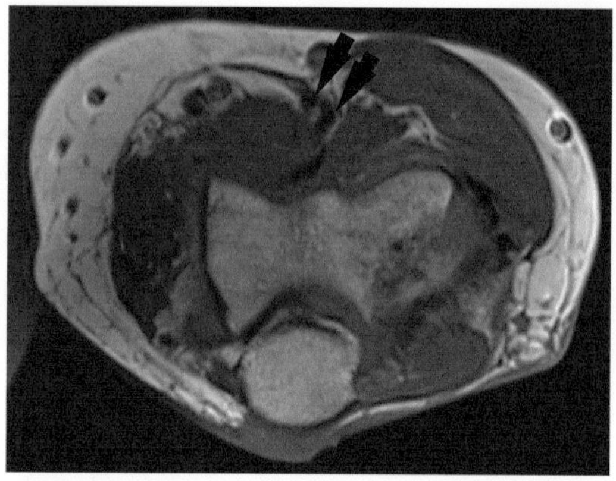

Fig. 2.6 AX T1 illustrating a bifurcated long head biceps tendon (black arrows). Unlike a torn tendon, the bifurcated tendons descend in parallel and insert normally

The elongated morphology and course of the DBT are well appreciated on MRI, although the fact that some tendon fibers also attach to the overlying edge of the bicipital aponeurosis is typically described only upon anatomic dissection [5]. However, it is important to be aware of this accessory attachment formed between the biceps aponeurosis and the DBT because this relationship provides the distal tendon with increased positional stability and explains why injury to one structure often presents with a coexisting injury to the other. The biceps aponeurosis (also known as

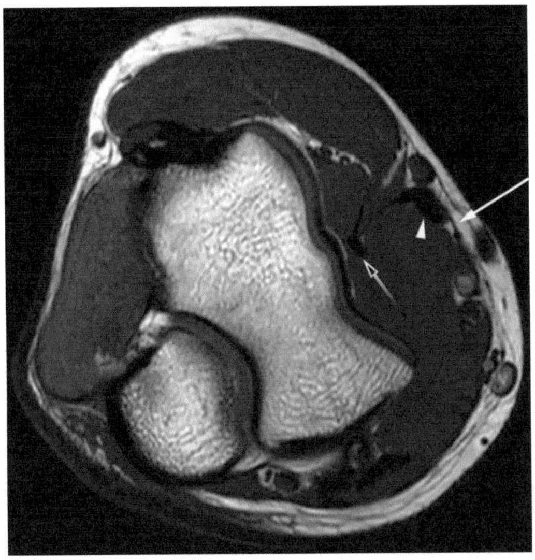

Fig. 2.7 AX T1 shows the biceps aponeurosis as a thin hypointense band (white arrow) superficial to the distal biceps tendon (white arrowhead) and the brachialis (black gradated arrow)

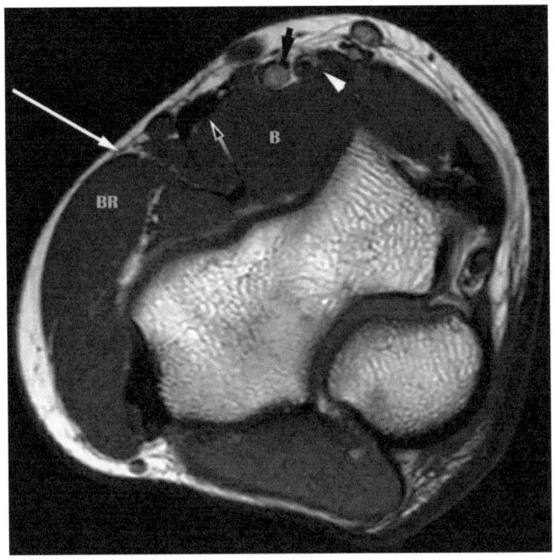

Fig. 2.8 AX T1, the musculocutaneous nerve (white arrow), is located lateral to the DBT (black gradated arrow). Both the median nerve (white arrowhead) and the brachial artery (black arrowhead) are superficial to the brachialis muscle belly and tendon (B) and medial to the brachioradialis (BR)

the lacertus fibrosus) extends from the myotendinous junction of the distal biceps to the medial aspect of the deep fascia of the forearm (Fig. 2.7) [1, 5, 13]. The biceps aponeurosis serves to hold the DBT in place and prevent proximal retraction in the setting of a distal biceps tendon tear. Thus, when proximal retraction of the DBT is in evidence, this implies a co-injury of the aponeurosis which may alter subsequent treatment.

As stated previously, the biceps brachii muscle is innervated by the musculocutaneous nerve that arises from the C5, C6 and C7 cervical nerve roots and receives its primary blood supply via the muscular branches of the brachial artery. The distal biceps tendon can be helpful in identifying the musculocutaneous nerve, median nerve, and brachial artery. As the tendon descends through the anterior compartment, it separates the musculocutaneous nerve laterally, from the median nerve and brachial artery medially, while remaining superficial to the brachialis muscle (Fig. 2.8) [5].

Although there is a bicipitoradial bursa that partially encircles the distal tendon, this bursa is only discernible on the rare occasion the bursa becomes distended with fluid [4]. Thus, visualization of the bursa on medical imaging typically reflects an underlying pathology resulting in inflammatory or traumatic fluid accumulation within the bursa. Furthermore, a distended bicipitoradial bursa may cause secondary compression of the radial nerve branches depending on the severity of fluid accumulation, leading to nerve entrapment syndromes of the forearm and hand [1, 5, 15].

The Brachialis

The second "B" anterior compartment muscle is the brachialis. The biceps brachii tendon and the distal brachialis are both located between the pronator teres medially and the brachioradialis laterally (Fig. 2.9) [5]. The brachialis muscle is the primary flexor of the arm irrespective of arm position and is located deep relative to the distal biceps tendon. Like the biceps brachii, the brachialis is innervated by the musculocutaneous nerve (C5, C6, C7) [14]. However, it also receives innervation from the radial nerve [1]. Similarly, the brachialis has two blood supplies, being supplied both by muscular branches of the brachial artery and the recurrent radial artery [13].

The brachialis originates from the mid to lower half of the anterior humeral diaphysis with fibers also attaching to the intermuscular septum [13, 16]. The broad footprint of this myotendi-

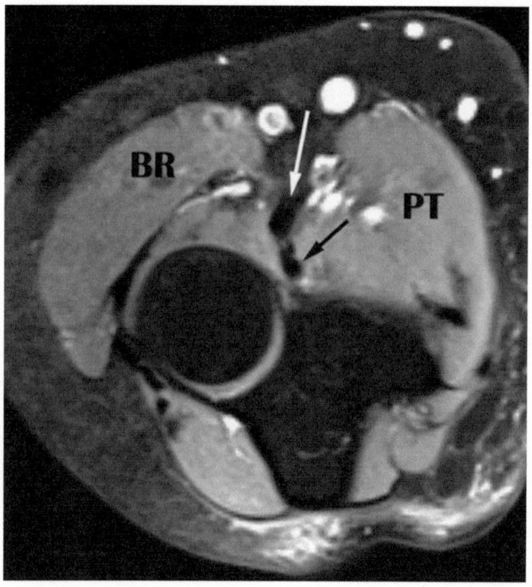

Fig. 2.9 AX PD showing the DBT (white arrow) and brachialis (black arrow) located between pronator teres (PT) medially and brachioradialis (BR) laterally

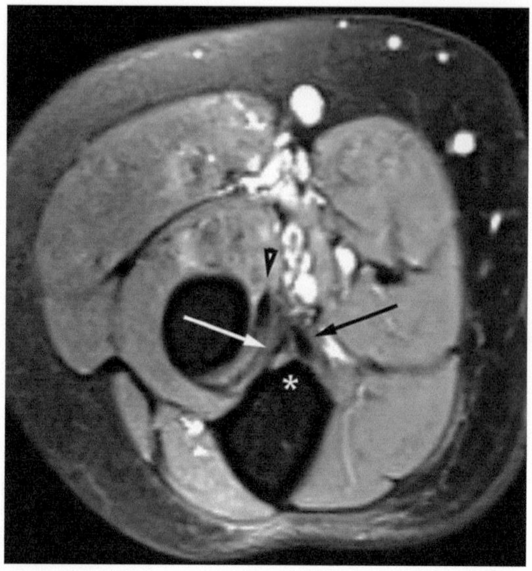

Fig. 2.10 AX PD showing the main distal brachialis tendon (black arrow) inserting upon the coronoid process (*), with the oblique cord extending toward the tuberosity inferiorly (white arrow). The DBT is approaching the radial tuberosity (arrowhead)

nous origin creates a strong stable attachment that is an uncommon site of injury. Distally, the brachialis inserts on the ulnar tuberosity and the neighboring coronoid process. Thus, in the setting of a coronoid process fracture, it is important to search for a coexisting injury to the distal brachialis [1, 13]. The distal tendon of the brachialis is typically smaller than the distal biceps tendon. As the tendon approaches the coracoid process, it gives off a minute oblique cord that inserts just inferiorly upon the ulnar tuberosity [17] (Fig. 2.10). Despite its small size, the distal brachialis tendon is enveloped and reinforced by muscle fibers. The degree of muscle encasement varies, so that the distal tendon can present as predominantly muscular, predominantly tendinous, or a mixture of the two. But the presence of these muscle fibers adds strength and protection to the tendon, explaining why brachialis tendon tears are less frequent than distal biceps tendon tears.

Anatomic dissection reveals that the distal insertion of the brachialis is comprised of a dominant superficial component and more diminutive deep component [13, 16]. The superficial brachialis muscle fibers arise from the anterolateral aspect of the middle third of the humerus and neighboring intermuscular septum. The deep fibers arise from the distal third of the anterior humeral diaphysis and distal intermuscular septum [1]. Both components insert upon the ulnar tuberosity; however, the superficial fibers insert more distal relative to the deep fibers [16]. It can be difficult on MRI to distinguish the superficial and deep components of the brachialis. It is more important to understand for the purposes of MRI interpretation and injury recognition that the proximal brachialis attaches to the majority of the mid and lower anterior humeral diaphysis and intermuscular septum and the distal components attach to the ulnar tuberosity.

The broad proximal origin of the brachialis and mixed myotendinous distal attachment make the brachialis a powerful arm flexor. The brachialis is able to flex the arm regardless of arm or elbow position, acting as the principle flexor of the upper extremity. An accessory brachialis muscle has been described, originating from the medial mid-diaphysis of the humerus rather than from the anterior cortex. Like the main brachialis, the accessory brachialis muscle also demonstrates an aponeurotic attachment with fibers blending with the medial aspect of the intermuscular septum [13]. Distally, the accessory muscle blends with the common flexor tendon [13]. When present, the accessory brachialis typically descends along the medial aspect of the elbow, crossing the median nerve and the brachial artery. At least one report has described a bifid distal tendon of the accessory brachialis [18]. If the distal tendon demonstrates a bifid appearance, the tendon fibers can encircle the median nerve resulting in median nerve impingement [13, 18].

The Brachioradialis

The third "B" anterior compartment muscle is the brachioradialis. The brachioradialis participates in *forearm* movements, consisting of forearm flexion at the elbow, and in both pronation and supination. The brachioradialis originates from the lateral supracondylar ridge of the humerus between the muscle bellies of the brachialis anteriorly and the lateral head of the triceps posteriorly. Distally, the muscle belly is found lateral to the biceps brachii and the brachialis muscles and anterior relative to the extensor carpi radialis longus muscle [5] (Fig. 2.11). The brachioradialis subsequently inserts upon the radial styloid process of the distal radius and is innervated by the deep branch of the radial nerve (C5, C6) while receiving its blood supply from the radial recurrent artery.

Arteries and Nerves

The Median Nerve

The principle nonmuscular contents of the anterior compartment include the median nerve, the radial nerve, and the brachial artery. The median nerve is formed from the brachial plexus spinal nerve roots of C5 to T1 and predominantly provides motor innervation to the muscles of the forearm and hand including the pronator teres, palmaris longus, flexor carpi radialis, and flexor digitorum superficialis muscles [5, 19]. The nerve also provides sensory innervation to the medial forearm, palm of the hand, and portions of multiple digits. The median nerve descends through the brachial canal located along the medial aspect of the arm in a neurovascular bundle with the brachial artery [20]. The nerve is located medial and parallel to the brachial artery as it enters the cubital fossa (Fig. 2.12).

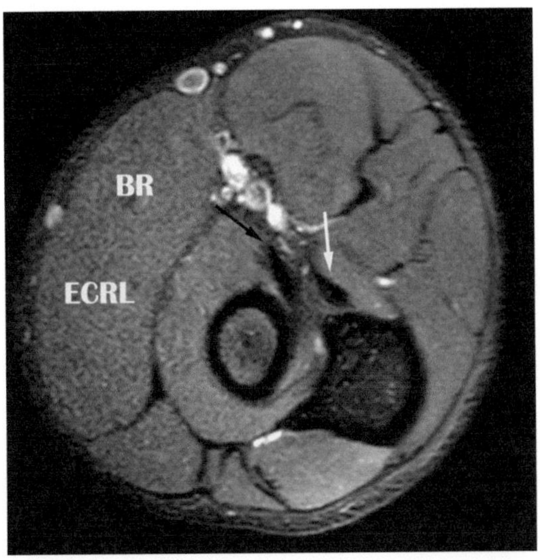

Fig. 2.11 AX PD the brachioradialis (BR) muscle is found lateral to the biceps brachii (black arrow), the brachialis (white arrow) tendons, and anterior to the extensor carpi radialis longus (ECRL) muscle

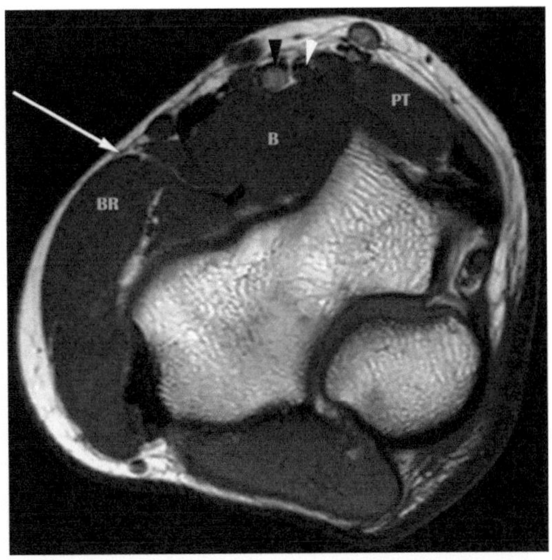

Fig. 2.12 AX T1 showing the median nerve (white arrowhead) runs medial and parallel to the brachial artery (black arrowhead). The musculocutaneous nerve (white arrow) courses in the superficial lateral anterior compartment relative to the brachioradialis (BR), brachialis (B), and pronator teres (PT) muscles

Distally, the median nerve travels between the superficial (humeral) and deep (ulnar) heads of the pronator teres muscle, remaining medial to both the ulnar and radial arteries throughout the proximal forearm [5, 19]. However, in up to 17% of individuals, the median nerve takes an intermuscular course between the brachialis muscle and the pronator muscle [1]. This is important to remember when the pronator teres is enlarged from edema, hypertrophy, or intramuscular mass, as the intermuscular course of the median nerve can become a site of neuronal impingement leading to pronator syndrome [5]. Median nerve entrapment can also occur at the level of the anteromedial distal humerus secondary to the varying presence of a *ligament of Struthers*. The ligament of Struthers is an accessory ligament that arises from a rudimentary supracondylar process of the medial epicondyle and attaches to the medial epicondyle [5]. Controversy exists as to the incidence of this anatomic variant, which was originally described by Struthers in the 1850s and is considered a developmental vestige of the supracondylar foramen found in reptiles [21, 22]. This should not be confused with the separate, but similarly named, "arcade of Struthers" which was described by Kane and colleagues in the 1970s and is a frequently occurring condensation of fascia along the medial elbow that connects the medial head of the triceps with the medial intermuscular septum and can result in ulnar nerve impingement [21, 22].

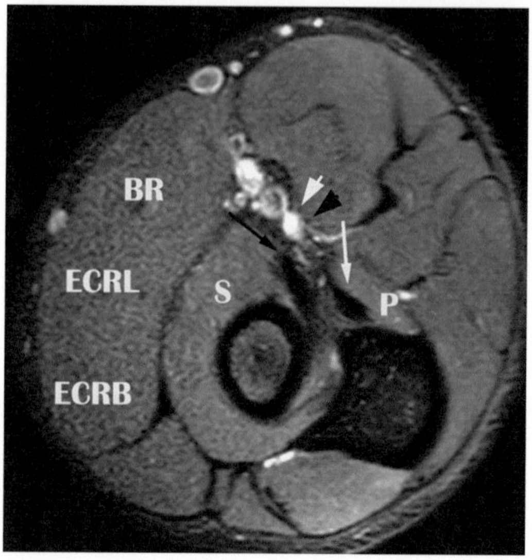

Fig. 2.13 AX T1 anterior interosseous nerve (AIN) (black arrowhead) arises from the median nerve (white arrowhead) at the level of the supinator muscle (S) and the ulnar head of the pronator teres muscle (P). Both nerves are T1 hypointense and are medial to the brachioradialis (BR), supinator and extensor carpi radialis longus (ECRL), and extensor carpi radialis brevis (ECRB) muscles. The biceps tendon (long black arrow) and the distal brachialis tendon (long white arrow) descend deep to the nerves

The Anterior Interosseous Nerve

At the level of the supinator muscle and the deep head of the pronator teres, the median nerve gives off a purely motor branch called the anterior interosseous nerve [19]. The anterior interosseous nerve innervates the pronator quadratus, flexor pollicis longus, and flexor digitorum profundus muscles. Compromise of the anterior interosseous nerve can lead to muscular atrophy of these muscles and the development of Kiloh-Nevin syndrome [1] (Fig. 2.13).

The Radial Nerve

The radial nerve (C5–T1) is a mixed motor and sensory nerve. The radial nerve and its motor branches supply motor function to the posterior compartment of the arm, forearm, and extensor muscles of the hand [23]. More specifically, the radial nerve proper provides motor innervation to the medial and lateral heads of the triceps, extensor carpi radialis longus, anconeus, brachioradialis, and lateral aspect of the brachialis muscle [5, 23]. It therefore supplies the muscles responsible for forearm, wrist, and elbow extension, along with elbow flexion, pronation, and supination [23].

The radial nerve and its sensory branches provide cutaneous sensory innervation to the anterolateral arm, the posterior distal arm and forearm, the dorsal aspects of the first through third fingers, and the lateral half of the fourth finger [23]. Although the radial nerve is a mixed nerve, its branches tend to be either purely motor or sensory.

In the proximal arm, the radial nerve has a posterior and lateral course relative to the humeral diaphysis, traveling within the spiral groove of the humerus, also termed the radial sulcus. This sulcus is a shallow concavity that extends obliquely down the lateral humerus between the humeral insertions of the lateral and medial heads of the triceps. This intimate arrangement between the radial nerve and humerus places the nerve at risk in the setting of a humeral diaphyseal fracture.

The radial nerve branches several times as it descends medially to laterally and posteriorly to anteriorly in the arm before reaching the level of the elbow. At the level of the mid-humeral diaphysis, the radial nerve gives off a major sensory branch called the posterior cutaneous nerve of the arm. The posterior cutaneous nerve supplies the skin of the anterolateral and posterior lower arm. While the posterior cutaneous nerve subsequently descends within the lateral arm, the radial nerve takes an anterior course between the brachialis, brachioradialis, and extensor carpi radialis longus muscles so that at the level of the distal arm and elbow, the nerve resides in the lateral aspect of the anterior compartment [1].

Some sources place the radial nerve in the lateral or posterior compartments due to the muscles it innervates. However, the radial nerve is included in the anterior compartment in this text which classifies structures purely by anatomic location in order to simplify identification on medical imaging. On MRI, a thin intermuscular fat plane best seen on axial nonfat-saturated imaging anterior to the lateral humeral epicondyle separates the brachioradialis and extensor carpi radialis longus muscles laterally from the brachialis muscle medially. Identifying this fat plane is a useful landmark as the fat outlines both the radial nerve and radial collateral artery (Fig. 2.14). When the radial nerve splits into superficial and deep branches at the level of the elbow, both of the proximal branches continue to course within the same fatty muscular fascial plane.

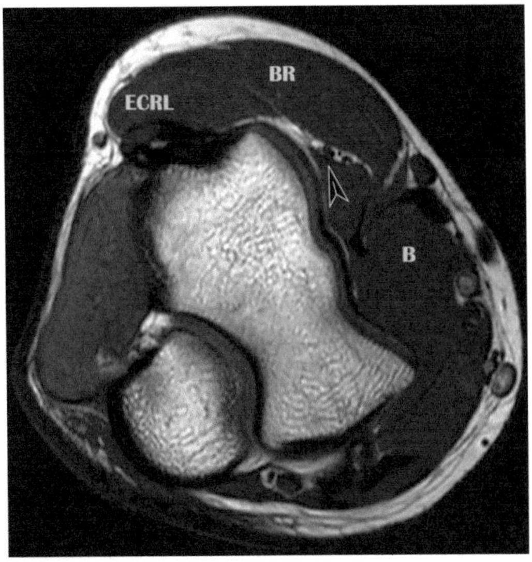

Fig. 2.14 AX T1 shows the radial nerve (arrowhead) in the thin fatty fascial plane between the extensor carpi radialis longus (ECRL), brachioradialis (BR), and brachialis (B)

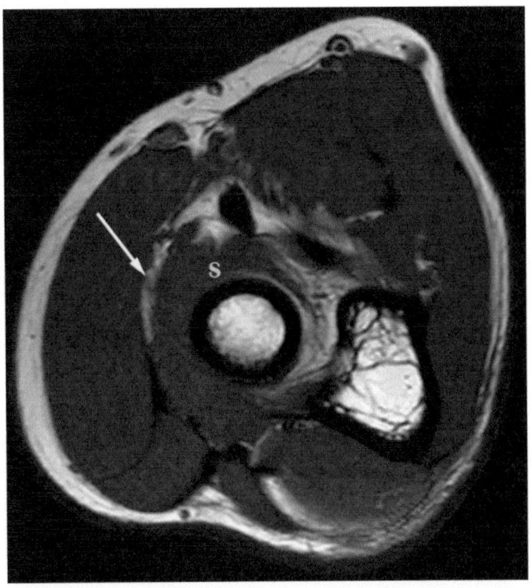

Fig. 2.15 AX T1 showing the deep branch of the radial nerve (white arrow). As the nerve descends, it courses posteriorly, passing between the heads of the supinator muscle (S) at the level of the distal radial neck, where it becomes the posterior interosseous nerve

Superficial and Deep Branches of the Radial Nerve and the Posterior Interosseous Nerve

At the elbow, the radial nerve is anterior to the radial head as it branches into its superficial sensory and deep motor branches (Fig. 2.15) [5, 24]. The superficial branch courses anteriorly and medially, residing within the fatty fascial plane anterior to the supinator muscle. The superficial branch is a sensory nerve providing sensation to the dorsal aspect to the first three and a half fingers. The deep branch also courses within the anterior forearm, but as its name implies, the nerve remains deep and lateral relative to the anterior branch.

The deep branch passes through the radial tunnel and between the heads of the supinator muscle after which it becomes the posterior interosseous nerve (Fig. 2.16) [5, 24]. This location, along the superior edge of the supinator muscle, is also termed the "arcade of Frohse" and can present as a potential site of nerve entrapment in the setting of a tendinous or thickened supinator attachment or any space-occupying lesion [25]. The posterior radial nerve provides motor innervation to the extensor carpi radialis brevis and supinator muscles, thereby contributing to forearm supination, and wrist extension and abduction [23]. The posterior interosseous nerve innervates the forearm extensors and abductor policies longus, abductor policies brevis, and extensor indicis proprius, thereby permitting wrist and finger extension and thumb abduction [5]. The posterior interosseous nerve courses along the posterior and lateral margin of the supinator muscle and is in close proximity to the radius, making it vulnerable to injury in the setting of a dislocated radial neck fracture [5, 26].

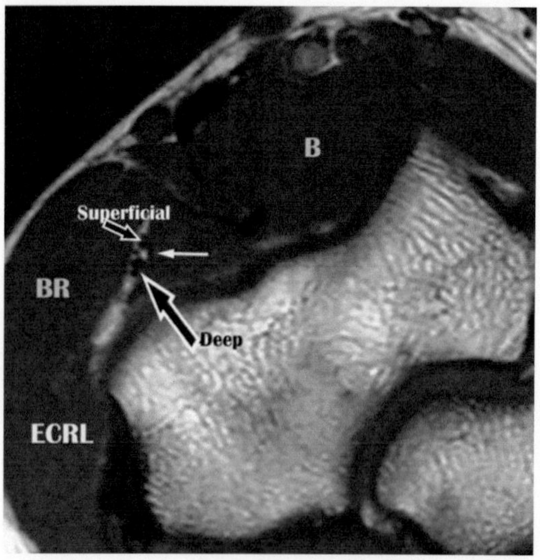

Fig. 2.16 AX T1 image at the level of the radial head where the radial nerve splits into a sensory superficial branch and a deep motor branch as annotated. The radial collateral artery (white arrow) is located in between them. The brachioradialis (BR), extensor carpi radialis longus (ECRL), and brachialis (B) are annotated for reference

The Musculocutaneous Nerve

The musculocutaneous nerve arises from the C5, C6, and (variable) C7 nerve roots but is often overlooked when discussing imaging elbow anatomy [14]. It is included in this chapter because the nerve provides motor innervation to the biceps brachii, the brachialis, and the coracobrachialis muscles of the anterior compartment of the arm with the biceps and brachialis continuing distally into the elbow [14] [27]. The nerve descends anteriorly within the arm until it reaches the level of the distal humeral metadiaphysis, where the nerve pierces the deep brachial fascia and becomes the lateral antebrachial cutaneous nerve (LABCN) [14, 27].

The LABCN is initially located in the anterior superficial distal arm lateral to the distal biceps and superficial to the brachialis. The nerve courses laterally and superficially as it descends into the forearm, eventually residing in the subcutaneous tissues overlying the extensor carpi radialis brevis. The nerve then splits into anterior and posterior components. The anterior branch continues on to innervate the radial aspect of the palmar forearm, while the posterior division supplies the radial aspect of the dorsal forearm. Trouble arises when hypertrophy of the biceps or the brachialis encroaches upon the LABCN at the distal arm and elbow. This can translate to intermittent nerve impingement when the arm is rotated through pronation and supination [14].

The Brachial Artery

The brachial artery follows an oblique course though the anterior subcutaneous tissues as it descends through the arm. At the level of the distal arm, the brachial artery crosses from the medial to the anterior subcutaneous soft tissues, running adjacent to the medial edge of the biceps muscle. When the vessel passes beneath the lacertus fibrosus, it is medial relative to the distal biceps tendon and superficial to the bra-

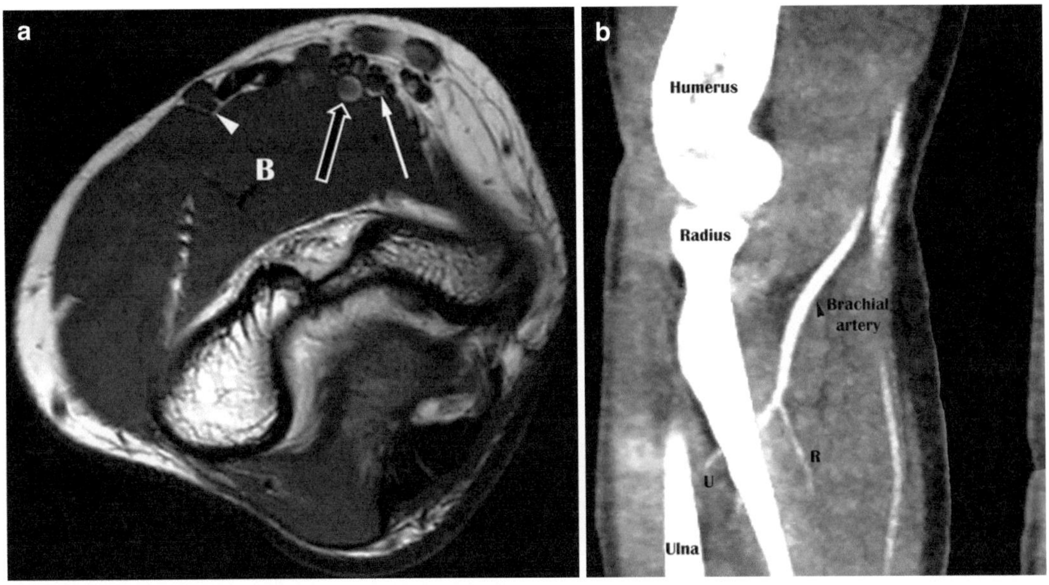

Fig. 2.17 (**a**) AX T1 illustrating the brachial artery (black arrow), the median nerve (white arrow), and the musculocutaneous nerve (white arrowhead) superficial to the brachialis muscle (B). (**b**) CT COR MIP demonstrating the radial artery (black arrowhead) bifurcating into the radial (R) and ulnar (U) arteries

chialis muscle (Fig. 2.17a). At the level of the radial head, the brachial artery splits into the radial and ulnar arteries of the forearm. Prior to its bifurcation, the brachial artery remains lateral and fairly parallel to the median nerve, making it a convenient means of identifying the nerve (Fig. 2.17b).

The Lateral Compartment

Lateral Compartment Muscles and Tendons

The lateral compartment consists of the radiocapitellar joint, the annular recess that encircles the radial neck, the common extensor tendon, and the underlying lateral collateral ligament complex [8]. A thin recess that exists between the lateral joint line and the overlying lateral collateral ligament is also considered part of the lateral joint but is typically appreciable only when filled with fluid such as following an arthrogram or trauma [8]. The lateral compartment is primarily the extensor compartment of the wrist and hand [5, 28]

The Common Extensor Tendon

The common extensor tendon is formed by the conjoined tendinous origin of the extensor carpi radialis brevis, extensor digitorum communes (EDC), extensor carpi ulnaris (ECU), and extensor digiti minimi (Fig. 2.18a). The common extensor tendon offers dynamic stability for the lateral elbow, reinforcing the static stabilization provided by the lateral collateral ligaments [10]. The common extensor tendon arises from the lateral humeral epicondyle deep to the brachioradialis muscle. The common extensor tendon is located on the anterolateral cortex of the lateral humeral epicondyle, immediately superficial and proximal relative to the insertion of the lateral collateral ligament complex [10]. The muscles that make up the common extensor tendon are arranged with the extensor digitorum located superficially and the extensor carpi radialis brevis located deeper [1]. At the origin of the common flexor tendon, the underlying humeral epicondyle has a fairly flat to gently concave morphology (Fig. 2.18a). Continuing distally the osseous morphology adopts a more acute angulated morphology from which the lateral capsular ligaments arise.

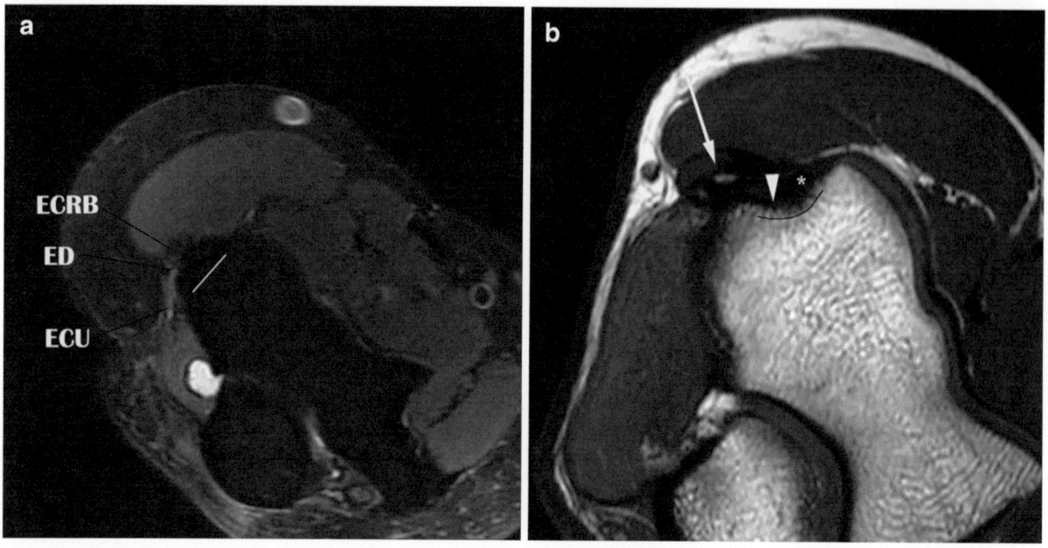

Fig. 2.18 (**a**) AX PDFS showing the proximal components of the common extensor tendon: extensor carpi ulnaris (ECU), extensor digitorum communes (ED), and extensor carpi radialis brevis (ECRB). At this level, the underlying humeral epicondyle has a flat to slightly concave morphology (white line). (**b**) AX T1 at the level of the olecranon process showing a more angulated, concave morphology of the lateral humeral epicondyle (black curvilinear line). This indicates the level of origin of the RCL (*) and the LUCL (white arrowhead). The common extensor tendon is located superficial to the ligaments (white arrow)

Lateral Compartment Ligaments

The lateral collateral ligament complex arises between the common extensor tendon and the deep joint capsule providing static varus stability to the radiocapitellar joint [1, 7, 29, 30]. These ligaments arise from the osseous concavity of the lateral humeral epicondyle immediately distal and deep to the common flexor tendon (Fig. 2.18b). The lateral collateral ligament complex is also referred to as the radial collateral ligament complex and is comprised of the radial collateral ligament (RCL), the lateral ulnar collateral ligament (LUCL), and the annular ligament [1, 5, 7, 31]. Some literary sources also describe an accessory lateral collateral ligament (ALCL), which is essentially an accessory slip of the annular ligament, arising from the annular ligament and inserting distally upon the tubercle of the supinator crest [9, 32]. When present, this accessory band is believed to stabilize the annular ligament, which in turn stabilizes the proximal radius. For the purposes of MRI interpretation, emphasis is placed on evaluating the integrity of the annular ligament, the radial collateral ligament, and the lateral ulnar collateral ligament as primary static stabilizers of the lateral elbow joint (Fig. 2.19a). The origins and insertions of the respective ligaments are so closely apposed that it can be difficult to differentiate one from the other without multiplanar triangulation; this is particularly true of the LUCL and RCL origins.

Proximally the RCL and LUCL fibers can be difficult to differentiate from each other and from the overlying tendon fibers of the common extensor tendon and muscular fascia [10]. Typically, the RCL is a thinner, more diminutive ligament compared with the thick band of the LUCL (Fig. 2.19b). However, even during cadaveric dissection, the proximal fibers of the LUCL may remain indistinguishable from the RCL [31]. Distinguishing one from the other requires awareness of the anteroposterior position of the acquired images. This entwined anatomical relationship between the lateral elbow structures explains why injury to one component often presents with concomitant injuries. For instance, the LUCL frequently tears near or at the level where it blends with the RCL, increasing the risk that an injury of one ligament will involve the other [31].

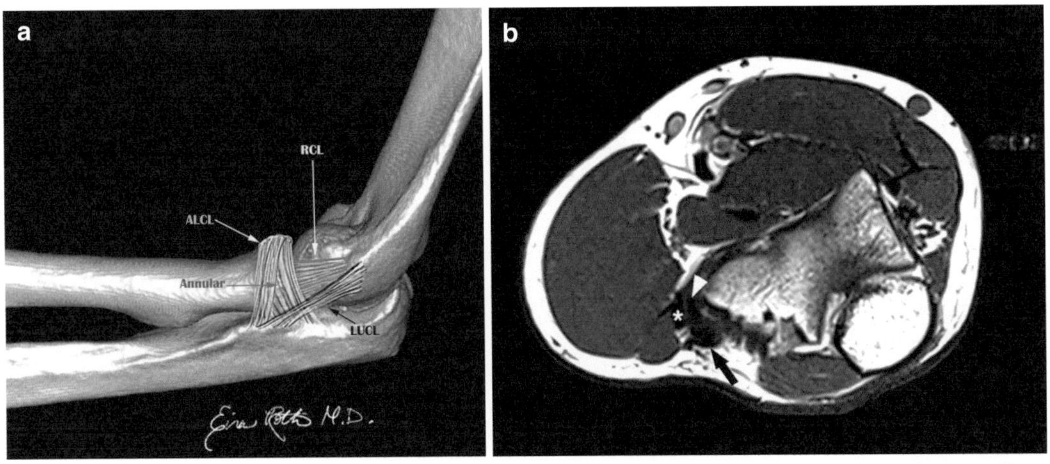

Fig. 2.19 (**a**) Illustration of the lateral elbow ligament complex demonstrating the radial collateral ligament (RCL), lateral ulnar collateral ligament (LUCL), and accessory lateral collateral ligament (ALCL). (**b**) Axial T1 shows hypointense origins of the LUCL posteriorly (black arrow) and RCL anteriorly (white arrowhead) which are located deep to the common extensor tendon (*)

The Radial Collateral Ligament

The radial collateral ligament (RCL) arises from the anterior-inferior aspect of the lateral epicondyle of the humerus and inserts upon the annular ligament at the radial head (Fig. 2.20) [5, 7, 9, 10, 31]. Anatomic dissection has revealed that some fibers also blend with the fascia of the supinator muscle; however, this is typically below the resolution of MR [10]. The resulting ligament has a fan- or funnel-shaped morphology that tapers distally deep to the common extensor tendon [1, 31]. An accessory RCL has been reported as a rare anatomic variant [31].

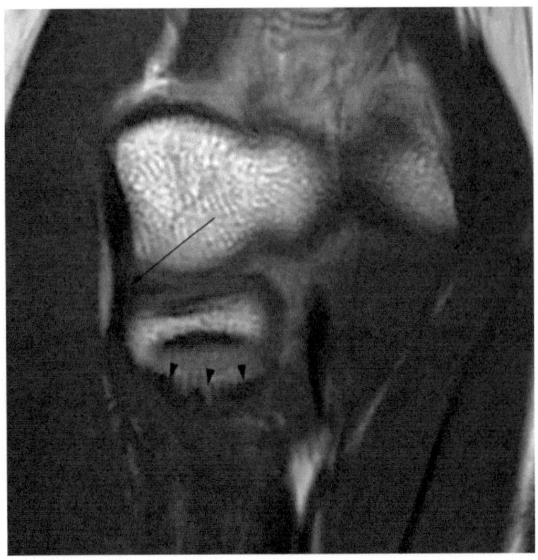

Fig. 2.20 COR T1 depicting radial collateral ligament (long black arrow) arising from the anteroinferior aspect of the lateral epicondyle and inserting on the annular ligament (black arrowheads)

The Lateral Ulnar Collateral Ligament

The lateral ulnar collateral ligament (LUCL) originates from the lateral epicondyle immediately posterior to the RCL origin (Fig. 2.21a). The LUCL then takes a posteromedial oblique course around the posterolateral edge of the radial head before inserting distally on the supinator crest of the proximal ulna (Fig. 2.21b) [5, 7, 10, 31].

The oblique course taken by the LUCL forms a sling around the proximal radius and provides protection against proximal radial subluxation [10, 33]. As the only component of the lateral collateral ligament complex to form a true bone-to-bone attachment, the LUCL has historically been considered as the primary posterolateral rotatory stabilizer of the lateral elbow against excess varus stress [1, 5, 7, 10, 33]. However, more recent studies have suggested that the annular ligament may play a greater role in elbow stability than was previously thought.

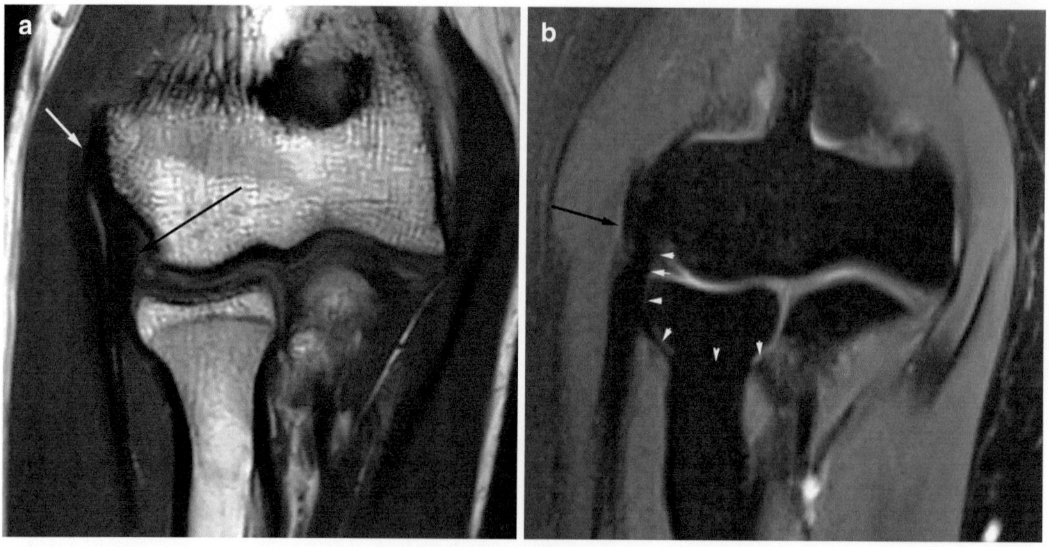

Fig. 2.21 (**a**) COR T1 depicting the proximal LUCL as a thick hypointense band (black arrow) immediately deep and distal to the common extensor tendon (white arrow). (**b**) COR PDFS showing the common extensor tendon (black arrow) superficial to the LUCL. The LUCL is evident curving around the radius to insert upon the supinator crest of the ulna (short white arrows)

The Annular Ligament

The annular ligament arises from the anterior margin of the lesser sigmoid notch of the ulna, also regarded as the radial notch [10]. The lesser sigmoid notch/radial notch is identified as a narrow depression on the lateral aspect of the coronoid process of the ulna that provides an osseous articulation with the proximal radius. The annular ligament then encircles the radial head and neck, securing the proximal radius to the posterior margin of the radial notch of the ulna (Fig. 2.22). In so doing, the annular ligament permits radial head rotation, which translates into forearm pronation and supination [7, 10].

Great anatomic variability exists in the morphology of the annular ligament. A broad conjoined insertion formed by the LUCL as it blends with the annular ligament has been observed in approximately 45% of the population, while a "bilobed" morphology was reported in 55% [10]. Although the anterior annular ligament attachment typically appears as a single band, the posterior attachment can consist of individual superior and inferior components [10, 34].

While the proximal annular ligament fits snuggly around the radial head, the inferior portion is more patulous, demonstrating a loose synovial attachment to the radial neck [10, 34]. This morphology permits the degree of radial head rotation necessary for pronation and supination, but the loose distal attachment also makes

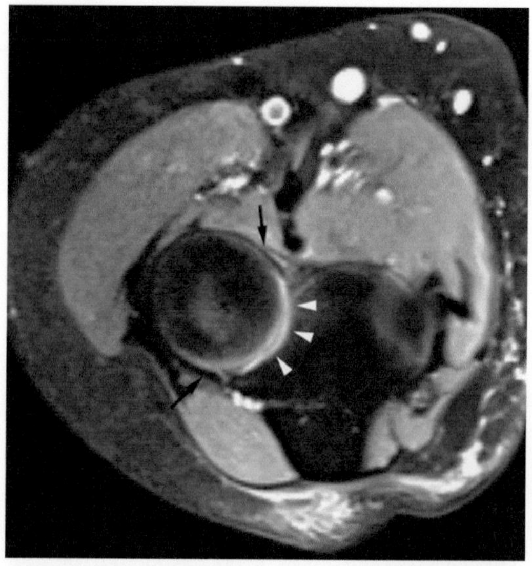

Fig. 2.22 AX PDFS demonstrates the hypointense annular ligament (black arrows) encircling the radial neck and inserting upon the radial notch (white arrowheads)

the ligament vulnerable to injury during elbow dislocation, particularly in the pediatric population. Frank disruption of the annual ligament has been found to coincide with posterolateral elbow instability in the form of increased anteroposterior and mediolateral radial head movement [10]. This has led some to consider the annular ligament as an important stabilizer of the radioulnar joint despite its anatomic variability.

The composition of the annular ligament is complex. The ligament receives contributions from the LUCL, overlying supinator muscle, and elbow joint synovium [34]. In some individuals, the synovial contribution can be accentuated, resulting in an accessory synovial fold emanating from the lateral joint capsule above the level of the annular ligament and extending into the periphery of the radiocapitellar joint [34]. Since the annular ligament receives contributions from its neighbors, injuries of the annular ligament are typically seen in combination with an injury to other lateral collateral ligament complex components. This anatomic relationship is important to consider following elbow dislocation, as torn annular ligament fibers can interpose within the joint, preventing successful restoration of radiocapitellar alignment which can lead to chronic elbow pain and secondary osteoarthritis [10].

The Medial Compartment

Medial Compartment Muscles

The medial compartment is considered the flexor-pronator compartment of the forearm. It contains the pronator teres, flexor carpi radialis (FCR), flexor carpi ulnaris (FCU), flexor digitorum superficialis (FDS), palmaris longus (PL), and flexor digitorum profundus (FDP) muscles. The FCR, FCU, FDS, and PL converge to share the same origin on the lateral humeral epicondyle. This common tendon is referred to as the common flexor tendon (Fig. 2.23a–c). The common flexor tendon reinforces the underlying ulnar collateral ligament (UCL) and functions as a dynamic stabilizer against excess valgus stress [1]. Due to the insertion site upon the medial humeral epicondyle, the included flexor muscles are considered the "epicondylar muscles" of the forearm.

The Pronator Teres

The pronator teres originates from the medial epicondyle along with the common flexor tendon and also has some fibers originating from the medial aspect of the coronoid process (Fig. 2.24) [5]. The pronator teres inserts on the lateral surface of the mid-radial diaphysis and assists with forearm pronation and elbow flexion [35]. Thus, the resulting tendon complex formed between the origin of the pronator teres and the common flexor tendon is termed the *common flexor-pronator mass* and provides dynamic resistance against excess valgus stress [7, 36]. The pronator teres is supplied by both the ulnar and the radial arteries and is innervated by the median nerve.

The Flexor Carpi Radialis

The flexor carpi radialis (FCR) arises from the medial epicondyle as part of the common flexor tendon before inserting on the base of the second and third metacarpals. It participates in hand flexion and radial deviation (hand abduction) at the wrist and is supplied by the ulnar artery and the median nerve.

The Flexor Carpi Ulnaris

The flexor carpi ulnaris (FCU) originates from the common flexor tendon but also has fibers arising from the medial aspect of the ulnar olecranon process and proximal dorsal ulnar shaft. This places the muscle at risk for injury in the setting of an olecranon process and proximal ulnar fracture [35, 37]. The muscle inserts on the pisiform, the hook of hamate, and the fifth metacarpal. The insertion on the pisiform and hamate blends with the pisohamate ligament, just as the attachment upon the base of the fifth metacarpal involves the pisometacarpal ligament [37].

The FCU is supplied by the ulnar artery and the muscular branches of the ulnar nerve (C7, C8, and T1). The muscle acts to flex and adduct the hand at the wrist [35, 37]. The interdigitating anatomic relationship between the distal inserting FCU tendon fibers and the underlying inter-

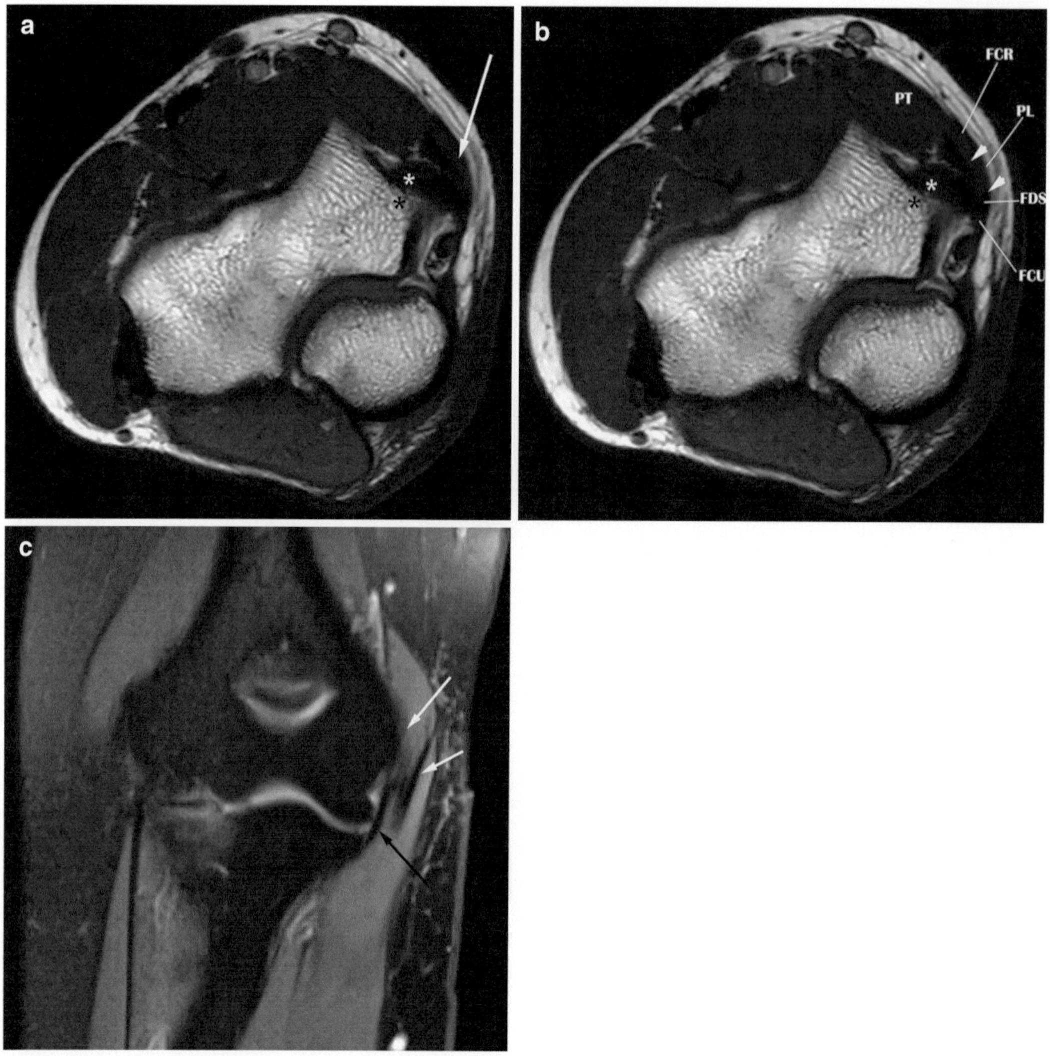

Fig. 2.23 (**a**) AX T1 depicts the common flexor tendon (white arrow) arising from the medial humeral epicondyle (black *). The common flexor tendon is comprised of the FCR, FCU, FDS, and PL origins. The tendon arises superficial and slightly proximal to the UCL (white *). (**b**) AX T1 depicts the common flexor tendon (white arrowhead) arising from the medial humeral epicondyle (black *). The common flexor tendon is comprised of the FCR, FCU, FDS, and PL. The tendon arises superficial and slightly proximal to the UCL (white *). (**c**) COR PDFS showing the common extensor tendon (white arrows) arising superficial to the anterior band of the UCL (black arrow)

carpal ligaments is important to recognize as an injury to the underlying carpal bones or ligaments can affect the FCU integrity. Similarly, most muscles of the arm and forearm have tendon fibers that attach to the nearby intermuscular fascia. Thus, fascial injuries can also involve the compartmental musculature.

The Flexor Digitorum Superficialis

The flexor digitorum superficialis (FDS) primarily originates as part of the common flexor tendon with some fibers attaching to the medial ridge of the coronoid process, the ulnar collateral ligament, and the antebrachial fascia. Some sources cite fibers also originating from the

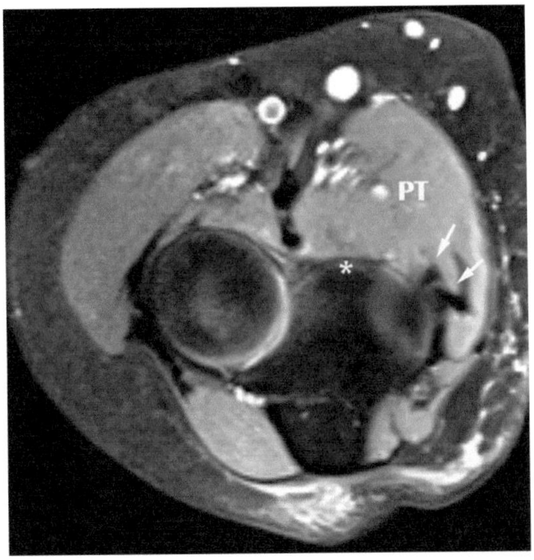

Fig. 2.24 AX PDFS showing the pronator teres (PT) muscle arising from the medial humeral epicondyle with the common flexor tendon, forming the "common flexor-pronator mass" (white arrows). A small contribution of fibers arise from the coronoid process of the ulna (white *)

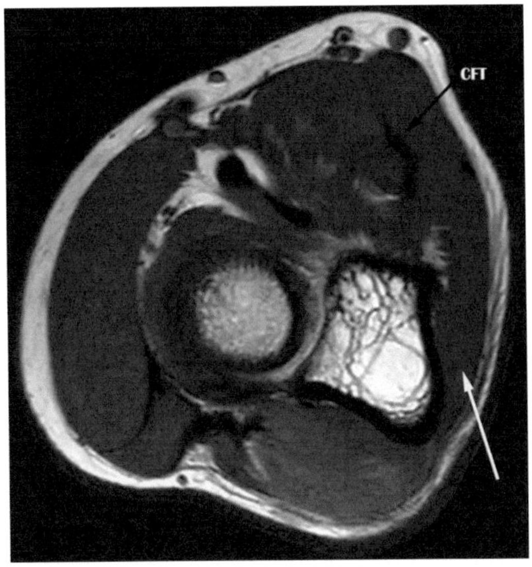

Fig. 2.25 AX T1 showing the FDP (white arrow) arising posterior and separate from the common flexor tendon (CFT). The FDP arises from the proximal ulnar shaft and interosseous membrane

superior-anterior aspect of the radial head [35]. The muscle inserts distally on the diaphysis of the middle phalanges of the second through fifth digits. The FDS flexes the middle phalanges of these fingers at the level of the proximal interphalangeal joints. With additional effort, the FDS also flexes the proximal phalanges of the same fingers at the level of the metacarpophalangeal joints and participates in wrist flexion when fingers are extended [17, 35, 38].

The Palmaris Longus

The palmaris longus (PL) originates from the medial humeral epicondyle as part of the common flexor tendon. The PL inserts on the flexor retinaculum and upon the superficial portion of the palmar aponeurosis to aid in hand flexion at the wrist. It is supplied by the median nerve (C7, C8) and the ulnar artery [6, 35].

The Flexor Digitorum Profundus

The flexor digitorum profundus (FDP) does not arise as part of the common flexor tendon or flexor-pronator mass. The FDP arises from the proximal 3/4 of the anteromedial ulna and the interosseous membrane and may include fibers originating from the coronoid process as well (Fig. 2.25) [1, 35, 37, 38]. The muscle inserts upon the distal phalanges of the second through fifth digits and participates in hand flexion at the interphalangeal joints and with wrist flexion when the fingers are extended [6, 35, 37, 38]. The muscle receives dual innervation, with the medial aspect supplied by the ulnar nerve (C8, T1) and the lateral part supplied by the interosseous branch of the median nerve (C8, T1). The corresponding ulnar and anterior interosseous arteries provide the respective blood supply [35].

The Flexor Pollicis Longus

Although the flexor pollicis longus (FPL) does not arise at the level of the elbow, it is commonly considered a lateral compartment muscle. The FPL arises from the anterior aspect of the mid-radius just inferior to the anterior oblique line and the FDS. The FPL arises proximal to the pronator quadratus muscle, with some fibers of the FPL originating from the neighboring interosseous membrane. Distally the FPL tendon passes beneath the flexor retinaculum to insert upon the base of the distal phalanx of the first digit to enable flexion of the thumb [13, 35]. The muscle is innervated by the anterior interosseous nerve, a branch of the median nerve, and is supplied by the anterior interosseous artery [35].

A common anatomic variant is an accessory head of the FPL that is also termed the "Gantzer muscle." This variation has a prevalence that ranges in the literature from 45% to 66% [13]. The origin of the Gantzer muscle varies, with the medial humeral epicondyle and the capitellum being the most reported. However, a Gantzer muscle originating from the actual muscle belly of the FDS has also been reported, as has a "dual origin" from the coronoid process and medial humeral epicondyle [13]. The accessory Gantzer muscle typically inserts distally onto the ulnar aspect of the FPL and is innervated by the anterior interosseous nerve [13]. Anatomic variability of the Gantzer muscle can result in close proximity with either the anterior interosseous nerve or the median nerve, thereby increasing the risk for compressive neuropathy. Compression of *either* nerve can lead to anterior interosseous syndrome or pronator syndrome, respectively [13].

Medial Compartment Ligaments

The Ulnar Collateral Ligament

The principle ligament of the medial compartment is the ulnar collateral ligament (UCL), which lies just deep to the common flexor tendon. The UCL is considered the main static stabilizer against valgus stress, as defined when the elbow is flexed greater than 20° [5]. The UCL is also referred to as the medial collateral ligament, with both terms used interchangeably, and is comprised of three bundles: the anterior, posterior, and transverse or oblique bands (Fig. 2.26a) [7, 39–41]. The ligament complex is commonly injured in overhead-throwing athletes which can result in valgus instability particularly during the late cocking and early acceleration phases of throwing [42].

The Anterior Bundle of the Ulnar Collateral Ligament

Mechanically, the anterior bundle is the most important bundle as it participates most in resisting valgus stress [7]. The anterior bundle arises from the anteroinferior aspect of the medial epicondyle and inserts on the sublime tubercle of the coronoid process (Fig. 2.26b, c) [1, 5, 43, 44]. The ligament has a linear morphology and is best visualized in the coronal plane due to its orientation and demonstrates the expected low T1 and T2 signal of ligaments. However, it is not uncommon to see subtle increased signal at the medial epicondylar attachment site on nonfat-saturated images due to normal infiltration of "fibrofatty slips" between the ligament fibers (Fig. 2.26d) [7]. Distally, the ligament can insert 1–3 mm beyond the articular cartilage forming a "pseudo-T sign" where trace joint fluid or intra-articular contrast insinuates between the bone and inserting ligament fibers (Fig. 2.27) [7]. The pseudo-T sign should not be confused with a true injury, and as such should not extend beyond 3 mm in craniocaudal length.

The role of the anterior bundle in resisting valgus stress appears most pronounced when the elbow is flexed between 50° and 70° [44]. In surgical and anatomic literature, the insertional footprint of the anterior bundle is described as being more substantial upon the ulna than previously believed, possibly contributing to its status as the principle restraint against valgus and rotational forces [42, 43, 45].

The Posterior Bundle of the Ulnar Collateral Ligament

As the name implies, the posterior bundle arises from the inferior aspect of the medial humeral epicondyle immediately posterior and slightly inferior to the anterior bundle and remains posterior as it descends to its ulnar insertion (Figs. 2.26c and 2.28). The posterior band has a somewhat fan-like morphology as it tapers to insert on the posteromedial aspect of the ulnar trochlear notch. The band provides resistance against excess internal elbow rotation [1]. The slightly different anatomical positioning between the anterior and posterior bands enables them to offer opposing function, with the anterior band tightening during elbow extension and the posterior band tightening with elbow flexion [41, 42]. These reciprocal actions not only create stability but also place

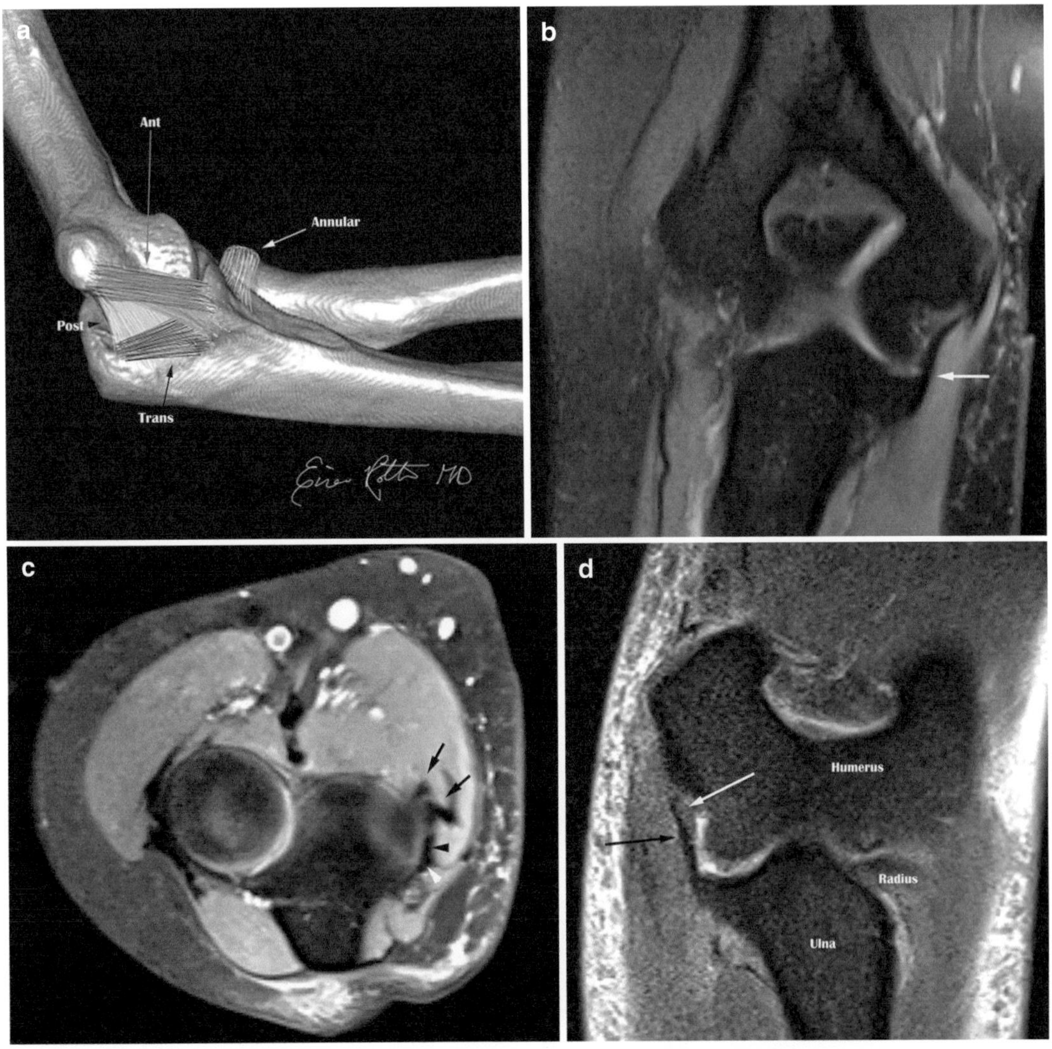

Fig. 2.26 (**a**) 3D volume rendering of the medial elbow with an illustration of the anterior (ant), posterior (post), and transverse (trans) bands of the UCL. (**b**) COR PDFS depicting the anterior band of the UCL (white arrow). (**c**) AX PDFS showing the proximal portions of the anterior (black arrowhead) and posterior bands (white arrowhead) of the UCL. The ligamentous bundles are deep to the common flexor tendon (black long arrows). (**d**) COR PDFS showing the proximal fibrofatty slips (white arrow) within a normal UCL (black arrow). The macroscopic fat is saturated on this image just as fat elsewhere in the elbow

both bundles at risk for injury secondary to repetitive elbow flexion and extension such as is seen with overuse injuries in overhead-throwing athletes [42].

The Transverse or Oblique Ligament of the Ulnar Collateral Ligament

Unlike the anterior and posterior bundles, the transverse bundle is often considered separately and is referred to by some as the "transverse or oblique ligament." The ligamentous band originates and inserts posterior and distal relative to the anterior and posterior bands. The morphology of the band ranges from linear to fanlike and is oriented anterior-posteriorly so that it originates and inserts on the ulna, failing to cross the ulnohumeral joint [7, 39]. Unfortunately, the orientation of the ligament means that the ligament is largely out of plane on conventional MR imaging, making it difficult to fully appreciate.

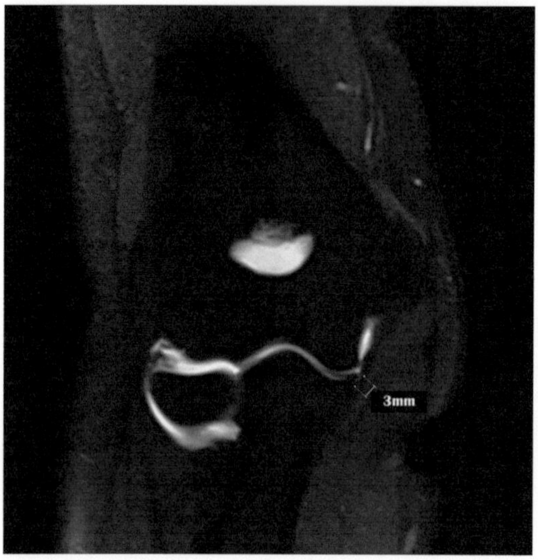

Fig. 2.27 "Pseudo-T sign": COR PDFS shows a low intact insertion of an intact anterior band of the UCL onto the ulna, immediately distal to the hyaline cartilage

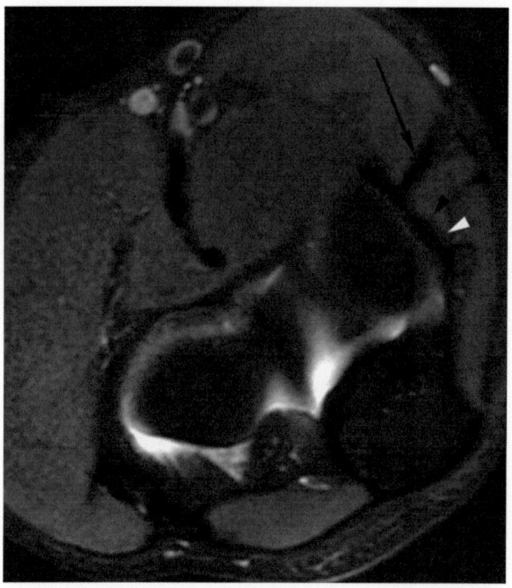

Fig. 2.28 AX PDFS at the level of the olecranon process demonstrating the anterior (black arrowhead) and posterior (white arrowhead) bands of the UCL as they descend toward their ulnar insertions. The bands of the UCL remain deep to the common flexor tendon (black arrow)

Historically this has been of limited concern, because the transverse ligament was thought to not participate in elbow stabilization due to its failure to cross the joint. However, a more recent investigation in the anatomic literature suggests that fibers of the transverse ligament may blend with fibers of the anterior bundle [42, 45]. Thus, it is possible that the transverse ligament does participate to some degree in elbow stability, possibly by reinforcing other bundles; however, the biomechanical significance remains unclear and merits further assessment [7].

The Posterior Compartment

Posterior Compartment Muscles

The Triceps

The triceps muscle gets its name from having three proximal origins and muscle bellies. The long head originates from the infraglenoid tubercle of the scapula. The medial and lateral heads both originate from the proximal humerus, with the lateral head arising from the upper half of the posterior humeral diaphysis and the medial head arising from the posteromedial humeral diaphysis. The medial head originates distal to other triceps origins and deep and medial relative to both the lateral and the long heads of the triceps [6]. Together the three muscle bellies converge to form a single thick distal tendon that inserts upon the olecranon process of the ulna [6, 7]. The distal triceps tendon does not insert directly on the tip of the olecranon process, where there is limited surface area, but approximately 1 cm distal to the olecranon tip (Figs. 2.29 and 2.30). This greater surface area permits a stronger tendon insertion, believed to translate into increased triceps strength and stability [1]. All three heads of the triceps are innervated by the radial nerve, while the blood supply is derived from the brachial artery, the superior ulnar collateral artery, and the profunda also referred to as the deep brachial artery [1, 7].

The Anconeus

The anconeus is a short, transversely oriented muscle that arises from the posterior lateral humeral epicondyle and inserts on the lateral aspect of the olecranon process and the superlateral aspect of the ulna in close proximity to the

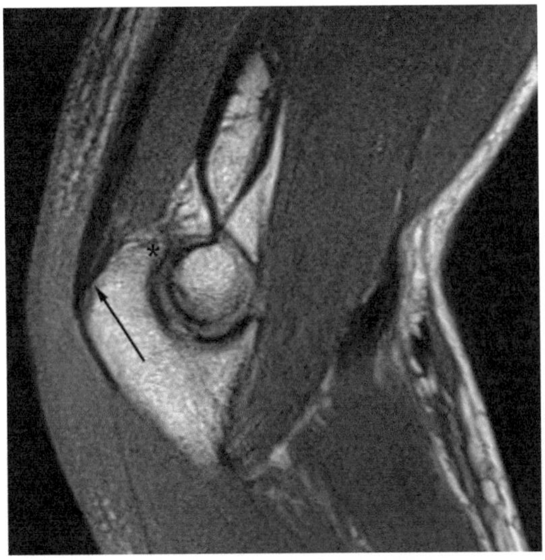

Fig. 2.29 SAG T1 demonstrating the triceps insertion (black arrow) approximately 1 cm distal to the tip of the olecranon process (*)

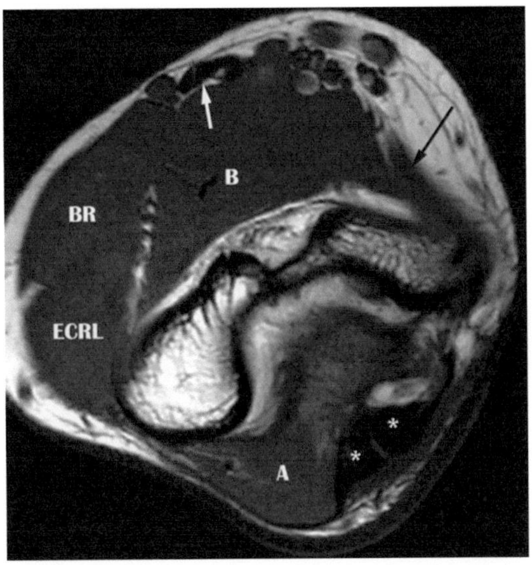

Fig. 2.30 AX T1 shows a normal triceps insertion (*). Fibrofatty slips can interdigitate between the tendon fibers. Other muscles identified at the same level include anconeus (A), extensor carpi radialis longus (ECRL), brachioradialis (BR), brachialis (B), distal biceps tendon (white arrow), and superficial head of the pronator teres (black arrow)

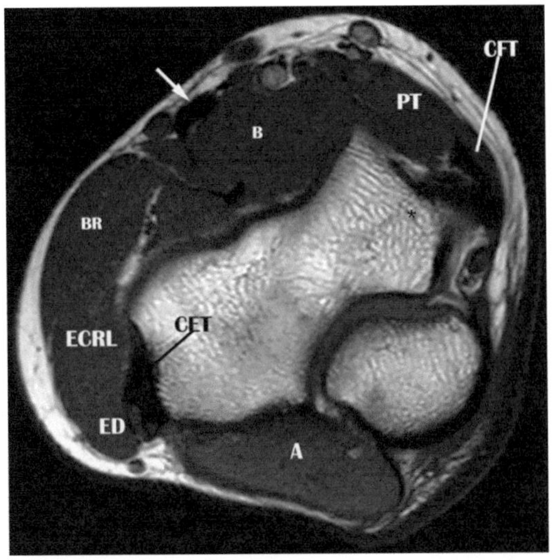

Fig. 2.31 AX T1 shows the anconeus (A) muscle posterior to the common extensor tendon (CET) and extensor digitorum (ED) muscle. Other anatomy identified at this level include the extensor carpi radialis longus (ECRL), brachioradialis (BR), brachialis (B), distal biceps tendon (white arrow), pronator teres (PT), and common flexor tendon (CFT)

edge of the distal triceps tendon (Fig. 2.31) [35]. The close anatomic relationship suggests the function of the anconeus, which is to assist the triceps with elbow extension, while also providing dynamic reinforcement for the lateral ulnar collateral ligament that lies deep to it [1]. The anconeus is innervated by the radial nerve (C7, C8) and receives its blood supply from the middle collateral branch of the profunda brachial artery.

A common anatomical variant is an accessory anconeus muscle called the anconeus epitrochlearis (Fig. 2.32a, b). The reported prevalence of this muscle ranges greatly in the literature from 1% to 34% [1]. This muscle extends from the olecranon to the medial epicondyle, following the same obliquity as the cubital tunnel retinaculum. This has led some to consider the muscle to be a failure of developmental regression during the formation of the cubital tunnel retinaculum [1, 13]. However, the muscle acts in tandem with the triceps, contracting during arm extension, leading others to postulate that the epitrochlearis may instead be an accessory component of the medial head of the triceps [1]. The clinical significance of this muscle is the association with cubital tunnel syndrome due to ulnar nerve compression.

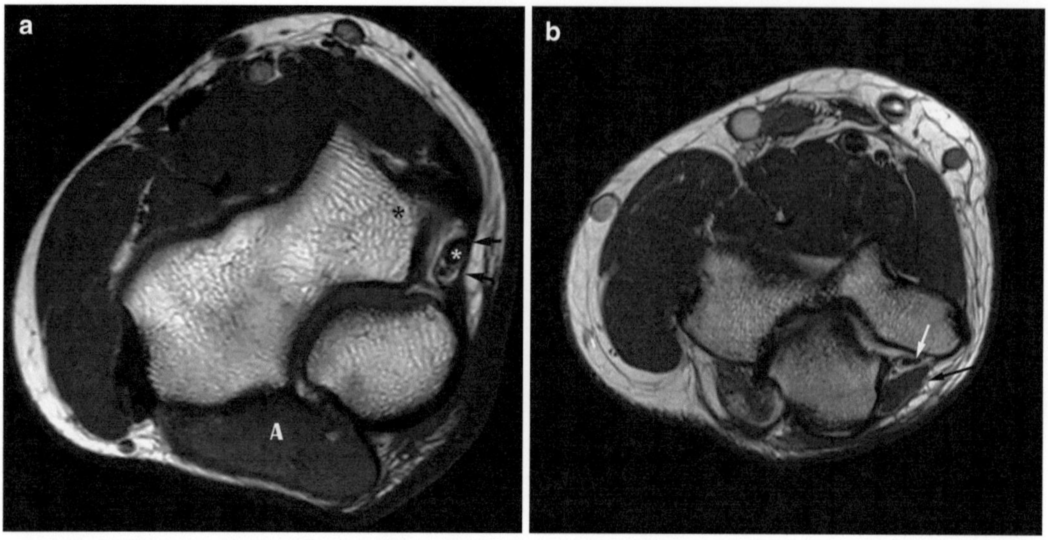

Fig. 2.32 (**a**) AX T1 shows a normal cubital tunnel at the level of the anconeus muscle (A) and the medial humeral epicondyle (black *). The tunnel is bounded by a thin hypoechoic retinaculum (black arrows). The ulnar nerve (white *) is located within the anterior tunnel. Adjacent to the nerve and also within the cubital tunnel are branches of the superior and inferior ulnar collateral and posterior ulnar recurrent arteries. (**b**) AX T1 an accessory anconeus muscle is located deep to the cubital tunnel retinaculum (black arrow). Normally there is no muscle above the ulnar nerve (white arrow)

The Ulnar Nerve and Cubital Tunnel

The ulnar nerve (C8–T1) is a mixed motor and sensory nerve to the upper extremity [19]. It supplies sensation to the dorsal and volar aspects of the digital tips of the fourth and fifth fingers. The nerve also supplies the volar aspect of the fifth finger and the lateral half of the fourth finger, along with sensation to the superficial soft tissues of the medial forearm, wrist, and palm [19]. The ulnar nerve also provides proprioception to the elbow joint and motor innervation to much of the hand and to the medial forearm. In the forearm, there are muscular motor branches of the ulnar nerve that supply the flexor carpi ulnaris and the flexor digitorum profundus. Distally, motor branches of the ulnar nerve innervate the hypothenar muscles, third and fourth lumbricals, dorsal and palmar interossei, adductor pollicis brevis, and palmaris brevis muscles [46].

The ulnar nerve descends along the medial arm, gradually adopting a more posteromedial course after piercing through the medial intermuscular septum at the level of the arcade of Struthers, an aponeurotic condensation that connects the medal head of the biceps to the medial intermuscular septum [19, 22, 46, 47]. At the distal arm, the ulnar nerve is within the superficial subcutaneous tissues directly posterior to the medial humeral epicondyle. At the elbow and proximal forearm, the nerve passes beneath the cubital tunnel retinaculum that spans the two heads of the extensor carpi ulnaris, entering the fibromuscular channel called the cubital tunnel [48]. Here, there is typically no overlying protective muscle present, and this leaves the nerve relatively exposed to direct trauma. Distally, the nerve runs between the flexor digitorum profundus and superficialis muscles of the forearm.

The cubital tunnel is distinct from the cubital fossa of the anterior elbow. The cubital tunnel is located along the posteromedial elbow and serves as a fibromuscular fat-filled conduit through which the ulnar neurovascular bundle passes into the proximal forearm. The roof is formed by

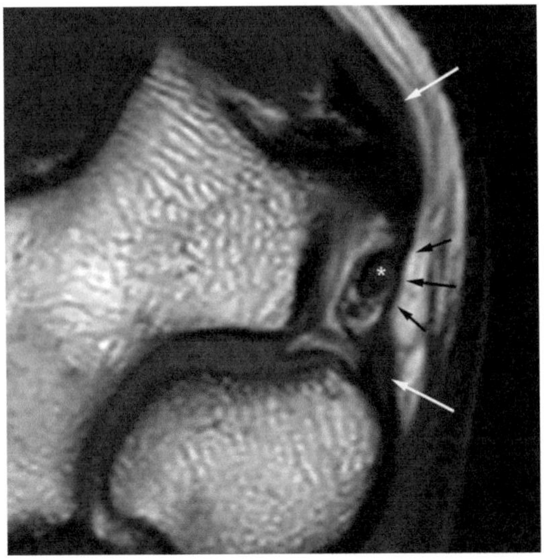

Fig. 2.33 AX T1 showing a close-up of the linear T1 hypointense cubital tunnel retinaculum (black arrows) between the ulnar and humeral heads of the extensor carpi ulnaris muscle (white arrows). The ulnar nerve (*) is adjacent to the posterior ulnar recurrent artery and vein

cubital tunnel retinaculum, which has several names. Most commonly this ligament is referred to as the cubital tunnel retinaculum, Osborne's ligament, the arcuate ligament of Osborne, or simply the arcuate ligament [48]. The floor is comprised of the posterior bundle of the UCL and joint capsule [7, 48]. The tunnel contains the ulnar nerve and the posterior ulnar recurrent artery and vein (Fig. 2.33) [1].

There is considerable anatomic variability associated with the cubital tunnel. The cubital tunnel retinaculum may be indiscernible in 10–25% of the general population, possibly predisposing those individuals to excessive ulnar nerve subluxation [7]. Varying degrees of cubital tunnel retinacular thickening have been reported without symptom correlation.

Since the cubital tunnel is a fat-filled space bordered by connective tissue, arm position results in a dramatic change in the tunnel's cross-sectional area and the subsequent pressure within the tunnel [1, 49]. Furthermore, because the cubital tunnel is a tight anatomic space, any space-occupying structure can cause impingement. Examples include a developmentally low origin of the medial triceps crowding the proximal cubital tunnel, or the presence of an accessory anconeus muscle can cause ulnar nerve impingement and the development of cubital tunnel syndrome [7].

Anatomic variants affecting the ulnar nerve exist beyond the morphology of the cubital tunnel. One variant located at the level of the elbow and proximal forearm is an anastomosis between the median and ulnar nerve that can occur anywhere between the medial epicondyle to the hand. This variation is referred to as a "Martin-Gruber anastomoses" [48, 50]. As a consequence of this variation, patients can have preserved motor function to their hand despite ulnar nerve injury because the motor innervation is maintained by branches from the median nerve.

The Olecranon Process and the Olecranon Fossa

The protuberant olecranon process of the ulna is the chief bony landmark of the posterior elbow. The olecranon articulates with a smooth depression located on the posterior distal humerus that is referred to as the olecranon fossa. The elongated shape of the olecranon provides static stability to the subsequent ulnohumeral joint. The fossa is filled with a fat pad that usually insinuates between the fossa and olecranon process, and normally is not readily discernible on imaging. However, the fat pad can become lifted superiorly by a joint effusion or traumatic hemarthrosis, making it visible on cross-sectional imaging and radiography.

The Olecranon Bursa

Superficial relative to the olecranon process, there is a synovial-lined space called the olecranon bursa. The bursa is interspersed between the posterior skin, ~~the~~ distal triceps, and ~~the~~ tip of the olecranon process. The purpose of the bursa is to allow smooth motion of the triceps and olecranon beneath the skin during elbow flexion and extension [3]. Typically, the bursa is collapsed and not readily visible on imaging unless it becomes distended by fluid from an inflammatory, infectious, or posttraumatic entity.

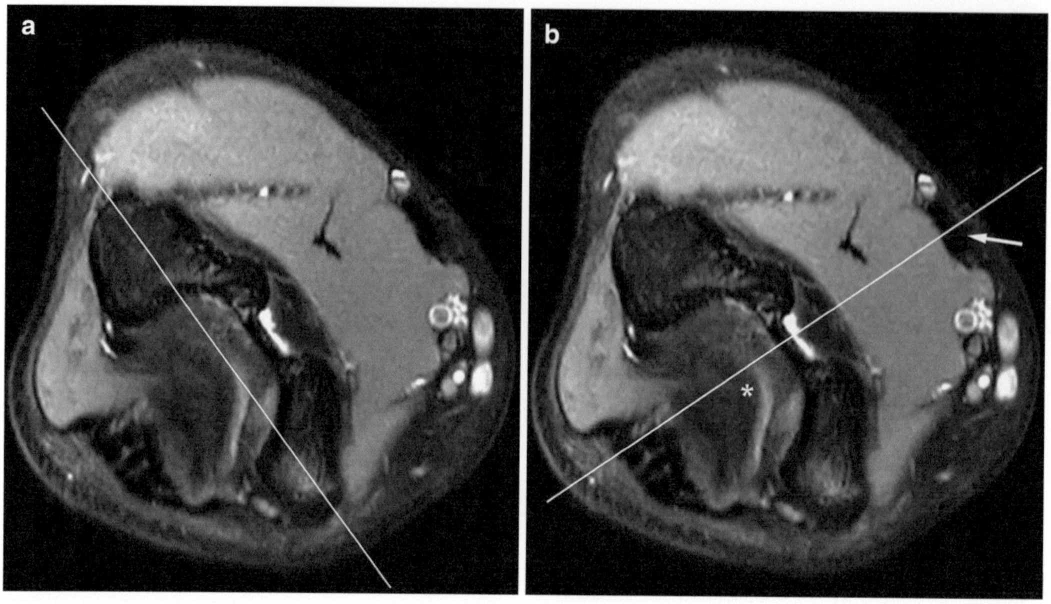

Fig. 2.34 (**a**) AX PDFS axis of image for coronal acquisition (white line) oriented parallel to the humeral epicondyles. (**b**) AX PDFS axis of image acquisition for sagittal imaging (white line), bisecting the distal biceps tendon (arrow) and olecranon tip (*)

MRI Optimization of the Elbow

Due to the complexity of the elbow joint, multiplanar imaging is crucial in order to best interrogate the various ligaments and tendons that stabilize and act on the joint. The slightly oblique course followed by most of the ligaments and the tendons necessitates that images in all planes be acquired slightly oblique relative to the proximal ulna and radius (Fig. 2.34a, b) [7]. Regardless of the plane of image acquisition, the field of view should begin above the level of the humeral epicondyles in order to include the origins of the common flexor and extensor tendons. Imaging should continue distally beyond the radial tuberosity to ensure the entire course of the distal biceps is imaged (Fig. 2.35).

All imaging planes and sequences assess bone marrow signal and muscular bulk. The axial plane of imaging is useful for evaluating short-axis, cross-sectional anatomy. Axial nonfat-saturated imaging is chiefly to evaluate anatomy as it displays the morphology, bulk and signal of the muscle bellies, tendons, and integrity of the muscular fascial planes and the perineuronal fat

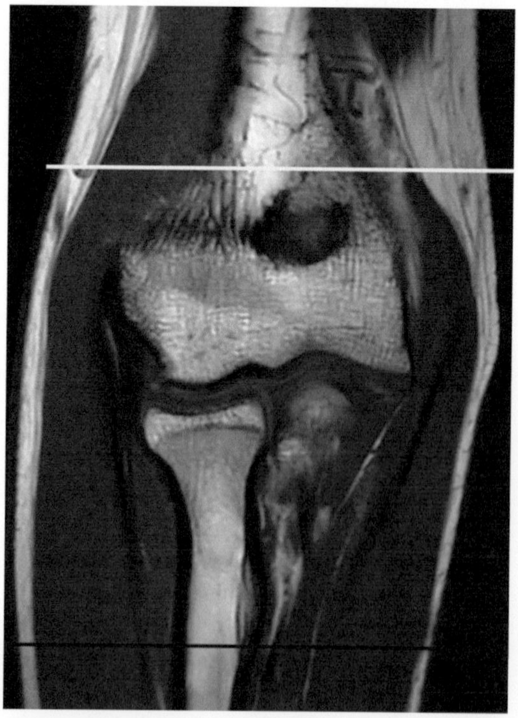

Fig. 2.35 COR image showing the AXIAL craniocaudal field of view that should extend from the humeral epicondyles proximally (white line) to the radial tuberosity inferiorly (black line)

planes [29]. Axial imaging is particularly crucial for evaluating the integrity of the annular ligament, which lies almost entirely in the axial plane [10, 34]. Adding axial fluid-sensitive, fat-saturated imaging assists in detecting pathology such as muscle fiber replacement or edematous obscuration of the normal muscular fascial planes and the perineuronal fat. Thus, in some facilities, the routine elbow MRI protocol includes both an axial T1 or PD nonfat-saturated sequence along with an axial fluid-sensitive fat-saturated sequence.

Conventional coronal plane imaging should be oriented in plane relative to the distal humeral condyles. Obtaining a coronal-oblique plane of imaging is accomplished by angling the localizer lines approximately 20–30° relative to the longitudinal axis of the ulna when the imaged arm is in full extension. This obliquity optimizes evaluation of the collateral ligaments, particularly the longitudinal course of the lateral ulnar collateral ligament, and is in-plane with the joint capsule [51]. Coronal or coronal-oblique imaging complements axial-plane imaging for better assessment of anatomic ligamentous integrity, since both the radial- and ulnar-sided ligaments are largely oriented in a coronal-oblique plane. This alignment is particularly true of the LUCL and RCL, which are both best evaluated on coronal/coronal-oblique images [10]. Coronal imaging is also ideal as a supplemental view in conjunction with axial imaging to evaluate the integrity of the common flexor and extensor tendon origins, underlying epicondylar marrow signal, and articular cartilage of the distal humerus, radial head, and proximal ulna [9]. Thus, the inclusion of T1- or PD-weighted nonfat-saturated coronal or coronal-oblique imaging along with coronal fluid-sensitive fat-saturated imaging should be considered.

A least one sequence acquired along the sagittal plane should be included in imaging evaluation of the elbow. Sagittal imaging is particularly useful for evaluating the craniocaudal longitudinal morphology of the triceps tendon and the integrity of its distal insertion. This plane of imaging is also useful when evaluating a joint effusion, fat pad displacement, olecranon bursal distention, and torn DBT retraction. Sagittal imaging helps assess the long-axis extent of marrow-replacing lesions, integrity of articular cartilage, morphology of the radial neck, and visualization of the inferior margin of the annular ligament, which adopts a fanlike or funnel-shaped appearance, as it tapers toward the radial neck [10, 34].

Special Considerations

If a study is being performed specifically to assess the DBT integrity, evaluation is optimized by placing the patient prone in the scanner and positioning the affected arm so that it is abducted over the patient's head with the elbow flexed and forearm supinated, resulting in a "thumb up" position [9]. This position has the advantage of laying out the oblique course of the DBT so that it is better captured in the plane of imaging [9].

If a study is being performed specifically to evaluate the integrity of the ligamentous joint capsule or to characterize a partial tendon tear, then MR arthrography is preferred over conventional MR imaging. The heightened contrast-to-noise ratio, accomplished with the installation of intra-articular contrast for the purpose of MR arthrography, has been shown to increase detection of ligament tears and partial tendon tears [31]. MR arthrography is also used to assess the stability of osteochondral defects and the presence of joint bodies and to evaluate postsurgical elbows [7, 9]. CT arthrography can be performed to better assess the elbow capsular integrity, cartilage, and intra-articular anatomy in patients for whom MRI is clinically contraindicated.

Intravenous gadolinium contrast with fat-saturated, multiplayer post-contrast imaging should be added when malignancy, inflammation, or a marrow-replacing process is suspected. Pre-contrast, fat-saturated T1-weighted imaging should also be included for comparison purposes in at least one plane, in order to distinguish true enhancement from intrinsically T1 bright tissue [9]. Regardless of the imaging plane selected, it is also beneficial to demarcate the area of clinical concern with a vitamin E capsule on the overlying skin surface. This ensures inclusion of the area in the field of view. If a superficial mass is suspected, care should be taken when applying the capsule so as not to compress and obviate the area of concern. In some institutions, the proximal and distal margins of a palpable mass are marked rather than the epicenter of the mass itself. This decreases the risk of compression as well as obscuration by artifact due to the intrinsic T2 relaxation time of the oily vitamin E capsule.

Technical Imaging Parameters

The technical parameters for image acquisition should be tailored with the aim of optimizing spatial resolution in order to offer the best delineation of the delicate ligaments and neurovascular bundles of the elbow. This is accomplished by using a small FOV of 10–12 cm, multiple acquisitions (≥1), use of an extremity coil, and imaging performed on a 1.5T or higher, with 3T being preferred at some institutions [8, 9, 31]. Image slice thickness should be thin, with minimal anatomic gapping [4, 52]. This translates to a slice thickness that is 3–4 mm or less and an image gap of less than 1 mm, with a common selection of 0.3–0.5 mm and some advocating for a gap of 0.3 mm or less [7, 31]. Thin image slice thickness and narrow gapping are recommended for both conventional MR imaging and MR arthrography [7, 9].

Patient positioning is somewhat determined by the patient's condition, size, and MRI coil selection. For the conventional elbow MRI exam, patients can be imaged either prone, prone-oblique, or supine. However, supine positioning, with the affected arm at the patient's side, appears to be more comfortable and better tolerated, resulting in less potential motion artifact [7, 9, 52]. This position is made possible when a phased array multichannel extremity coil is available [8]. Unfortunately, this position places the elbow outside of the MRI magnetic isocenter, causing field inhomogeneity and incomplete fat saturation (Fig. 2.36a, b) [7, 53]. In instances where there is significant artifact degradation, the use of STIR imaging may result in improved fat suppression but at the cost of decreasing the signal-to-noise ratio [7, 54]. Manual shimming has also been suggested as a means of decreasing field inhomogeneity artifact [8].

Conversely, when the arm is raised over the patient's head and the patient is placed either prone or prone-oblique, the arm becomes closer to the MRI isocenter with improved signal homogeneity and subsequent fat saturation [7–9, 51]. Accommodating large patients may necessitate imaging with the arm extended above the patient's head while the patient is lying obliquely in the

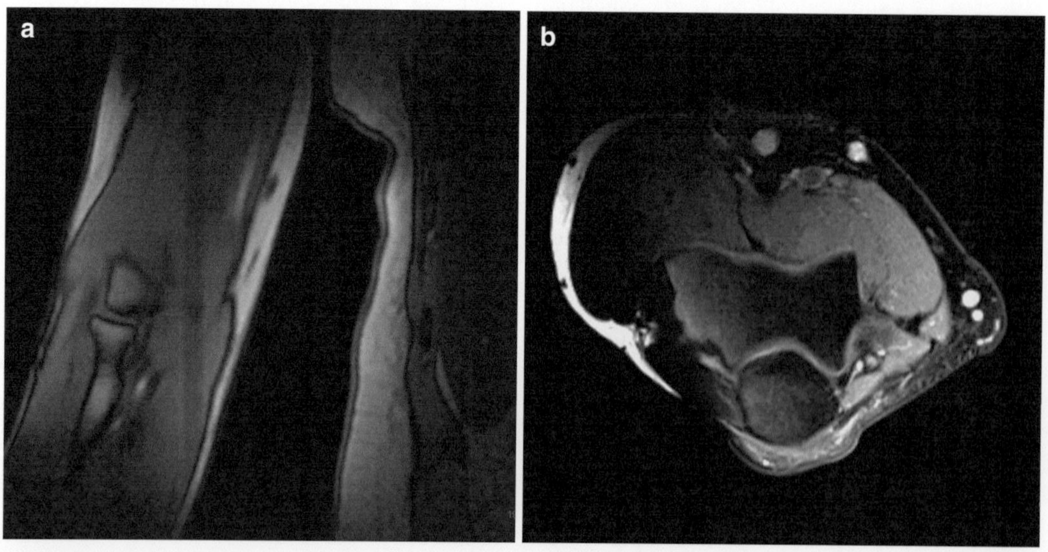

Fig. 2.36 (**a**) Localizer demonstrating arm positioned at the patient's side. (**b**) AX T2FS demonstrating the subsequent failed fat saturation of the lateral subcutaneous tissues

bore. However, these positions are often less comfortable increasing the likelihood of motion degradation [7–9].

Tailoring the MRI for the purpose of evaluating the DBT may necessitate patient repositioning. As state previously, some advocate for imaging with the patient prone or oblique in the bore with their arm raised above their head and their elbow flexed while the forearm is partially supinated resulting in a “thumb up” position. This position, called the FABS technique, an acronym for *f*lexed *ab*ducted *s*upinated view, captures the entire length of the tendon in one imaging plane often on a single image [9, 55]. However, this position may be difficult to maintain if patients have pain or limited mobility. Options include beginning the examination with conventional patient positioning and then repositioning the patient into FABS positioning for final sequences.

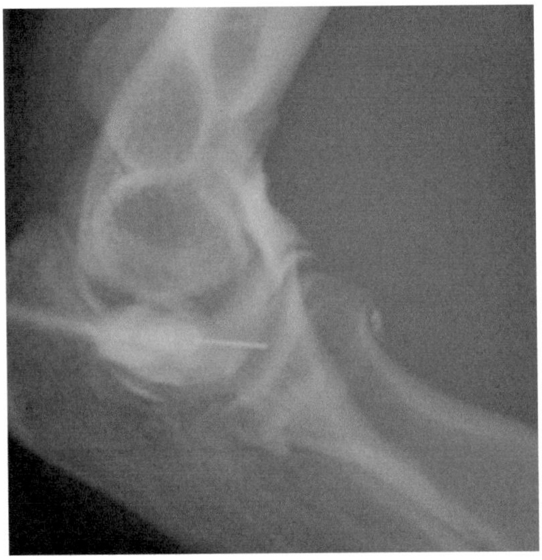

Fig. 2.37 Fluoroscopic image documenting the needle directed into the radiocapitellar joint from a lateral approach with the needle aimed just above the central articular surface of the radial head

MR Elbow Arthrography

The instillation of contrast into the elbow joint can be performed using a lateral, posterior, or posterolateral approach under fluoroscopic or ultrasound guidance for a subsequent MR or CT arthrogram [7]. To perform a lateral approach injection, the patient is placed with the arm extended overhead, and the elbow is flexed 90°. After the skin is cleaned, prepped, and draped, local anesthetic is given, and a 22-gauge needle is advanced into the radiocapitellar joint just above the central articular surface of the radial head (Fig. 2.37) [7, 56]. This approach is the most commonly used, particularly in institutions where injection is performed on a standard fluoroscopy unit without the advantage of a C-arm. This approach is possible to perform within the fixed space between the fluoroscopy table and camera intensifier and is advantageous if there is suspected injury to the triceps tendon or posterior compartment.

A posterior approach aims the needle tip between the olecranon process, the humeral olecranon fossa, and the radial head [7]. This approach has the advantage of completely avoiding the radial collateral ligament, which may be of particular interest if the patient presents with lateral elbow symptoms. The patient’s elbow is placed in a 90-degree flexion, and the needle is advanced between the humeral condyles just cranial relative to the tip of the olecranon process (Fig. 2.38) [7, 8]. This approach is particularly useful if a C-arm is available that enables multiplanar guidance in order to assess needle depth during needle advancement.

The posterolateral approach begins with the patient placed with their elbow at 90 degrees of flexion. However, the needle is advanced between the olecranon process, the posterior lateral distal humerus, and the radial head so as to miss both the radial collateral ligament complex anteriorly and the triceps tendon posteriorly [7]. This final approach is less frequently used than the lateral and posterior techniques, as the obliquity of the needle can make it difficult to assess needle depth.

Regardless of the needle approach, once intra-articular needle tip placement is confirmed, a total of 5–10 cc of dilute gadolinium contrast is instilled into the joint. The degree of contrast administered varies greatly across institutions with the most common quantity appearing to fall between 5 and 8 cc [8, 9, 40, 51]. The contrast should distend the joint capsule, filling the posterior olecranon recess, anterior humeral recess,

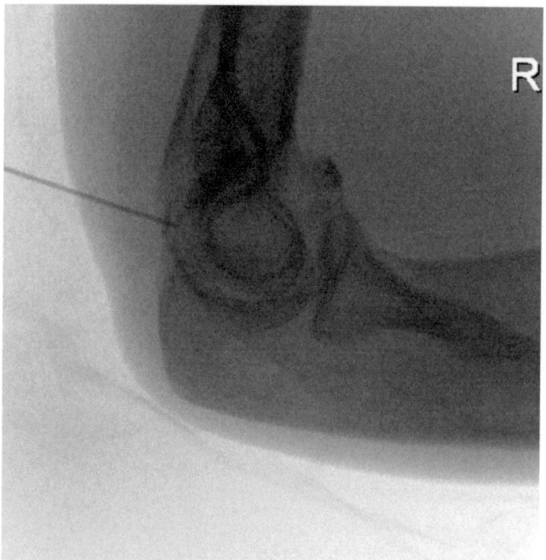

Fig. 2.38 Fluoroscopic image illustrating the posterior approach with the needle aiming between the humeral condyles, just above the tip of the olecranon process

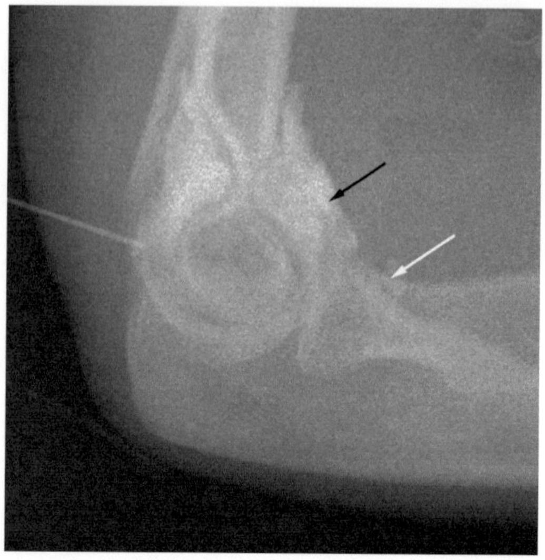

Fig. 2.39 Posterior postinjection radiograph showing the needle directed into the olecranon recess, and contrast in the anterior humeral recess (black arrow) and the annular recess (white arrow)

Table 2.1 Example of MR protocol parameters for 1.5T

Elbow routine	Ax T1	Ax T2 FS	Cor T1	Cor T2 FS	Sag T2 FS
FOV (mm)	120–140	120–140	140	140	140
Thickness (mm)	3	3	3	3	3
Spacing	0.5–0.8	0.5–0.8	0.5–0.8	0.5–0.8	0.5–1
Matrix	230/256	230/256	250/384	208/384	250/384
Voxel size (mm^3)	≤1	≤1	<1	<1	<1
TR	400–750	3000–4750	400–750	3000–4750	3000–4750
TE	<30	60–70	<30	60–70	60–80
Total scan time (min)	14–17				

and annular recess that encircle the radial neck (Fig. 2.39) [8].

The most common contrast concentration utilized for MRI arthrogram is 1 in 200 dilution of gadolinium. This ratio is obtained by drawing up 0.1 cc of gadolinium and diluting into a 20 cc mixture. The mixture often contains a combination of saline, iodinated contrast, and anesthetic such as lidocaine, bupivacaine, or ropivacaine. Contents and amounts can vary between institutions but the gadolinium dilution is constant.

Post-arthrogram imaging should be obtained less than 1 hour following contrast injection to prevent absorption or extra-articular extravasation of contrast resulting in a non-arthrographic imaging study [51]. An example arthrography protocol consists of T1 fat-suppressed triplanar imaging in axial, coronal, and sagittal planes, followed by fat-suppressed fluid-weighted coronal imaging and sagittal imaging that is either T1- or T2-weighted without fat suppression [9]. Some institutions advocate for two imaging planes such axial and sagittal being performed *with* T1 fat saturation, while the coronal plane is T1-weighted without fat saturation, followed by triplane fluid-sensitive imaging all with fat saturation (Tables 2.1 and 2.2) [7].

Table 2.2 Example of MR arthrography parameters for 1.5T

Elbow arthrogram	Ax T1*	Cor T1*	Ax T2 FS	Cor T2 FS	Cor T1 FS	Sag T2 FS
FOV (mm)	140	140	140	140	140	140
Thickness (mm)	3	3	3	2–3	2–3	3–4
Spacing	.5–0.8	0.5–0.8	0.5–0.8	0.5–0.8	0.5–0.8	0.5–1
Matrix	230–256/256	256/256	230–256/256	224–256/150–256	224–256/128	208–256/256
Voxel size (mm^3)	≤1	<1	≤1	<1	<1	1–1.2
TR	400–750	400–750	2000–4000	2000–4000	400–750	2000–4000
TE	<20	<30	60	60	<30	60
Total scan minutes	20–27					
Choose one to be without fat saturation	*	*				

Image Optimization

Image optimization largely centers on maximizing the signal-to-noise ratio (SNR) and anatomic detail in order to adequately assess the small and intricate anatomy of the elbow. This is predicated on appropriate coil selection, with preference for dedicated extremity phased array coils that are capable of functioning as both send and receive coils.

Choosing an appropriate field of view (FOV) requires optimizing patient position so that the elbow is located as close to the magnetic isocenter as possible, as well as excluding unnecessary peripheral detail and extra-anatomic dead space [4]. Selecting a FOV that is too large can increase the likelihood of inhomogeneous fat saturation, while selecting one that is too small, particularly in a large patient, can accentuate anatomic wrap artifact [54, 57]. Maximizing SNR is particularly important for fat-saturated fluid-sensitive sequences which due to their acquisition parameters have less intrinsic signal relative to noise to begin with [57]. To compensate, SNR can be optimized by decreasing the time to echo (TE), thereby increasing the time for signal detection by the MR unit [57]. Increasing voxel size can be accomplished by reducing the matrix size or increasing the FOV [54, 57]. For larger joints or larger patients, SNR can also be improved by increasing slice thickness.

Another hurtle in quality image acquisition is an inability to apply satisfactory post-contrast fat saturation due to metal artifact or old equipment. Such a failure degrades visualization of administered contrast that is intrinsically T1 bright similar to the neighboring fat. To improve anatomic conspicuity, consider increasing the number of signal averages (NEX) to increase available signal and subsequently improve SNR. Unfortunately, this technique lengthens overall imaging time and therefore may not be a popular option for sites with busy MR schedules [57]. For conventional non-orthographic MR studies, fat saturation can be improved by replacing traditional T2-weighted sequences with STIR imaging. In addition, some MR vendors have released metal artifact reduction software that is specifically intended to decrease susceptibility artifact for MR and MR arthrography exams using parameter modification such as manipulations in acquisition bandwidth [54]. These software packages may be worth considering if a large percentage of the patient population present with orthopedic hardware.

Overall, the small size and anatomic complexity of the elbow result in special considerations that affect the physical imaging and subsequent radiologic interpretation of the joint. Familiarity with the off-axis alignment of the joint is crucial when orienting the planes of imaging in order to acquire satisfactory images. Awareness of the close anatomic relationship that exists between the bones, ligaments, and tendons of the joint is imperative for competent assessment of elbow integrity and the recognition of injury patterns, many of which will be presented in the following chapters.

References

1. Tagliafico AS, Bignotti B, Martinoli C. Elbow US: anatomy, variants, and scanning technique. Radiology. 2015;275(3):636–50.
2. Alcid JG, Ahmad CS, Lee TQ. Elbow anatomy and structural biomechanics. Clin Sports Med. 2004;23(4):503–17, vii.
3. Fowler KA, Chung CB. Normal MR imaging anatomy of the elbow. Magn Reson Imaging Clin N Am. 2004;12(2):191–206, v.
4. Helms CA, Major NM, Anderson MW, Kaplan PA, Dussault R. Musculoskeletal MRI. 2nd ed. Philadelphia: Saunders; 2009. p. 224–43.
5. Konin GP, Nazarian LN, Walz DM. US of the elbow: indications, technique, normal anatomy, and pathologic conditions. Radiographics. 2013;33(4):E125–47.
6. ASCM. Bushman BA, Battista R, Swan P, Ransdell L, Thompson WR, editors. ACSM'S resources for the personal trainer. 4th ed. Baltimore: Wolters Kluwer/ Lippincott Williams & Wilkins. p. 70–3.
7. Bucknor MD, Stevens KJ, Steinbach LS. Elbow imaging in sport: sports imaging series. Radiology. 2016;280(1):328.
8. Johnson D, Stevens KJ, Riley G, Shapiro L, Yoshioka H, Gold GE. Approach to MR imaging of the elbow and wrist: technical aspects and innovation. Magn Reson Imaging Clin N Am. 2015;23(3):355–66.
9. Berquist TH, Bancroft LW. In: Berquist TH, editor. MRI of the musculoskeletal system. 5th ed. Philadelphia: Lippincott Williams & Wilkins; 2006. p. 657–717.

10. Mak S, Beltran LS, Bencardino J, Orr J, Jazrawi L, Cerezal L, et al. MRI of the annular ligament of the elbow: review of anatomic considerations and pathologic findings in patients with posterolateral elbow instability. AJR Am J Roentgenol. 2014;203(6):1272–9.
11. Wells J, Ablove RH. Coronoid fractures of the elbow. Clin Med Res. 2008;6(1):40–4.
12. Chung CB, Chew FS, Steinbach L. MR imaging of tendon abnormalities of the elbow. Magn Reson Imaging Clin N Am. 2004;12(2):233–45, vi.
13. Sookur PA, Naraghi AM, Bleakney RR, Jalan R, Chan O, White LM. Accessory muscles: anatomy, symptoms, and radiologic evaluation. Radiographics. 2008;28(2):481–99.
14. Nguyen ML, Rosenthal J, Umpierrez M, Lourie GM, Singer AD. MRN findings of lateral antebrachial cutaneous nerve impingement in a collegiate athlete. Skelet Radiol. 2020;49(5):809–14.
15. Spinner RJ, Lins RE, Collins AJ, Spinner M. Posterior interosseous nerve compression due to an enlarged bicipital bursa confirmed by MRI. J Hand Surg Br. 1993;18(6):753–6.
16. Sanal HT, Chen L, Negrao P, Haghighi P, Trudell DJ, Resnick DL. Distal attachment of the brachialis muscle: anatomic and MRI study in cadavers. AJR Am J Roentgenol. 2009;192(2):468–72.
17. Gray H. The muscles and fascia of the arm. In: Lewis W, editor. Anatomy of the human body. 20th ed. Philadelphia: Lea & Febiger; 1918.
18. Loukas M, Louis RG Jr, South G, Alsheik E, Christopherson C. A case of an accessory brachialis muscle. Clin Anat. 2006;19(6):550–3.
19. Bordalo-Rodrigues M, Rosenberg ZS. MR imaging of entrapment neuropathies at the elbow. Magn Reson Imaging Clin N Am. 2004;12(2):247–63, vi.
20. Soubeyrand M, Melhem R, Protais M, Artuso M, Creze M. Anatomy of the median nerve and its clinical applications. Hand Surg Rehabil. 2020;39(1):2–18.
21. Tubbs RS, Deep A, Shoja MM, Mortazavi MM, Loukas M, Cohen-Gadol AA. The arcade of Struthers: an anatomical study with potential neurosurgical significance. Surg Neurol Int. 2011;2:184.
22. Caetano EB, Sabongi Neto JJ, Vieira LA, Caetano MF. The arcade of Struthers: an anatomical study and clinical implications. Rev Bras Ortop. 2017;52(3):331–6.
23. Glover NM, Murphy PB. Anatomy, shoulder and upper limb, radial nerve. Treasure Island (FL): StatPearls; 2020.
24. Wheeless C. June 23 2016 [cited 8-25-2020]. In: Wheeless' textbook of orthopaedics [Internet]. Duke Orthopaedics. June 23 2016. [cited 8-25-2020]. Available from: http://www.wheelessonline.com/ortho/posterior_interosseous_nerve.
25. Kinni V, Craig J, van Holsbeeck M, Ditmars D. Entrapment of the posterior interosseous nerve at the arcade of Frohse with sonographic, magnetic resonance imaging, and intraoperative confirmation. J Ultrasound Med. 2009;28(6):807–12.
26. Terra BB, Sassine TJ, Lima GF, Rodrigues LM, Padua DV, Nadai A. Radial head fracture associated with posterior interosseous nerve injury. Rev Bras Ortop. 2016;51(6):725–9.
27. Desai SJ, Lalone E, Athwal GS, Ferreira LM, Johnson JA, King GJ. Hemiarthroplasty of the elbow: the effect of implant size on joint congruency. J Shoulder Elb Surg. 2016;25(2):297–303.
28. Kachrimanis G, Papadopoulou O. Acute partial rupture of the common extensor tendon. J Ultrasound. 2010;13(2):74–5.
29. Porrino JA, Monroe EJ. Practical approach musculoskeletal MRI: MRI of the elbow [eBook]. Bare Bones Books; 2013.
30. Chung C. MRI of the upper extremity. Lippincott Williams & Wilkins/ Wolterz Kluwer; 2010. p. 541–75.
31. Carrino JA, Morrison WB, Zou KH, Steffen RT, Snearly WN, Murray PM. Lateral ulnar collateral ligament of the elbow: optimization of evaluation with two-dimensional MR imaging. Radiology. 2001;218(1):118–25.
32. Bozkurt M, Acar HI, Apaydin N, Leblebicioglu G, Elhan A, Tekdemir I, et al. The annular ligament: an anatomical study. Am J Sports Med. 2005;33(1):114–8.
33. Camp CL, Sanchez-Sotelo J, Shields MN, O'Driscoll SW. Lateral ulnar collateral ligament reconstruction for posterolateral rotatory instability of the elbow. Arthrosc Tech. 2017;6(4):e1101–e5.
34. Sanal HT, Chen L, Haghighi P, Trudell DJ, Resnick DL. Annular ligament of the elbow: MR arthrography appearance with anatomic and histologic correlation. AJR Am J Roentgenol. 2009;193(2):W122–6.
35. University of Washington Muscle Atlas [Internet]. University of Washington. 1997 [cited 7-29-2020]. Available from: https://rad.washington.edu/muscle-atlas/.
36. Karbach LE, Elfar J. Elbow instability: anatomy, biomechanics, diagnostic maneuvers, and testing. J Hand Surg Am. 2017;42(2):118–26.
37. Muscle Tables [Internet]. 2001 [cited 2-14-2020]. Available from: http://www.ptcentral.com/muscles.
38. e-Anatomy [Internet]. Available from: www.imaios.com.
39. Beckett KS, McConnell P, Lagopoulos M, Newman RJ. Variations in the normal anatomy of the collateral ligaments of the human elbow joint. J Anat. 2000;197(Pt 3):507–11.
40. Peterson JJ, Fenton DS, Czervionke LF. Image-guided musculoskeletal intervention [internet]. Philadelphia: Saunders Elsevier; 2008; [48-62].
41. Fuss FK. The ulnar collateral ligament of the human elbow joint. Anatomy, function and biomechanics. J Anat. 1991;175:203–12.
42. Labott JR, Aibinder WR, Dines JS, Camp CL. Understanding the medial ulnar collateral ligament of the elbow: review of native ligament anatomy and function. World J Orthop. 2018;9(6):78–84.

43. Clark NJ, Desai VS, Dines JD, Morrey ME, Camp CL. Nonreconstruction options for treating medial ulnar collateral ligament injuries of the elbow in overhead athletes. Curr Rev Musculoskelet Med. 2018;11(1):48–54.
44. Tribst MF, Zoppi A, Camargo JC, Sassi D, de Carvalho AE. Anatomical and functional study of the medial collateral ligament complex of the elbow. Acta Ortop Bras. 2012;20(6):334–8.
45. Camp CL, Jahandar H, Sinatro AM, Imhauser CW, Altchek DW, Dines JS. Quantitative anatomic analysis of the medial ulnar collateral ligament complex of the elbow. Orthop J Sports Med. 2018;6(3):2325967118762751.
46. Becker RE, Manna B. StatPearls. Treasure Island (FL): StatPearls Publishing; 2018. Available from: https://www.ncbi.nlm.nih.gov/books/NBK499892/.
47. Andrews K, Rowland A, Pranjal A, Ebraheim N. Cubital tunnel syndrome: Anatomy, clinical presentation, and management. J Orthop. 2018;15(3):832–6.
48. Granger A, Sardi JP, Iwanaga J, Wilson TJ, Yang L, Loukas M, et al. Osborne's ligament: a review of its history, anatomy, and surgical importance. Cureus. 2017;9(3):e1080.
49. Gelberman RH, Yamaguchi K, Hollstien SB, Winn SS, Heidenreich FP Jr, Bindra RR, et al. Changes in interstitial pressure and cross-sectional area of the cubital tunnel and of the ulnar nerve with flexion of the elbow. An experimental study in human cadavera. J Bone Joint Surg Am. 1998;80(4):492–501.
50. Cavalheiro CS, Filho MR, Pedro G, Caetano MF, Vieira LA, Caetano EB. Clinical repercussions of Martin-Gruber anastomosis: anatomical study. Rev Bras Ortop. 2016;51(2):214–23.
51. Steinbach LS, Chung CB, Yoshioka H. In: Chung CB, Steinbach LS, editors. MRI of the upper extremity. Philadelphia: Lippincott Williams & Wilkins/ Wolterz Kluwer; 2010. p. 190–1, 8–9.
52. Kaplan LJ, Potter HG. MR imaging of ligament injuries to the elbow. Magn Reson Imaginsg Clin N Am. 2004;12(2):221–32, v–vi.
53. Sampath SC. Magnetic resonance imaging of the elbow: a structured approach. Sport Health. 2013;5(1):34–49.
54. Roth E, Hoff M, Richardson ML, Ha AS, Porrino J. Artifacts affecting musculoskeletal magnetic resonance imaging: their origins and solutions. Curr Probl Diagn Radiol. 2016;45(5):340–6.
55. Giuffrè BM, Moss MJ. Optimal positioning for MRI of the distal biceps brachii tendon: flexed abducted supinated view. AJR Am J Roentgenol. 2004;182(4):944–6.
56. Lungu E, Moser TP. A practical guide for performing arthrography under fluoroscopic or ultrasound guidance. Insights Imaging. 2015;6(6):601–10.
57. Morrison W, Sanders T. In: Elsevier M, editor. Optimization of clinical musculoskeletal imaging. Philadelphia; 2008. p. 3–34.

Elbow Pathology: Traumatic

3

Lindsay Stratchko, Lauren Ladd,
and Donna G. Blankenbaker

Osseous Fractures

Radiographs are the imaging method of choice for evaluation of patients with traumatic elbow pain. Magnetic resonance (MR) imaging plays a role in the identification of subtle or radiographically occult fractures and characterizes associated soft tissue injuries of the elbow. Additional advantages of MR imaging include the ability to image patients in a cast without significant reduction in image quality.

Radial Head/Neck Fractures

Etiology and Clinical Presentation

Radial head fractures are the most common elbow fractures, accounting for approximately 33% of elbow fractures [1]. Patients often present following fall on an outstretched hand with the elbow in extension and forearm in pronation. This position results in longitudinal force transmission from the wrist to the radial head. Isolated radial head or neck fractures occur if the integrity of the interosseous membrane and the distal radioulnar joint (DRUJ) are maintained; however, Essex-Lopresti fractures result when a radial head fracture is combined with interosseous membrane and DRUJ compromise. The constellation of injuries associated with Essex-Lopresti fractures impairs longitudinal stability of the forearm, often requiring operative management to restore axial strength and prevent proximal migration of the radius.

Approximately one third of radial head fractures are associated with additional elbow or wrist fractures, elbow dislocation, or ligament injuries [1]. Patients often present with lateral elbow pain and limited forearm pronation and supination. Additionally, the presence of an elbow effusion may inhibit full elbow flexion and extension.

Imaging/Classification

While radiographs are first-line imaging in patients with suspected radial head fracture, MR imaging has been shown to be a useful tool in detecting radiographically occult fractures in adult patients with elbow effusion on radiographs following trauma [2]. The best diagnostic clue is a positive fat pad sign on lateral radiograph

L. Stratchko (✉) · D. G. Blankenbaker
University of Wisconsin School of Medicine and Public Health, Madison, WI, USA
e-mail: LStratchko@uwhealth.org; DBlankenbaker@uwhealth.org

L. Ladd
Indiana University School of Medicine, Indianapolis, IN, USA
e-mail: LMLadd@iupui.edu

B. U. Casagranda (ed.), *MRI of the Upper Extremity*, https://doi.org/10.1007/978-3-030-81612-4_3

(Fig. 3.1). Radial head fractures are typically a longitudinal fracture line located in the lateral aspect of the radial head, while radial neck fractures are seen as buckling or angulation of the radial head/neck junction and typically oriented in the transverse plane.

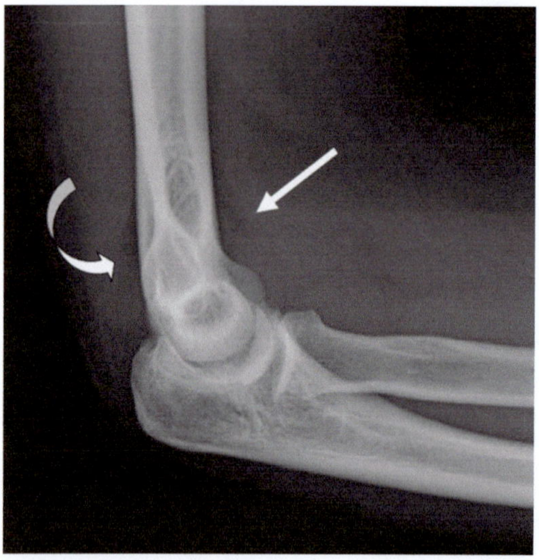

Fig. 3.1 Elbow joint effusion. A 54-year-old female presents with elbow pain after a fall. Lateral elbow radiograph shows elevation of the anterior (arrow) and posterior (curved arrow) fat pads consistent with an elbow effusion

Mason Classification

The most widely used classification for radial head fractures is the Mason classification (Fig. 3.2) which describes the degree of displacement, comminution, and the presence or absence of elbow dislocation [3]:

- Type I fractures are displaced less than 2 mm and lack a mechanical block to motion (Fig. 3.3).
- Type II fractures are displaced greater than 2 mm, and restricted range of motion may or may not be present.
- Type III fractures are comminuted and displaced greater than 2 mm. A mechanical block to motion is present.
- Type IV fractures include a radial head fracture in the setting of elbow dislocation.

Treatment

Isolated nondisplaced radial head fractures with preserved range of motion may be managed conservatively with immobilization. In the event of fracture displacement, comminution, or additional elbow fractures, operative intervention is often required. Options for management include radial head resection for low-demand patients at

Fig. 3.2 Mason classification of radial head fractures

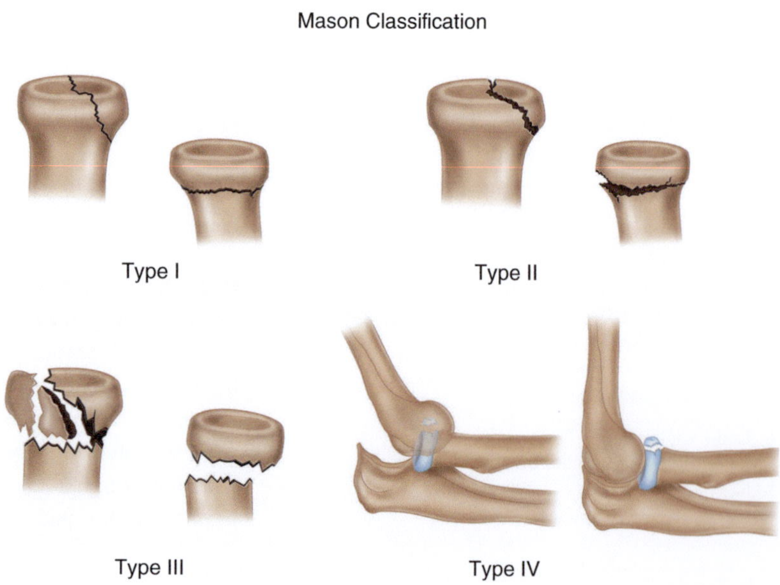

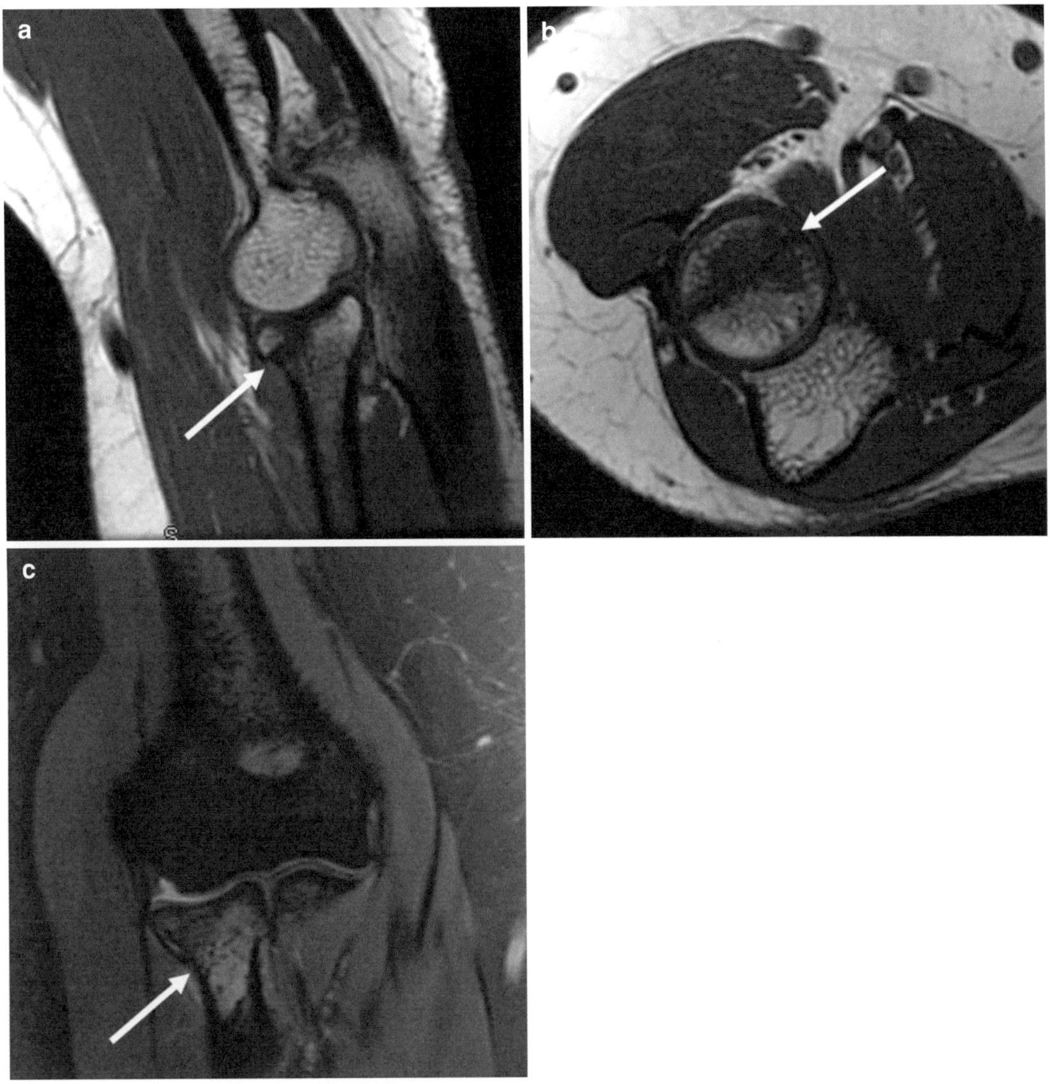

Fig. 3.3 Radial head fracture. A 56-year-old woman presents with elbow pain after a fall. Sagittal T1 image (**a**) shows a minimally depressed intra-articular radial head fracture (arrow). Axial T1 image (**b**) details articular surface involvement of the low-signal fracture line (arrow). Coronal T2 fat-suppressed image (**c**) demonstrates the extent of bone marrow edema within the proximal radius (arrow)

the time of injury or if the patient experiences continued pain after failed trial of conservative management. Open reduction and internal fixation (ORIF) is indicated in Mason type II or III fractures where fragment reduction and fixation are feasible. In the event of highly comminuted fractures where anatomic reduction is not achievable or elbow fracture dislocations (including Essex-Lopresti injuries), radial head arthroplasty is an option to restore radial length and range of motion [4].

Olecranon Fractures

Etiology and Clinical Presentation

Various forces upon the elbow produce different types of olecranon fractures, including transverse, oblique, and comminuted fractures. Contraction of the triceps muscle during elbow extension or eccentric contraction during throw deceleration generally results in transverse olecranon fractures. Repeated contact of the olecranon process with the olecranon fossa in valgus extension produces oblique fractures. Comminuted fractures often follow direct blow injuries. Olecranon fractures occur in a bimodal distribution with young, athletic individuals suffering fractures from high-energy injuries, while elderly patients are more susceptible to low-energy mechanisms such as falls [5].

Imaging/Classification

Colton Classification

Multiple olecranon fracture classification systems have been described without universal acceptance of a single system. The Colton classification was initially outlined in 1973, which was based on mechanism of injury, fracture morphology, and elbow stability [6]. According to the Colton classification, olecranon fractures are categorized as either nondisplaced (type I) or displaced (type II) (Fig. 3.4). Nondisplaced fractures are considered those who have less than 2 mm of displacement, and the degree of displacement does not increase with elbow flexion. Displaced fractures are further subcategorized based on fracture morphology:

- Type I: Nondisplaced fractures with less than 2 mm displacement (Fig. 3.5)
- Type II: Displaced fractures:
  - a: Avulsion fractures involving the triceps insertion
  - b: Oblique or transverse fractures
  - c: Comminuted fractures
  - d: Olecranon fracture in combination with elbow dislocation

AO Classification

AO is the acronym for *Arbeitsgemeinschaft für Osteosynthesefragen* which translates in German to "working group for bone fusion issues." The AO classification was designed as a comprehensive long bone fracture classification system. Originally introduced in 1987, the AO classification remains in use today after validation [7]. The first component of the AO method includes the specific bone as well as the involved segment of bone. The proximal ulna is denoted "2U1" in the AO scheme (Fig. 3.6). Once the bone and segment are established, the joint involvement is detailed as either extra-articular (A), partial articular (B), or complete articular (C). Further subdivisions are as follows:

- Extra-articular fractures (A)
  - 1: Avulsion of the triceps insertion
  - 2: Simple proximal metaphyseal fracture
  - 3: Multifragmentary proximal metaphyseal fracture
- Partial articular fractures (B)
  - 1: Olecranon fracture
  - 2: Coronoid fracture
- Complete articular fractures (C)
  - 3: Complex articular fracture involving both the olecranon and coronoid

Mayo Classification

The Mayo classification was first described in 1993 by Cabanela and Morrey to simplify prior olecranon classification systems [8]. This system characterizes fractures based on displacement, comminution, and stability of the ulnohumeral joint, which implies the condition of the ligament stabilizers (Fig. 3.7):

- Type I fractures are nondisplaced.
- Type II fractures are displaced; however, the ulnohumeral joint remains stable. Type II fractures are the most common type of olecranon fractures.
- Type III fractures are displaced fractures with joint dislocation or instability during valgus and/or varus stress, indicating collateral ligament tears. Type III fractures are often associated with additional elbow fractures of the radial head or coronoid process.

Each fracture type is further subdivided into noncomminuted (A) or comminuted (B) fractures [9]. The Mayo classification has been shown to have poor reproducibility in the clinical setting, and several studies have shown the fracture types

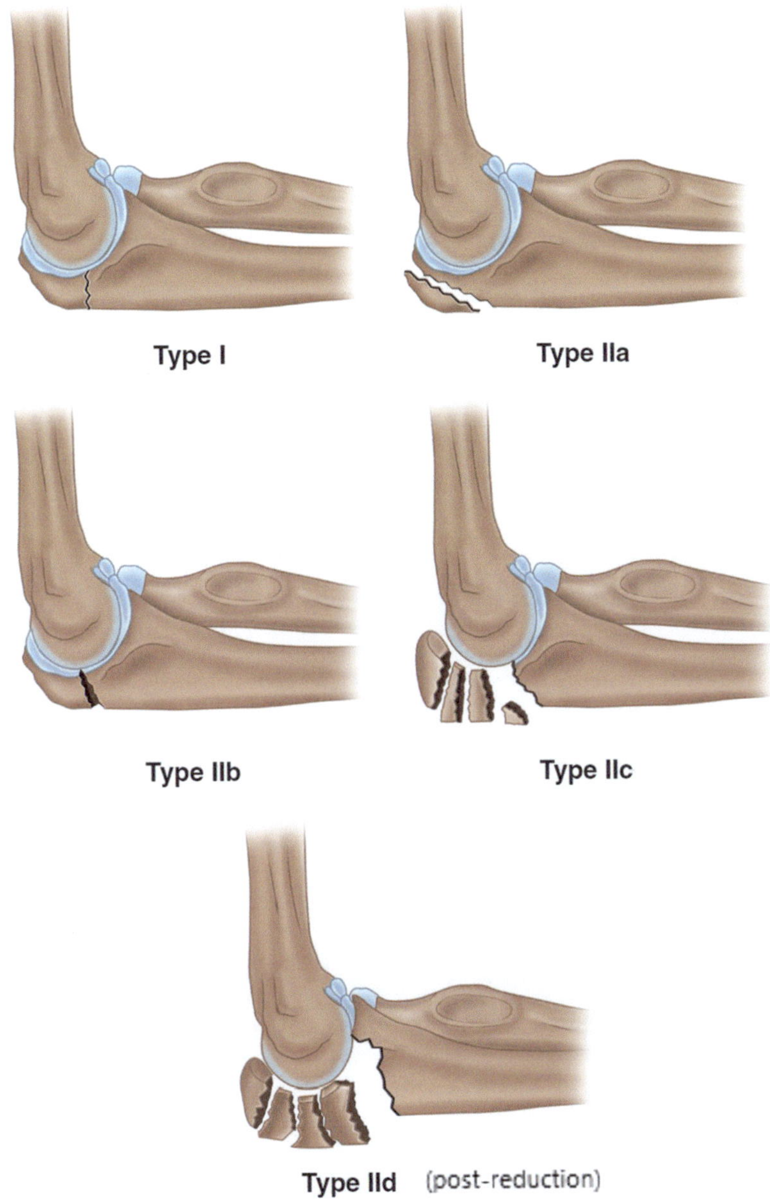

Fig. 3.4 Colton classification of olecranon fractures

did not demonstrate differences in outcomes [10, 11]. Despite these limitations, the Mayo classification system is commonly used in clinical and research applications.

Schatzker Classification

The Schatzker classification system is based on fracture pattern and takes into consideration the type of fixation required (Fig. 3.8) [12]:

- Transverse fractures occur at or near the apex of the sigmoid notch and are often associated with an avulsion mechanism.
- Transverse-impacted fractures are typically comminuted and result in depression of the articular surface.
- Oblique fractures result from abnormal contact between the olecranon process and the olecranon fossa during elbow hyperextension.

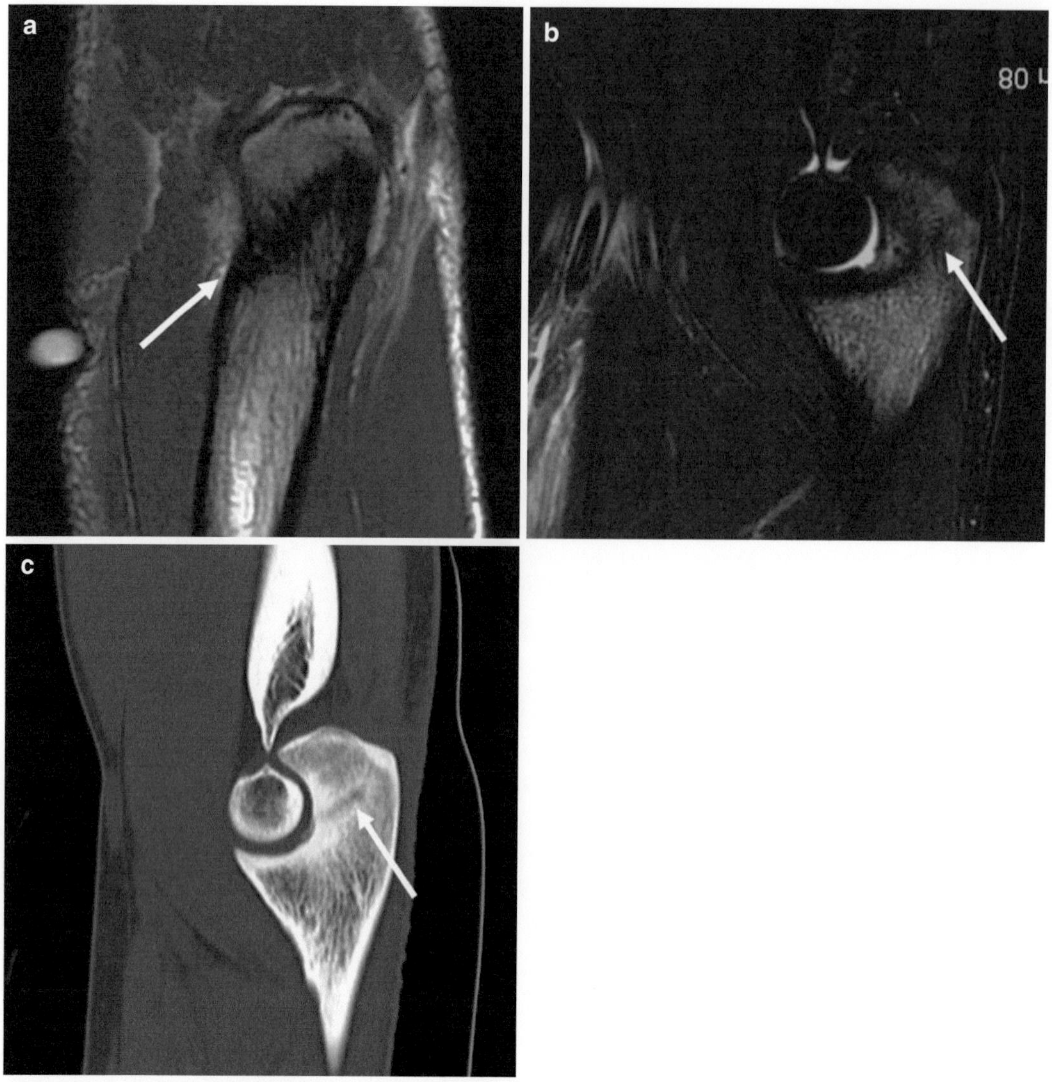

Fig. 3.5 Colton type I olecranon fracture. A 64-year-old man presents with elbow pain after a fall. Coronal T1 (**a**) and sagittal T2 fat-suppressed (**b**) images show the low-signal fracture line (arrow), which corresponds with the nondisplaced intra-articular fracture (arrow) on sagittal CT (**c**)

These fractures often originate at the sigmoid notch and extend distally.

- Comminuted fractures typically follow high-energy trauma and are associated with additional elbow injuries.
- Oblique-distal fractures extend distal to the coronoid process and often alter elbow stability.
- Fracture dislocations are generally a result of severe elbow trauma and are associated with concomitant injury to the static and dynamic elbow stabilizers as well as additional fractures.

Treatment

Conservative management can often be trialed in nondisplaced fractures or elderly patients with low demand. Operative management consists of one of the four techniques, including fragment excision, tension band fixation, plate fixation,

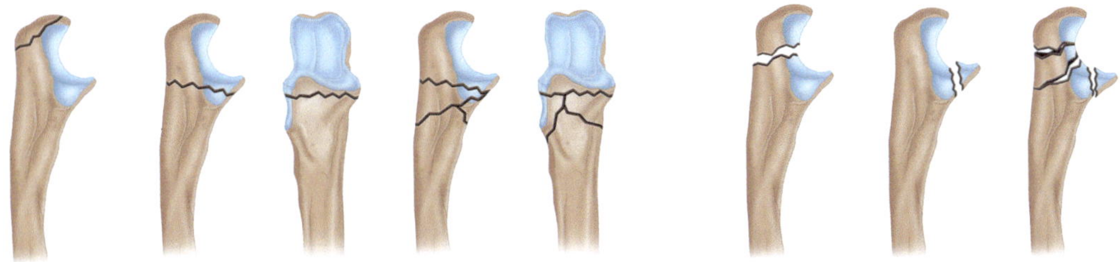

Fig. 3.6 AO classification. The proximal olecranon is designated bone "2U1" in this classification Scheme. *A* extra-articular, *B* partial articular, *C* complete articular. Further subdivision with numbers designates the location of the fracture as discussed in this chapter

and intramedullary fixation. Fragment excision is preferred in patients with small fracture fragments or poor bone quality that could impede adequate healing, such as patients with osteoporosis. The principle of the tension band technique involves conversion of distracting forces into dynamic compression across the fracture (Fig. 3.9). Intramedullary fixation can be used alone or in combination with tension bands to treat simple transverse or oblique olecranon fractures. Finally, comminuted fractures often require plate stabilization, which can support bone graft material in the event of articular surface depression [13].

Coronoid Fractures

Etiology and Clinical Presentation

The presence of a coronoid process fracture signifies an episode of elbow instability, often following posterior subluxation or dislocation of the olecranon resulting in shear injury of the coronoid process. Elbow stability is related to the size of the coronoid process fracture fragment as the anterior joint capsule inserts approximately 6 mm distal to the coronoid tip. Another major elbow stabilizer, the anterior band of the ulnar collateral ligament, inserts approximately 18 mm from the coronoid tip. Coronoid fractures can occur in isolation or in association with posteromedial rotatory instability (PMRI) and posterolateral rotatory instability (PLRI) or in the terrible triad of elbow injuries which consists of coronoid and radial head fractures in combination with elbow dislocation. The anteromedial coronoid facet is involved during varus stress associated with PMRI, which can also result in lateral collateral ligament complex injuries. Alternatively, coronoid tip fractures are seen in valgus PLRI as well as radial head fractures and lateral collateral ligament complex tears, particularly with involvement of the lateral ulnar collateral ligament.

Imaging/Classification

Regan-Morrey Classification

The Regan-Morrey classification was developed in 1989 and is based on the percentage of coronoid height involvement [14]. Increased size of coronoid process fractures has been associated with concomitant elbow injuries, necessity of operative intervention, as well as greater loss of long-term range of motion [15]. Fracture type involves the size of the fracture fragment, and A or B designations correspond with those without and with associated dislocation, respectively (Fig. 3.10):

- Type I fractures are avulsion fractures of the coronoid tip
- Type II fractures are either simple or comminuted fractures involving less than 50% of the coronoid process height.
- Type III fractures involve greater than 50% of the coronoid (Fig. 3.11).

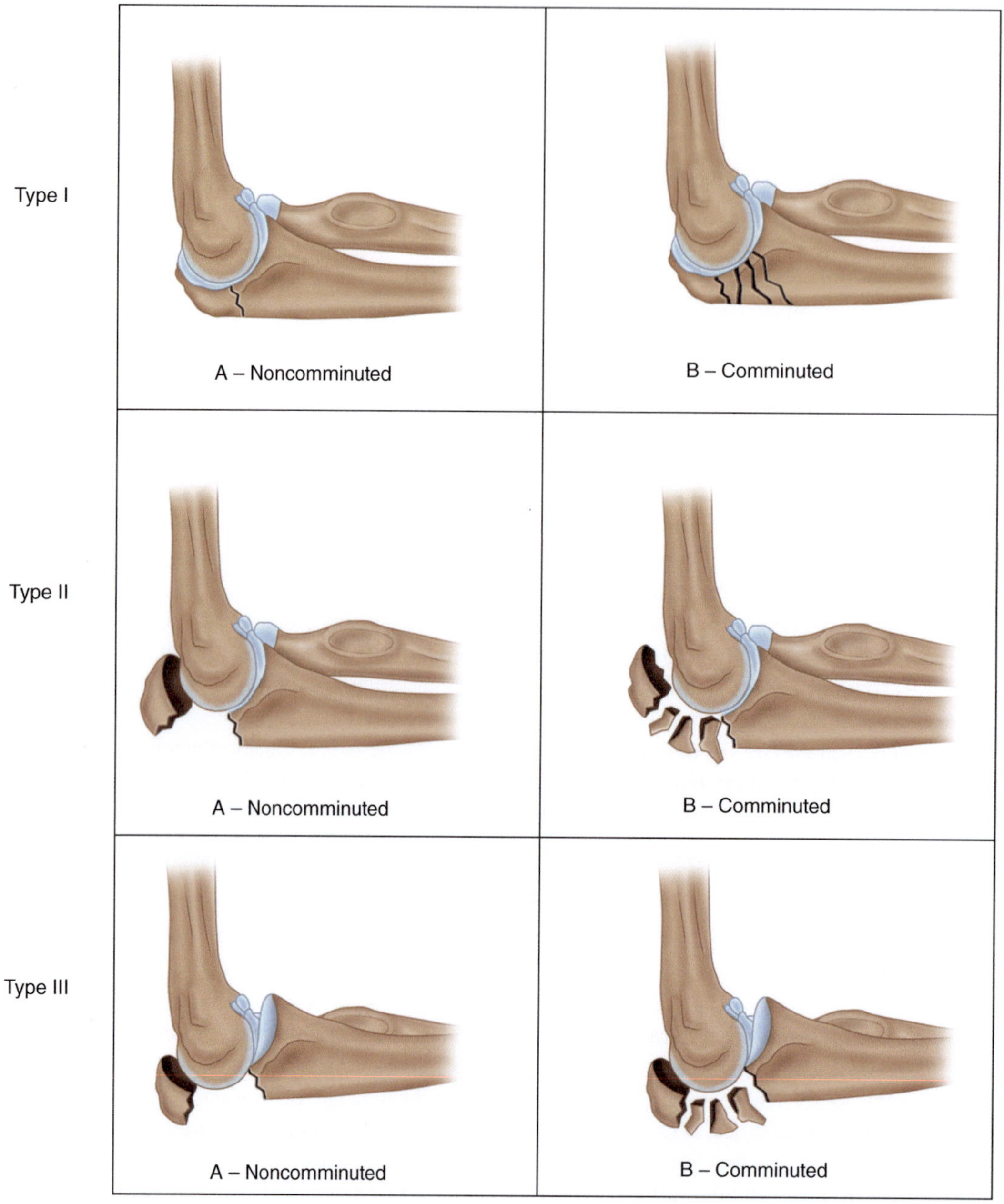

Fig. 3.7 Mayo classification of olecranon fractures

Type I injuries are typically shear-type fractures associated with episodes of subluxation or dislocation. Often, type I injuries are proximal to the capsular attachment, whereas type II injuries often involve the anterior capsular insertion. Type II fractures have been associated with terrible triad elbow injuries as well as PMRI-associated elbow dislocations. Type III coronoid fractures result in destabilization of the elbow as the brachialis and the anterior bundle of the ulnar collateral ligament attach at the coronoid base [16].

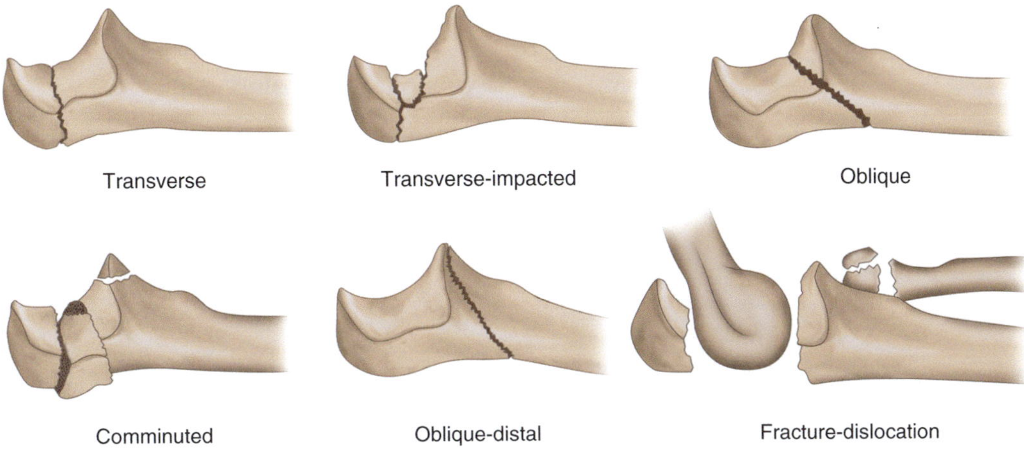

Fig. 3.8 Schatzker classification of olecranon fractures

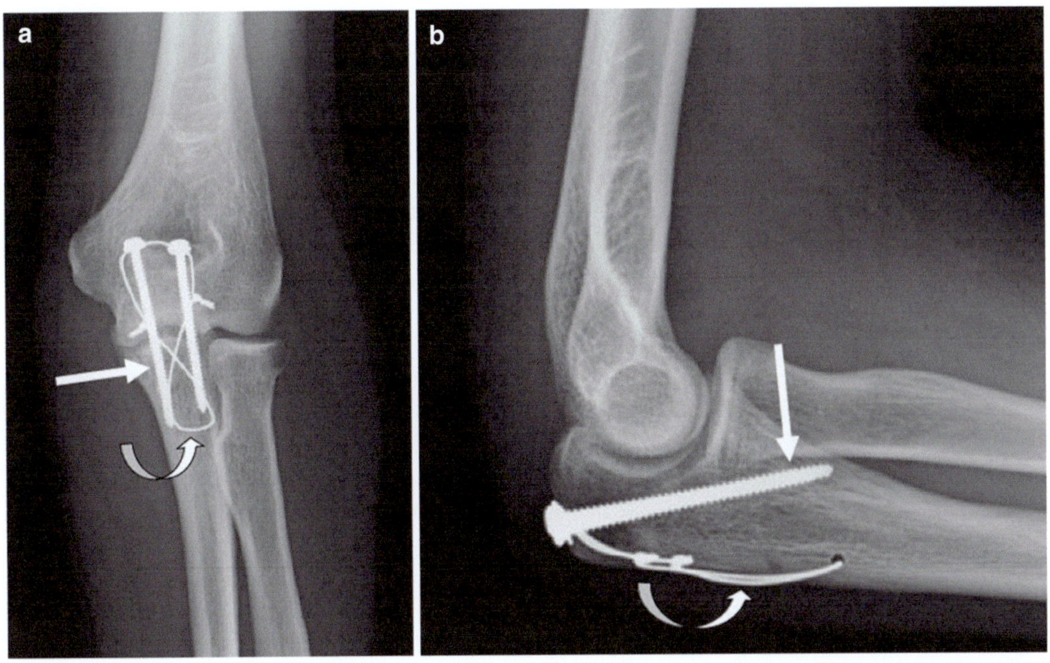

Fig. 3.9 Olecranon fracture fixation. A 27-year-old male status postsurgical treatment for olecranon fracture. AP (**a**) and lateral (**b**) elbow radiographs show fixation screws (arrow) and figure-of-eight tension bands (curved arrow) across a healed olecranon fracture

O'Driscoll Classification

The O'Driscoll classification system was later developed around common mechanisms of injury, fracture patterns, and additional injuries that accompany coronoid process fractures [17]. In addition to coronoid tip and base fractures, the O'Driscoll classification recognizes the anatomic importance of the anteromedial facet and its role

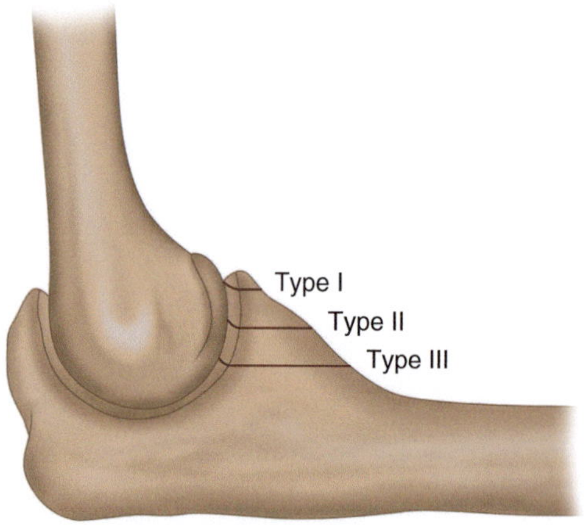

Fig. 3.10 Regan-Morrey classification of coronoid fractures

in varus elbow stability. Injuries are subdivided based on location and number of fracture fragments (Fig. 3.12):

- Type I injuries involve the coronoid tip and are further subdivided into fractures that involve less than or equal to 2 mm of coronoid height (subtype 1) versus those involving greater than 2 mm (subtype 2).
- Type II fractures include the anteromedial facet. Three subtypes include those that involve the anteromedial rim only (subtype 1), the anteromedial rim and coronoid tip (subtype 2), and the anteromedial rim and sublime tubercle (subtype 3).
- Type III injuries occur at the coronoid base either through the coronoid body and base (subtype 1) or through the olecranon (subtype 2).

Treatment

In the event of nondisplaced fractures and elbow stability on physical exam, conservative management with immobilization is indicated. Open reduction and internal fixation is reserved for patients with an unstable exam or for those following a terrible triad elbow injury. Finally, external fixation can be used in patients with poor bone stock or with large fracture fragments.

Intra-articular

Osteochondral Lesion

Etiology and Clinical Presentation

"Osteochondral lesion" is a general term used for any disruption or injury to the articular cartilage and underlying bone. This broad term encompasses both osteochondroses, typically seen in pediatric and young adult patients, as well as acute osteochondral fractures. Both types of osteochondral lesions are commonly due to trauma, and most frequently involve the capitellum [18–20].

There are two main types of osteochondroses of the elbow: Panner disease and osteochondritis dissecans. Panner disease is osteochondrosis of the entire capitellum epiphysis in a child with unfused physes and will be detailed further in the "Pediatric Pathology" section. Osteochondritis dissecans (OCDs) occurs in older children and young adults, typically in the teen years, with closed capitellar physes.

Although the etiology is debated, it is generally accepted that overuse or repetitive trauma coupled with limited blood supply of the capitellum may contribute to repetitive damage of the cartilage and bone [21]. Specifically, the capitellum is supplied by posterior extraosseous perforating vessels, including from the radial recurrent, radial collateral, and interosseous recurrent arteries, which traverse the epiphysis. The lack of intraosseous supply from the metaphysis places the capitellum at risk for vascular compromise and/or impaired healing after trauma [22]. OCDs of the elbow most often occur in throwing athletes, such as baseball players, and athletes with high compressive forces, such as gymnasts. For throwing athletes, the late cocking and early acceleration phases of overhead throwing result in tensile forces and distraction through the medial elbow and, consequently, osteochondral compression of the radiocapitellar joint laterally [21, 23]. Much less commonly, OCDs may be seen in the superoposterior trochlear groove in athletes with force against the elbow while in hyperextension (such as swimmers or basketball players) [24]. Patients

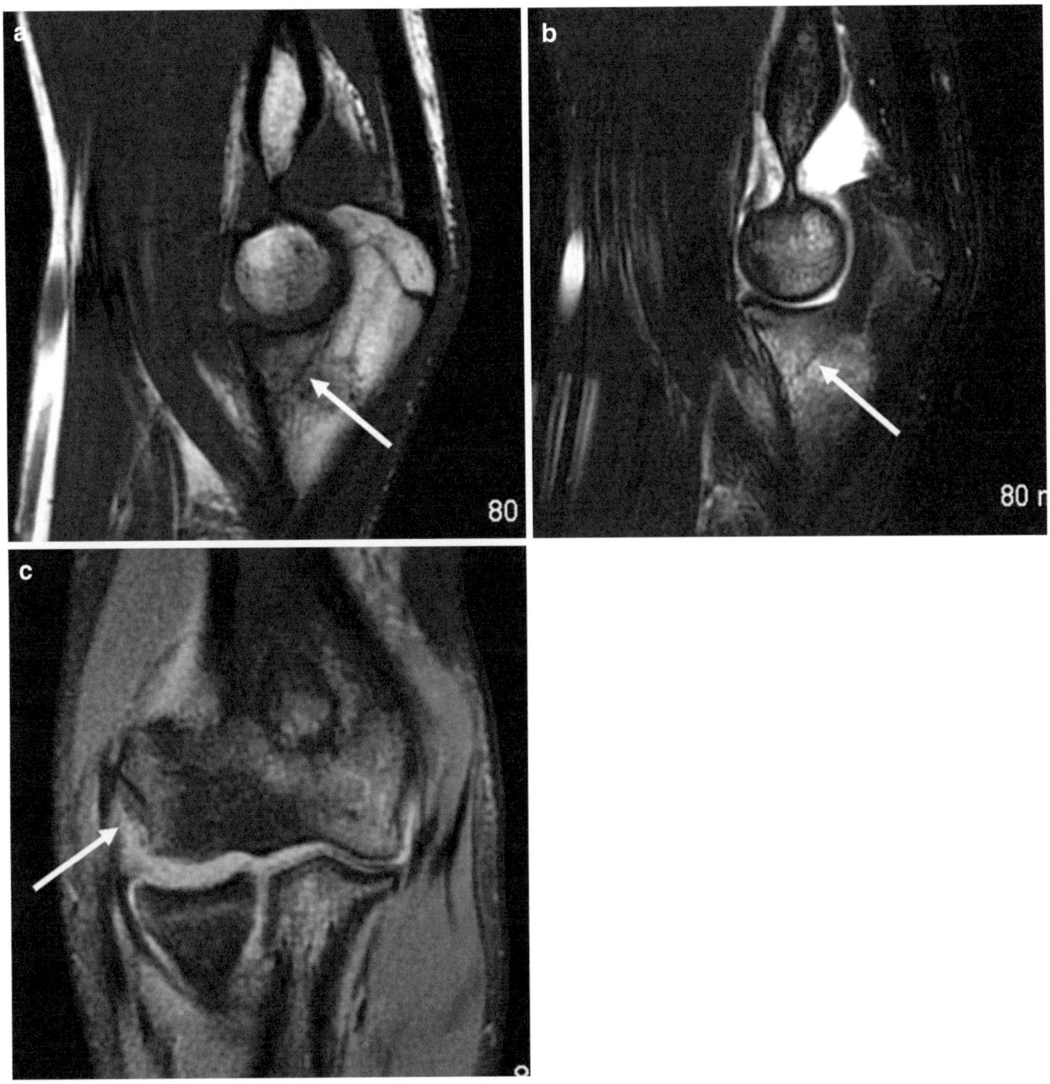

Fig. 3.11 Type III coronoid process fracture. A 16-year-old male basketball player presents with radial sided wrist pain after a fall. Sagittal T1 (**a**) and T2 fat-suppressed (**b**) images show the low-signal nondisplaced coronoid base fracture (arrows) with surrounding bone marrow edema. Coronal PD fat-suppressed image (**c**) shows an associated proximal RCL and LUCL tear (arrow)

may be asymptomatic or present with lateral elbow pain, swelling, restricted range of motion, or instability, depending on the acuity and stability of the lesion [21, 24].

Clinical exam and radiographs both are limited in sensitivity and specificity for diagnosing osteochondroses due to variable presentation and small nondisplaced osseous abnormality. Therefore, MR imaging, with sensitivity up to 100% for detection of OCDs in the elbow of children, is the mainstay in evaluating and characterizing osteochondral lesions [19]. Chondral irregularity and fissuring with subjacent low T1 and increased T2 osseous signal intensity – with or without flattening of the subchondral bone plate – at the classic location in the anterolateral capitellum help establish the diagnosis [21, 24]. Once the diagnosis is made, lesion size, location, stability, and viability are key imaging characteristics to report to help guide management.

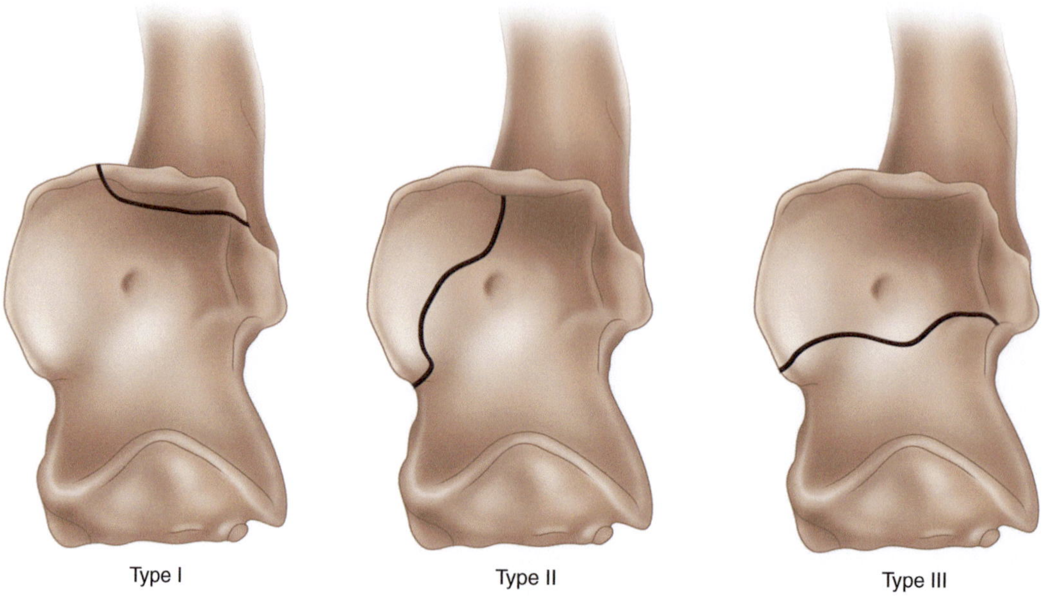

Fig. 3.12 O'Driscoll classification of coronoid fractures

Imaging

The hallmark features of unstable OCD lesions, which typically require surgical treatment, are the following: rim of high-signal intensity (fluid or granulation tissue) at the interface of the lesion and adjacent normal bone (Fig. 3.13a), cysts at the lesion margin, associated overlying articular cartilage defect at the lesion margins (Fig. 3.13b), discontinuity in the subchondral bone plate with fluid-filled cleft (Fig. 3.14), osteochondral void filled with fluid, and presence of an osteochondral joint body [21, 24–26]. These characteristics have been identified in other large joints for decades and have recently also been confirmed in the elbow of adolescents [27]. Lesions without fluid signal intensity at the interface of the abnormal bone with more normal medullary signal are considered stable, though chondral irregularity may result in production of joint bodies [19], which may result in locking or pain and often need surgical intervention. The MR classification system for osteochondral defects, generalized from large joints and not specific to the elbow, can be found in Table 3.1.

Some studies have shown improved accuracy in detecting instability with MR arthrography as contrast extends through the unstable cleft [29], although if the cleft is filled with granulation tissue fluid may not fill the defect. Additionally, MR imaging with intravenous contrast has also been shown to help determine stability and viability. When contrast enhancement is seen at the interface between the lesion and normal bone, this indicates granulation tissue and is inherently unstable. Further, enhancement of the fragment, either homogeneously or incompletely throughout the fragment, indicates viability, whereas marginal or no enhancement is often seen with unstable fragments and poorer clinical outcomes [30].

Osteochondral Fracture

Acute osteochondral fractures are less common than osteochondrosis and occur at any age. These are attributable to trauma, which are most commonly sudden compressive impact and high shear stress at the bone-cartilage interface. They

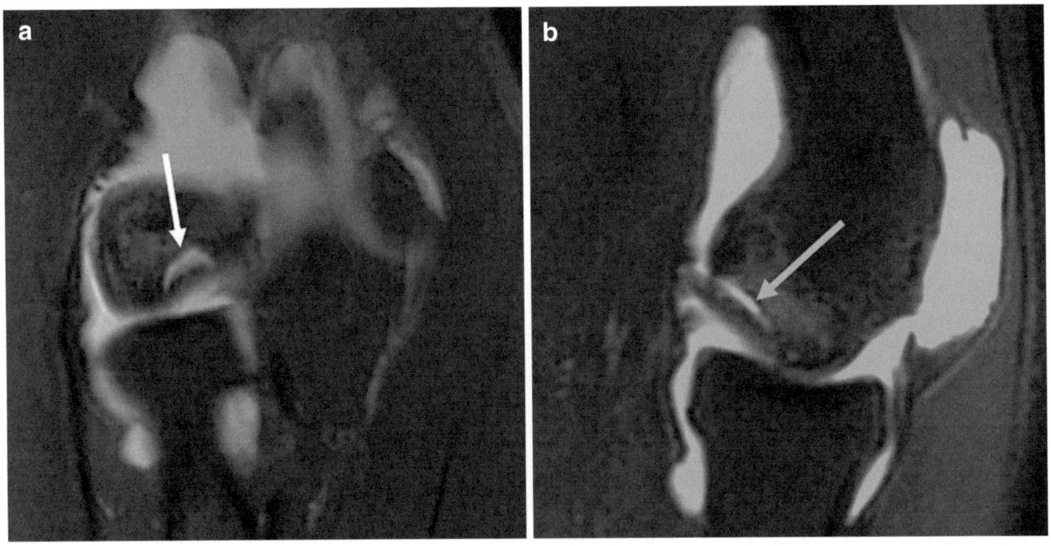

Fig. 3.13 Unstable osteochondral lesion. A 14-year-old male pitcher. Sagittal (**a**) and axial (**b**) T2 fat-suppressed images show an unstable OCL within the capitellum (arrows). The joint effusion helps to determine the status of the lesion to be unstable

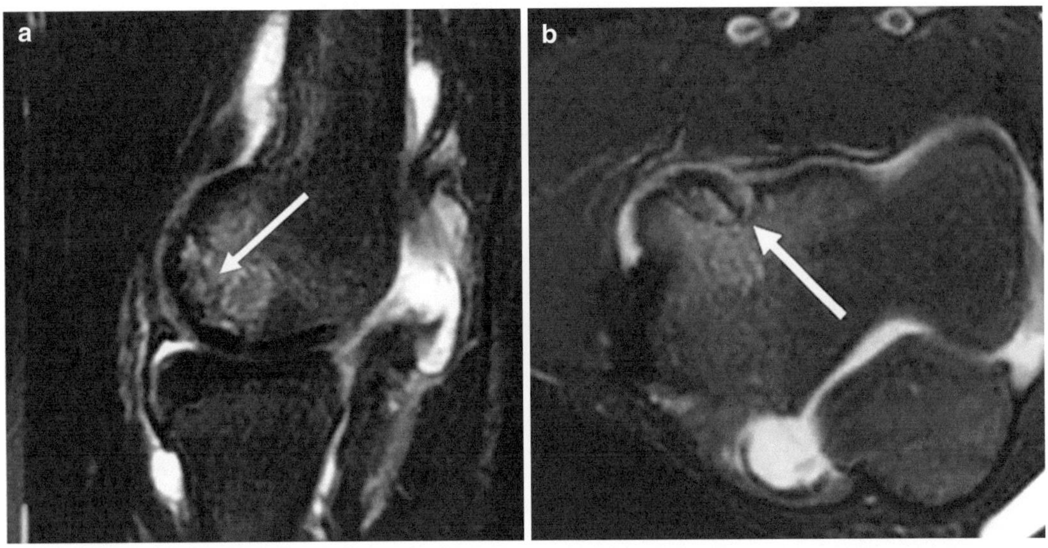

Fig. 3.14 Unstable osteochondral lesion. A 17-year-old male pitcher presents with elbow pain. Coronal (**a**) and sagittal (**b**) T1 fat-suppressed MR arthrogram images show an unstable OCL of the capitellum (arrows). Note the fluid surrounding the lesion with incongruity along the anterior capitellum in which the fragment is slightly displaced

may be a consequence of valgus stress with compression and shear forces through the radiocapitellar joint or as sequela of subluxation or dislocation [18, 21]. Two specific osteochondral fractures may result in serious negative consequences including coronal shear fractures of the distal humerus and the Osborne-Cotterill lesion of the posterolateral capitellum.

Table 3.1 MR osteochondral defect grading [28]

Grade	Imaging findings
I	Intact cartilage with abnormal underlying bone marrow signal intensity
II	High-signal breach of cartilage overlying bone marrow signal change
III	Thin, high-signal rim extending behind the osteochondral fragment
IV	Mixed or low-signal joint body in the center of the lesion or in the joint space

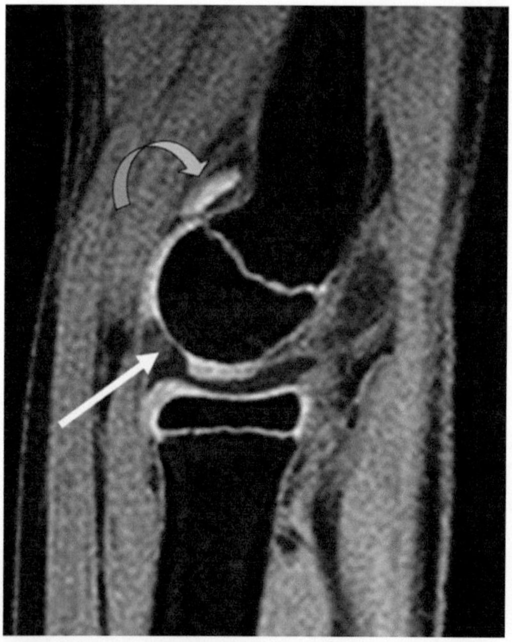

Fig. 3.15 Kocher-Lorenz coronal shear fracture. Sagittal T2* gradient echo image in a 14-year-old boy shows a cartilage fracture involving the anterior capitellum (arrow) with displaced chondral fragment in the radial fossa (curved arrow)

Coronal shear osteochondral fractures of the distal humerus are a well-studied group of acute osteochondral fractures that may be difficult to diagnose radiographically, particularly in the immature skeleton. Specifically, type 2 (Kocher-Lorenz) coronal shear fracture involves the anterior capitellar cartilage and a thin fragment of subchondral bone plate and rapidly leads to joint degeneration if not treated surgically in a timely manner (Fig. 3.15) [31, 32].

The Osborne-Cotterill lesion is a posterolateral capitellum osteochondral fracture that is easy to overlook but of great importance due to associated injury of key elbow stabilizers. This fracture typically occurs after elbow dislocation and is often associated with a defect of the posterolateral radial head (Fig. 3.16) [33, 34]. There may be vague discomfort or more significant symptoms with locking of the joint, pain and clicking with physical activity, or recurrent dislocation. Physical examination may result in radial head dislocation [33]. If not accurately identified, long-term complications include posterolateral rotatory instability due to involvement and effective avulsion of the lateral ulnar collateral ligament (LUCL), which originates at the posterolateral capitellum. Because the LUCL can be difficult to accurately identify on MR imaging, visualized in only 50% of asymptomatic elbows in a study by Terada and colleagues, diagnosis of this lesion is better made on CT examination [34]. Regardless of imaging method, accurate diagnosis is key to help direct the patient to surgical fixation, which is most successfully achieved by LUCL reconstruction and cortical bone graft in the capitellum defect [35].

Pitfalls

The ability to accurately diagnose the above-described entities depends on understanding of normal elbow anatomy that may present as pitfalls in MR imaging. The most important of these pitfalls is the capitellum pseudodefect. This is a normal groove at the junction of the capitellum and lateral epicondyle and partly aligns (though does not articulate) with the posterior radial head in extension (Fig. 3.17). As a consequence, this rough-appearing, nonarticular "defect" is commonly mistaken for an osteochondral lesion of the posterior capitellum on axial and coronal MR images [36]. Key features to help distinguish this from a true osteochondral lesion are as follows: location (posterior capitellum), lack of signal abnormality of the underlying bone, and identification of this normal anatomic region on sagittal MR images.

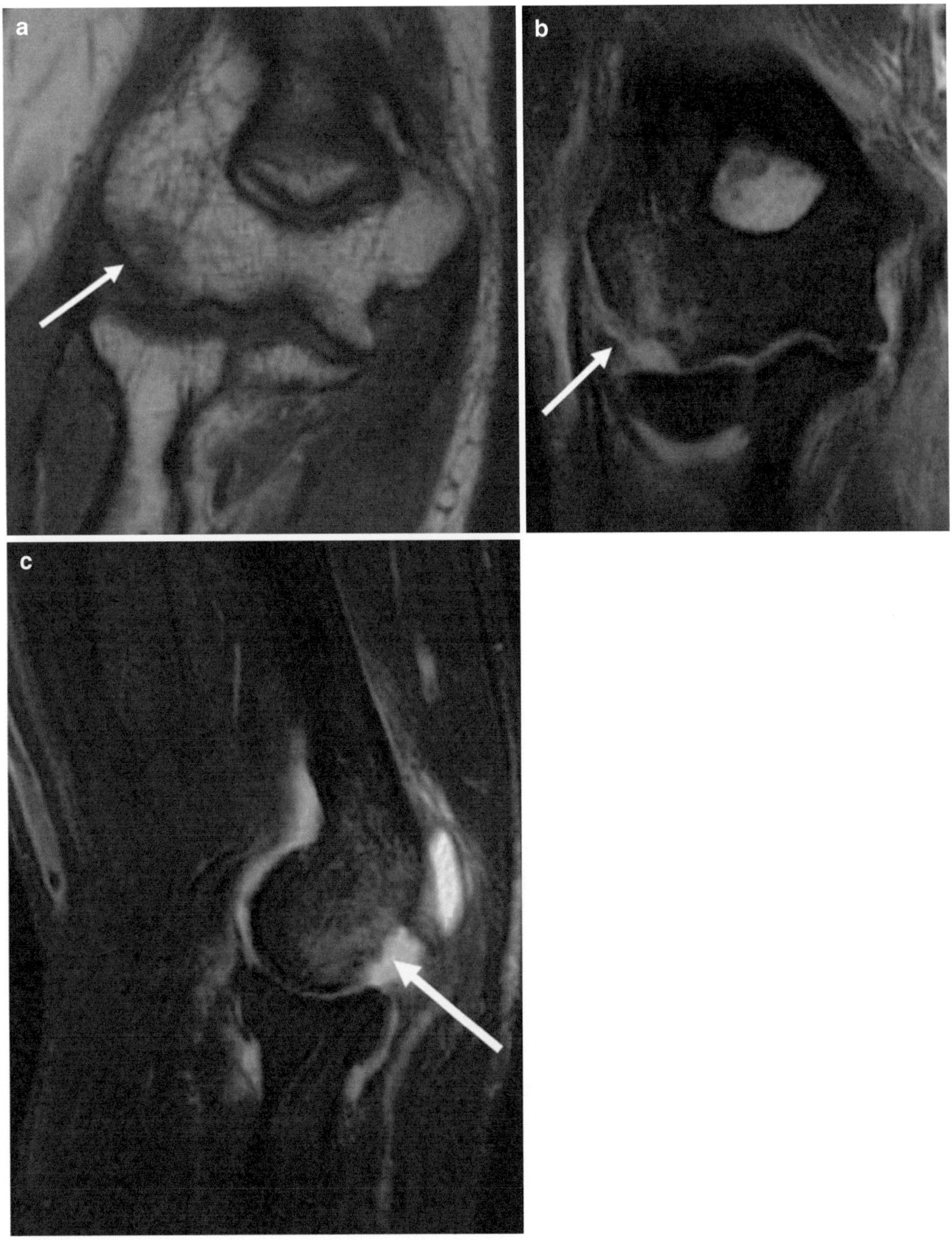

Fig. 3.16 Osborne-Cotterill lesion. Coronal T1 (**a**), coronal T2 fat-suppressed (**b**), and sagittal T2 fat-suppressed (**c**) images in a 24-year-old woman show a subtle impaction fracture with associated bone marrow edema involving the posterolateral capitellum (arrows)

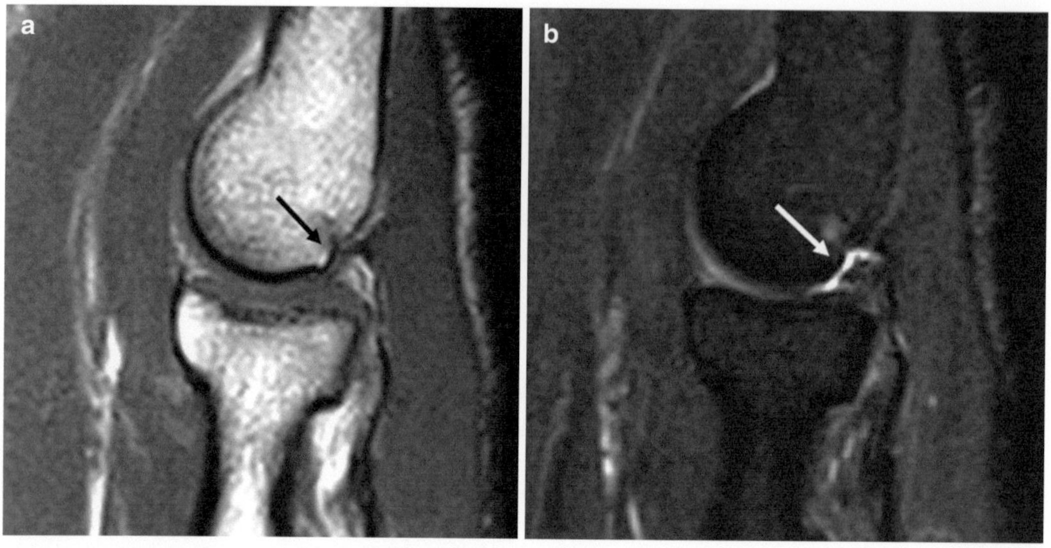

Fig. 3.17 Capitellum pseudodefect. Sagittal T1 (**a**) and T2 fat-suppressed (**b**) images in an asymptomatic 36-year-old woman show a focal concavity devoid of articular cartilage consistent with a capitellum pseudodefect (arrow)

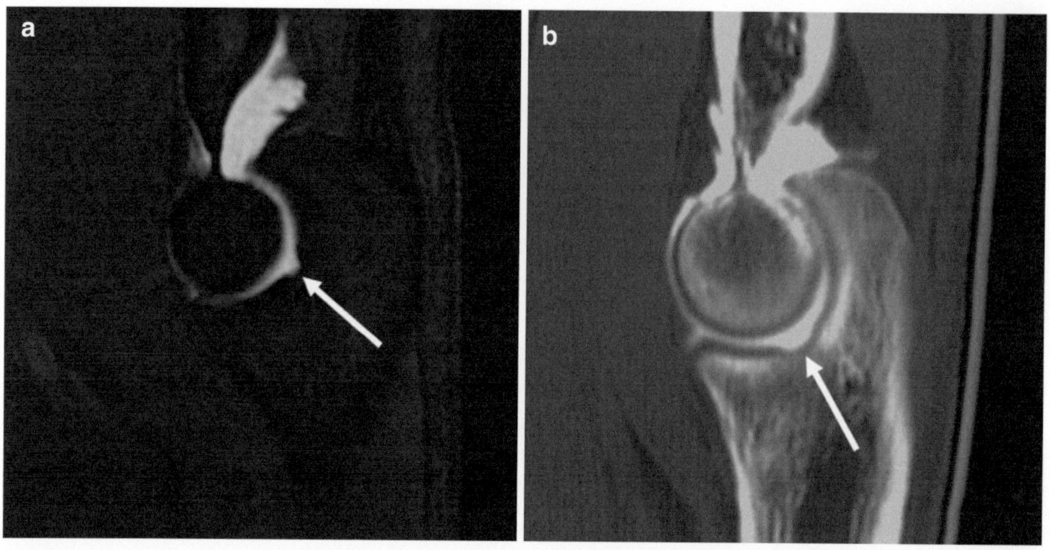

Fig. 3.18 Trochlear groove pseudodefect of the ulna. A 27-year-old man with lateral elbow pain has a prominent trochlear groove pseudodefect incidentally noted during MR imaging. Sagittal T2 fat-suppressed image (**a**) shows a bare area (arrow) involving the central olecranon without overlying articular cartilage, which is similar in appearance to a different 36-year-old woman with a shallow trochlear pseudodefect (arrow) on sagittal CT arthrogram (**b**)

Another potential pseudolesion that could be mistaken for an osteochondral lesion or joint body is the transverse trochlear ridge (Fig. 3.18). This is the non-articulating, rough central aspect of the trochlear ridge between the olecranon and coronoid portions of the proximal ulna. It is sometimes called the "trochlear pseudodefect" with a bare area lacking overlying cartilage [37]. Also in this region, there may be a bony prominence that can be mistaken for a joint body [36].

Understanding the normal anatomy and these anatomic variants is essential to avoid overcalling pathology.

Treatment

For all varieties of osteochondral lesions, early diagnosis and treatment may prevent the need for surgery and/or chronic complications [19]. Ultimately, the size, stability, and viability of these lesions are the determining factors to guide management. If less than 50% of the capitellum is involved, the lesion is stable and viable, and there are no mechanical symptoms; conservative treatment with activity modification and nonsteroidal anti-inflammatory medications is the first-line treatment [21, 27]. If conservative treatment fails (up to 50% of cases) or the lesion is unstable or nonviable, operative management is necessary. Treatment options in these cases include resection of joint bodies, reattachment of fragments, chondroplasty, mosaicplasty with autograft from the knee, allograft, or valgus wedge humeral osteotomy to unload the radiocapitellar joint [38]. Acute osteochondral fractures nearly always require open reduction and internal fixation, though this may be difficult in small fragments due to the lack of adequate bone volume to fixate [31]. Return to activity is then based on clinical symptoms as imaging may lag or be abnormal for years.

Synovial Fringe

Etiology and Clinical Presentation

Intra-articular synovial folds, otherwise known as plicae, form during embryonal development. Mesenchymal cavitation occurs at the radiohumeral, ulnohumeral, and radioulnar locations whereby these cavities combine, and septal remnants can form as a result of this process. Synovial folds are variably present and often asymptomatic in most individuals. In certain patients, synovial fold hypertrophy, inflammation, and the development of adjacent chondral damage can lead to mechanical symptoms and discomfort [39]. The radiohumeral plica is located along the margin of the radiocapitellar joint, proximal to the annular ligament. Symptomatic patients complain of lateral elbow pain and varying degrees of locking or catching during elbow range of motion.

Imaging

The radiohumeral synovial fold is divided based on anatomic location, including the anterior, lateral, posterolateral, and lateral olecranon portions. The anterior fold is present in approximately 67% of individuals and averages 2.3 mm in thickness. The lateral fold is least common in incidence, seen in approximately 5–20%. This fold is curvilinear and typically measures 1.7 mm in thickness, often with free-edge irregularity. The posterolateral synovial fold is the most commonly identified, seen in up to 100% of cadaveric specimens (Fig. 3.19). Additionally, the posterolateral plica was found to be the thickest in asymptomatic individuals, measuring 3 mm. Finally, the lateral olecranon plica is described in up to 33% of individuals and measures up to 1.9 mm in thickness [40, 41].

Elbow synovial fold syndrome can result following a direct blow to the elbow or as a consequence of repetitive elbow flexion/extension or forearm pronation/supination. Local synovitis is produced when plicae become stretched or compressed between the radiocapitellar articular surfaces. Evaluation of synovial folds is best accomplished on coronal fluid-sensitive sequences. Normal plicae are hypointense with well-defined margins, often outlined by elbow joint fluid. Abnormal synovial fold thickening greater than 3 mm has been shown to correlate with elbow symptoms [42, 43]. Plicae irregularity or nodularity is a less specific sign of synovial fold syndrome; however, the presence of focal synovitis in the posterolateral elbow and cartilage loss along the anterolateral aspect of the radial head are secondary signs of synovial fold abnormalities [39, 44].

Treatment

A short course of conservative management with activity cessation, anti-inflammatory medications, and physical therapy is preferred initially. If nonoperative management fails, arthroscopic

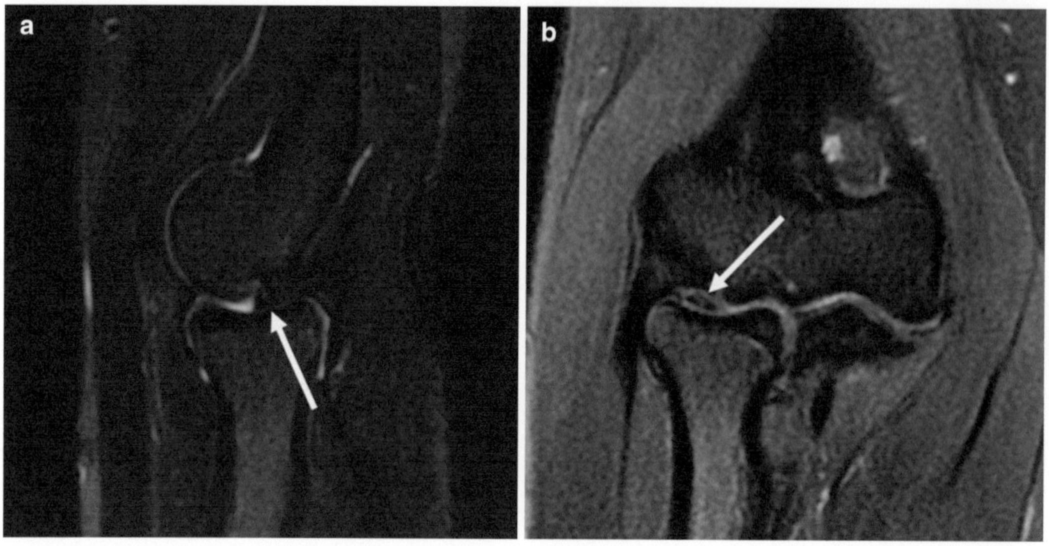

Fig. 3.19 Posterolateral synovial fold. A 22-year-old woman presents with intermittent catching during elbow range of motion. Sagittal (**a**) and coronal (**b**) T2 fat-suppressed images show a thickened posterolateral synovial fold extending into the posterior radiocapitellar joint (arrow)

resection of pathologic plicae is pursued to improve pain and restore range of motion. Arthroscopy has been shown to have excellent symptomatic and functional outcomes, and delay in surgery should be avoided to minimize articular cartilage damage due to prolonged synovial fold impingement [45].

Intra-articular Bodies

Etiology and Clinical Presentation

Intra-articular bodies may occur as a result of trauma, degenerative joint disease, osteonecrosis, and neuropathic arthropathy or due to benign synovial proliferation associated with primary synovial chondromatosis. Symptoms are typically slow to progress and often begin with pain and joint swelling. Progression to limited range of motion, elbow locking, catching, and stiffness can result depending on the size, number, and location of intra-articular bodies.

Primary synovial chondromatosis is seen in a younger age group, typically in the fourth or fifth decades. Men are affected more frequently with a 2:1 male-to-female ratio. Foci of cartilaginous bodies develop within the synovium, and over time with progressive growth, they separate and form intra-articular bodies [46]. Approximately two thirds of intra-articular bodies undergo ossification and can be seen radiographically, while the remaining persist nonossified. The intra-articular bodies seen in primary synovial chondromatosis are more uniform in size and shape compared to intra-articular bodies resulting from other etiologies.

Imaging

Small intra-articular bodies are more conspicuous in the presence of a joint effusion or intra-articular contrast administration (Fig. 3.20). The composition of intra-articular bodies determines the MR imaging appearance. Calcified intra-articular bodies are hypointense on all pulse sequences and generally demonstrate blooming artifact on gradient echo sequences, while those consisting of cartilage demonstrate intermediate proton density or T1 signal and increased T2 signal. Large ossified intra-articular bodies containing internal bone marrow will show increased T1 and T2 signal with subsequent signal dropout on fat-suppressed imaging. As stated previously, intra-articular bodies associated with primary

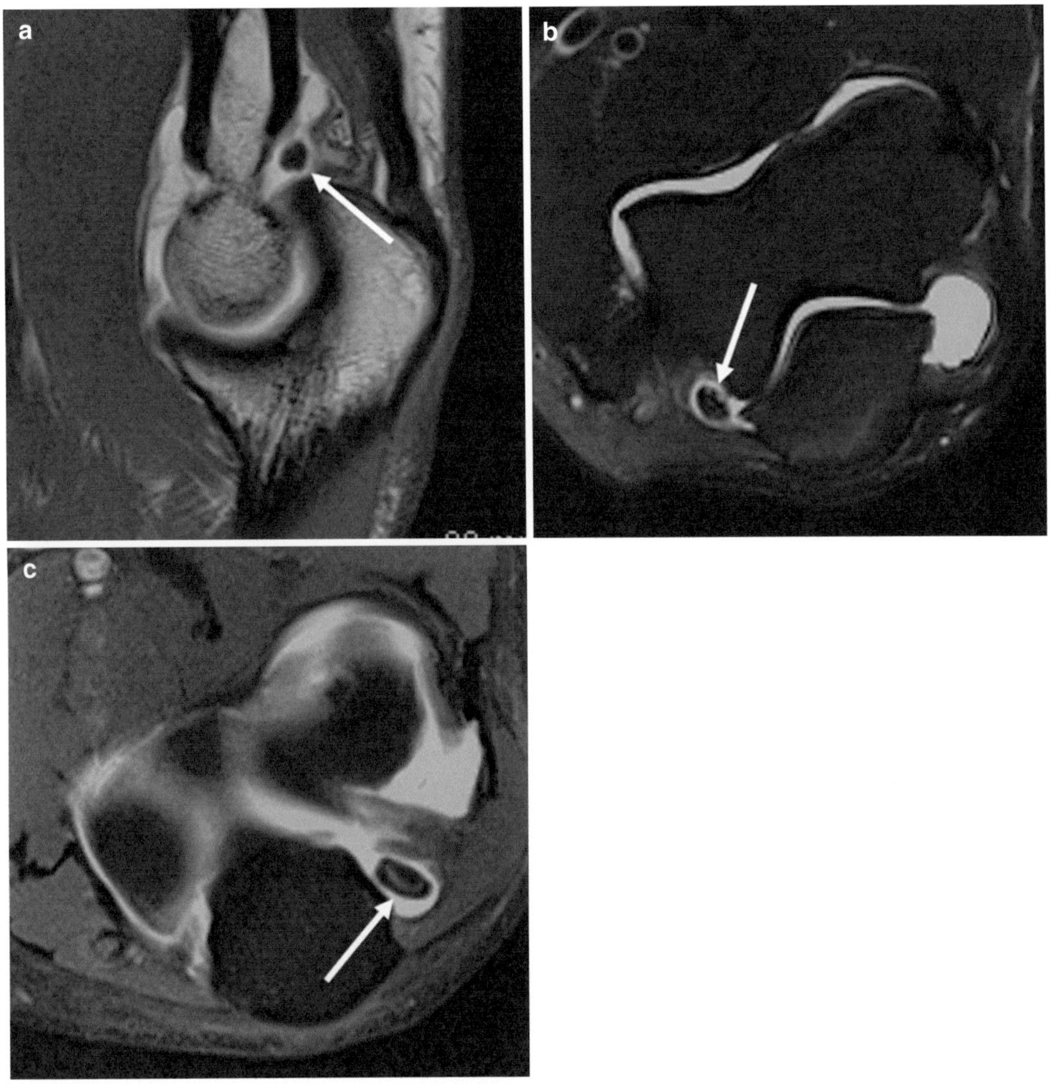

Fig. 3.20 Intra-articular bodies. A 67-year-old man complains of mechanical symptoms. Sagittal T1 arthrogram image (**a**) shows a low-signal intra-articular body in the olecranon recess (arrow). Axial T1 fat-suppressed arthrogram images (**b**, **c**) show additional low-signal intra-articular bodies along the medial and lateral aspect of the olecranon (arrows)

synovial chondromatosis are uniform in size, shape, and signal, while secondary intra-articular bodies may vary [47].

Classification/Staging

Milgram described three phases of primary synovial chondromatosis in 1977 based on clinical and pathologic variations during disease progression [48]:

- Stage I involves synovial inflammation in the absence of intra-articular bodies. Patients may complain of pain or swelling during stage I; however, individuals in this phase may remain asymptomatic.
- Stage II disease is characterized by transitional loose bodies that are in the process of separating from the synovium and forming

intra-articular bodies. On imaging, synovial proliferation and loose bodies are seen.
- Stage III includes multiple intra-articular bodies without associated synovial inflammation or proliferation.

Treatment

Surgical resection is the management of choice for patients with primary synovial chondromatosis with variable rates of recurrence. In secondary forms of chondromatosis, observation is considered in patients with minimal symptoms and preserved range of motion. Arthroscopy with loose body resection is reserved for patients presenting with mechanical symptoms that affect elbow range of motion or severe pain.

Pediatric Pathology

Pediatric overhead athletes are subject to elbow injuries due to repeated microtrauma to the skeletally immature elbow during critical periods of development. Similarly, gymnasts are at increased risk of elbow pathology due to compressive forces from upper extremity weight-bearing.

Panner Disease

Etiology and Clinical Presentation

Panner disease is a type of osteochondrosis involving the humeral capitellum, which is thought to result secondary to recurrent valgus stress. Due to the vascular anatomy of the skeletally immature chondroepiphysis described previously, repetitive compression at the radiocapitellar joint may result in disordered endochondral ossification secondary to vascular insult at the pliant cartilage matrix [49]. Debate exists as to whether Panner disease is an entirely separate entity from osteochondritis dissecans versus a spectrum of lateral elbow epiphyseal injury, and some consider age at onset and severity of symptoms to be the greatest predictors of functional outcomes [50].

Clinically, Panner disease may be difficult to distinguish from capitellar osteochondritis dissecans. Useful differentiating features include age of onset and the presence or absence of mechanical symptoms. Panner disease affects a younger age group, typically between the ages of 5 and 10 years old, while OCD often occurs in adolescents older than 12 years of age. Due to the lack of discrete osteochondral defects or fragments, patients with Panner disease will often lack elbow catching or locking, which is common in OCD. Presenting symptoms include insidious onset lateral elbow pain and stiffness, typically including an extension deficit [51].

Imaging

Radiographs can have variable appearance in Panner disease depending on the stage of disease. Early on, radiographs may be normal or may show decreased size, fragmentation, lucency, or fissuring involving the capitellum. Contralateral comparison radiographs are useful in detecting subtle abnormalities and asymmetry of the epiphysis. Subsequent radiographs may show sclerosis and persistent irregularity or flattening of the capitellum; however, reconstitution often occurs, and radiographs normalize over time. MR imaging shows diffuse edema in the capitellum as demonstrated by decreased T1 signal and hyperintensity on fluid-sensitive sequences (Fig. 3.21). No associated cartilage abnormalities or intra-articular bodies accompany the bone marrow signal changes [49].

Treatment

Symptomatic treatment is the mainstay of management of Panner disease. Rest, immobilization, and anti-inflammatory medications often result in significant symptomatic relief. Surgical intervention is rarely indicated, and long-term outcomes are excellent in the patient population [52].

Little League Elbow

Etiology and Clinical Presentation

The term “Little League elbow” refers to a spectrum of elbow injuries that occur as a result of medial elbow traction during the acceleration phase of pitching in skeletally immature athletes.

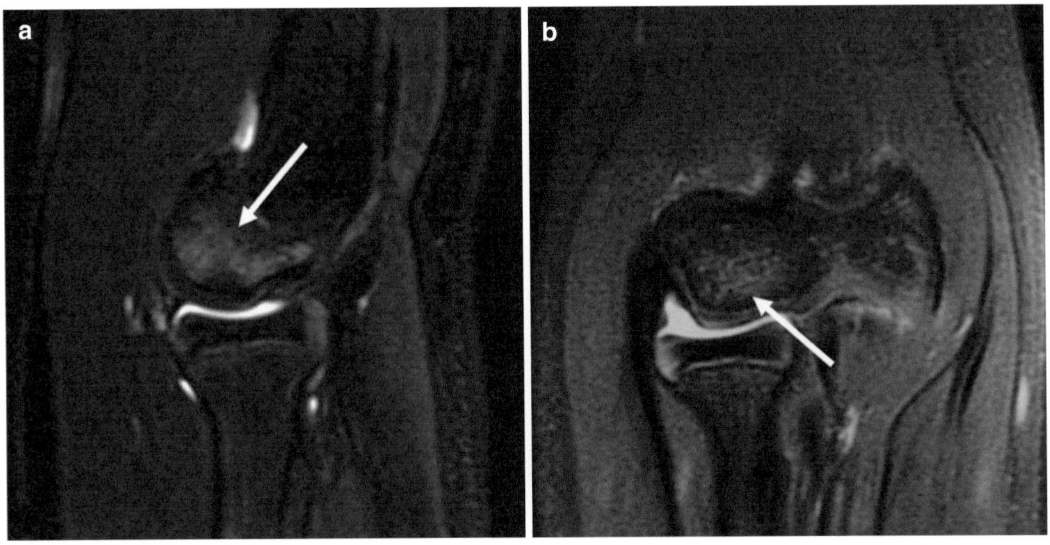

Fig. 3.21 Panner disease. An 8-year-old boy complains of generalized elbow pain. Sagittal (**a**) and coronal (**b**) T2 fat-suppressed images show diffuse bone marrow edema (arrow) involving the capitellum without associated fracture or chondral abnormality

Increase in pitch count and breaking pitches are risk factors for the development of Little League elbow. Due to these risks, the USA Baseball Medical and Safety Advisory Committee recommends pitch count limits based on age as well as avoidance of breaking pitches until the age of 14–16 years [53]. Patients typically present with medial elbow pain centered over the apophysis with decrease in strength and pitch velocity.

Imaging

Radiographs are frequently normal in the pediatric overhead throwing athlete with elbow pain. When repetitive elbow trauma persists, apophyseal fragmentation, displacement, and overgrowth may develop. Patient age and skeletal maturity determine imaging findings associated with valgus overload in overhead throwers. The medial epicondyle apophysis begins to ossify at the age of 5–6 years old and usually fuses by age 15–16. In early childhood, the apophysis is weakest and prone to displacement or fragmentation. The apophysis strengthens as the pediatric skeleton matures, which leads to increased incidence of physeal fractures as the physeal cartilage becomes the weakest link. Once the medial epicondyle fuses, pediatric mechanics more closely reflect those of adults, leading to ulnar collateral ligament and common flexor tendon injuries. MR imaging findings of medial epicondyle apophysitis include bone marrow edema of the apophysis on fluid-sensitive sequences. Apophyseal displacement, fragmentation, and fluid signal within the physis signify abnormal traction on the medial epicondyle (Fig. 3.22). Extra-osseous injuries such as tendinopathy or tears of the common flexor tendon as well as thickening or tearing of the underlying ulnar collateral are also on the spectrum of medial elbow injuries associated with valgus extension overload injuries in the pediatric throwing athlete.

Treatment

Conservative management with an emphasis on rest is the mainstay of treatment in patients with Little League elbow in the absence of an open fracture, intra-articular fragment displacement, or significant displacement in the setting of apophyseal avulsion. There is debate on the degree of displacement necessary to benefit from operative intervention. Some believe displacement greater than 5 mm should proceed to surgery, while others endorse conservative management for displacement up to 15 mm [54, 55].

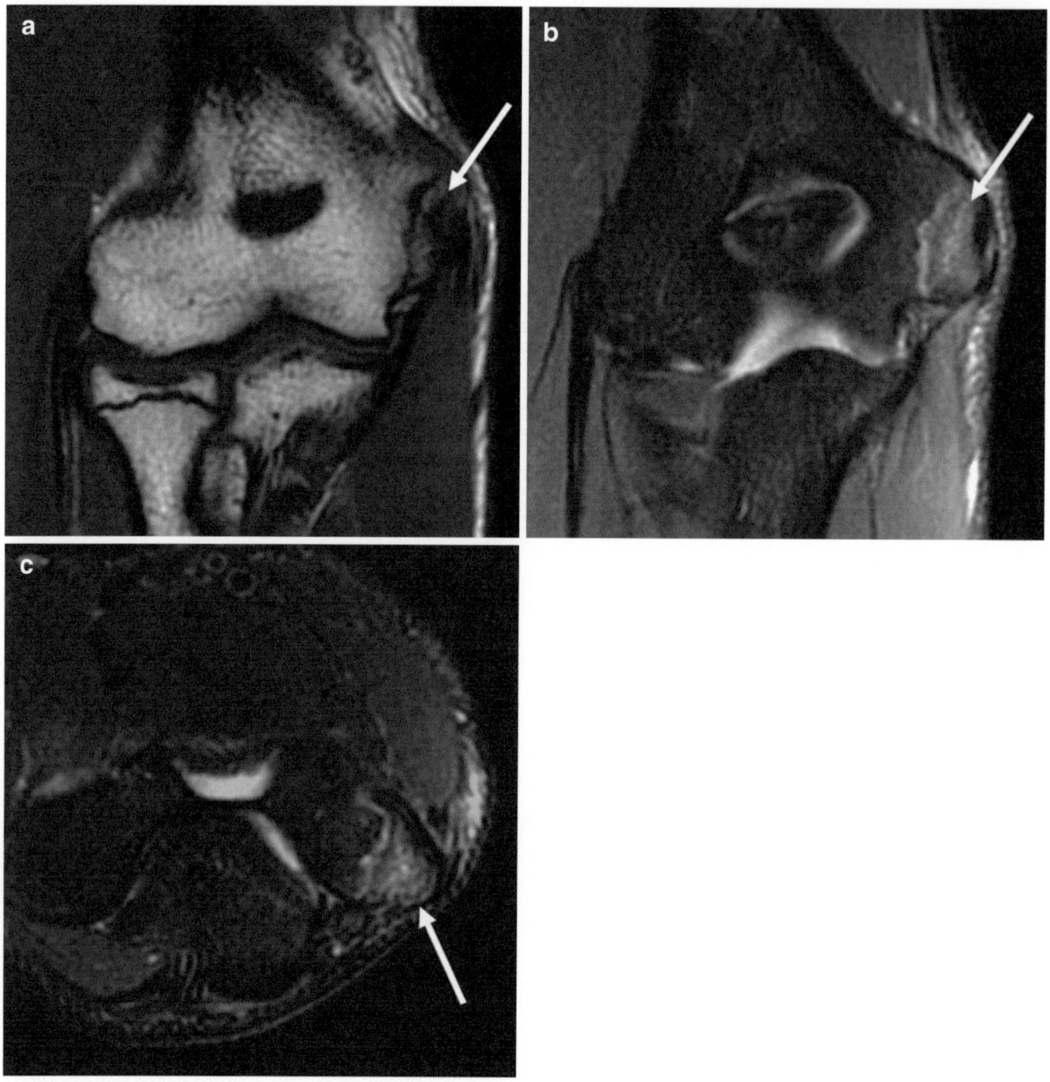

Fig. 3.22 Little League elbow in a 12-year-old baseball pitcher. Coronal T1 image (**a**) shows mild widening of the medial epicondyle physis (arrow) as well as subtle low signal within the medial epicondyle apophysis, which corresponds with bone marrow edema (arrow) on coronal T2 fat-suppressed image (**b**). Axial T2 fat-suppressed image (**c**) demonstrates apophyseal marrow edema (arrow) as well as adjacent soft tissue edema about the medial epicondyle

Ligaments

There are many passive and active stabilizers of the elbow, including the bones and joint congruity, tendons and muscles, and ligaments. The stability of the elbow relies heavily on ligament integrity, which are two of the main passive stabilizers. Thus, an in-depth understanding of the anatomy of these crucial structures, as well as the constellations of imaging findings with injuries of both the medial and lateral elbow ligaments, is important to ensure accurate interpretation of MR imaging of the elbow. Given the wide range of surgical treatment approaches, both arthroscopically and open procedures, as well as differing arthroscopic port placement and patient positioning, accurate diagnosis is crucial prior to treatment [56].

Medial

Etiology and Clinical Presentation

The ulnar collateral ligament (UCL) is comprised of three components: the anterior, posterior, and transverse bands. The anterior band arises from the anterior aspect of the medial epicondyle and inserts on the medial aspect of the coronoid. The posterior band arises from the posteroinferior medial epicondyle and inserts on the medial olecranon. The transverse band courses from the coronoid to olecranon aspect of the proximal ulna and is not a significant stabilizer of the elbow [23].

Of these, the anterior band of the UCL is most important for medial elbow stability as the primary restraint to valgus stress from 30- to 120-degree flexion [57–59]. The midportion of the anterior band remains tense throughout the entire range of motion, and the posterior band contributes some to stability in extreme of flexion [57].

Injury of the ulnar collateral ligament ranges from sprain to partial or complete tear. These injuries may occur as consequence of elbow dislocation from fall onto an outstretched hand with elbow in extension or, more commonly, chronic repetitive trauma from valgus stress at the elbow. Chronic valgus stress is classically seen and described in baseball players but can be seen in any overhead throwing athlete. During late cocking and early acceleration of the action of overhead throwing, excessive tensile force is placed on the medial elbow and ulnar collateral ligament [18, 56]. Over time, this may result in chronic sprain, partial tear (which may be adaptive in throwers without symptoms), or complete tear of the UCL. On physical exam, there is laxity with valgus stress and possibly pain at the medial elbow with extension and/or the milking maneuver, where the patient places valgus stress on the joint by reaching beneath the affected arm with the contralateral hand and pulling on affected arm's thumb [58].

Imaging

Similar to most soft tissue injuries in the elbow, radiographs may be normal. Thus, MR imaging is the gold standard for identification and characterization of ligament injuries. The anterior bundle of the UCL (aUCL) is best seen on coronal images as a hypointense band of tissue that is broad at its origin at the medial humeral epicondyle and courses distally to insert narrowly at the anteromedial aspect of the coronoid process (also called the sublime tubercle). Although previously it was believed that the normal insertion was at the articular margin of the coronoid, newer anatomic studies have revealed that the distal insertion may be up to 3 mm distal to the joint margin on the ulnar ridge [23, 60]. With sprains, the ligament may become ill-defined with increased signal of the ligament on T1- and T2-weighted images from hemorrhage and edema. Partial tears of the aUCL are identified when there is partial discontinuity of the ligament, often filled with joint fluid (Fig. 3.23). This may result in the classic "T sign," originally used to describe a partial thickness undersurface tear at the distal insertion (Fig. 3.24). However, this sign is not specific for partial tears as it can be seen in asymptomatic individuals and is thought to be adaptive from chronic stress or sequel of remote injury at this insertion. Thus, a T sign with cleft >3 mm – and correlation with symptoms and surrounding bone marrow and soft tissue edema – is considered more accurate evidence of partial tear than variant anatomy [61]. Finally, complete tears are typically more discrete with a fluid-filled gap through the full thickness of the ligament with or without redundancy of the torn ligament stump and extracapsular extension of joint fluid (Fig. 3.25) [62]. These injuries are reportedly most commonly seen at the midsubstance from chronic repetitive microtrauma, though avulsion of the sublime tubercle and aUCL attachment can be seen with acute injury [23].

Ulnar collateral ligament insufficiency may also lead to additional injuries. In some throwing athletes, the aforementioned excessive tensile force at the medial elbow causes UCL attenuation or failure. This, then, accentuates valgus overload and increases lateral joint compressive forces and posterior joint shear forces [56]. This constellation of injuries is referred to as valgus extension overload syndrome (VEOS). MR findings of these

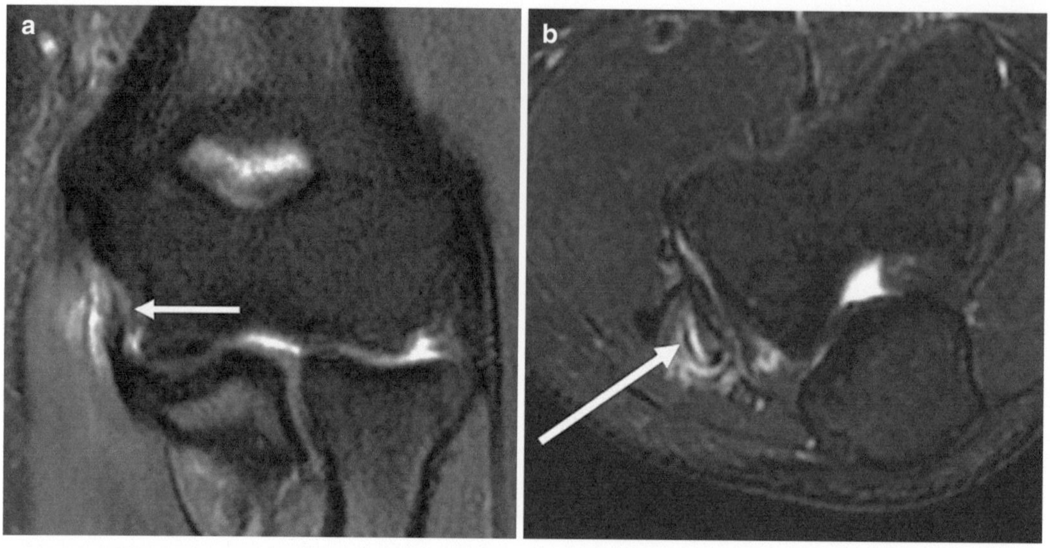

Fig. 3.23 Ulnar collateral ligament tear in a 19-year-old man. Coronal PD fat-suppressed image (**a**) shows a high-grade partial tear of the mid-UCL (arrow). Axial T2 fat-suppressed image (**b**) shows the concomitant partial tear of the common flexor tendon unit (arrow)

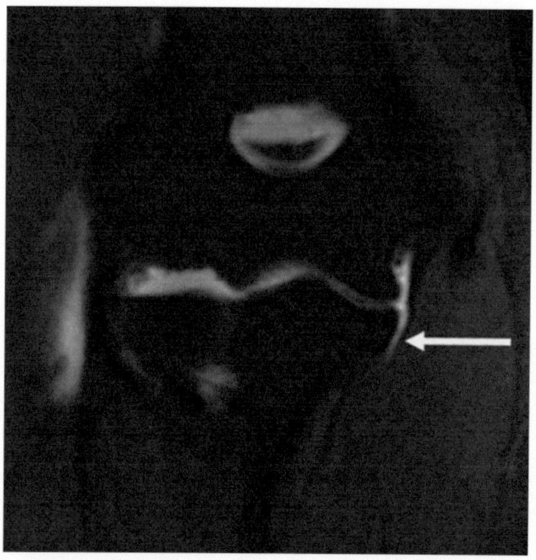

Fig. 3.24 T-sign in a 19-year-old male baseball pitcher. Coronal T1 fat-suppressed arthrogram image demonstrates contrast extension deep to the ulnar attachment of the ulnar collateral ligament (arrow) consistent with a partial undersurface tear

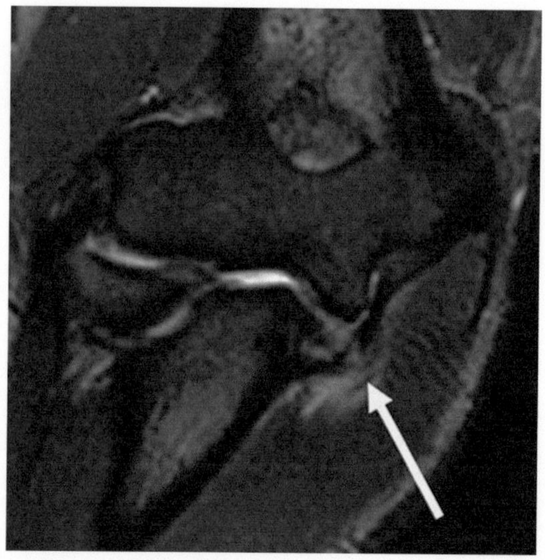

Fig. 3.25 Complete tear UCL in a 17-year-old pitcher. Coronal PD fat-suppressed image shows fluid tracking across the anterior band UCL and focal defect (arrow)

additional injuries include chondral injury, osteophytes, and possibly joint bodies at the radiocapitellar joint, as well as posteromedial olecranon osteophytes with corresponding bone marrow edema and/or osteophytes at the articulating olecranon fossa and posteromedial trochlea (Fig. 3.26) [56]. Further valgus stress after UCL failure in this syndrome may also stress the medial elbow soft tissues, resulting in ulnar neuritis or flexor-pronator tendinopathy or myotendinous strain. These are both best characterized on fat-suppressed T2-weighted sequences where there is increased caliber and fluid signal intensity of the ulnar nerve near the cubital tunnel in ulnar neuritis and intermediate signal intensity of a thickened proximal common flexor tendon or feathery edema within the proximal flexor and pronator muscles in the setting of flexor-pronator pathology [63].

Treatment

The management of UCL tears depends largely on the patient's level of activity or sporting and type of sport. Nonoperative management, including bracing and rehabilitation, is recommended for sprains and may be considered for partial tears or even complete tears in non-throwing athletes, such as gymnasts, or those who are not athletes [58]. However, Rettig and colleagues found that only 42% of baseball players were able to

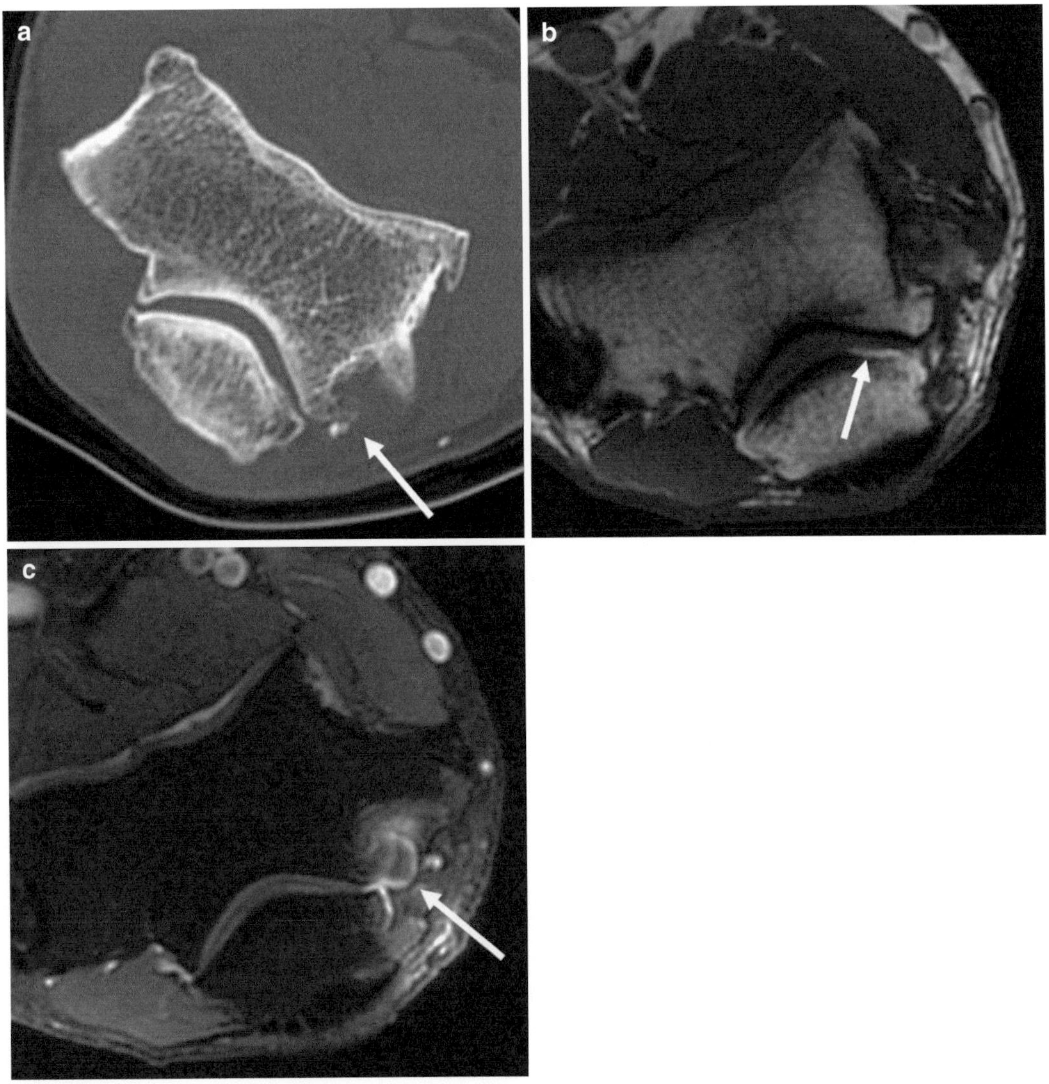

Fig. 3.26 Posteromedial impingement. A 63-year-old male presents with chronic medial elbow pain. Axial CT (**a**), T1 (**b**), and T1 fat-suppressed contrast-enhanced MR (**c**) images demonstrate posteromedial osteophyte formation at the ulnotrochlear articulation (**a**, arrow) and corresponding area of localized cartilage loss (**b**, arrow) on MRI. There is focal synovial enhancement (**c**, arrow) adjacent to the posteromedial olecranon osteophytes

return to play at prior activity level when treated nonoperatively [64]. Thus, surgical reconstruction is favored in athletes, particularly those wanting to return to play in overhead throwing sports, and has been demonstrated to have great success with more than 90% of such athletes reporting excellent long-term results [65].

The commonest surgical technique is graft reconstruction and also well known as the Tommy John surgery originally performed by Dr. Frank Jobe in 1974. An autograft is harvested from the palmaris longus or semitendinosus tendon and is fixed via distal humeral and proximal ulnar osseous tunnels in the same alignment as a native aUCL to restore its stabilizing function [23]. This may also be performed for partial thickness tears that involve the more posterior distal insertion of the aUCL on the proximal ulna, which has been shown to contribute most to rotational stability [65]. In valgus extension overload syndrome, surgery is the mainstay treatment to prevent further associated injuries detailed above. During the ligament graft reconstruction, however, it is also important to remove joint bodies and posteromedial olecranon osteophytes, the latter of which is the commonest cause of reoperation in these patients [56].

Lateral Collateral Ligament Complex

Etiology and Clinical Presentation

The lateral collateral ligament complex is comprised primarily of three components, including the radial collateral ligament (RCL), lateral ulnar collateral ligament (LUCL), and annular ligament. Both the RCL and LUCL originate from the anteroinferior aspect of the lateral epicondyle, where there is close apposition of and difficulty identifying separation from the overlying common extensor tendon [23]. The RCL extends in a fan-like fashion to insert on the annular ligament circling the radial head. Because the insertion is not on the margin of the radial head itself, a cleft of fluid between the distal RCL and the margin of the radial head is normal. The LUCL courses posterior to the radial head and neck to insert on the supinator crest of the posterolateral ulna. Finally, the annular ligament courses around the circumference of the radial head, attaching to the adjacent anterior and posterior margins of the proximal ulnar radial notch. This ligament is the primary stabilizer of the proximal radioulnar joint, which is most important when skeletally immature [23, 57]. Of the lateral collateral ligament complex, the lateral ulnar collateral ligament is the most important stabilizing ligament. This is the primary constraint against ulnar rotation away from the trochlea as is seen in posterolateral rotatory instability [57].

Chronic varus stress at the elbow, as is seen in racquet sports, may lead to common extensor origin tendinopathy at the lateral epicondyle (otherwise known as "tennis elbow" or "lateral epicondylitis"). This varus stress and degeneration of the overlying tendon may lead to excessive tensile force on the RCL and/or LUCL, which, in turn, can cause ligament sprain, partial tear, or complete tear, similar to the aUCL described above. If a complete tear occurs, particularly of the LUCL, the patients are at risk for posterolateral rotatory instability (PLRI).

PLRI is the commonest instability of the elbow and is a clinical syndrome of painful clicking or locking and recurrent instability of the elbow, particularly in extension [66]. This occurs due to LUCL deficiency – from trauma or degeneration as detailed above with excessive varus stress, generalized ligamentous laxity, or iatrogenic injury as a complication from lateral elbow surgeries – that allows external rotation of the radius and ulna with respect to the distal humerus and consequent posterior radial head dislocation [67, 68]. Although it may be seen as a consequence of lateral epicondylitis, it is much more commonly seen as a complication of traumatic dislocation (Fig. 3.27) [33]. One particularly problematic fracture seen in traumatic dislocation is the Osborne-Cotterill lesion (previously described in "osteochondral lesions") or posterolateral capitellar osteochondral fracture. The fragment may seem somewhat insignificant initially on imaging as it is a small cortical avulsion; however, it involves the LUCL origin and may result in PLRI. Ultimately, the mechanism

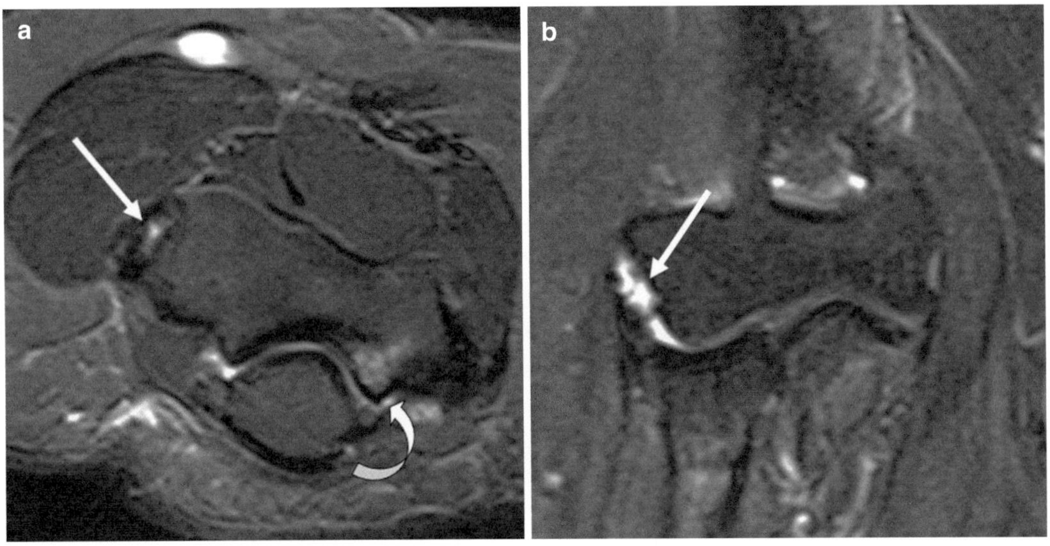

Fig. 3.27 Posterolateral rotatory instability. Axial T2 fat-suppressed (**a**) image in a 50-year-old man demonstrates a partial tear of the deep fibers of the common extensor tendon (straight arrow) as well as bone marrow edema along the posteromedial aspect of the ulnotrochlear joint (curved arrow). Coronal T2 fat-suppressed (**b**) image shows a high-grade partial tear of the proximal radial collateral ligament (arrow)

of injury is a predictable pattern of soft tissue and/or bone injury, referred to as the circle of Horii (Fig. 3.28). First, stage 1 begins with partial or complete disruption of the LUCL (or both RCL and LUCL), resulting in posterolateral rotational subluxation of the ulna on the humerus. In stage 2, there is progressive stress on and injury of the anterior and posterior capsule, resulting in incomplete posterior elbow dislocation with a "perched" ulna on the humeral trochlea. Lastly, in stage 3, further ligament rupture of the medial elbow occurs, resulting in complete posterior elbow dislocation. Stage 3 is subdivided into the initial tear of the posterior band of the UCL and eventually the anterior band of the UCL, when the humerus is finally stripped of its soft tissue attachments to the proximal radius and ulna [69].

Imaging

The RCL and LUCL are best visualized on coronal MR images as vertical and oblique hypointense bands, respectively, coursing from the lateral epicondyle to their above-described distal insertions [57]. The course of the LUCL creates challenges in clearly identifying this structure in its entirety on MR imaging. One study reports only 50% were identified in participants with asymptomatic elbows [34]. Potter and colleagues, however, report success in identifying the LUCL in 100% of a series of 9 symptomatic and 9 asymptomatic individuals as well as LUCL pathology using thin sections or 3D sequences [66]. Since the commonest site of tear is at the proximal origin at the lateral epicondyle, coronal images are key in evaluating these tears (Fig. 3.29) [70]. Careful observation will reveal posterior decentering of the radial head with respect to the capitellum on sagittal images as the LUCL loses its ability to be a posterior stabilizing sling for the radius. Care should be taken to search for associated fractures of the radial head and/or capitellum or lateral humeral epicondyle.

Treatment

Treatment for lateral collateral ligament complex tears, similar to UCL tears, is often surgical reconstruction. This is particularly important for the LUCL given its tremendous impact on elbow stability and in prevention of developing PLRI. Reconstruction is performed with a free

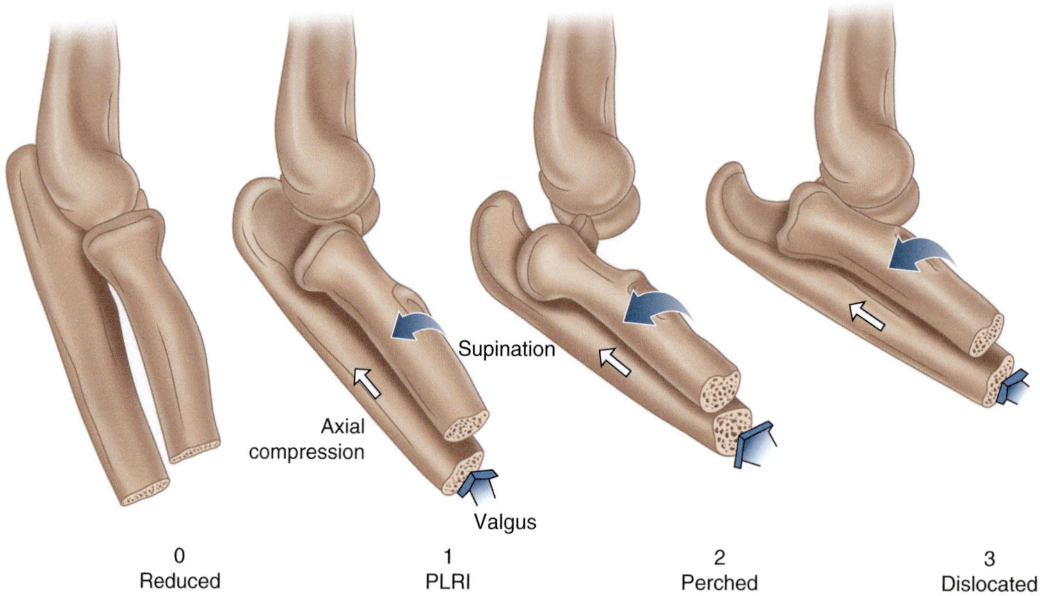

Fig. 3.28 Circle of Horii. Illustration shows the predictable progression through the stages of injury involving the supporting structures of the elbow

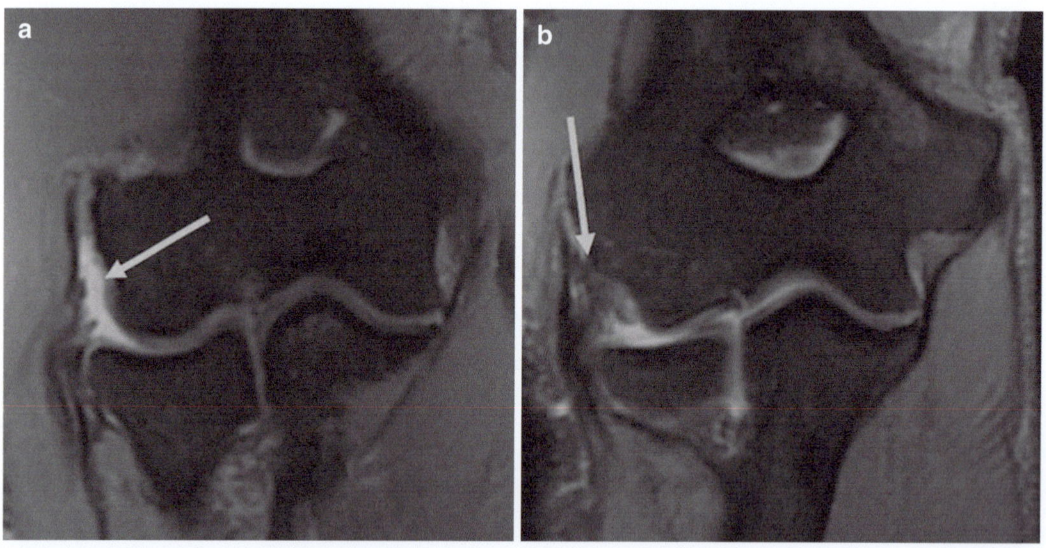

Fig. 3.29 Radial collateral ligament tear. Coronal PD fat-suppressed images in a 49-year-old-man show a tear of the radial collateral ligament (**a**-arrow) and partial tearing of the lateral ulnar collateral ligament (**b**-arrow)

tendon graft from the palmaris longus or gracilis tendon and is fixed via osseous tunnels in the lateral humeral epicondyle proximally to the sublime tubercle of the ulna distally, ensuring orientation that simulates an anatomic LUCL [23]. Correcting radial head and/or capitellum bony deficiencies, as well as correcting excessive varus alignment of the distal humerus with a corrective osteotomy, may also be performed for optimal reconstruction success.

Muscles and Tendons

The spectrum of musculotendinous injuries about the elbow results from repetitive overuse injury to acute trauma or a combination of factors. Clinically, muscle and tendon abnormalities may be identified on the basis of physical exam, but MR imaging helps delineate the extent of injury as well as coinciding pathology.

Distal Biceps Tendon Rupture

Etiology and Clinical Presentation

Injuries of the distal biceps tendon occur less frequently compared to tears of the proximal biceps tendon, comprising only 3% of all biceps tendon injuries [71]. Complete or partial rupture of the distal biceps typically occurs following forced extension of a flexed elbow. Distal biceps tendon injuries often present in the dominant arm of middle-aged men. Smoking and anabolic steroid use have been associated with increased risk of rupture [72, 73]. Complete biceps tendon ruptures present with a palpable tendon defect in the antecubital fossa on physical exam. Proximal retraction of the myotendinous unit results in caliber change and muscle prominence known as the "reverse Popeye" sign. Partial ruptures are more challenging to detect clinically and often require imaging to determine the location and extent of tendon injury.

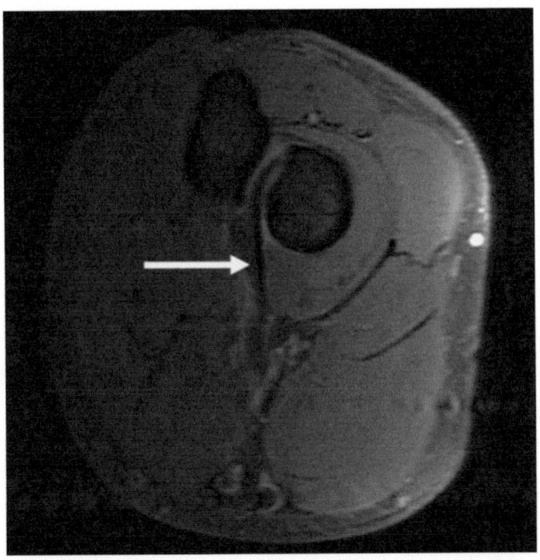

Fig. 3.30 Normal biceps insertion with FABS technique. FABS PD fat-suppressed image of the elbow in an asymptomatic volunteer delineates the distal biceps tendon at the radial insertion (arrow)

Imaging

Typically, the biceps tendon is evaluated on MR imaging in axial and sagittal planes performed with the elbow in full extension. Due to the oblique course of the distal biceps tendon, MR imaging in elbow flexion, shoulder abduction, and forearm supination (FABS position) can be used as an adjunct to standard MR sequences to optimize visualization of the distal biceps tendon from the musculotendinous junction to the insertion [74]. With the patient lying prone in the FABS position, imaging is performed perpendicular to the radial shaft to allow evaluation of the distal biceps tendon on a single image (Fig. 3.30).

Complete Tear

On fluid-sensitive sequences, a hyperintense fluid-filled tendon gap is seen in the acute setting following complete biceps tendon rupture. The degree of tendon retraction and, likewise, the size of the fluid gap are determined by the integrity of the lacertus fibrosus. When intact, the lacertus fibrosus limits the degree of biceps retraction and can simulate an intact tendon on clinical exam. The proximal tendon stump is often thickened, redundant, and increased in signal intensity. Additionally, intramuscular and soft tissue edema and hemorrhage are common in the acute setting, which can also be seen as increased signal on fluid-sensitive sequences (Fig. 3.31) [75].

Partial Tear

Partial biceps rupture presents with tendon thinning or attenuation on MR imaging. Fluid signal clefts and partial fiber discontinuity without complete disruption are consistent with partial rupture (Fig. 3.32). Secondary signs of partial tendon tears include bicipitoradial bursitis as well as radial tuberosity bone marrow edema, which is seen in approximately 50% of cases [71].

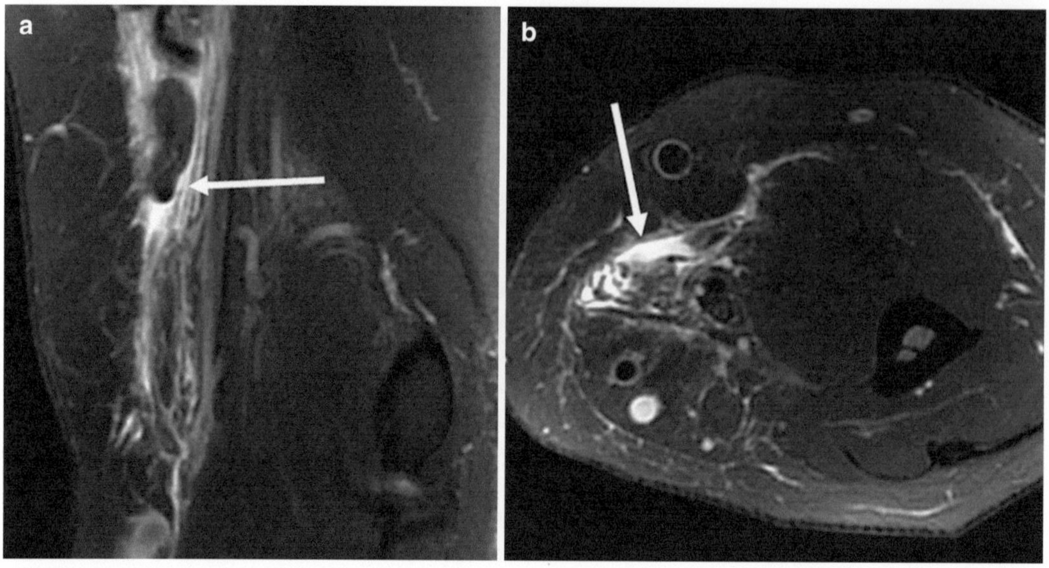

Fig. 3.31 Biceps rupture in a 52-year-old man. Sagittal (**a**) and axial (**b**) T2 fat-suppressed images show complete rupture of the biceps tendon (arrows) with retraction of the tendon end and fluid/hematoma filling the tendon gap. Measurements should be described from the retracted tendon to the radial tuberosity

A less common subset of partial tears includes single-head ruptures. The short and long heads of the biceps tendon insert separately at the radial tuberosity. Proximal to the elbow joint, the long and short head tendons are oriented side-by-side with the short head located medially and the long head laterally. The lacertus fibrosis consistently arises from the short head tendon and can aid in its identification. Distally, the short head tendon extends superficial to the long head and has an ovoid footprint along the distal aspect of the radial tuberosity. The long head travels deep to the short head and inserts proximally with a round footprint [76]. The short head tendon is more susceptible to isolated single-head rupture compared to the long head tendon. Isolated single-head rupture of the short or long head tendons can be mistaken clinically for partial tendon tears; however, it is crucial to distinguish these pathologies due to implications in management (Fig. 3.33) [77].

Classification/Staging

Established on prior MR evidence, Fuente et al. developed an injury classification based on both MR imaging and ultrasound findings [78]. Different tendon injuries are defined as one of the following:

- Major injuries require surgical management, which include complete tears of the distal biceps tendon or high-grade partial tears involving greater than 50% of the tendon attachment. Complete tears are further subdivided based on the status of the lacertus fibrosus:
  - Intact lacertus fibrosus is associated with tendon retraction less than or equal to 8 cm.
  - Torn lacertus fibrosus is associated with tendon retraction greater than 8 cm.
- Minor injuries are those that do not require surgical management, such as low-grade partial tears involving less than 50% of the tendon attachment as well as tendinopathy.

Treatment

Partial biceps tendon ruptures or complete tendon ruptures in low-demand patients are usually managed nonoperatively, while those that fail conservative management or injuries in young or

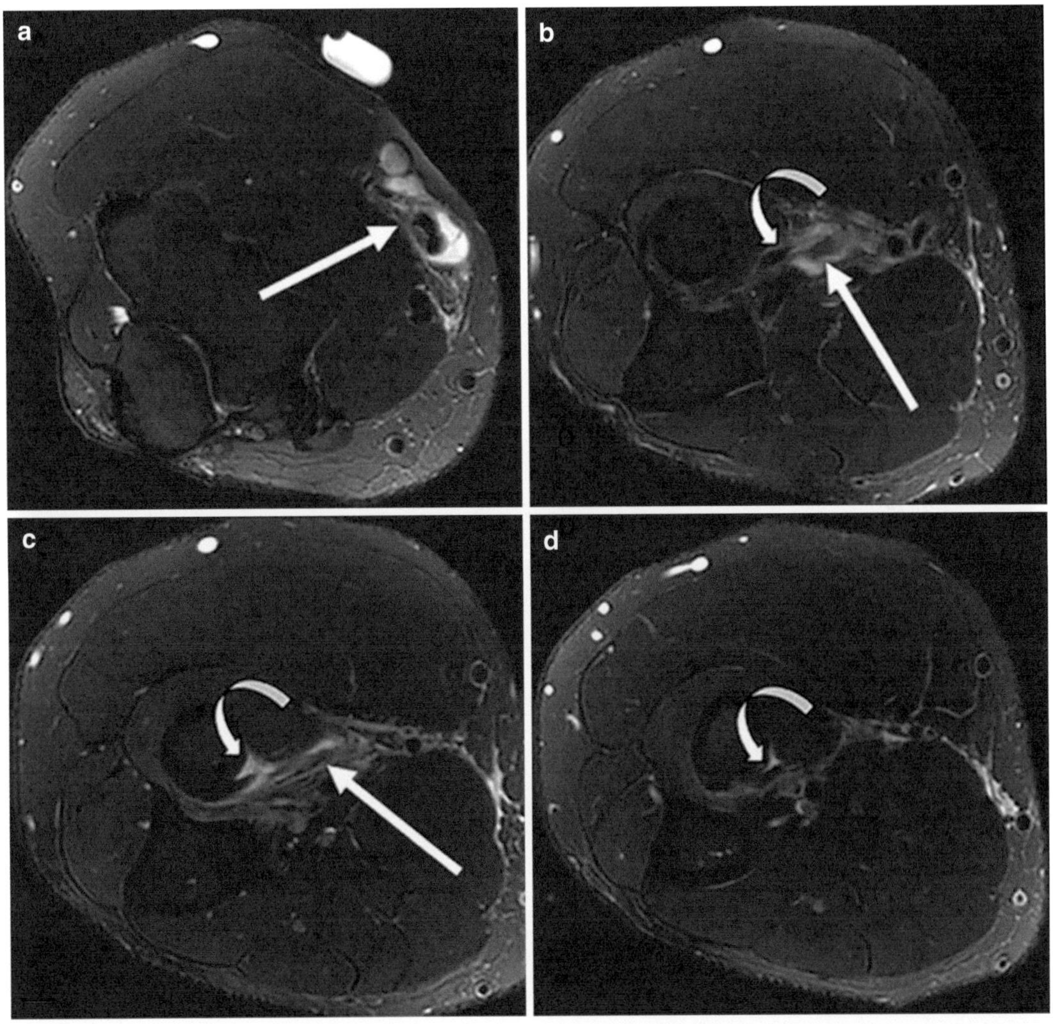

Fig. 3.32 Partial biceps tendon tear. Axial T2 fat-suppressed images proximal to distal (**a–d**) in a 37-year-old man show a partial tear of the biceps tendon. Fluid surrounds the biceps tendon with irregularity and high-grade partial tearing of the short head (straight arrows). The long head of the biceps tendon is intact (curved arrows) and attaches onto the radial tuberosity

active patients often require surgery to restore strength in flexion and supination [79]. Minimally invasive single incision techniques have become the operative approach of choice to minimize the risk of developing heterotopic ossification. This method limits surgical exposure and requires accurate diagnosis of distal tendon involvement in the setting of single-head tears as the separate footprints of the long and short head tendons can be challenging to differentiate operatively [77].

Tendinopathy

Tendinopathy occurs 1–2 cm proximal to the insertion of the distal biceps tendon. This region has relatively decreased perfusion and elasticity over time and is subsequently slower to heal fol-

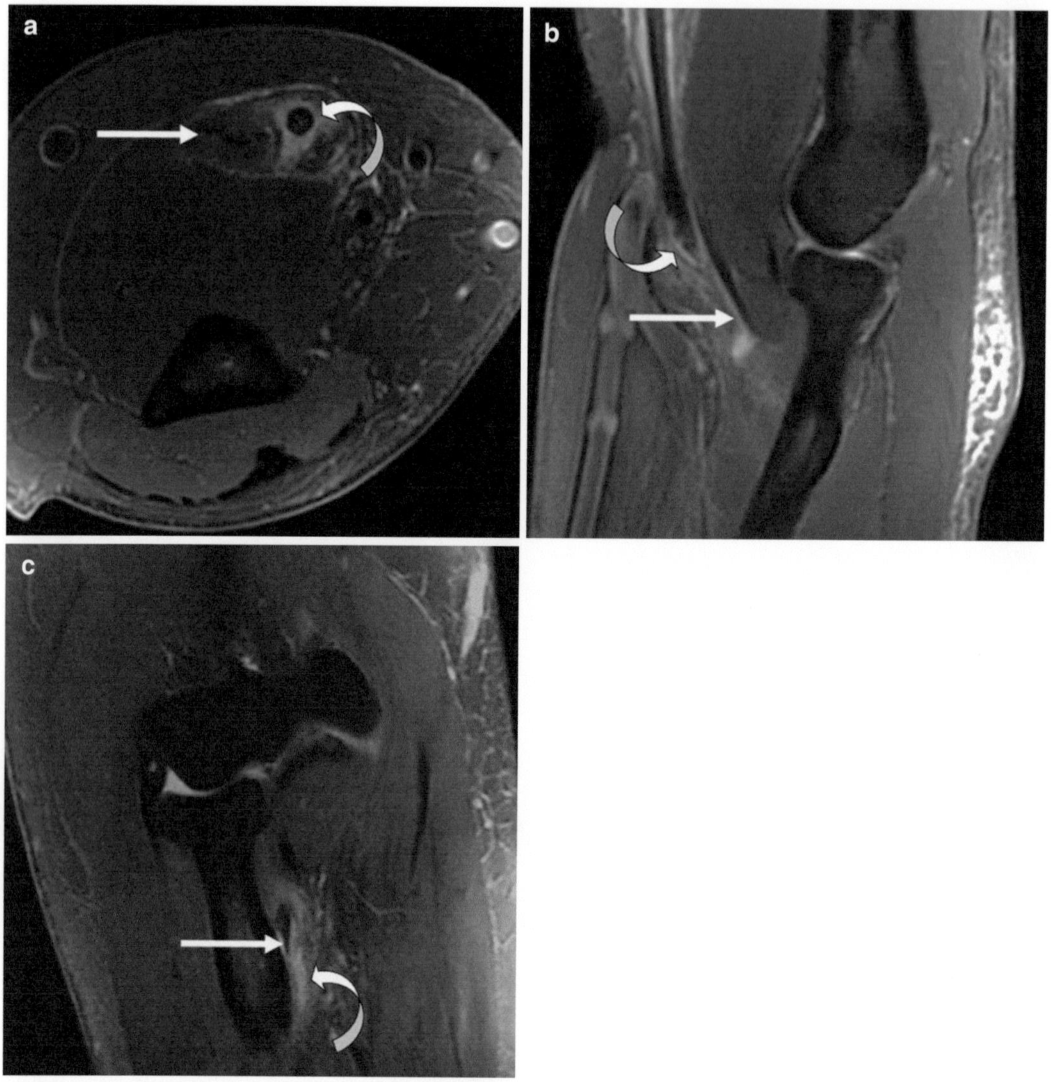

Fig. 3.33 Isolated short head biceps rupture. A 57-year-old man presents with anterior elbow pain after lifting. Axial T2 fat-suppressed (**a**) image above the level of the elbow shows thickening of the distal short head tendon (curved arrow) with surrounding fluid signal adjacent to a normal-appearing long head distal biceps myotendinous junction (straight arrow). Sagittal T2 fat-suppressed (**b**) image demonstrates an intact distal long head tendon (straight arrow) beneath a torn and retracted short head tendon (curved arrow). Coronal T2 fat-suppressed (**c**) image at the radial tuberosity shows an intact long head tendon (arrow) proximal to a fluid-filled tendon gap at the short head tendon footprint (curved arrow)

lowing traumatic insult. Degeneration associated with hypoxic tendinopathy can be worsened when combined with impingement during repetitive pronation or secondary to enthesophytes at the radial tuberosity [80]. Imaging features of biceps tendinopathy includes tendon thickening and increased signal without fiber disruption or fluid clefts to suggest tear [81].

Distal Triceps Tendon Rupture and Tendinopathy

Etiology and Clinical Presentation

Distal triceps tendon ruptures occur infrequently, accounting for approximately 0.8% of tendon ruptures. Men are more commonly affected, and tendon rupture typically follows a traumatic event such as a direct blow, fall on outstretched hand, or forced eccentric contraction. Local and systemic factors have been associated with reduction in tendon strength and greater risk of tendon injury. Local factors including corticosteroid injections, olecranon bursitis, and prior operations can result in attritional changes of the triceps tendon. Systemic factors such as rheumatoid arthritis, quinolone therapy, hyperparathyroidism, anabolic steroid use, and diabetes mellitus have been shown to increase tendon vulnerability [82]. Complete triceps tendon rupture is less common than partial tendon rupture, occurring less than 1% [83].

Imaging

Familiarity with distal triceps tendon anatomy aids in classifying tendon injuries. The triceps tendon consists of the lateral, medial, and long heads, which form deep and superficial layers proximal to the olecranon insertion. The superficial layer is comprised of the lateral and long heads, which form a central tendon. Additionally, a lateral expansion extends from the superficial layer over the anconeus and blends with the forearm fascia distally [84]. The lateral expansion functions similarly to the lacertus fibrosus, providing a small amount of elbow extension and limiting the degree of tendon retraction in the event of tendon rupture. The deep layer is formed from the muscular medial head with a small tendon that extends to the olecranon [83].

Complete tendon tears typically occur at the olecranon insertion and may be accompanied by an avulsed fracture fragment or enthesophyte. Often in these injuries, the lateral and long heads are torn, while the medial head attachment remains. MR imaging is useful in determining the location and extent of tendon involvement. Sagittal sequences can be used to identify avulsed osseous fragments and delineate the degree of tendon retraction (Fig. 3.34). Fluid-sensitive sequences detect peritendinous and intramuscular edema and hemorrhage, while T1-weighted imaging can identify the presence and severity of fatty muscle replacement in chronic tendon injuries. Predisposing conditions to triceps rupture such as olecranon bursitis are readily identified on MRI [85].

Treatment

Management of distal triceps tendon injuries is determined by muscle and tendon integrity as well as strength of elbow extension on physical

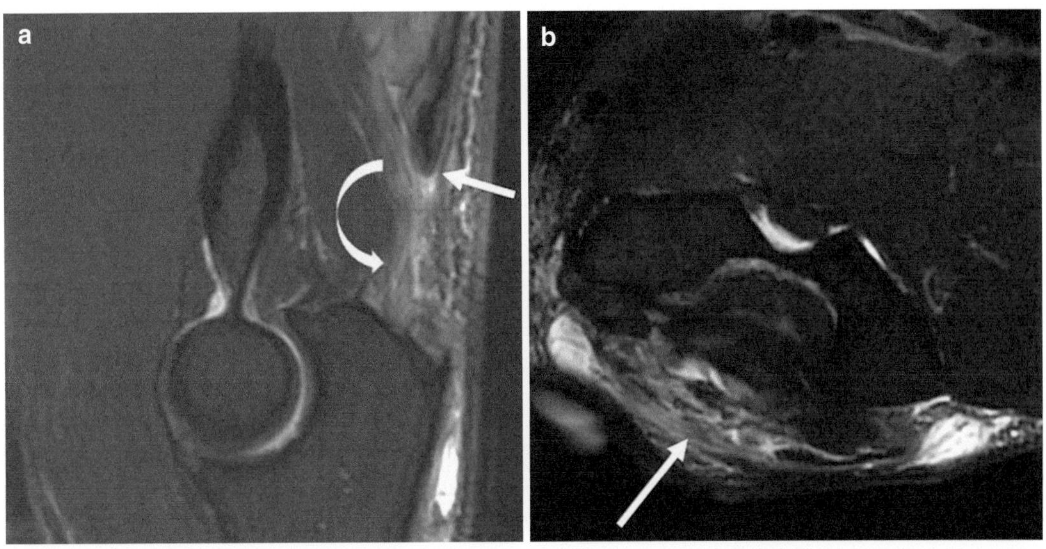

Fig. 3.34 Triceps tear in a 53-year-old man. Sagittal (**a**) and axial (**b**) T2 fat-suppressed images show complete tears of both the long and lateral heads of the triceps tendon (straight arrow). There is edema within the medial head of the triceps due to muscle strain/partial tearing (curved arrow). Injuries of the triceps tendon usually result in partial tears of the long and lateral heads, as the medial head is mostly muscle and attaches on the more anterior aspect of the olecranon

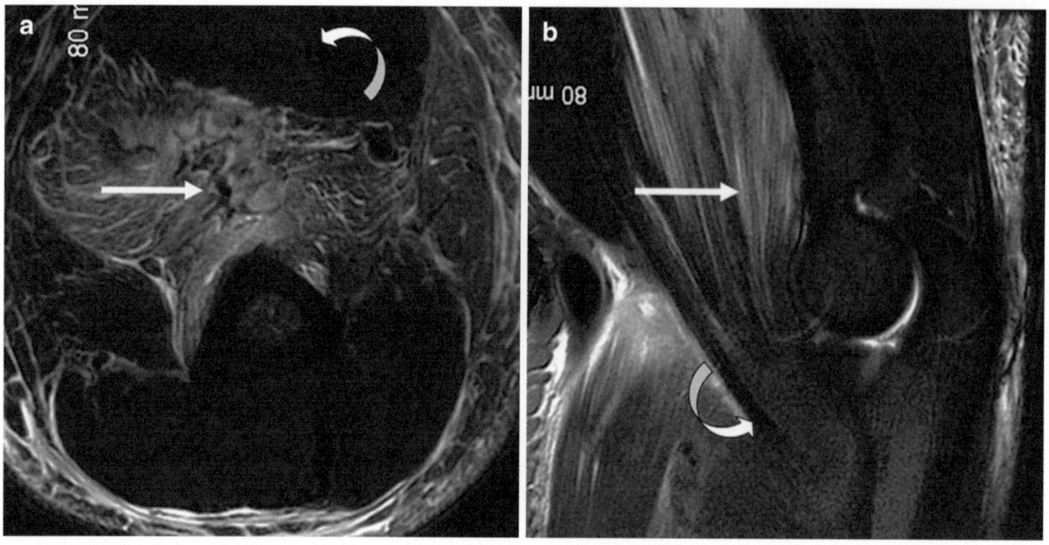

Fig. 3.35 Brachialis injury in a 19-year-old football player. Axial (**a**) and sagittal (**b**) T2 fat-suppressed images demonstrate diffuse edema and T2 signal hyperintensity of the brachialis muscle (straight arrow) deep to the distal biceps muscle (curved arrow)

exam. Early surgical repair is indicated in complete triceps tendon rupture as well as high-grade partial tendon rupture involving greater than 50% tendon thickness. Low-grade partial tears, particularly in patients with limited mobility, are managed with several weeks of splint immobilization followed by physiotherapy to restore functional range of motion [86].

Brachialis

Distal brachialis muscle and tendon injuries are quite rare with only several reports in the literature. Anatomic studies of the brachialis demonstrate two discrete heads of the distal tendon, the superficial and the deep head. The superficial head inserts distally on the coronoid process, providing stability as well as mechanical advantage when the elbow is in a flexed position. The deep head inserts proximally and aids in the initiation of flexion when the elbow is in the extended position [87]. Forced eccentric contraction and hyperextension can lead to injury, which have similar symptoms to distal biceps tendon rupture, including pain and swelling of the anterior arm distally. A palpable tendon defect is not appreciated in isolated brachialis tendon injuries due to the intact overlying biceps brachii tendon. Radiographs are often normal in cases of brachialis muscle or tendon injuries. MR imaging is useful in detecting the integrity of the distal tendon as well as identification of muscle strain and hematoma (Fig. 3.35) [88, 89].

Lateral Epicondylosis (Common Extensor Tendinopathy)

Etiology and Clinical Presentation

Tennis elbow, or lateral epicondylosis, received its name due to the high prevalence of lateral elbow pain attributable to common extensor tendon pathology in tennis players, affecting over 50% [90]. Additionally, common extensor tendinopathy affects nonathletes, including laborers and those who perform repetitive lifting or gripping. Symptoms result from incomplete healing of microscopic and macroscopic trauma to the common extensor tendon during repeated wrist extension [91]. Common extensor tendinopathy is often a clinical diagnosis with focal pain at the lateral epicondyle, exacerbated by wrist extension; however, imaging is occasionally performed to evaluate the severity of injury or identify alternate etiologies for persistent lateral-sided elbow pain.

Imaging

The deep fibers of the common extensor tendon are comprised of the extensor carpi radialis brevis (ECRB), which is most frequently affected in common extensor tendinopathy. MR imaging shows thickening as well as increased signal on T1- and T2-weighted imaging, characteristically involving the undersurface of the proximal common extensor tendon at the humeral epicondyle origin. Areas of signal abnormality of the common extensor tendon correspond to regions of fibroblast proliferation and collagen degeneration [92]. Tendon thinning, fiber disruption, and fluid signal within the common extensor tendon represent tendon tears (Fig. 3.36). Secondary signs of common extensor tendinopathy include bone marrow edema involving the lateral epicondyle as well as high T2 signal within the anconeus muscle [93]. The severity of common extensor tendinopathy has been associated with the integrity of the underlying LUCL. In a study evaluating the LUCL in patients with symptoms of lateral epicondylosis, the LUCL was typically normal in cases of mild common extensor tendinopathy. In contrast, the LUCL in patients with moderate or severe common extensor tendinopathy was frequently abnormal. Approximately 73% of patients with moderate common extensor tendinopathy on MR imaging showed thickening of the LUCL. All patients with severe lateral epicondylosis were found to have LUCL pathology; specifically, almost 90% of patients were found to have partial or complete LUCL tears [94]. As such, it is essential to determine the integrity of the lateral collateral ligament complex on MR as conservative management has a greater likelihood of failure when an associated ligamentous injury is present [95].

Classification

Baker et al. described an arthroscopic classification system for lateral epicondylosis in 1998. The classification system focuses on the condition of the ECRB tendon as well as the joint capsule [96]:

- Type I involves inflammation and fraying of the ECRB tendon.
- Type II consists of linear tears involving the undersurface of the ECRB tendon.
- Type III includes an avulsion injury of the tendon and joint capsule.

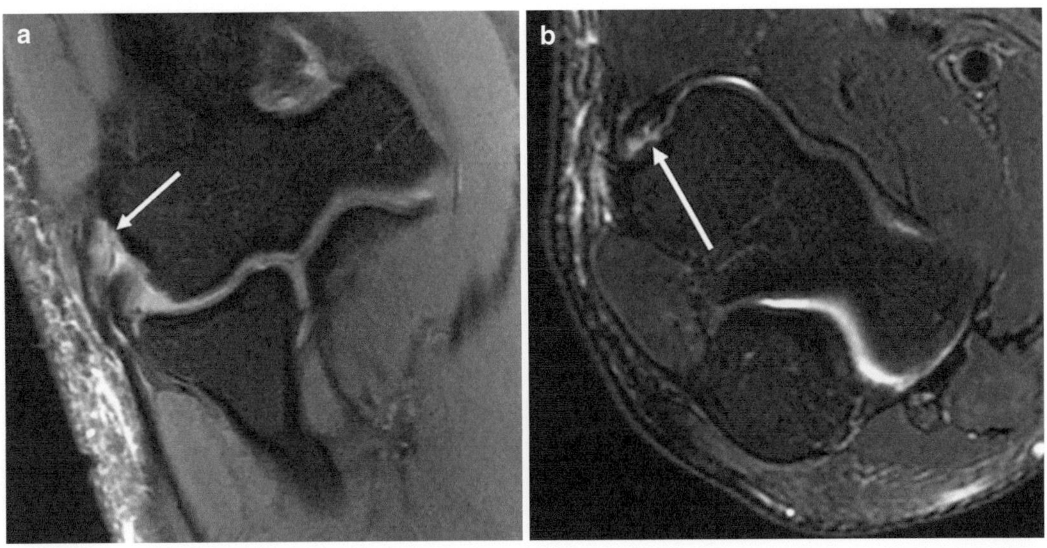

Fig. 3.36 Common extensor tendinopathy. Coronal PD (**a**) and axial T2 (**b**) fat-suppressed images in a 42-year-old man show thickening and increased signal within the common extensor tendon origin (arrows)

Treatment

In isolated common extensor tendinopathy, nonoperative management is initially favored, including rest, activity modification, and physical therapy. Corticosteroid injections are controversial in the management of common extensor tendinopathy as studies have shown that steroids may weaken the common extensor tendon and predispose it to complete rupture [97]. When conservative measures fail, ECRB debridement or release is the operative intervention of choice [98]. Patients with underlying lateral collateral ligament complex compromise are at higher risk of elbow instability following ECRB tendon release due to loss of both static and dynamic lateral elbow stabilizers, increasing the likelihood of surgical failure and reoperation [99].

Medial Epicondylosis (Common Flexor Tendinopathy)

Etiology and Clinical Presentation

Medial epicondylosis, or tendinopathy of the flexor-pronator mass, is far less common than lateral epicondylosis, occurring five to ten times less frequently. Men and women are equally affected, and the majority of cases involve the dominant arm of athletes or patients in their fourth and fifth decades. Repetitive wrist flexion and forearm pronation result in microtrauma of the common flexor tendon, which leads to inflammation, fibroblast proliferation, and subsequent fibrosis. Additionally, valgus elbow stress during early throw acceleration is antagonized by the common flexor tendon predisposing it to injury. On examination, patients describe point tenderness at the medial epicondyle which is exacerbated by resisted forearm pronation and wrist flexion.

Imaging

Acute or chronic common flexor tendon tears, avulsion fractures of the medial epicondyle, and tendinopathy can produce medial elbow pain, and cross-sectional imaging may be necessary to differentiate these pathologies. MR imaging is useful in distinguishing these processes and clarifying the etiology of medial elbow pain. The common flexor tendon is normally hypointense on all pulse sequences and is optimally assessed in axial and coronal planes. Tendinopathy (or medial epicondylosis) results in thickening and increased T1 and T2 signal within the common flexor tendon; however, the most specific MR findings include intratendinous T2 hyperintensity as well as peritendinous soft tissue edema (Fig. 3.37) [100]. The MR

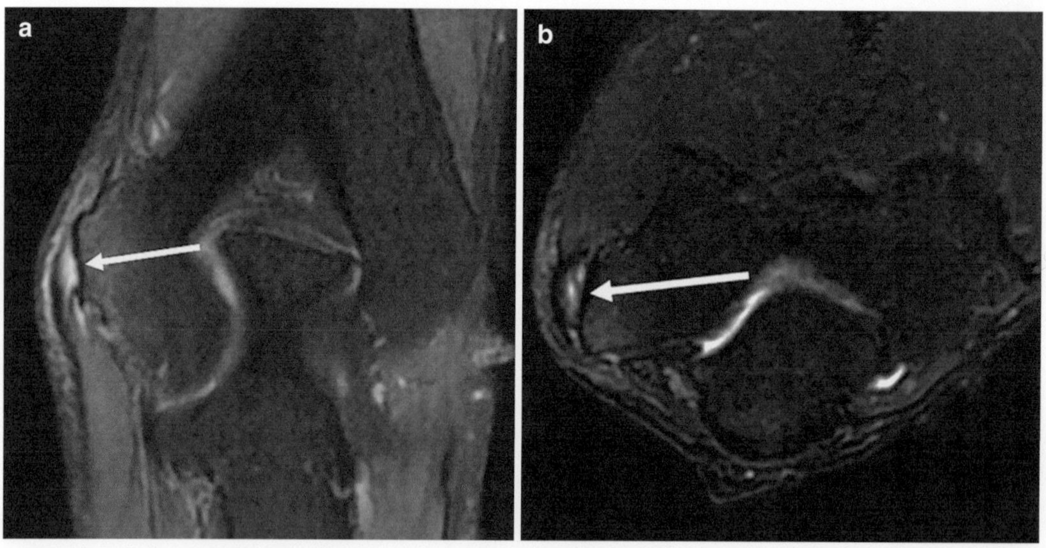

Fig. 3.37 Common flexor tendinopathy. Coronal PD (**a**) and axial T2 (**b**) fat-suppressed images in a 28-year-old man show thickening and increased signal within the common flexor tendon origin (arrows). Often there is coexisting partial tearing in these individuals as seen in this patient

appearance of common flexor tendon tear includes fluid signal within or traversing the tendon as well as partial or complete fiber disruption. Tendinopathy of the flexor-pronator mass is associated with additional ulnar-sided elbow pathology, including ulnar neuropathy and ulnar collateral ligament injury, and MR imaging plays an important role in identifying affiliated elbow injuries [101].

Treatment

Conservative treatment is preferred in the management of common flexor tendinopathy and is effective in the majority of cases. Activity modification, bracing, and stretching are often sufficient to alleviate symptoms; however, operative intervention is indicated in refractory symptoms. Surgical treatment includes open debridement versus reattachment or repair of the common flexor tendon.

Soft Tissues

Nerves

Traction injuries and entrapment neuropathies comprise traumatic elbow pathology. MR imaging provides a detailed evaluation of nerve course and signal as well as information on secondary signs of nerve impingement including muscle edema and atrophy (Fig. 3.38).

Ulnar Nerve

Cubital Tunnel Syndrome

Etiology and Clinical Presentation

Ulnar neuropathy secondary to cubital tunnel syndrome is a common upper extremity entrapment neuropathy, second in incidence to carpal tunnel syndrome. Traction of the ulnar nerve within the confinement of the cubital tunnel during valgus stress predisposes it to injury, particularly if there is failure of static restraint of the ulnar collateral ligament. Posteromedial osteophyte formation can also result in extrinsic compression of the ulnar nerve (Fig. 3.26). Repeated elbow flexion and hypermobility predispose patients to ulnar neuropathy at the elbow. Alternate locations of ulnar nerve compression have been established, including the

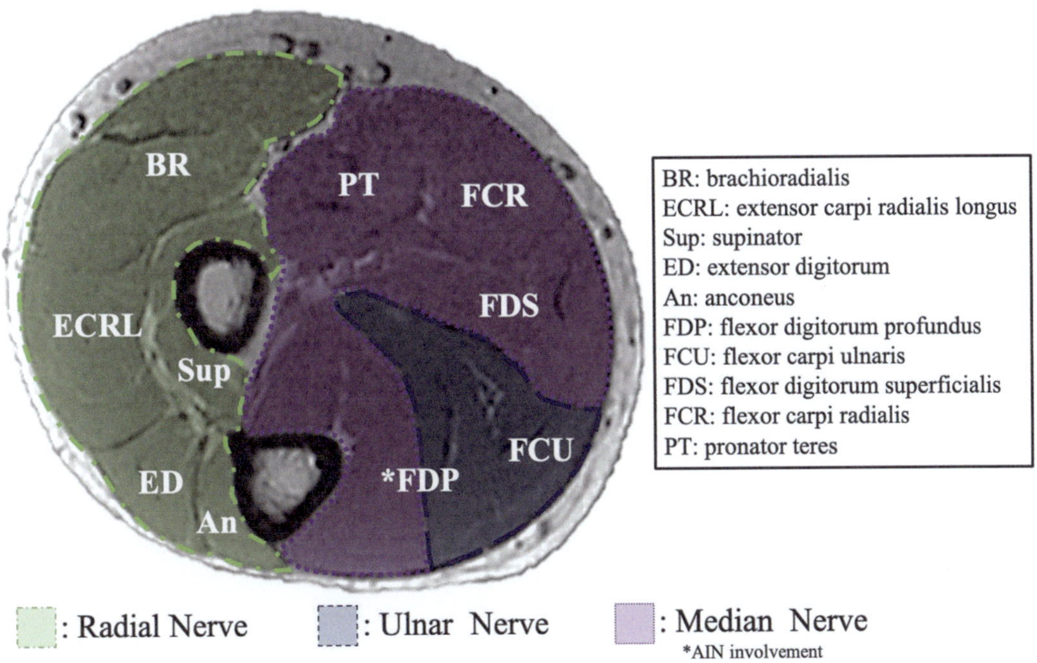

Fig. 3.38 Muscle innervation diagram of the proximal forearm

arcade of Struthers, between the humeral and ulnar heads of the flexor carpi ulnaris, the medial epicondyle, and the deep flexor aponeurosis. Anatomic variations can also predispose individuals to the development of cubital tunnel syndrome. An accessory anconeus epitrochlearis muscle is present in almost 25% of the population. A low-lying medial head of the triceps may also compress the ulnar nerve within the cubital tunnel. The cubital tunnel retinaculum has been shown to be thickened in 22% of patients, which may result in mass effect on the ulnar nerve. Alternatively, the cubital tunnel retinaculum is absent in up to 10% of the population, and this may predispose patients to ulnar nerve subluxation or dislocation, either of which may cause ulnar neuropathy [102]. Symptoms of cubital tunnel syndrome include paresthesias involving the ulnar aspect of the forearm and hand, including the ring and small fingers. A claw deformity of the fourth and fifth digits can also occur from chronic compression of the ulnar nerve.

Imaging

In addition to the ability to detect anatomic variants within and around the cubital tunnel, MR imaging plays an important role in evaluating the size, signal, and course of the ulnar nerve at the elbow. Cross-sectional area of 0.08 cm^2 has an established 95% sensitivity and 80% specificity for detecting ulnar neuropathy. Additionally, obliteration of perineural fat can be seen in combination with focal or diffuse nerve enlargement (Fig. 3.39). Subtle increase in ulnar nerve signal on fluid-sensitive MR sequences can be challenging to detect; however, the use of short-tau inversion recovery images or high spatial resolution neurography sequences can provide more accurate evaluation of the ulnar nerve [103]. Secondary signs of cubital tunnel syndrome include denervation muscle changes in the distribution of the ulnar nerve. Hyperintensity on fluid-sensitive sequences within the flexor carpi ulnaris as well as the medial half of the flexor digitorum profundus muscles may be seen followed by fatty muscle replacement in long-standing nerve compromise.

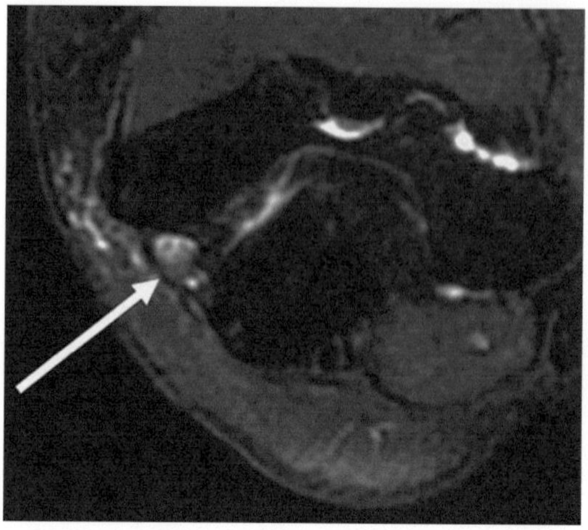

Fig. 3.39 Ulnar neuritis. A 65-year-old woman presents with lateral elbow pain and paresthesias in her ring and small fingers. Axial T2 fat-suppressed image shows enlargement and increased signal of the ulnar nerve (arrow) at the level of the cubital tunnel

Treatment

In patients with mild symptoms, activity modification, nonsteroidal anti-inflammatory medication, and nocturnal bracing with elbow in extension are used to improve symptoms of cubital tunnel syndrome. In severe symptoms or when conservative measures fail, operative interventions include ulnar nerve decompression with or without nerve transposition or medial epicondylectomy. Ulnar nerve transposition is favored when osteophytes, heterotopic ossification, fracture, or tumor compromises the cubital tunnel. Additionally, greater success with transposition is seen in throwing athletes due to repetitive flexion and valgus stress.

Median Nerve

Pronator Syndrome

Etiology and Clinical Presentation

Pronator syndrome is a result of median nerve compression at the level of the elbow. Multiple locations of entrapment have been reported, including a supracondylar process, which is an osseous eminence along the anteromedial aspect of the distal humeral diaphysis. The ligament of

Struthers extends from the supracondylar process to the medial epicondyle and may compress the median nerve proximal to the elbow. The lacertus fibrosus, or bicipital aponeurosis, travels over the median nerve and brachial artery within the antecubital fossa. Distal to the elbow joint, the median nerve can become entrapped between the humeral (superficial) and ulnar (deep) heads of the pronator teres or at the flexor digitorum superficialis aponeurosis. Symptoms of pronator syndrome can be difficult to distinguish from carpal tunnel syndrome; however, characteristic symptoms include forearm pain as well as a positive Tinel sign at the proximal forearm with a negative Tinel sign at the wrist [104]. The most common site of nerve compression is at the pronator teres, and symptoms can often be elicited by resisted pronation.

Imaging

Radiographs are often the initial imaging method of choice in patients with suspected pronator syndrome to evaluate for the presence of a supracondylar process. MR imaging can aid in identifying the location of median nerve compression; however, it may appear normal on imaging. Denervation muscle changes affect the anterior compartment of the forearm excluding the flexor muscles innervated by the ulnar nerve (flexor carpi ulnaris and the medial half of the flexor digitorum profundus) [105].

Treatment

Conservative management of pronator syndrome is often trialed over a course of 3–6 months with rest from offending activity, splinting, and use of nonsteroidal medication. This is followed by median nerve decompression if nonoperative management fails.

Anterior Interosseous Nerve Syndrome

Etiology and Clinical Presentation

The anterior interosseous nerve (AIN) is a branch of the median nerve that begins approximately 5 cm beyond the elbow joint. It passes between the humeral and ulnar heads of the pronator teres before extending along the palmar aspect of the forearm interosseous membrane. The lateral half of the flexor digitorum profundus as well as the deep forearm compartment including the flexor pollicis longus as well as the pronator quadratus muscles. AIN syndrome can result from iatrogenic trauma from venous puncture, extrinsic compression from an accessory flexor pollicis longus muscle (known as Gantzer muscle), or radial diaphysis trauma. Symptoms of AIN syndrome include motor deficits with preservation of sensation as the AIN is a motor branch. Patients present with decreased grip strength and inability to form the "OK sign" due to weakness of the flexor digitorum profundus and flexor pollicis longus [105].

Imaging

While enlargement or increased signal of the nerve on fluid-sensitive sequences can be seen in the setting of AIN syndrome, the most predictable sign of AIN compression is diffuse T2 signal hyperintensity within the pronator quadratus muscle (Fig. 3.40). Rupture of the flexor pollicis longus or flexor digitorum profundus tendons can mimic symptoms of AIN syndrome, and MR imaging can easily differentiate between these entities [106].

Treatment

Many patients respond to nonoperative management of AIN syndrome; however, an extended course of rest and physical therapy may be required. Nerve decompression is reserved for cases where a cyst or mass is compressing the AIN or when a conservative management fails.

Radial Nerve

Posterior Interosseous Nerve Syndrome

Etiology and Clinical Presentation

The posterior interosseous nerve (PIN) is a continuation of the deep branch of the radial nerve after it extends through the supinator muscle. The

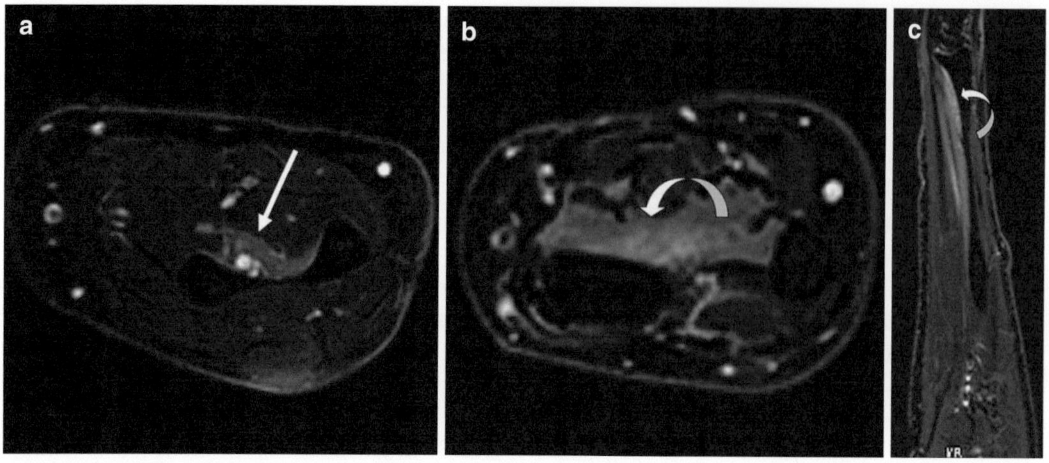

Fig. 3.40 AIN in a 44-year-old woman. Axial T2 fat-suppressed images at the proximal (**a**) and distal (**b**) forearm show denervation edema in the flexor digitorum profundus (straight arrow) and pronator quadratus (curved arrow) muscles, which is also seen on sagittal T2 fat-suppressed image (**c**)

PIN travels around the radial neck and along the posterior aspect of the forearm interosseous membrane to innervate the common and deep extensor muscle groups. Multiple areas of compression have been established, including the radial tunnel, which is formed by the radiocapitellar joint capsule posteriorly, the biceps and brachialis tendons medially, and the brachioradialis and extensor carpi radialis muscles laterally. Recurrent branches from the radial artery can cross and impinge the posterior interosseous nerve, termed the leash of Henry. The ECRB as well as the supinator muscles can also result in symptomatic compression of the PIN. Lastly, the arcade of Frohse is a fibrous arch proximal to the supinator muscle and is the most common cause of PIN entrapment [104]. The close proximity of the PIN to the radial neck increases its vulnerability in the event of radial neck fractures or radial head dislocation. Symptoms of PIN syndrome include forearm and wrist pain as well and weakness in wrist extension.

Imaging

PIN syndrome is typically diagnosed clinically based on physical exam; however, MR imaging is useful in determining the level of compression as well as whether or not the symptoms are due to extrinsic compression from a mass lesion [107]. Denervation edema or atrophy can be seen in the common and deep extensor muscles of the forearm (Fig. 3.41).

Treatment

Surgery is indicated for treatment of a compressive mass affecting the PIN. Similar to other entrapment neuropathies, operative nerve release is pursued when conservative measures fail to alleviate symptoms.

Bursae

Normal bursae are synovial-lined potential spaces located between apposing structures in areas subject to motion that function to reduce friction in these areas. Bursitis can result secondary to many etiologies, but mechanical trauma and overuse are common causes of bursitis about the elbow. The two main bursae about the elbow are the bicipitoradial and olecranon bursae.

Bicipitoradial Bursitis

Etiology and Clinical Presentation

The bicipitoradial bursa is located between the radial tuberosity and the distal biceps tendon. The most common cause of bicipitoradial bursitis is repetitive trauma, but additional etiologies including inflam-

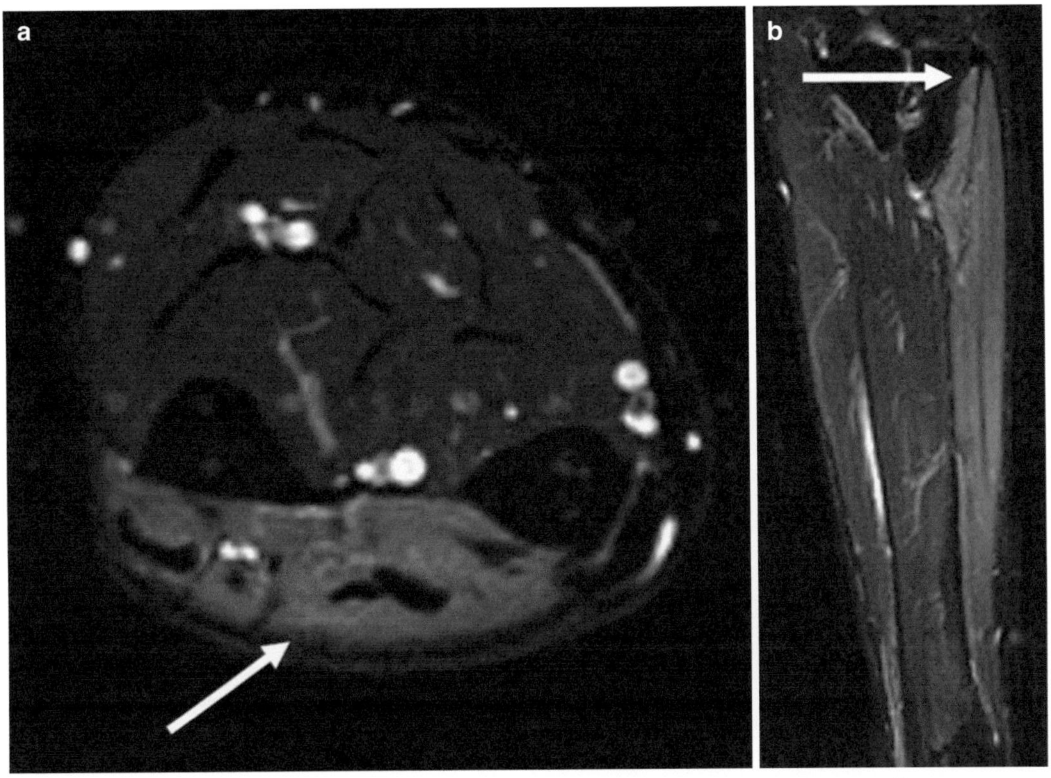

Fig. 3.41 PIN syndrome. A 39-year-old man complains of forearm pain and weakness with wrist extension. Axial (**a**) and coronal (**b**) T2 fat-suppressed images show denervation edema within the extensor tendons (arrows) along the posterior aspect of the interosseous membrane (**a**), extending from the lateral epicondyle (**b**)

matory arthropathies, infection, and synovial chondromatosis can lead to bursal expansion. Distention of the bicipitoradial bursa can limit elbow flexion and extension. If adjacent radial nerve compression is present, symptoms are determined by the specific branch involved. The superficial branch of the radial nerve is a sensory branch that innervates the dorsal and radial aspect of the hand and if impinged can lead to numbness in this distribution. The deep branch of the radial nerve is a motor branch that controls the forearm extensors, and the supinator muscle and weakness in forearm extension may occur if bursal mass effect involves the deep branch. If significantly enlarged, bicipitoradial bursitis can be a palpable antecubital mass [108].

Imaging

MR imaging in bicipitoradial bursitis shows fluid distention of the bursa interposed between the deep fibers of the distal biceps tendon and the anterior cortex of the proximal radius and best assessed on axial images (Fig. 3.42). The mean size of the bicipitoradial bursa is 1.8 × 2.5 cm, and the configuration may be teardrop-shaped during forearm pronation due to compression of the biceps tendon against the radial cortex or U-shaped around the distal biceps tendon during supination. Typically, there is no articular communication with the bicipitoradial bursa. The bursa may change shape depending on whether the forearm is supinated or pronated. If enlargement leads to nerve compression, denervation muscle edema or atrophy can be identified in the supinator and forearm extensors [109]. Bicipitoradial bursitis can also be associated with biceps tendinopathy or tear, and therefore careful evaluation of the tendon is crucial.

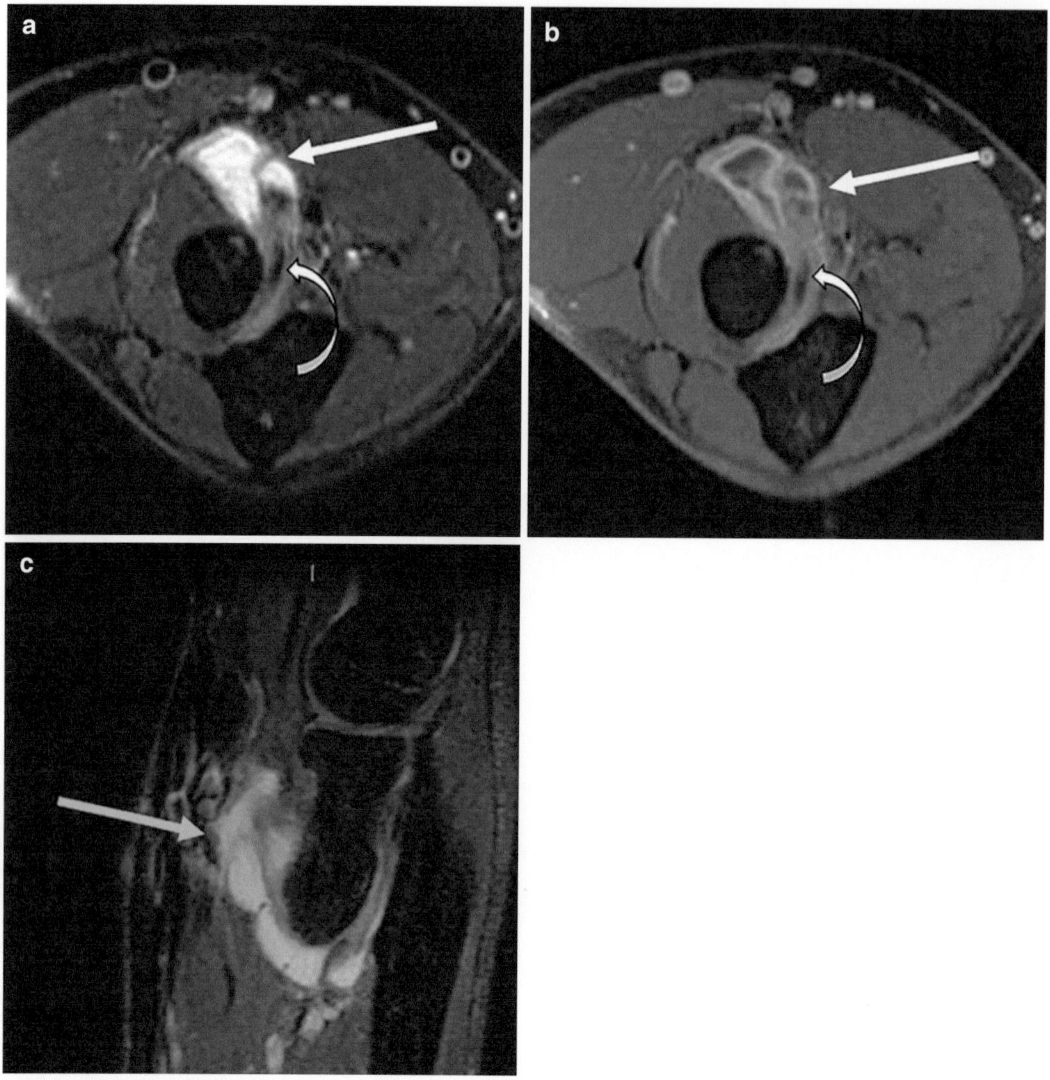

Fig. 3.42 Bicipitoradial bursitis in a 42-year-old woman. Axial (**a**) and sagittal (**b**) T2 fat-suppressed images show a lobulated mass (straight arrows) fluid equivalent in signal along the anterior forearm. This fluid collection is anterior and wraps around the biceps tendon (curved arrows). Axial T1 fat-suppressed post-contrast image (**c**) shows peripheral enhancement

Treatment

Conservative management including aspiration and corticosteroid injection has been implicated in bicipitoradial bursitis. If significant bursal enlargement recurs or results in limited range of motion or neurologic symptoms, surgical resection may be required for symptom management.

Olecranon Bursitis

Etiology and Clinical Presentation

The olecranon bursa is a potential space lined with a synovial membrane, which functions to reduce friction between the soft tissues and the olecranon process [110]. Olecranon bursitis is a

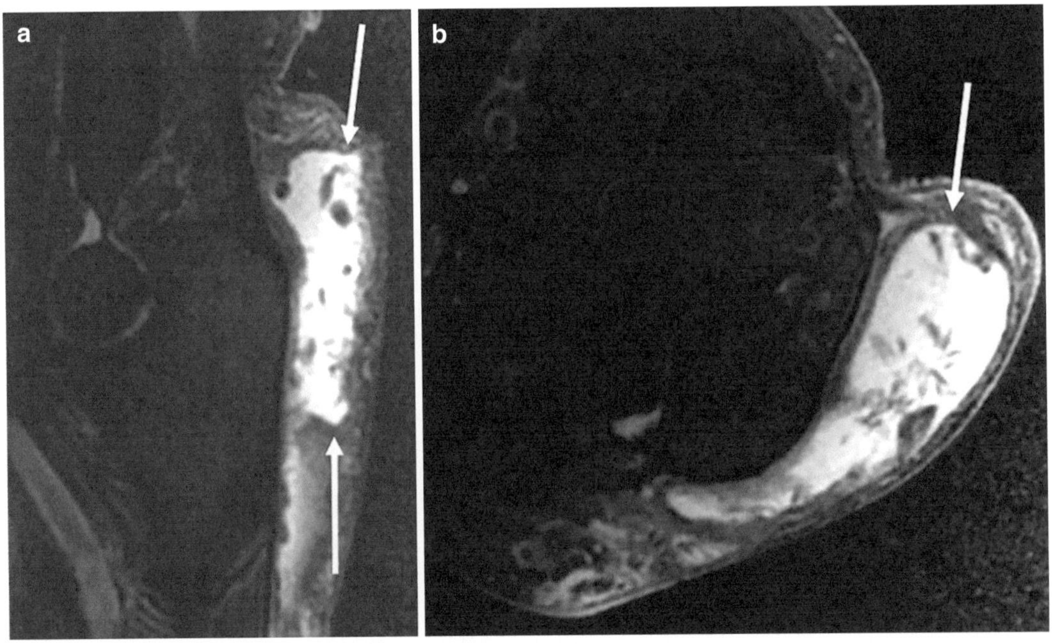

Fig. 3.43 Olecranon bursitis in a 62-year-old man. Sagittal (**a**) and axial (**b**) T2 fat-suppressed images show a large olecranon bursa with associated internal debris (arrows). There are many causes for bursitis including posttraumatic, inflammatory, crystalline, inflammatory, or infectious etiologies

clinical diagnosis with focal pain and swelling along the posterior aspect of the elbow, localized over the olecranon. Repetitive trauma or prolonged pressure to the elbow can result in inflammation and accumulation of fluid within the olecranon bursa. Other causes include systemic inflammatory conditions (rheumatoid arthritis, gout) or infection. If the bursitis is bilateral, the presumptive diagnosis is gout until proved otherwise.

Imaging

MR imaging features of olecranon bursitis include a T2 hyperintense fluid collection in the posterior elbow subcutaneous fat with or without marginal lobulation, internal septations, or complexity (Fig. 3.43). Soft tissue and olecranon bone marrow edema are associated findings of olecranon bursitis. Reactive triceps tendon thickening and muscle edema can be seen with olecranon bursitis, which can predispose patients to distal triceps tendon rupture. If bursal and soft tissue enhancement are absent on MR, septic bursitis can be excluded; however, many imaging findings of septic and nonseptic olecranon bursitis overlap, and fluid sampling should be pursued if there is concern for infection [111].

Treatment

Treatment of olecranon bursitis is dependent on the presence or absence of infection. Septic olecranon bursitis is treated with antibiotic therapy with or without bursectomy depending on the severity of infection. Nonseptic bursitis is managed with conservative management and intermittent aspiration with bursectomy reserved for refractory cases [112].

References

1. Kovar FM, Jaindl M, Thalhammer G, Rupert S, Platzer P, Endler G, et al. Incidence and analysis of radial head and neck fractures. World J Orthop. 2013;4(2):80–4.

2. Major NM, Crawford ST. Elbow effusions in trauma in adults and children: is there an occult fracture? Am J Roentgenol. 2002;178(2):413–8.
3. Mason ML. Some observations on fractures of the head of the radius with a review of one hundred cases. Br J Surg. 1954;42(172):123–32.
4. Swensen SJ, Tyagi V, Uquillas C, Shakked RJ, Yoon RS, Liporace FA. Maximizing outcomes in the treatment of radial head fractures. J Orthop Traumatol. 2019;20(1):15.
5. Wiegand L, Bernstein J, Ahn J. Fractures in brief: olecranon fractures. Clin Orthop Relat Res. 2012;470(12):3637–41.
6. Colton CL. Fractures of the olecranon in adults: classification and management. Injury. 1973;5(2):121–9.
7. Meinberg EG, Agel J, Roberts CS, Karam MD, Kellam JF. Fracture and dislocation classification compendium-2018. J Orthop Trauma. 2018;32:S1–170.
8. Cabanela M, Morrey BF. The elbow and its disorders. 2nd ed. Philadelphia: WB Saunders; 1993.
9. Sullivan CW, Desai K. Classifications in brief: Mayo classification of olecranon fractures. Clin Orthop Relat Res. 2019;477(4):908–10.
10. Bailey CS, MacDermid J, Patterson SD, King GJW. Outcome of plate fixation of olecranon fractures. J Orthop Trauma. 2001;15(8):542–8.
11. Erturer RE, Sever C, Sonmez MM, Ozcelik IB, Akman S, Ozturk I. Results of open reduction and plate osteosynthesis in comminuted fracture of the olecranon. J Shoulder Elb Surg. 2011;20(3):449–54.
12. Schatzker J, Tile M. The rationale of operative fracture care. 3rd ed. Berlin/Heidelberg: Springer; 1987.
13. Newman SDS, Mauffrey C, Krikler S. Olecranon fractures. Injury. 2009;40, Injury:575–81.
14. Regan W, Morrey BF. Classification and treatment of coronoid process fractures. Orthopedics. 1992;15(7):845–8.
15. Adams JE, Hoskin TL, Morrey BF, Steinmann SP. Management and outcome of 103 acute fractures of the coronoid process of the ulna. J Bone Joint Surg Br. 2009;91(5):632–5.
16. Cage N, Dori J, Abrams R, Callahan J, Botte M. Soft tissue attachments of the ulnar coronoid process: An anatomic study with radiographic correlation. Clin Orthop Relat Res. 1995;320(November):154–8.
17. O'Driscoll S, Jupiter J, Cohen M, Ring D, McKee M. Difficult elbow fractures: pearls and pitfalls - PubMed [Internet]. Instr Course Lect. 2003 [cited 2020 Oct 31]:113–34. Available from: https://pubmed.ncbi.nlm.nih.gov/12690844/.
18. Hayter CL, Giuffre BM. Overuse and traumatic injuries of the elbow. Magn Reson Imaging Clin N Am. 2009;17:617–38.
19. Jans LBO, Ditchfield M, Anna G, Jaremko JL, Verstraete KL. MR imaging findings and MR criteria for instability in osteochondritis dissecans of the elbow in children. Eur J Radiol. 2012;81(6):1306–10.
20. Kan H. Osteochondral abnormalities: pitfalls, injuries, and osteochondritis dissecans. In: Imaging of the active lifestyle: from the weekend warrior to the pro athlete; 2011. p. 149–52.
21. Bancroft LW, Pettis C, Wasyliw C, Varich L. Osteochondral lesions of the elbow. Semin Musculoskelet Radiol. 2013;17(5):446–54.
22. Yamaguchi K, Sweet FA, Bindra R, Morrey BF, Gelberman RH. The extraosseous and intraosseous arterial anatomy of the adult elbow. J Bone Joint Surg Am. 1997;79(11):1653–62.
23. Beltran LS, Bencardino JT, Beltran J. Imaging of sports ligamentous injuries of the elbow. Semin Musculoskelet Radiol. 2013;17(5):455–65.
24. Ouellette H, Kassarjian A, Tretreault P, Palmer W. Imaging of the overhead throwing athlete, Seminars in musculoskeletal radiology, vol. 9. Berlin/Heidelberg: Thieme Medical Publishers, Inc.; 2005. p. 316–33.
25. Kijowski R, Blankenbaker DG, Shinki K, Fine JP, Graf BK, De Smet AA. Juvenile versus adult osteochondritis dissecans of the knee: appropriate MR imaging criteria for instability. Radiology. 2008;248(2):571–8.
26. Jans L, Van Praet L, Elewaut D, Van Den Bosch F, Carron P, Jaremko JL, et al. MRI of the SI joints commonly shows non-inflammatory disease in patients clinically suspected of sacroiliitis. Eur J Radiol. 2014;83(1):179–84.
27. Nguyen JC, Degnan AJ, Barrera CA, Hee TP, Ganley TJ, Kijowski R. Osteochondritis dissecans of the elbow in children: MRI findings of instability. Am J Roentgenol. 2019;213(5):1145–51.
28. Nelson DW, Dipaola J, Colville M, Schmidgall J. Osteochondritis dissecans of the talus and knee: prospective comparison of MR and arthroscopic classifications. J Comput Assist Tomogr. 1990;14(5):804–8.
29. Steinbach LS, Palmer WE, Schweitzer ME. Special focus session: MR arthrography. In: Radiographics. Berlin/Heidelberg: Radiological Society of North America Inc.; 2002. p. 1223–46.
30. Peiss J, Adam G, Casser R, Urhahn R, Günther RW. Gadopentetate-dimeglumine-enhanced MR imaging of osteonecrosis and osteochondritis dissecans of the elbow: initial experience. Skelet Radiol. 1995;24(1):17–20.
31. McKee MD, Jupiter JB, Bamberger HB. Coronal shear fractures of the distal end of the humerus. J Bone Joint Surg A. 1996;78(1):49–54.
32. Frank JM, Saltzman BM, Garbis N, Cohen MS. Articular shear injuries of the capitellum in adolescents. J Shoulder Elb Surg. 2016;25(9):1485–90.
33. Vargas DG, Woodcock S, Porto GF, Gonzalez JC. Osborne-Cotterill lesion a forgotten injury: review article and case report. Clin Shoulder Elb. 2020;23(1):27–30.
34. Jeon IH, Micic ID, Yamamoto N, Morrey BF. Osborne-cotterill lesion: an osseous defect of the capitellum associated with instability of the elbow. Am J Roentgenol. 2008;191(3):727–9.
35. Jeon IH, Min WK, Cho HS, Kim PT. Surgical treatment and clinical implication for posterolateral rotatory instability of the elbow: Osborne-Cotterill lesion of the elbow. J Trauma. 2011;71(3):E45–9.

36. Rosenberg ZS, Beltran J, Cheung Y, Broker M. MR imaging of the elbow: normal variant and potential diagnostic pitfalls of the trochlear groove and cubital tunnel. Am J Roentgenol. 1995;164(2):415–8.
37. Totlis T, Otountzidis N, Papadopoulos S, Piagkou M, Natsis K. Ulnar trochlear notch articular surface has three morphological patterns: a neglected major anatomical feature. Surg Radiol Anat. 2019;41(11):1333–6.
38. Mihara K, Tsutsui H, Nishinaka N, Yamaguchi K. Nonoperative treatment for osteochondritis dissecans of the capitellum. Am J Sports Med. 2009;37(2):298–304.
39. Cerezal L, Rodriguez-Sammartino M, Canga A, Capiel C, Arnaiz J, Cruz A, et al. Elbow synovial fold syndrome. AJR Am J Roentgenol. 2013;201(1):W88–96.
40. Koh S, Morris RP, Andersen CL, Jones EA, Viegas SF. Ultrasonographic examination of the synovial fold of the radiohumeral joint. J Shoulder Elb Surg. 2007;16(5):609–15.
41. Isogai S, Murakami G, Wada T, Ishii S. Which morphologies of synovial folds result from degeneration and/or aging of the radiohumeral joint: an anatomic study with cadavers and embryos. J Shoulder Elb Surg. 2001;10(2):169–81.
42. Husarik DB, Saupe N, Pfirrmann CWA, Jost B, Hodler J, Zanetti M. Ligaments and plicae of the elbow: normal MR imaging variability in 60 asymptomatic subjects. Radiology. 2010;257(1):185–94.
43. Awaya H, Schweitzer ME, Feng SA, Kamishima T, Marone PJ, Farooki S, et al. Elbow synovial fold syndrome: MR imaging findings. Am J Roentgenol. 2001;177(6):1377–81.
44. Antuna SA, O'Driscoll SW. Snapping plicae associated with radiocapitellar chondromalacia. Arthroscopy. 2001;17(5):491–5.
45. Steinert AF, Goebel S, Rucker A, Barthel T. Snapping elbow caused by hypertrophic synovial plica in the radiohumeral joint: a report of three cases and review of literature. Arch Orthop Trauma Surg. 2010;130(3):347–51.
46. Neumann JA, Garrigues GE, Brigman BE, Eward WC. Synovial chondromatosis. JBJS Reviews. Journal of Bone and Joint Surgery Inc. 2016;4:1–7.
47. Murphey MD, Vidal JA, Fanburg-Smith JC, Gajewski DA. From the archives of the AFIP: imaging of synovial chondromatosis with radiologic-pathologic correlation. Radiographics. 2007;27:1465–88.
48. Milgram J. Synovial osteochondromatosis: a histopathological study of thirty cases. J Bone Joint Surg Am. 1977;59(6):792–801.
49. Kobayashi K, Burton KJ, Rodner C, Smith B, Caputo AE. Lateral compression injuries in the pediatric elbow: Panner's disease and osteochondritis dissecans of the capitellum. J Am Acad Orthop Surg. 2004;12:246–54.
50. Ruch DS, Poehling GG. Arthroscopic treatment of Panner's disease. Clin Sports Med. 1991;10:629–36.
51. Wong TT, Lin DJ, Ayyala RS, KazAm JK. Elbow injuries in pediatric overhead athletes. AJR Am J Roentgenol. American Roentgen Ray Society. 2017;209:849–59.
52. Smith MG. Osteochondritis of the humeral capitulum. J Bone Joint Surg Br. 1964;46:50–4.
53. Benjamin HJ, Briner WW. Little league elbow. Clin J Sport Med. 2005;15:37–40.
54. Gottschalk HP, Eisner E, Hosalkar HS. Medial epicondyle fractures in the pediatric population. J Am Acad Orthop Surg. 2012;20:223–32.
55. Josefsson PO, Danielsson LG. Epicondylar elbow fracture in children: 35-year follow-up of 56 unreduced cases. Acta Orthop. 1986;57(4):313–5.
56. O'Holleran JD, Altchek DW. The Thrower's elbow: arthroscopic treatment of valgus extension overload syndrome. HSS J. 2006;2(1):83–93.
57. Martin S, Sanchez E. Anatomy and biomechanics of the elbow joint. Semin Musculoskelet Radiol. 2013;17(5):429–36.
58. Nicolette GW, Gravlee JR. Ulnar collateral ligament injuries of the elbow in female division I collegiate gymnasts: a report of five cases. Open Access J Sports Med. 2018;9:183–9.
59. Rosas HG, Lee KS. Imaging acute trauma of the elbow. Semin Musculoskelet Radiol. 2010;14(4):394–411.
60. Farrow LD, Mahoney AJ, Stefancin JJ, Taljanovic MS, Sheppard JE, Schickendantz MS. Quantitative analysis of the medial ulnar collateral ligament ulnar footprint and its relationship to the ulnar sublime tubercle. Am J Sports Med. 2011;39(9):1936–41.
61. Lin DJ, Kazam JK, Ahmed FS, Wong TT. Ulnar collateral ligament insertional injuries in pediatric overhead athletes: are MRI findings predictive of symptoms or need for surgery? Am J Roentgenol. 2019;212(4):867–73.
62. Potter HG. Imaging of posttraumatic and soft tissue dysfunction of the elbow. In: Clinical orthopaedics and related research. Lippincott Williams and Wilkins; 2000. p. 9–18.
63. Cain EL, Ryan MK. Traumatic instability: treatment options and considerations for recurrent posttraumatic instability. Sports Med Arthrosc Rev. Lippincott Williams and Wilkins. 2018;26:102–12.
64. Rettig AC, Sherrill C, Snead DS, Mendler JC, Mieling P. Nonoperative treatment of ulnar collateral ligament injuries in throwing athletes. Am J Sports Med. 2001;29(1):15–7.
65. Frangiamore SJ, Bigart K, Nagle T, Colbrunn R, Millis A, Schickendantz MS. Biomechanical analysis of elbow medial ulnar collateral ligament tear location and its effect on rotational stability. J Shoulder Elb Surg. 2018;27(11):2068–76.
66. Potter HG, Weiland AJ, Schatz JA, Paletta GA, Hotchkiss RN. Posterolateral rotatory instability of the elbow: usefulness of MR imaging in diagnosis. Radiology. 1997;204(1):185–9.
67. O'Driscoll S, Morrey B, Korinek S, An K. Elbow subluxation and dislocation. A spectrum of instability - PubMed [Internet]. Clin Orthop Relat Res. 1992 [cited 2020 Oct 31]:186–97. Available from: https://pubmed.ncbi.nlm.nih.gov/1611741/.

68. Pringle L, Burt A, Chang E, Resnick D. Posteromedial rotatory instability of the elbow. Radsource MRI Web Clinic. 2019.
69. O'Driscoll SW, Jupiter JB, King GJ, Hotchkiss RN, Morrey BF. The unstable elbow. Instr Course Lect. 2001;50:89–102.
70. Timmerman LA, Andrews JR. Histology and arthroscopic anatomy of the ulnar collateral ligament of the elbow. Am J Sports Med. 1994;22(5):667–73.
71. Williams BD, Schweitzer ME, Weishaupt D, Lerman J, Rubenstein DL, Miller LS, et al. Partial tears of the distal biceps tendon: MR appearance and associated clinical findings. Skelet Radiol. 2001;30(10):560–4.
72. Safran M, Graham S. Distal biceps tendon ruptures: incidence, demographics, and the effect of smoking. Clin Orthop Relat Res. 2002:275–83.
73. Schneider A, Bennett JM, O'Connor DP, Mehlhoff T, Bennett JB. Bilateral ruptures of the distal biceps brachii tendon. J Shoulder Elb Surg. 2009;18(5):804–7.
74. Giuffrè BM, Moss MJ. Optimal positioning for MRI of the distal biceps brachii tendon: flexed abducted supinated view. Am J Roentgenol. 2004;182(4):944–6.
75. Chew ML, Giuffrè BM. Disorders of the distal biceps brachii tendon. Radiographics. 2005;25(5):1227–37.
76. Eames MHA, Bain GI, Fogg QA, Van Riet RP. Distal biceps tendon anatomy: a cadaveric study. J Bone Joint Surg A. 2007;89(5):1044–9.
77. Koulouris G, Malone W, Omar IM, Gopez AG, Wright W, Kavanagh EC. Bifid insertion of the distal biceps brachii tendon with isolated rupture: magnetic resonance findings. J Shoulder Elb Surg. 2009;18(6):e22.
78. de la Fuente J, Blasi M, Martínez S, Barceló P, Cachán C, Miguel M, et al. Ultrasound classification of traumatic distal biceps brachii tendon injuries. Skelet Radiol. 2018;47(4):519–32.
79. Tarallo L, Lombardi M, Zambianchi F, Giorgini A, Catani F. Distal biceps tendon rupture: advantages and drawbacks of the anatomical reinsertion with a modified double incision approach 11 Medical and Health Sciences 1103 Clinical Sciences. BMC Musculoskelet Disord. 2018;19(1):364.
80. Seiler JG, Parker LM, Chamberland PDC, Sherbourne GM, Carpenter WA. The distal biceps tendon. Two potential mechanisms involved in its rupture: arterial supply and mechanical impingement. J Shoulder Elb Surg. 1995;4(3):149–56.
81. Nguyen ML, Rosenthal J, Karas S, Gottschalk M, Daly C, Wagner E, et al. A comprehensive review of the normal, abnormal, and post-operative MRI appearance of the distal biceps brachii. Skeletal Radiol. Springer Science and Business Media Deutschland GmbH. 2020;49:1695–707.
82. Van Riet RP, Morrey BF, Ho E, O'Driscoll SW. Surgical treatment of distal triceps ruptures. J Bone Joint Surg A. Journal of Bone and Joint Surgery Inc. 2003;85:1961–7.
83. Negrão JR, Mogami R, Ramirez Ruiz FA, Wagner FV, Haghighi P, Ward SR, et al. Distal insertional anatomy of the triceps brachii muscle: MRI assessment in cadaveric specimens employing histologic correlation and Play-doh® models of the anatomic findings. Skelet Radiol. 2020;49(7):1057–67.
84. Barco R, Sánchez P, Morrey ME, Morrey BF, Sánchez-Sotelo J. The distal triceps tendon insertional anatomy—implications for surgery. JSES Open Access. 2017;1(2):98–103.
85. Koplas MC, Schneider E, Sundaram M. Prevalence of triceps tendon tears on MRI of the elbow and clinical correlation. Skelet Radiol. 2011;40(5):587–94.
86. Khiami F, Tavassoli S, De Ridder BL, Catonné Y, Sariali E. Distal partial ruptures of triceps brachii tendon in an athlete. Orthop Traumatol Surg Res. 2012;98(2):242–6.
87. Leonello DT, Galley IJ, Bain GI, Carter CD. Brachialis muscle anatomy: a study in cadavers. J Bone Joint Surg A. 2007;89(6):1293–7.
88. Wasserstein D, White L, Theodoropoulos J. Traumatic brachialis muscle injury by elbow hyperextension in a professional hockey player. Clin J Sport Med. 2010;20(3):211–2.
89. Winblad JB, Escobedo E, Hunter JC. Brachialis muscle rupture and hematoma. Radiol Case Rep. 2008;3(4):251.
90. Maylack F. Epidemiology of tennis, squash, and racquetball injuries. Clin Sports Med. 1988;7:233–8.
91. Coonrad RW, Hooper WR. Tennis elbow: its course, natural history, conservative and surgical management. J Bone Joint Surg A. 1973;55(6):1177–82.
92. Regan W, Wold LE, Coonrad R, Morrey BF. Microscopic histopathology of chronic refractory lateral epicondylitis. Am J Sports Med. 1992;20(6):746–9.
93. Coel M, Yamada CY, Ko J. MR imaging of patients with lateral epicondylitis of the elbow (tennis elbow): importance of increased signal of the anconeus muscle. Am J Roentgenol. 1993;161(5):1019–21.
94. Bredella MA, Tirman PFJ, Fritz RC, Feller JF, Wischer TK, Genant HK. MR imaging findings of lateral ulnar collateral ligament abnormalities in patients with lateral epicondylitis. Am J Roentgenol. 1999;173(5):1379–82.
95. Morrey B. Re-operation for failed tennis elbow surgery. J Shoulder Elb Surg. 1992:47–9.
96. Baker CL, Cummings PD. Arthroscopic management of miscellaneous elbow disorders. Oper Tech Sports Med. 1998;6(1):16–21.
97. Unverferth LJ, Olix ML. The effect of local steroid injections on tendon. Am J Sports Med. 1973;1(4):31–7.
98. Nirschl R, Pettrone F. Tennis elbow and the surgical treatment of lateral epicondylitis. J Bone Joint Surg Am. 1979;61:832–9.
99. Morrey BF. Reoperation for failed surgical treatment of refractory lateral epicondylitis. J Shoulder Elb Surg. 1992;1(1):47–55.

100. Kijowski R, De Smet AA. Magnetic resonance imaging findings in patients with medial epicondylitis. Skelet Radiol. 2005;34(4):196–202.
101. Vangsness CT, Jobe FW. Surgical treatment of medial epicondylitis. Results in 35 elbows. J Bone Joint Surg Br. 1991;73(3):409–11.
102. Bucknor MD, Stevens KJ, Steinbach LS. Elbow imaging in sport: sports imaging series. Radiology. Radiological Society of North America Inc. 2016;279:12–28.
103. Keen NN, Chin CT, Engstrom JW, Saloner D, Steinbach LS. Diagnosing ulnar neuropathy at the elbow using magnetic resonance neurography. Skelet Radiol. 2012;41(4):401–7.
104. Miller TT, Reinus WR. Nerve entrapment syndromes of the elbow, forearm, and wrist. AJR Am J Roentgenol. 2010;195:585–94.
105. Linda DD, Harish S, Stewart BG, Finlay K, Parasu N, Rebello RP. Multimodality imaging of peripheral neuropathies of the upper limb and brachial plexus. Radiographics. 2010;30(5):1373–400.
106. Dunn AJ, Salonen DC, Anastakis DJ. MR imaging findings of anterior interosseous nerve lesions. Skelet Radiol. 2007;36(12):1155–62.
107. Kim S, Choi JY, Huh YM, Song HT, Lee SA, Kim SM, et al. Role of magnetic resonance imaging in entrapment and compressive neuropathy - what, where, and how to see the peripheral nerves on the musculoskeletal magnetic resonance image: part 2. Upper extremity. Eur Radiol. 2007;17(2):509–22.
108. Kegels L, Van Oyen J, Siemons W, Verdonk R. Bicipitoradial bursitis a case report. Acta Orthop Belg. 2008;72:362–5.
109. Skaf AY, Boutin RD, Dantas RWM, Hopper AW, Muhle C, Chou DS, et al. Bicipitoradial bursitis: MR imaging findings in eight patients and anatomic data from contrast material opacification of bursae followed by routine radiography and MR imaging in cadavers. Radiology. 1999;212(1):111–6.
110. Shell D, Perkins R, Cosgarea A. Septic olecranon bursitis: recognition and treatment. J Am Board Fam Pract. 1995;8(3):217–20.
111. Floemer F, Morrison WB, Bongartz G, Ledermann HP. MRI characteristics of olecranon bursitis. Am J Roentgenol. 2004;183(1):29–34.
112. Baumbach SF, Lobo CM, Badyine I, Mutschler W, Kanz KG. Prepatellar and olecranon bursitis: literature review and development of a treatment algorithm. Arch Orthop Trauma Surg. 2014;134:359–70.

Elbow Pathology: Nontraumatic

4

Sara M. Bahouth and Connie Chang

Arthritis

Osteoarthrosis

Primary osteoarthrosis is usually described as age-related wear and tear of the cartilage occurring predominantly in weight-bearing joints [1]. Elbow primary osteoarthrosis is uncommon, affecting 1–3% of the population, and most common among middle-aged men who report heavy manual labor or elbow overuse [2–4].

In the early stages of the disease, patients often present with pain on extension and flexion. It is thought that the reason for the pain is primarily the friction of the osteophytes at the tips of the coronoid and olecranon with their respective fossae [4]. Pain, in the later stages of the disease, is thought to be secondary to diffuse articular degeneration [4]. Another manifestation of elbow osteoarthrosis is stiffness or a "locking sensation." Osteoarthritis is the second most frequent cause of elbow stiffness after previous trauma [5]. As the osteophytes enlarge, they become space-occupying and result in rigidity of the elbow joint [4]. All of these manifestations may severely affect a patient's activity of daily living and quality of life.

S. M. Bahouth · C. Chang (✉)
Division of Musculoskeletal Imaging and Intervention, Massachusetts General Hospital, Boston, MA, USA
e-mail: sbahouth@mgh.harvard.edu; cychang@mgh.harvard.edu

Radiologic evaluation of elbow osteoarthrosis should begin with radiographs that can offer most of the information needed for diagnosis and treatment planning [6]. Computed tomography (CT) is used to identify osteophytes and loose bodies not well visualized on radiographs and to delineate heterotopic ossification [6]. Magnetic resonance imaging (MRI) is utilized to best assess the articular cartilage and to evaluate for infection.

MRI provides full assessment of the bone, articular cartilage, synovium, and soft tissues. If elbow osteoarthrosis is present, the following findings may be identified (Fig. 4.1):

1. Osteophytes: Bone marrow signal on T1- and T2-weighted images.
2. Subchondral sclerosis: Hypointense signal on T1-weighted images and fluid-sensitive sequences.
3. Subchondral cyst formation: Hypointense signal on T1-weighted images and hyperintense signal on T2-weighted images.
4. Subchondral edema and effusion in the setting of high-grade cartilage loss.
5. Loose bodies.
6. Nonuniform loss of joint space with preservation of the joint space centrally and degenerative changes anteriorly and posteriorly.
7. Distribution: Involvement of the radiocapitellar joint alone is uncommon. There is usually concomitant degenerative changes of the ulnohumeral joint [4].

B. U. Casagranda (ed.), *MRI of the Upper Extremity*, https://doi.org/10.1007/978-3-030-81612-4_4

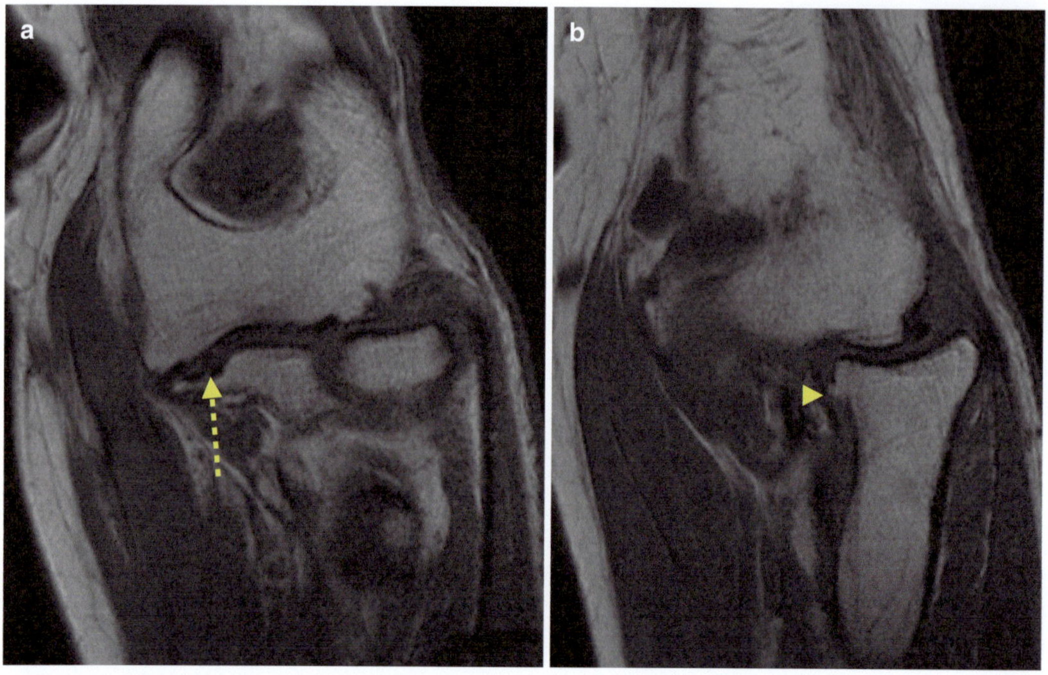

Fig. 4.1 Primary osteoarthrosis in a 62-year-old female. (**a**, **b**) Coronal T1-weighted MR images show severe joint space narrowing, osteophytosis (arrow head), and subchondral sclerosis (dashed arrow)

Neuropathic Arthropathy

Neuropathic arthropathy, also known as Charcot joint, is a progressive, destructive arthritis that rarely affects the elbows. Among patients with neuropathic arthropathy, only 3% of the cases involve the elbow [7]. It is associated with cervical spine pathology such as syringomyelia or diabetes. Twenty-five percent of patients with syringomyelia will develop neuropathic arthropathy with 80% occurring in the upper extremity [8]. Patients usually present with painless joint swelling, joint instability, or elbow dysfunction.

There are three phases of the neuropathic joint: the destructive/atrophic phase, reparative/hypertrophic phase, and quiescent phase. During the destructive phase, the joint is swollen and there is extensive bone erosion. As for the reparative phase, there is dense fibrous tissue formation with coalescence of the debris. The quiescent phase is mainly depicted by osseous sclerosis. The atrophic changes are mainly seen in the hip, shoulder, and foot, while the hypertrophic changes are described more in the elbow [8].

Usually radiographs are adequate for evaluation of neuropathic arthropathy. However, if an MRI is needed for confirmation, the following findings are expected:

1. Osseous destruction of both sides of the joint best seen on T1-weighted images
2. Bone production including sclerosis and heterotopic ossification
3. Intramuscular edema surrounding the joint
4. Joint effusion, hyperintense on fluid-sensitive sequences and hypointense on T1 sequence, intra-articular debris

A cervical MRI study should be considered to evaluate for cervical spine pathology, especially in the setting of bilateral abnormalities.

Rheumatoid Arthritis

Rheumatoid arthritis (RA) is an autoimmune multisystemic inflammatory condition with a prevalence of 1% [9]. It may affect multiple joints.

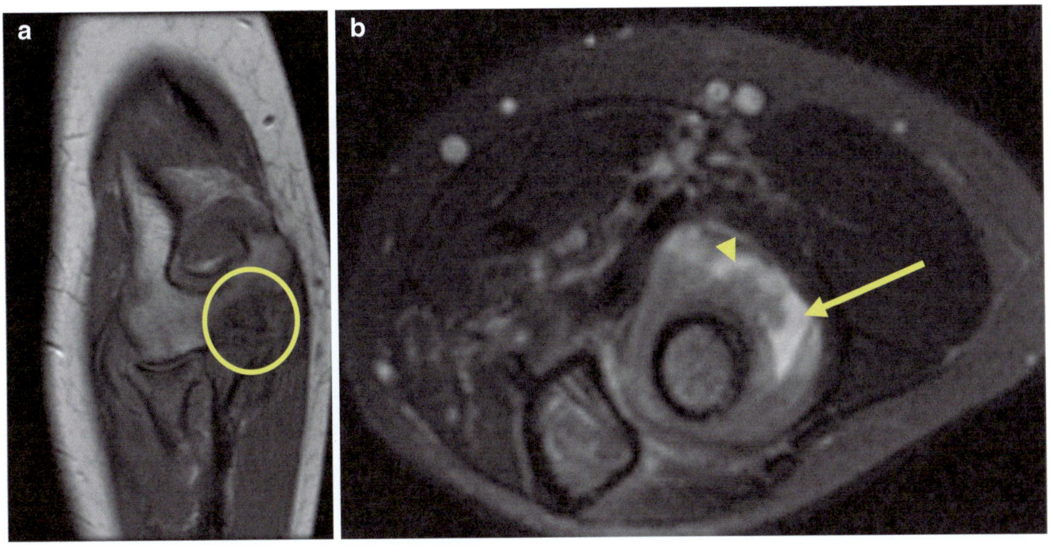

Fig. 4.2 A 43-year-old woman with rheumatoid arthritis. (**a**) Coronal T1-weighted MR image shows bone erosions and edema at the ulnotrochlear articulation (circle). (**b**) Axial T2-weighted MR image demonstrates elbow effusion (arrow) and marked synovitis (arrow head)

20–50% of RA patients will demonstrate elbow involvement [10]. The disease is more common in women and can occur at any age but has a peak onset in the fourth and fifth decades of life [9].

Rheumatoid arthritis is the most common source of inflammatory symptoms of the elbow [11]. Its clinical manifestation parallels the pathology occurring in the joint. The initial presentation in nearly half of patients with RA is elbow synovitis manifesting as pain and restriction of motion [10]. If the synovitis does not resolve, secondary changes can occur, such as flexion contracture caused by loss of extension ability due to pain. Synovitis can affect the elbow ligaments leading to instability and can cause joint capsule distention leading to neurovascular compression symptoms [12]. Chronic synovitis can damage the articular cartilage resulting in secondary osteoarthritis [10].

The first step in the radiographic evaluation of RA should be AP and lateral radiographs. Findings may include symmetric joint space narrowing, periarticular erosions, and disuse osteopenia [13]. Additional workup with MRI has proved to have its advantages. MRI is the most sensitive modality to diagnose early RA which is important in the setting of early treatment with disease-modifying antirheumatic drugs [9]. MRI also plays a role in assessing for RA activity by detecting effusions, capsular distention, and bone marrow edema.

Some of the findings seen on MRI in the setting of elbow RA include (Fig. 4.2):

1. Bone erosions are more specific for RA than synovitis. They equally involve the capitellum, trochlea, ulna, and radial head/neck.
2. Bone marrow edema can be predictive of future erosion sites. It appears hyperintense on fluid-sensitive sequences and hypointense on T1 sequence [14].
3. Joint effusion. Hyperintense on fluid-sensitive sequences and hypointense on T1 sequence. Absence of enhancement. Rice bodies, which have a hypointense signal on fluid-sensitive sequences, may be seen within the effusion.
4. Thickened and inflamed synovium (synovitis): hypointense on T1 sequence, hyperintense on fluid-sensitive sequence, and early enhancement, which differentiates it from adjacent effusion [9].
5. Cartilage – decreased thickness and irregularity.

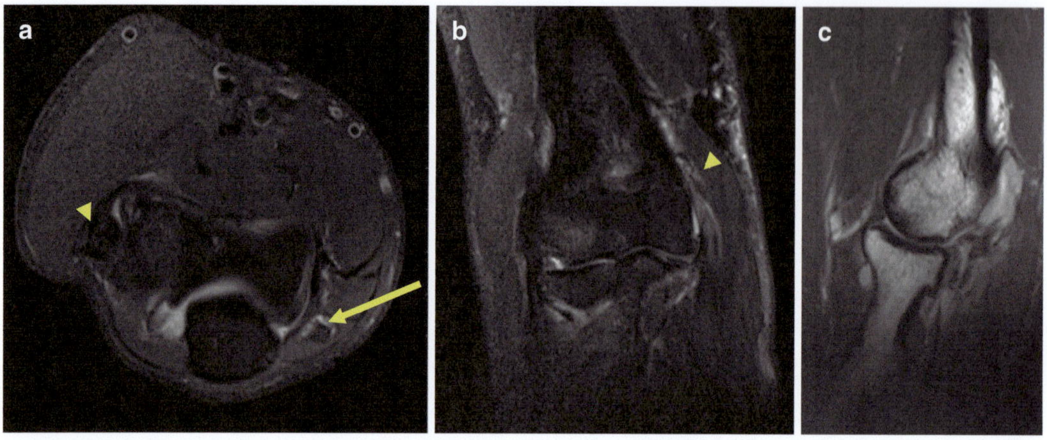

Fig. 4.3 A 51-year-old male with psoriatic arthritis. (**a**) Axial PD fat-saturated (FS) weighted MR image shows thickening and edema of the common extensor (arrow) and flexor tendons (arrow head) and the adjacent soft tissues. (**b**) Coronal T2 FS-weighted MR image demonstrates enthesitis of the common flexor tendon (arrow head). (**c**) Sagittal PD-weighted MR image shows bone erosion, subchondral sclerosis, a joint effusion, and synovitis

6. Olecranon bursitis: Bursal fluid appears hypointense on T1 and hyperintense on fluid-sensitive sequences.

Psoriatic Arthritis

Another inflammatory condition that affects the elbow is psoriatic arthritis. Its prevalence is between 2% and 3% [15]. It occurs equally in men and women and is more common in Caucasians [15]. Enthesitis is the hallmark of psoriatic arthritis. Some studies suggest that it is the initial site of inflammation that may ultimately lead to marginal bone erosions [16]. Elbow enthesitis was described as the sixth most common site of enthesopathy in patients with psoriatic arthritis after the Achilles tendon, plantar fascia, patellar tendon, quadriceps tendon, and great trochanter [15]. It mainly involves the olecranon process and the bicipital insertion of the proximal radius.

Similar to RA, radiographic evaluation should begin with radiographs which may show ossific enthesopathy, periostitis, bone proliferation, and joint subluxation. Further workup with MR imaging is helpful to detect early stages of the disease and help differentiate between active inflammation and chronic abnormalities when contrast is used.

Findings on MRI may include (Fig. 4.3):

1. Enthesitis which can have different imaging manifestations:
   (a) Soft tissue swelling of the entheseal area (hyperintense signal on fluid-sensitive sequences)
   (b) Increased bursal fluid adjacent to ligament/tendon insertions
   (c) Hyperintense signal on fluid-sensitive sequences at the insertions of ligaments and tendons [9]
   (d) Bone marrow edema at the tendon/ligament insertion site
2. Periostitis: Smooth or irregular cortical bone thickening
3. Synovitis which appears indistinguishable from that of rheumatoid arthritis: hypointense on T1 sequence, hyperintense on fluid-sensitive sequence, and early enhancement, which differentiates it from adjacent effusion [9]
4. Bone erosions: Hypointense T1 signal at the site of erosions

Gout Arthropathy

Gout arthropathy is a crystalline arthropathy caused by monosodium urate crystal deposition in joints. The prevalence of gout ranges from 1% to 4% [17]. It is generally more common in men, the

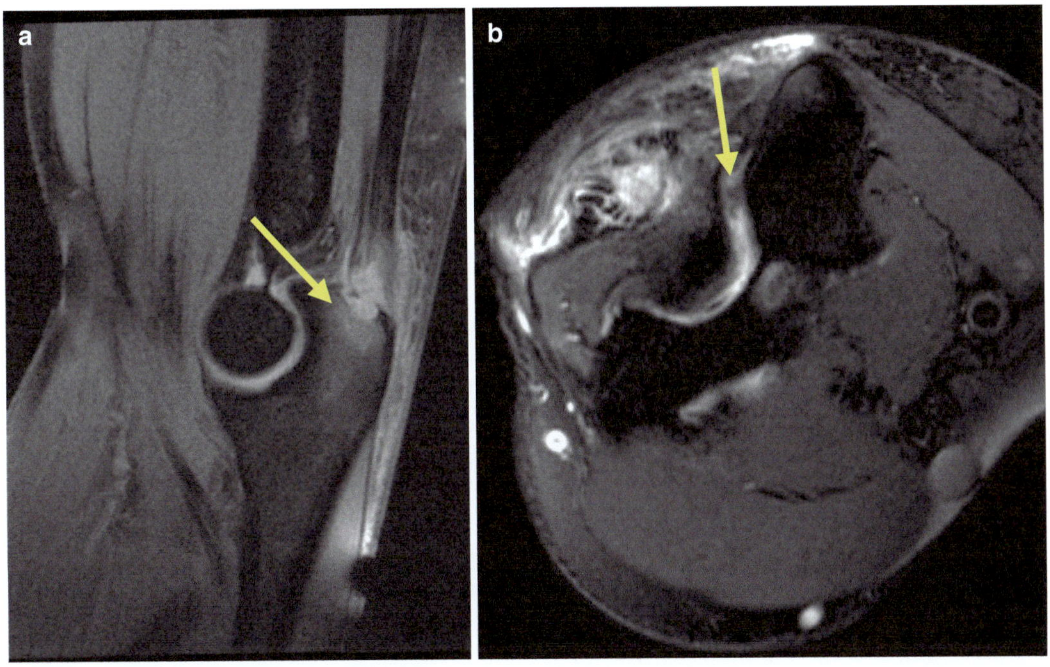

Fig. 4.4 A 59-year-old male with gout arthropathy. (**a**) Sagittal PD FS-weighted MR image shows an olecranon bone erosion (arrow) with underlying bone marrow edema. (**b**) Axial T2 FS-weighted MR image demonstrates joint effusion with synovial thickening (arrow) as well as triceps tendinopathy with surrounding soft tissue edema

elderly, and patients from Oceanian islands [17]. However, studies have shown that the incidence of gout in postmenopausal women and women above the age of 60 becomes similar to that of men [18]. Patients usually present with intermittent acute episodes of inflammation. Elbow involvement occurs in 30% of patients with gout, and the main presenting symptom is olecranon bursitis [19]. When a patient presents with bilateral olecranon bursitis, gout is favored to be the culprit over an infectious process or trauma [19].

The radiographic evidence of gout is usually delayed and manifests 6–8 years after initial attack [19]. Radiographic findings depend on the location of the urate crystal deposition. If it deposits in the soft tissues, tophi develop and are described as hyperdense soft tissue masses. The most classical radiographic presentation of gout is punched out juxta-articular erosions with sclerotic margins, overhanging edges, and preserved joint spaces [19].

Additional workup with MRI may be performed to evaluate gout at unusual locations and if other modalities are equivocal [20]. It can also be utilized to exclude osteomyelitis and septic arthritis. MRI has a better sensitivity than radiographs to identify erosions and detect early changes such as bone marrow edema and synovitis [20]. Findings seen with elbow gout arthropathy include (Fig. 4.4):

1. Olecranon bursitis: Hyperintense fluid collection on fluid-sensitive sequences over the extensor surface of the elbow
2. Chronic gouty tophi are a mixture of crystals, hemosiderin, protein, and fibrous tissue: Varying signal intensities on MR but are usually low signal on T1 sequence, low- intermediate signal on fluid-sensitive sequences and demonstrate homogeneous intense enhancement
3. Bone erosions: Juxta-articular, eccentrically located bone erosions
4. Thickened and inflamed synovium (synovitis): hypointense on T1 sequence, hyperintense on fluid-sensitive sequence, positive early enhancement, which differentiates it from adjacent effusion

Calcium Pyrophosphate Deposition Disease

Calcium pyrophosphate deposition disease (CPPD) is another crystal arthropathy that is characterized by deposition of pyrophosphate crystals into tendons, ligaments, cartilage, and synovium [21]. It is estimated that CPPD affects 4–7% of the adult population in Europe and the United States and predominately occurs in older individuals [22]. It can be idiopathic or of metabolic, hereditary, or posttraumatic etiology [23].

Clinical presentation of CPPD ranges from asymptomatic joint disease to pseudogout syndrome which is defined as CPPD with synovitis. Chondrocalcinosis is a nonspecific feature of some CPPD cases and is best depicted on radiographs and CT. Chondrocalcinosis is the deposition of CPPD crystals into fibrous and/or hyaline cartilage, with or without arthropathy. The imaging findings of CPPD arthropathy are similar to osteoarthritis. However, CPPD typically involves non-weight-bearing joints like the elbow and shoulder, whereas osteoarthrosis usually involves the weight-bearing joints like the knees and hips.

Advanced imaging with MRI may be useful to detect CPPD disease in some cases but remains insensitive to tissue calcification which is more common in CPPD when compared to other arthropathies [19]. MRI findings include (Fig. 4.5):

1. Chondrocalcinosis may not be conspicuous on MR and its signal is variable: hypointense or hyperintense on T1 sequences and fluid-sensitive sequences.
2. Productive arthropathy characterized by osteophytes, subchondral sclerosis, subchondral cyst formation, and subchondral edema.

Hydroxyapatite Crystal Deposition Disease

Hydroxyapatite crystal deposition disease (HADD) is a self-limited condition also known as calcific tendinosis. Women are more often affected than men with a peak incidence in the fourth through sixth decade of life [24]. Other groups affected include those routinely raising

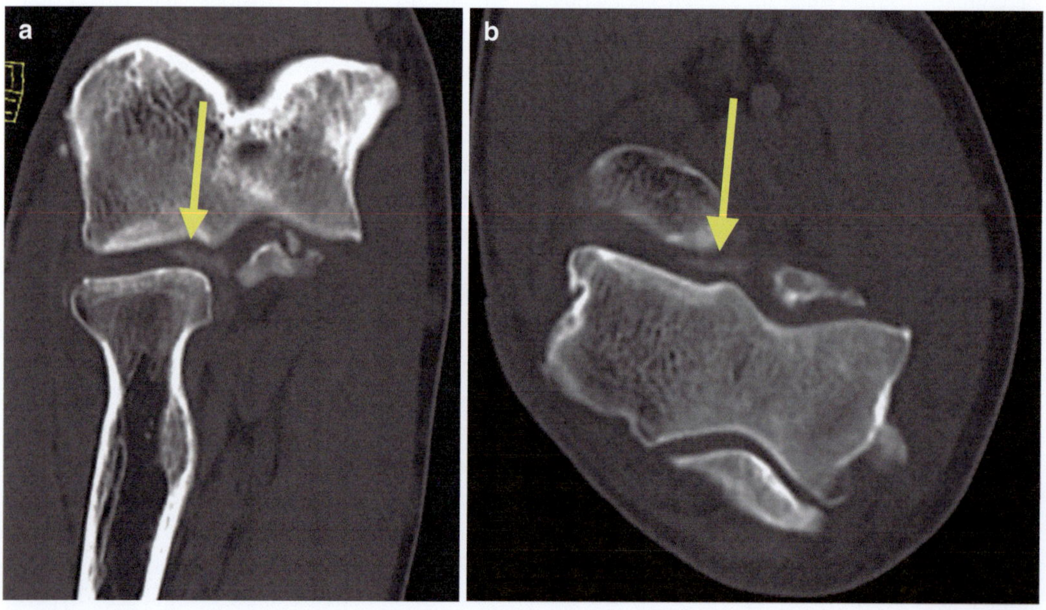

Fig. 4.5 A 69-year-old male with CPPD. (**a**) Coronal and (**b**) axial CT images show chondrocalcinosis within the radiocapitellar joint (arrow)

their arms up and down whether during sport or work. HADD causes periarticular disease in the form of tendinitis or bursitis and rarely causes true articular disease [19]. It can affect any joint but is most common in the shoulder followed by the hip and elbow. Elbow HADD mainly involves the medial epicondyle, lateral epicondyle, and olecranon process [25].

Uhthoff and Sarkar broadly classified HADD into the formative and resorptive phases [26]. During the formative phase where the fibrocartilage is replaced with calcific deposits, patients are usually asymptomatic. However, during the resorptive phase, the calcific deposits can rupture to nearby tissue and result in acute inflammation which manifests as acute joint pain.

Imaging evaluation of HADD ideally begins with radiography because of its high sensitivity to detect calcifications [25]. Further workup with MRI is not necessarily needed but can be advantageous when detecting the pattern of crystal deposit migration during the resorptive phase. MRI is also helpful in evaluating the inflammatory response triggered by HADD in the resorptive phase. Some of the MRI findings include (Fig. 4.6):

1. Periarticular calcium hydroxyapatite depositions: hypointense on all pulse sequences, which can make it difficult to identify without correlative radiographs. The crystal deposits do not enhance.
2. Local inflammatory changes: bursal fluid, soft tissue edema, or bone marrow edema around the deposit(s).

Hemophilia

Hemophilia is a congenital disease characterized by deficit or absence of clotting factors [27]. One of its major complications if not treated correctly is hemophilic arthropathy [28]. The most common joint involved is the knee, followed by the elbow and the ankle [29]. Around 80–90% of patients with hemophilia without primary prophylaxis treatment present elbow arthropathy [27].

The arthropathy is a result of repeated intra-articular hemorrhage that leads to synovial hypertrophy and inflammation which in turn is prone to more bleeding [30]. Patients usually present with elbow pain, limited range of motion, and decreased muscle strength. Extension is the first movement of the elbow joint affected [27].

Early osteochondral damage secondary to small intra-articular bleeds may be subclinical and undetectable on physical exam [31]. Diagnostic imaging is helpful in diagnosis of subclinical arthropathy which may impact prophylactic treatment [31]. A radiograph is only effective in assessment of late arthropathy [28]. The most commonly observed radiographic signs are enlargement of the epiphysis and osteoporosis. Less commonly observed findings include soft tissue swelling, enlargement of the radial head, and joint space irregularity with narrowing. MR imaging is more sensitive for evaluation of hemophilic arthropathy and detection of early changes [28]. Some findings seen on MR imaging include (Fig. 4.7):

1. Effusion/hemarthrosis: heterogeneous on T1 and fluid-sensitive sequences due to blood products at different stages
2. Synovial hypertrophy and inflammation: hypointense on T1 sequence, hyperintense on fluid-sensitive sequence, and early enhancement
3. Hemosiderin deposits along the synovium: hypointense on T1 and fluid-sensitive sequences. Susceptibility or “blooming” artifact on gradient-echo sequence
4. Cartilage loss
5. Subchondral erosions and cysts
6. Hemophilic soft tissue pseudotumor is progressive cystic swelling of muscle due to repeated bleeding:
    (a) Soft tissue mass is heterogeneous on T1 and fluid-sensitive sequences due to blood products of various ages
    (b) Hemosiderin nodular deposits along capsule of lesion (low signal on all sequences, blooms on gradient-echo sequences)
    (c) Possible scalloping of adjacent bone

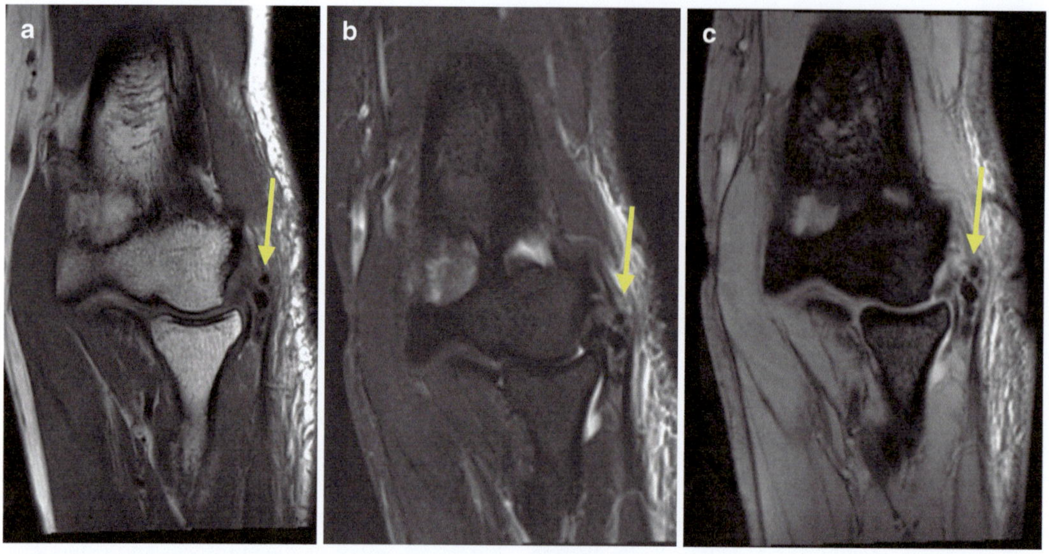

Fig. 4.6 A 33-year-old female with hydroxyapatite crystal deposition arthropathy. Images show multiple calcifications (arrows) along the proximal fibers of the common extensor tendon that appear hypointense on T1-weighted MR image (**a**) and hypointense on STIR MR image (**b**) and that demonstrate blooming artifact on susceptibility weighted MR image (**c**)

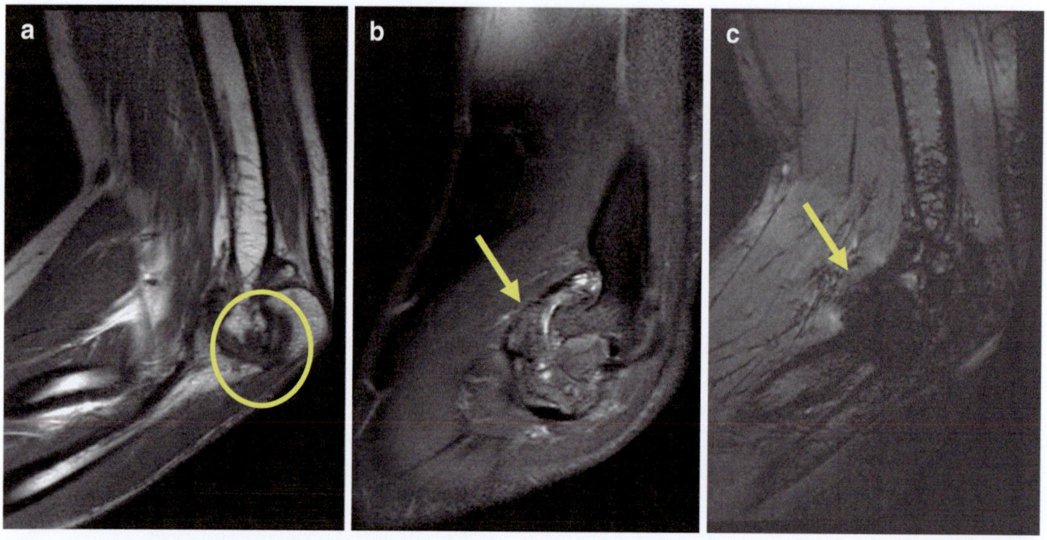

Fig. 4.7 A 20-year-old male with hemophilic arthropathy. (**a**) Sagittal T1-weighted MR image shows severe elbow joint space narrowing and extensive bone erosions (circle). (**b**) Sagittal T2 FS-weighted MR image demonstrates severe joint space narrowing, bone marrow edema of the distal humerus, and proximal ulna (arrow). (**c**) Marked blooming artifact is seen in the gradient-echo MR sequence around the elbow consistent with hemosiderin deposition (arrow)

Diffuse Idiopathic Skeletal Hyperostosis

Diffuse idiopathic skeletal hyperostosis (DISH) is a common condition characterized by ossification of the spinal and extraspinal entheses [32]. Elbow hyperostosis is seen in 49% of patients with extraspinal DISH with the olecranon being the most common site involved [19]. The prevalence of elbow hyperostosis is higher in patients with spinal DISH and in patients with shoulder DISH, illustrating the multifocal nature of the disease [33].

Clinically, patients usually present with pain and limited range of motion secondary to the ossifications [19]. Radiographically, hyperostotic spurs are present at the interface of strong muscles and bone, like triceps/olecranon, common extensors/lateral epicondyle, and common flexors/medial epicondyle [34]. It is important to remember that DISH is not an arthropathy and could be differentiated from osteoarthritis by lack of joint and articular involvement. Further evaluation with MRI is rarely necessary but findings include:

1. Ossific spurs: T1 hypointense in early stages and T1 hyperintense when the ossification gets bigger, hypointense on fluid-sensitive sequences unless large enough, minimal enhancement in absence of fractures
2. Normal joint space
3. Normal cartilage

Tumor

Osteochondroma

Osteochondroma is one of the most common benign bone tumors, accounting for 34.9% of all benign bone tumors, but they are rare around the elbow [35]. It is a cartilaginous neoplasm that occurs in the proximal metaphysis of long bones and grows away from the nearby joint [36]. Osteochondromas can be classified as either solitary or multiple where they can occur spontaneously or in an autosomal dominant disorder known as hereditary multiple exostoses (HME) [35].

Patients with osteochondromas located between the ulna and radius in the elbow usually do not have early symptoms, but as the tumor progresses, symptoms including pain, limited mobility, and skeletal deformities develop [36]. Radial head dislocation has been described in the pediatric HME population when the tumor involves the metaphysis of the ulna causing shortening of the ulna in comparison to the radius during growth. This leads to radial bowing and subsequent radial head dislocation [36].

Similar to other bone tumors, initial workup of osteochondromas begins with radiographs which may show a sessile or pedunculated lesion in the metaphyseal region typically projecting away from the joint. The lesion is usually composed of a stalk, marrow, and cortex, all continuous with normal underlying bone. As for the hyaline cartilage cap that is associated with osteochondromas, it is not always visualized with radiographs, but when it is, it appears as a rim of endochondral calcifications. MR is the best imaging modality to evaluate the cartilaginous cap, assess for malignant transformation of the tumor, and detect adjacent bone marrow and soft tissue edema. Findings on MR imaging include (Fig. 4.8):

1. A cartilage cap: Intermediate to hypointense on T1-weighted sequence, hyperintense on fluid-sensitive sequences, non-enhancing on post-contrast imaging. The cartilage cap thickness should not measure over 1.5 cm in thickness [37]. A thick (more than 1.5 cm) and/or enhancing cartilage cap is worrisome for malignant transformation.
2. Normal medullary bone extending into the exostoses with cortex continuous with parent bone.
3. Bone marrow and soft tissue edema may represent mechanical changes from impingement or trauma.

Fibrous Dysplasia

Fibrous dysplasia is a benign tumor-like bone lesion where normal bone is replaced with immature disorganized bone and a dense fibrotic stroma [12]. It is a rare disease accounting for 5–7% of all benign bone tumors; however, it is the most common benign bone tumor of the elbow constituting 20% of all benign elbow bone lesions [38]. Fibrous dysplasia usually presents in young adults.

Patients with fibrous dysplasia are usually asymptomatic, but if they are symptomatic, they present with pain which may be due to a pathologi-

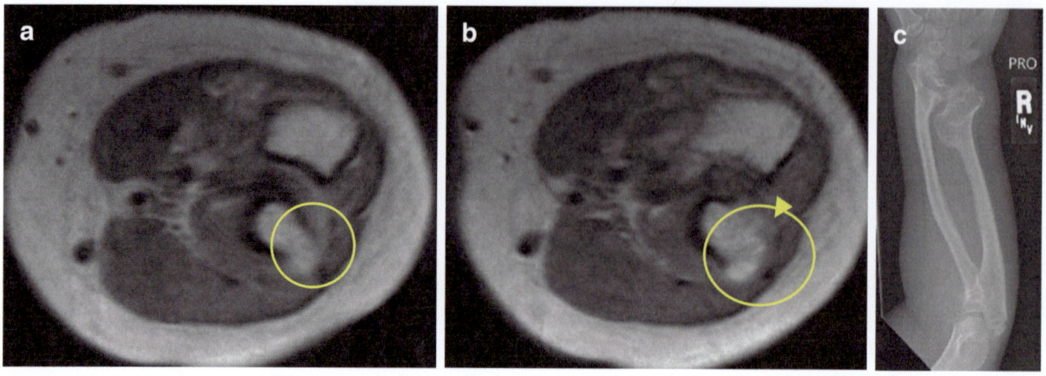

Fig. 4.8 A 21-year-old male with known osteochondromas of the forearm. (**a, b**) Axial PD-weighted MR images show a bone exostosis with medullary bone continuity arising from the proximal radius (arrow) and a thin cartilaginous cap (arrowhead). (**c**) Plain radiograph of the forearm shows multiple proximal and distal ulnar and radial osteochondromas with bone remodeling distally

cal fracture or with a bowing deformity [38]. Radiographically, fibrous dysplasia has a characteristic appearance of a lucent bone lesion with ground glass internal matrix and a thick sclerotic border [12]. MR imaging has a limited role in differentiating fibrous dysplasia from other bone lesions but may be useful in assessing for malignant transformation to osteosarcoma, fibrosarcoma, or chondrosarcoma. Findings of fibrous dysplasia described on MR imaging include (Fig. 4.9):

1. Solid lesion showing heterogeneity in different parts of the lesion: heterogeneous intermediate signal on T1 sequence, heterogeneous signal on fluid-sensitive sequences, heterogeneous contrast enhancement on post-contrast imaging. Active portions of the lesion avidly enhance, while inactive portions mildly enhance.
2. Bone lesion that results in expansion of the medullary cavity and thinning of the overlying cortex.
3. Aneurysmal bone cyst may be associated with the lesion: fluid-fluid level on fluid-sensitive sequences.

Enchondroma

Enchondroma is a common benign cartilaginous bone tumor that compromises around 7.7% of all bone tumors [39]. Peak incidence of enchondroma is childhood to early adulthood and most commonly arises in the small bones of the hand and in major long bones such as the femur, proximal humerus, and tibia [40]. Enchondromas around the elbow are rare.

Patients are typically asymptomatic unless there is a superimposed pathologic fracture. New pain at the site of known enchondroma may indicate malignant transformation, which is rare [41]. Radiographically, enchondromas most commonly appear as central metaphyseal lesions with intralesional "rings and arcs" calcifications and without a sclerotic border. Additional evaluation with MR imaging may be useful to assess for soft tissue extension and to confirm the diagnosis [39]. Of note, MR imaging plays a limited role in differentiating enchondromas from low-grade chondrosarcomas due to overlap in their radiological features. Findings associated with enchondromas include:

1. Lobulated lesion: Intermediate to low signal on T1 sequence, high signal on fluid-sensitive sequences (consistent with hyaline cartilage); peripheral or septal enhancement on post-contrast imaging.
2. Endosteal scalloping: Scalloping >2/3 cortical thickness or >2/3 length of central lesion should raise concern for transformation to chondrosarcoma [41].

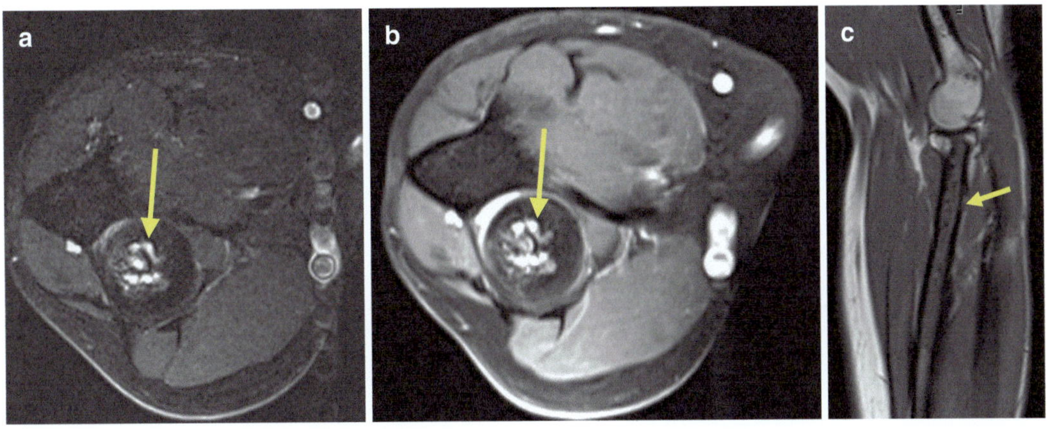

Fig. 4.9 A 34-year-old female with fibrous dysplasia. (**a**) Axial STIR-weighted MR image shows a heterogeneous predominantly STIR hyperintense lesion (arrow) in the radial head. (**b**) Axial T1 FS post-contrast weighted MR image demonstrates heterogeneous enhancement of the lesion with multiple areas of avid enhancement (arrow). (**c**) Sagittal T1-weighted image shows the extent of the T1 hypointense lesion spanning from the proximal radial head to the mid-radial diaphysis resulting in expansion of the medullary cavity (arrow)

Synovial Chondromatosis

Synovial chondromatosis is a benign proliferative condition of the synovial membrane which results in the formation of cartilaginous or osseous bodies within a joint or bursa [42]. It most commonly occurs in the posttraumatic setting and between the fourth and fifth decades of life. Men are more often affected than women [9]. The most common location is the knee followed by the elbow, hip, and shoulder [9].

Patients typically present with progressive loss of range of motion, pain, swelling, joint snapping, and locking [42]. Radiographically, the appearance of synovial chondromatosis depends on the degree of ossification of the cartilaginous bodies. However, in its most distinctive appearance, multiple small, calcific joint bodies of uniform size are present. If the cartilaginous bodies are not calcified, definitive diagnosis may require MR imaging [42]. Findings of elbow synovial chondromatosis seen on MR imaging include (Fig. 4.10):

1. Multiple uniformly sized loose bodies with different degrees of calcification are most commonly seen in one of the three locations in the elbow including the coronoid fossa, olecranon fossa, and annular recess [9]. The noncalcified portions of the cartilaginous bodies are intermediate to hypointense on T1 sequence and hyperintense on fluid-sensitive sequences. Areas of mineralization within the bodies are depicted as signal voids with blooming artifact on gradient-echo imaging.
2. Synovial thickening: Hypointense on fluid-sensitive sequences, enhances on post-contrast imaging, typically blooms on gradient-echo imaging.
3. Adjacent bone erosions are common.
4. Joint effusion. Hyperintense on fluid-sensitive sequences; hypointense on T1 sequence.

Intra-articular Tenosynovial Giant Cell Tumor

Intra-articular tenosynovial giant cell tumor (ITGCT), formerly known as pigmented villonodular synovitis, is a rare benign proliferative and hemorrhagic synovial disorder [43]. The disease presents in either a localized or diffuse form. ITGCT prefers large joints such as the knee and hip and less commonly occur in the ankle, shoulder, and elbow [9]. It usually affects adults in their third and fourth decades of life without gender predilection [43].

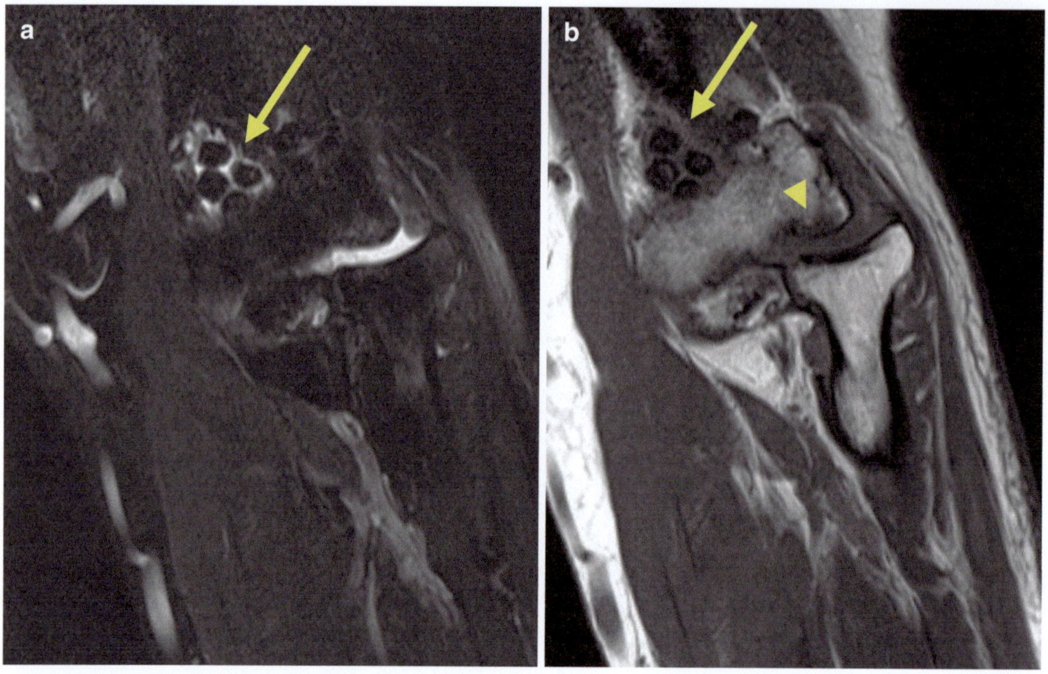

Fig. 4.10 A 47-year-old male with synovial chondromatosis. Coronal T2 FS- (**a**) and T1 (**b**)-weighted MR images show multiple T2 FS and T1 hypointense ossified loose bodies within the joint space, predominantly within the coronoid fossa (arrows). Bone erosions are also noted (arrow head)

Patients with ITGCT typically present with pain, stiffness, and recurrent effusions of the joint [43]. On radiographs, ITGCT can manifest as a large joint effusion without fracture, bone erosion due to direct pressure, or even bone invasion [44, 45]. Additional workup with MR imaging is useful to depict abnormalities of the joint and evaluate the extent of disease [45]. MR imaging findings of ITGCT include (Fig. 4.11):

1. Synovial-based masses: Low to intermediate signal on T1 sequence, low signal on fluid-sensitive sequences, blooming artifact on gradient-echo images, homogeneous or peripheral synovial enhancement on post-contrast imaging
2. Joint effusion. Hyperintense on fluid-sensitive sequences, hypointense on T1 sequence
3. Bone erosions

Osteosarcoma

Osteosarcoma is the second most common primary malignant bone tumor in adults with peak incidence in the second decade of life [46]. Its most common histologic subtype is conventional osteosarcoma representing 80% of all cases [47]. Elbow osteosarcoma is not as frequent as in the distal femur, proximal tibia, and proximal humerus [38].

Clinical presentation of elbow osteosarcoma is insidious with the most common presenting symptom being pain, worse with movement and swelling [38]. Initial workup with radiographs typically shows an aggressive mixed lytic/sclerotic metaphyseal lesion with reactive periosteal new bone formation and cortical bone erosion [46]. Additional workup with MR imaging is necessary to evaluate for local invasion into the adjacent soft tissues, level of bone marrow replacement, skip lesions, and extension into the joints and growth plate [47]. Findings of conventional elbow osteosarcoma on MR image include:

1. Heterogeneous lesion where ossified portions of the lesion appear hypointense on all sequences and non-ossified portions are hypointense on T1-weighted sequences and

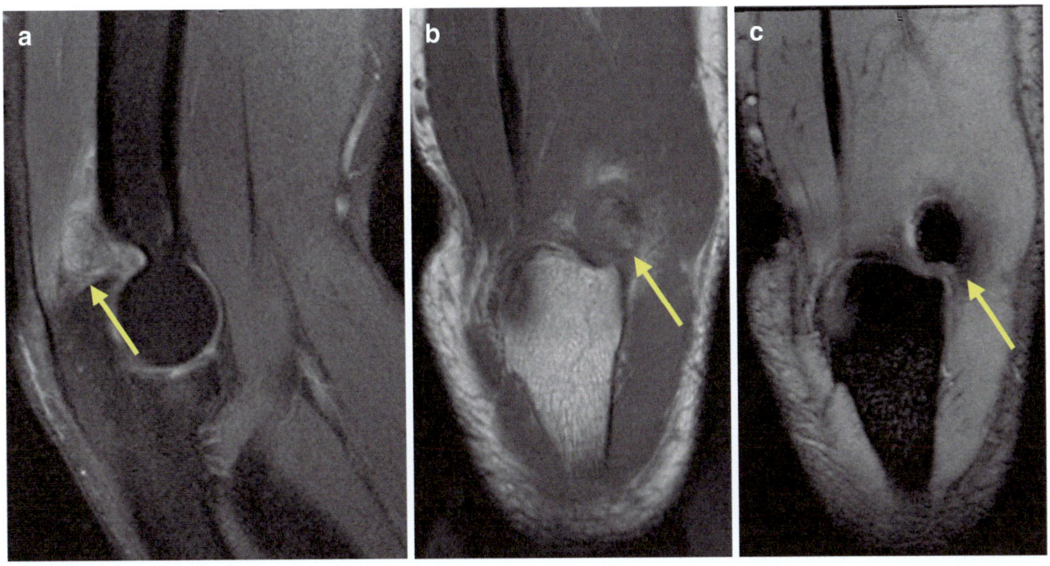

Fig. 4.11 A 23-year-old male with localized intra-articular tenosynovial giant cell tumor. Coronal and sagittal MR images show a heterogeneous T2 mildly hyperintense (**a**) and T1 isointense (**b**) rounded lesion in the posterior fat pad (arrows) that demonstrates blooming artifact on susceptibility weighted imaging (**c**)

hyperintense on fluid-sensitive sequences. Non-necrotic portions of the mass enhance on post-contrast imaging.

2. Associated soft tissue mass appears hyperintense on fluid-sensitive sequences.
3. Peritumoral edema in the bone and soft tissue.

Ewing Sarcoma

Ewing sarcoma is a malignant round cell tumor, typically arising from the metadiaphysis of long bones or less commonly from flat bones [48]. Ewing sarcoma can also arise from the soft tissues immediately adjacent to the bone. It is the second most common primary bone tumor in children [49]. The majority of Ewing's sarcomas of the bone are located in the lower extremities and pelvic girdle but rarely arise from the elbow [38, 50].

Patients with elbow Ewing sarcoma generally present with severe local bone pain, palpable soft tissue mass, and/or systemic symptoms such as fever [38]. On radiographs, Ewing sarcoma appears as a moth-eaten destructive lucent lesion with a large noncalcified soft tissue component and aggressive periosteal bone formation [48]. Further workup with MR imaging is warranted to evaluate for the local extent of the tumor and its relation with the neurovascular bundle [48]. The findings of elbow Ewing sarcoma seen on MR imaging include (Fig. 4.12):

1. Bone tumor: Low to intermediate signal on T1-weighted sequence, homogenous low to intermediate signal on fluid-sensitive sequence, heterogeneous but avid enhancement on post-contrast imaging
2. Adjacent bone marrow and soft tissue edema

Chondrosarcoma

Chondrosarcoma is a malignant hyaline cartilage tumor that arises in the fourth or fifth decade of life. It is the third most common primary malignant bone tumor. It can be classified as primary (de novo) or secondary, arising from a preexisting cartilaginous lesions, such as enchondroma or osteochondroma [51]. Common locations of chondrosarcoma in descending order are the long bones, pelvis, ribs, and spine [51]. However, it rarely occurs in the elbow [38].

Patients with chondrosarcoma of the elbow usually present with elbow pain and swelling,

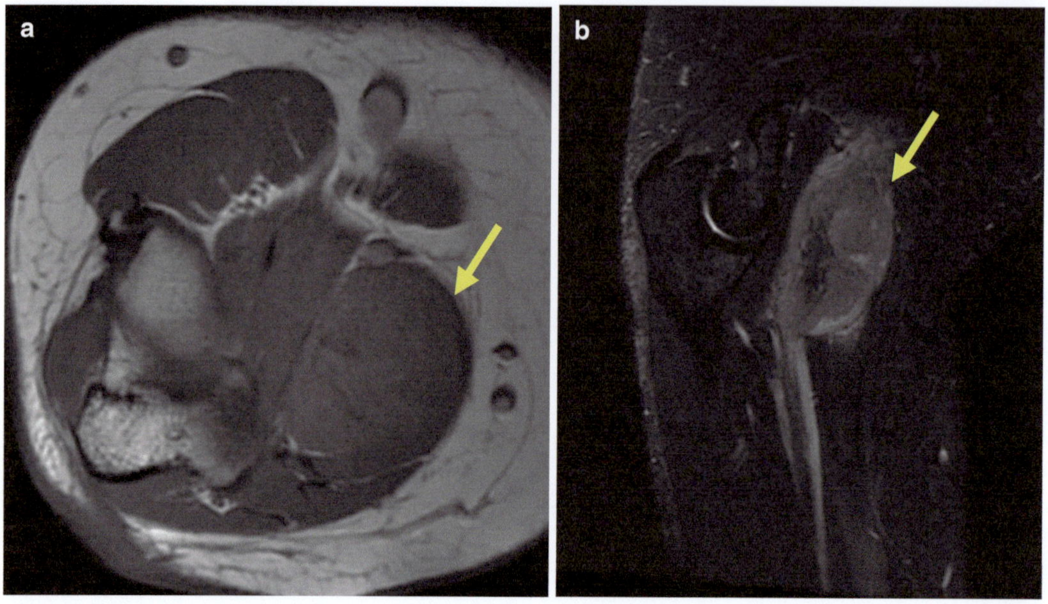

Fig. 4.12 A 20-year-old female with Ewing sarcoma. Axial and sagittal MR images show a T1 isointense (**a**) and heterogeneous T2 hyperintense (**b**) mass (arrows) in the anterior elbow soft tissues

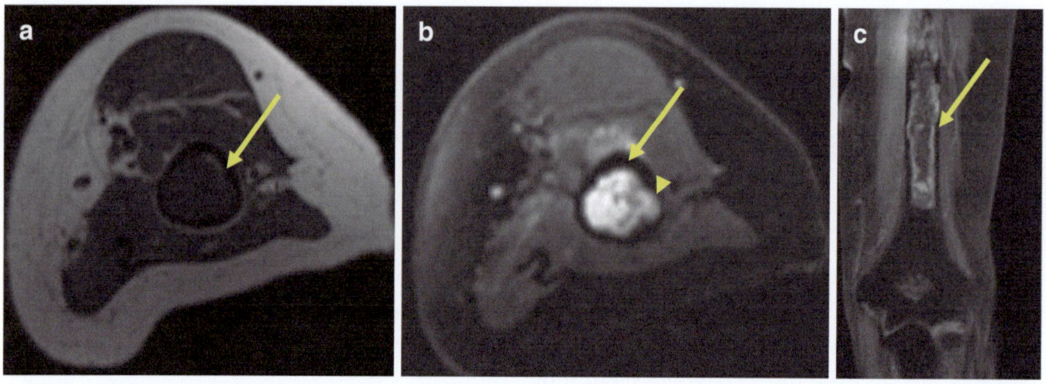

Fig. 4.13 A 57-year-old male with biopsy-proven chondrosarcoma of the distal humerus. Axial T1-weighted (**a**) and STIR (**b**) MR images show a lobulated T1 hypointense and STIR hyperintense lesion within the distal humeral diaphysis (arrows) resulting in endosteal scalloping (arrow head). The lesion demonstrates peripheral and septal enhancement (arrow) on coronal post-contrast T1-weighted image (**c**)

similar to many other malignant bone tumors. Radiographically, chondrosarcoma is demonstrated as an aggressive lytic lesion with internal "rings and arcs" calcifications (78% of cases) and endosteal scalloping [51]. Additional workup with MR imaging may be helpful to differentiate between low-grade and high-grade chondrosarcoma. It can also be useful to evaluate the extent of the intraosseous tumor. MR imaging features of chondrosarcoma include (Fig. 4.13):

1. Lobular bone lesion: Hypointense on T1 sequence with small areas of hyperintensity due to entrapped yellow marrow, hyperintense on fluid sequences with hypointense internal septa, septal and peripheral enhancement on post-contrast imaging:

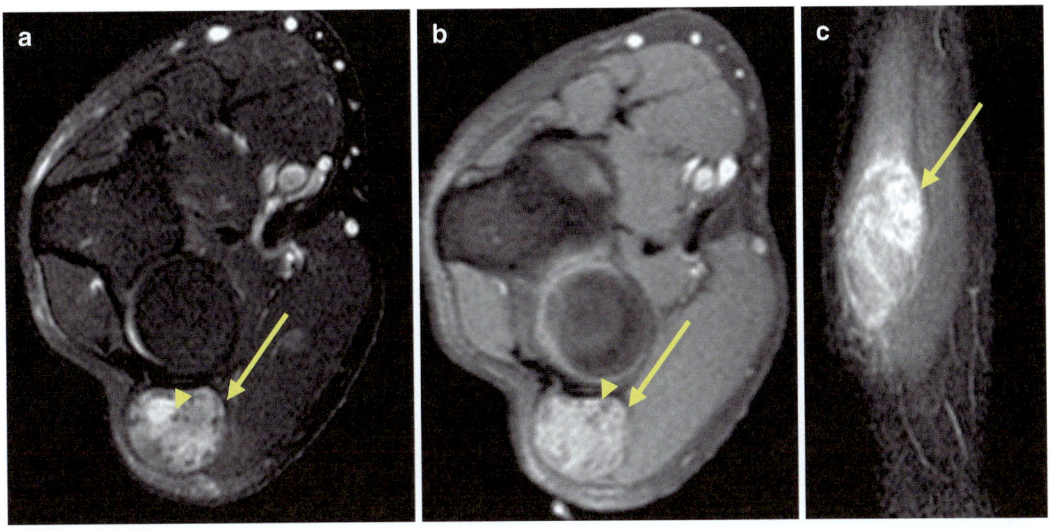

Fig. 4.14 A 33-year-old female with biopsy-proven synovial sarcoma. Axial T2 FS- (**a**) and T1-weighted (**b**) images of the proximal forearm demonstrates a heterogeneous T1 isointense and T2 FS hyperintense circumscribed mass (arrows) in the anterior proximal forearm with multiple internal calcifications (arrow head) and cystic changes consistent with the "triple sign." (**c**) Sagittal post-contrast T1-weighted image shows heterogeneous mass enhancement (arrow)

   (a) Internal mineralization: Signal void on T1 sequence and heterogeneous hypointense signal on fluid-sensitive sequences.
   (b) Low grade vs high grade: Entrapped fat within the lesion suggests low grade. Soft tissue extension suggests high grade [51].
2. Endosteal scalloping, reactive cortical changes, and extraosseous extension are all clearly observed.
3. Perilesional marrow edema is uncommon.

Synovial Cell Sarcoma

Synovial cell sarcoma is a malignant soft tissue tumor which represents 3–14% of all malignant soft tissue neoplasms [52]. It is more common in males and usually occurs in young adults [52]. The popliteal fossa is the most common location for synovial sarcoma. Approximately 20% occur at or distal to the elbow, usually on the flexor surface of the forearm [52].

Clinically, patients with synovial cell sarcoma typically present with a palpable mass, pain, or tenderness [52]. Dystrophic calcifications are seen in 30% of tumors [53]. MR imaging is the best modality to evaluate the tumor and its local extension. Findings seen on MR imaging include (Fig. 4.14):

1. Large soft tissue mass: Heterogeneous isointense signal on T1 sequence, heterogeneous hyperintense signal on fluid-sensitive sequences, diffuse or heterogeneous enhancement on post-contrast imaging
2. "Triple sign": Combination of necrosis and cystic degeneration (hyperintense), viable tumor (less hyperintense), and fibrotic bands and calcification (hypointense)
3. "Bowls of grapes": Multiloculated appearance of the mass
4. Fluid-fluid level on fluid-sensitive sequences

Inflammatory and Infectious

Olecranon Bursitis

Olecranon bursitis is the most common superficial bursitis. Inflammation of the olecranon bursa results in a distended fluid-filled bursa in the subcutaneous soft tissues posterior to the olecranon

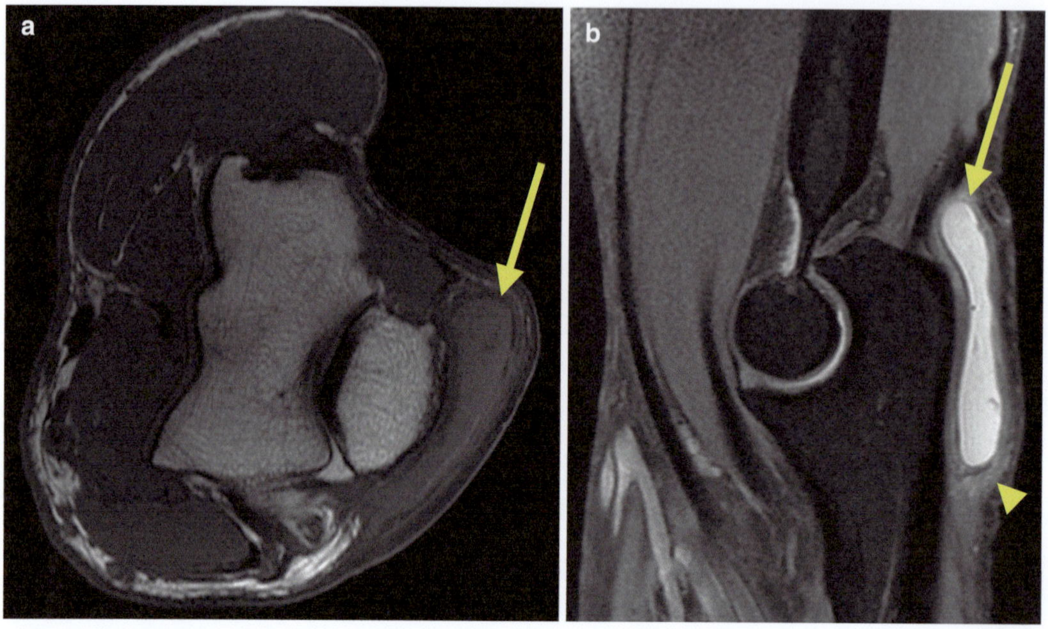

Fig. 4.15 A 47-year-old male with olecranon bursitis. Axial T1-weighted MR image (**a**) and T2 FS-weighted MR image (**b**) show moderate amount of T1 hypointense and T2 FS hyperintense olecranon bursal fluid collection (arrow). Mild subcutaneous edema is noted on axial T2 FS MR image (arrow head)

process [54]. Causes include overuse, repetitive trauma, inflammatory arthropathies like rheumatoid arthritis and gout, as well as prolonged sustained pressure against the elbow such as uremic patients undergoing dialysis [55].

Patients with olecranon bursitis usually present with posterior elbow pain and swelling without tenderness or redness [54]. Olecranon bursitis is a clinical diagnosis [55]. However, if radiographs are obtained, soft tissue swelling superficial to the olecranon is seen. MR imaging is reserved to evaluate for superimposed infection if clinically suspected [9].

Findings of olecranon bursitis on MR imaging are (Fig. 4.15):

1. Bursal fluid collection: Hypointense on T1 sequence, hyperintense on fluid-sensitive sequences, rim enhancement on post-contrast imaging. More complex fluid may be present with hemorrhage, infection, or gout.
2. Subcutaneous edema may be seen.
3. Joint effusion. Hyperintense on fluid-sensitive sequences and hypointense on T1 sequence.

Bicipitoradial Bursitis

Bicipitoradial bursitis is inflammation of the bicipitoradial bursa whose main role is to reduce friction between the biceps tendon and the radial tuberosity [56]. It is most commonly caused by chronic mechanical friction, low-grade infections such as tuberculosis, and inflammatory arthropathies such as rheumatoid arthritis [56].

Clinically, patients present with a mass or swelling at the antecubital fossa associated with pain and limited range of motion [57]. Most radiographs will show no abnormality in most cases [57]. Hence, the role of MR imaging in evaluation of bicipitoradial bursitis would reveal (Fig. 4.16):

1. Bicipitoradial bursa which is only visualized when distended either with fluid or synovial proliferation [57]: hypointense on T1 sequence, hyperintense on fluid-sensitive sequences, and rim enhancement on post-contrast imaging
2. Associated bicipital insertional tendinosis and tear
3. Bone marrow edema or erosion at the radial tuberosity

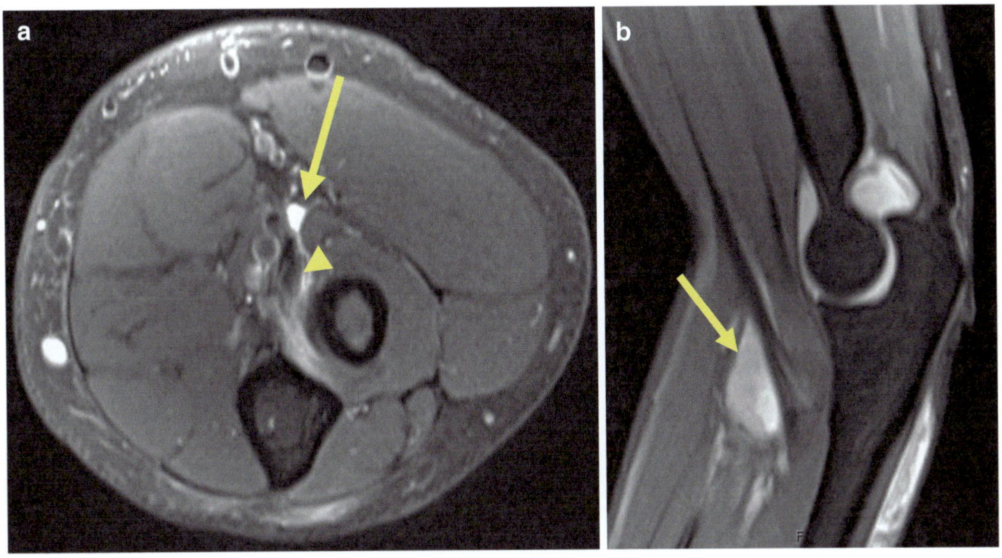

Fig. 4.16 A 42-year-old female with bicipitoradial bursitis. Axial (**a**) and sagittal (**b**) PD FS-weighted MR images show moderate amount of fluid within the bicipitoradial bursa (arrow). Insertional biceps tendinosis is seen on axial PD FS-weighted MR image (arrow head)

Septic Arthritis

Septic arthritis or infectious arthritis is an intra-articular infection which may lead to joint destruction. This common disease is mainly caused by the bacteria *Staphylococcus aureus* [9]. The elbow is involved in 6–9% of the cases [58].

Patients are usually immunocompromised or have a predisposing condition such as rheumatoid arthritis, diabetes, corticosteroid treatment, or intravenous drug abuse [9]. They usually present with pain, swelling, and decreased range of motion [9]. Early diagnosis of septic arthritis is crucial, because delay may result in increased morbidity and complications such as cartilage destruction and osteomyelitis [59].

On radiographs, the dominant finding of septic arthritis is a joint effusion. If left untreated, joint space narrowing and bone destruction may be seen. As for MR imaging, its main advantage is to evaluate for complications of septic arthritis such as osteomyelitis and soft tissue abscesses [9]. Findings of septic arthritis on MR imaging include (Fig. 4.17):

1. Joint effusion: hyperintense on fluid-sensitive sequences, hypointense on T1 sequence, shaggy rim enhancement on post-contrast imaging.
2. Synovitis is demonstrated by thickened synovium which appears T2 hyperintense and avidly enhancing on post-contrast imaging.
3. Cartilage destruction: irregular appearance of the cartilage with subchondral bone marrow edema.
4. Bone erosions.

Cat-Scratch Disease

Cat-scratch disease is a self-limited benign disease caused by *Bartonella henselae*, most commonly, as a result of a cat scratch [9]. In its most common form, it presents as epitrochlear lymphadenopathy in individuals between the ages of 5 and 21 years [60].

Patients initially present with a small skin lesion. After approximately 2 weeks, they start complaining of edema and tenderness related to regional lymphadenopathy [9]. Constitutional symptoms such as fever, anorexia, and myalgias are also common [60].

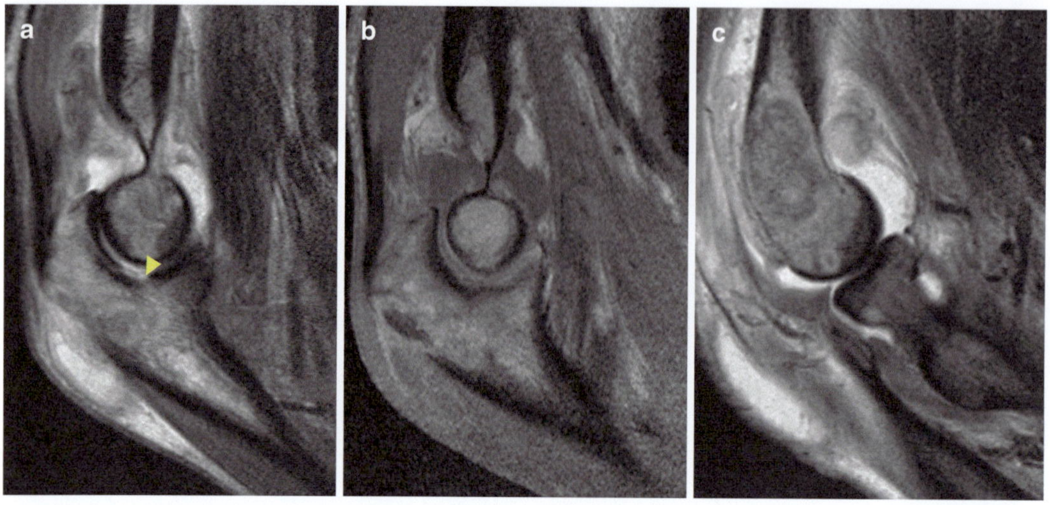

Fig. 4.17 A 63-year-old male with elbow septic arthritis. Sagittal PD FS-weighted (**a**), T1-weighted (**b**), and T1 FS post-contrast (**c**) MR images show a large PD FS hyperintense T1 hyperintense joint effusion with marked enhancement. Bone erosion involving the olecranon process is noted (arrow head)

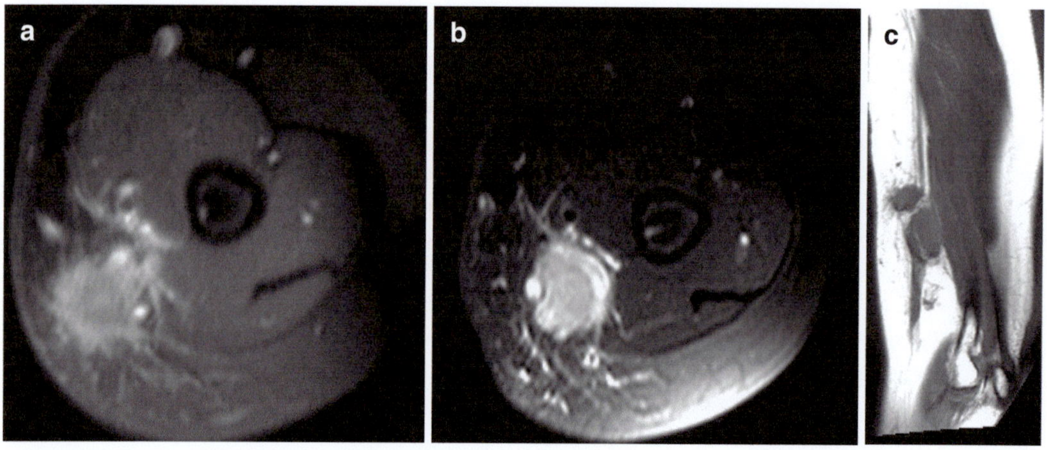

Fig. 4.18 An 18-year-old female with cat-scratch disease. Axial T1 FS post-contrast (**a**), axial STIR (**b**), and sagittal T1-weighted (**c**) MR images demonstrate findings consistent with epitrochlear lymphadenitis: There is an ovoid STIR hyperintense (**a**) and T1 isointense (**c**) enhancing (**a**) mass along the volar-medial aspect of the distal humeral metadiaphysis

Cat-scratch disease is a clinical diagnosis, making the role of imaging futile [60]. However, if radiographs are obtained, nonspecific soft tissue swelling corresponding to lymphadenopathy may be seen. On MR imaging, the classic findings of cat-scratch disease include (Fig. 4.18):

1. Enlarged epitrochlear/axillary lymph nodes with nonspecific nodular appearance: hyperintense on fluid-sensitive sequences, enhance on post-contrast imaging
2. Surrounding soft tissue edema

Congenital

Congenital Radial Head Dislocation

Congenital radial head dislocation is the most common congenital anomaly of the elbow; however, it is rare [61]. This presents as a posterior dislocation that can either be unilateral or more commonly bilateral [62]. It can occur in isolation or in association with a syndrome, gene mutation, or positive family history [62].

Clinical manifestations of congenital radial head dislocation are usually delayed and only present in late childhood when the patients present with limited range of motion, elbow pain, or deformity [61, 62]. Imaging workup initially includes radiographs and later possibly MR imaging. A set of diagnostic criteria has been proposed by McFarland that favors congenital head dislocation over posttraumatic ones. These findings can be seen on radiographs or MR imaging and include (Fig. 4.19) [62]:

1. Absent or hypoplastic capitellum
2. Prominent ulnar epicondyle
3. Dome-shaped radial head with elongated neck
4. Short ulna when compared to the radius (negative ulnar variance)

Congenital Radioulnar Synostosis

Congenital radioulnar synostosis is a rare malformation of the upper extremity that can be seen in association with syndromes and skeletal dysplasias but is also seen sporadically as an isolated finding [63]. This results from a failure of prenatal segmentation of the forearm bones and most commonly occurs at

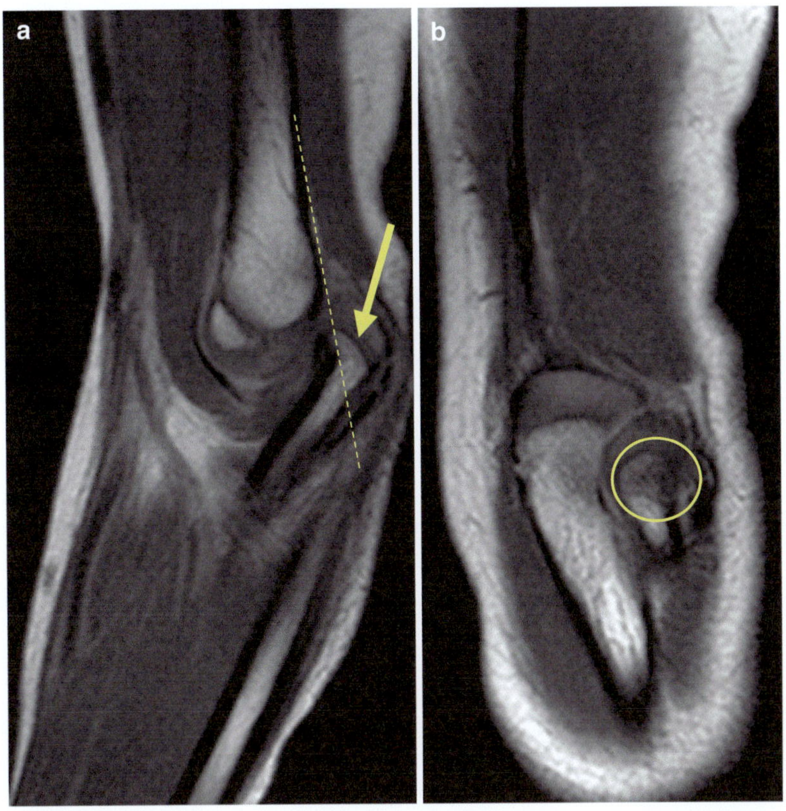

Fig. 4.19 An 8-year-old male with congenital radial head dislocation. T1-weighted sagittal (**a**) and coronal (**b**) MR images show a posteriorly dislocated (arrow) dome-shaped radial head with elongated neck (circle)

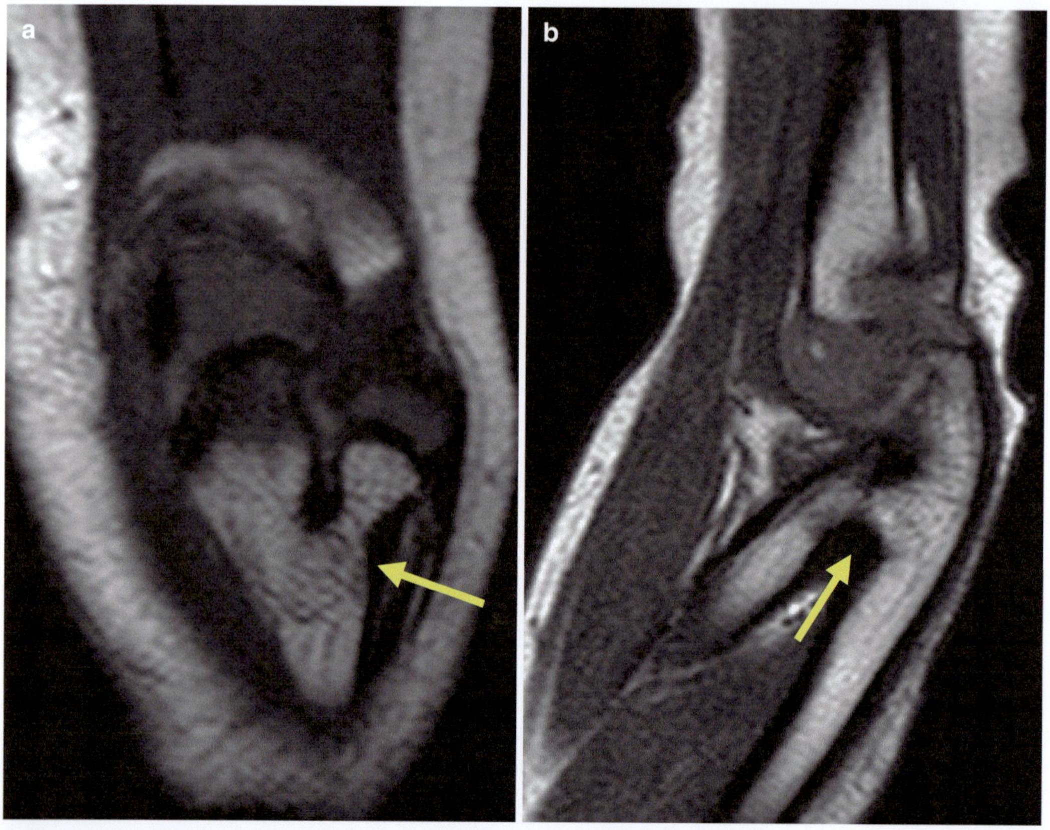

Fig. 4.20 A 6-year-old female with congenital radioulnar synostosis. T1-weighted coronal (**a**) and sagittal (**b**) MR images demonstrate fusion of the proximal radius and ulna (arrow)

the proximal portion of the forearm [64]. It is reported to be bilateral in 60–80% of patients [65].

Patients may be asymptomatic, present with cosmetic deformities, or have limited ability to pronate and supinate their forearms [64, 65]. Radiographs and advanced imaging will show (Fig. 4.20):

1. Fusion of the proximal radius to the ulna
2. Anterior bowing of the radius

Supracondylar Spur

Supracondylar spur is a congenital anatomic variant consisting of a beak-like bony projection arising from the anteromedial surface of the humerus, about 5 cm above the medial epicondyle [66, 67]. It is usually associated with the ligament of Struthers which is a fibrous structure that connects the spur to the medial epicondyle [67]. Supracondylar spurs occur in 0.4–2.7% of the population [67].

Patients are usually asymptomatic but may present with symptoms related to compression of the median nerve or brachial artery such as paresthesia, weakness, muscle atrophy, and ischemic pain. These compression symptoms are exacerbated with extension and pronation of the forearm [66, 68]. Typically, supracondylar spurs are incidentally discovered on radiographs [67]. They appear as bony projections arising from the anteromedial aspect of the humerus and pointing toward the elbow joint [67] (Fig. 4.21). Additional workup with MR imaging is useful to detect the ligament of Struthers and its anatomic relationship to the median nerve and brachial artery [68]. MR imaging is also helpful in detecting occult fracture of the spur.

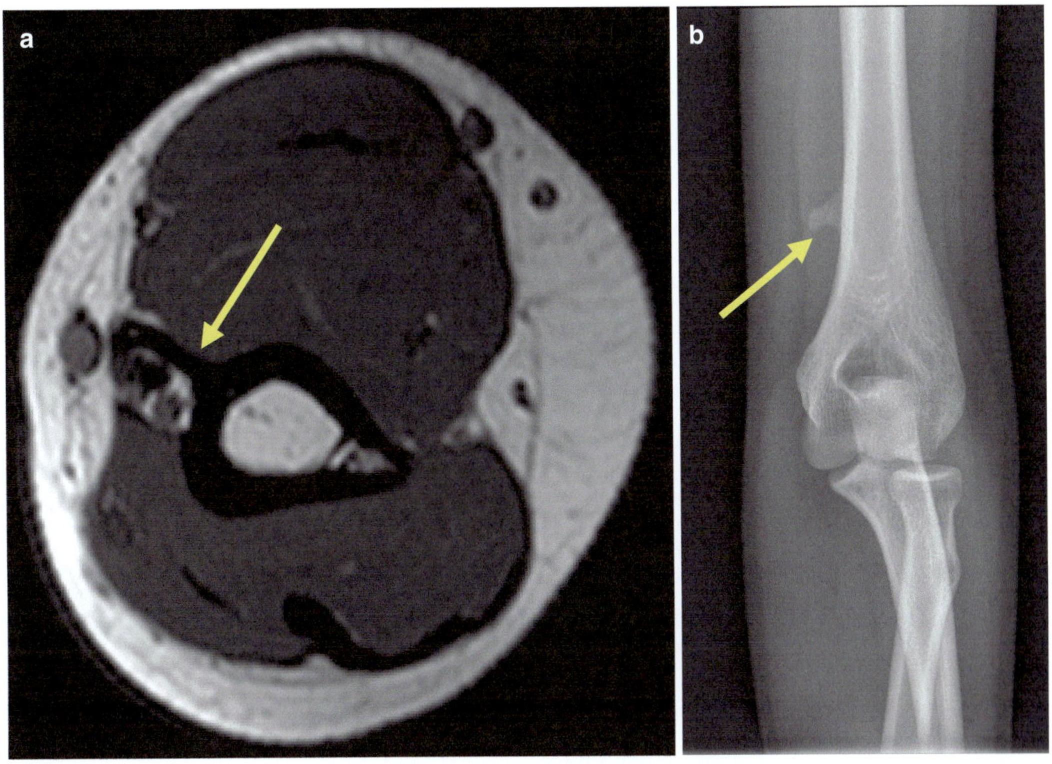

Fig. 4.21 An 11-year-old female with a supracondylar spur. Axial T1-weighted MR image (**a**) and AP plain radiograph of the elbow (**b**) show a supracondylar spur (arrow) arising from the anteromedial aspect of the distal humerus that follows normal bone signal

References

1. E. C. Huskisson, P A Dieppe, A. K. Tucker, AND L. B. Cannell. Another look at osteoarthritis. Ann Rheum Dis,. 1979;38:423–428.
2. Stanley D. Prevalence and etiology of symptomatic elbow osteoarthritis. J Shoulder Elb Surg. 1994;3(6):386–9.
3. Oya N, Tajika T, Ichinose T, Sasaki T, Yamamoto A, Kuboi T, et al. The prevalence of elbow osteoarthritis in Japanese middle-aged and elderly populations: the relationship between risk factors and function. J Shoulder Elb Surg. 2018;27(6):1086–91.
4. Wysocki RW, Cohen MS. Primary osteoarthritis and posttraumatic arthritis of the elbow. Hand Clin. 2011;27(2):131–7, v.
5. Carlier Y, Lenoir H, Rouleau DM, Mansat P, Vidil A, Ferrand M, et al. Arthroscopic debridement for osteoarthritis of the elbow: results and analysis of predictive factors. Orthop Traumatol Surg Res. 2019;105(8S):S221–S7.
6. Papatheodorou LK, Baratz ME, Sotereanos DG. Elbow arthritis: current concepts. J Hand Surg Am. 2013;38(3):605–13.
7. Stewart N, Karpik K. Syringomyelic neuropathic arthropathy of the elbow. N Z Med J. 2016;129(1443):87–91.
8. Snoddy MC, Lee DH, Kuhn JE. Charcot shoulder and elbow: a review of the literature and update on treatment. J Shoulder Elb Surg. 2017;26(3):544–52.
9. Jbara M, Patnana M, Kazmi F, Beltran J. MR imaging: Arthropathies and infectious conditions of the elbow, wrist, and hand. Radiol Clin N Am. 2006;44(4):625–42, ix.
10. Kauffman JI, Chen AL, Stuchin S, Di Cesare PE. Surgical management of the rheumatoid elbow. J Am Acad Orthop Surg. 2003;11(2):100–8.
11. Murphy MS. Management of inflammatory arthritis around the elbow. Hand Clin. 2002;18(1):161–8.
12. Kokkalis ZT, Jain S, Sotereanos DG. Fibrous dysplasia around the elbow. J Shoulder Elb Surg. 2010;19(1):e6–11.
13. Soojian MG, Kwon YW. Elbow arthritis. Bull NYU Hosp Jt Dis. 2007;65(1):61–71.
14. McGonagle D, Conaghan PG, O'Connor P, Gibbon W, Green M, Wakefield R, et al. The relationship between synovitis and bone changes in early untreated rheumatoid arthritis: a controlled magnetic resonance imaging study. Arthritis Rheum. 1999;42(8):1706–11.

15. Sakkas LI, Alexiou I, Simopoulou T, Vlychou M. Enthesitis in psoriatic arthritis. Semin Arthritis Rheum. 2013;43(3):325–34.
16. McGonagle D, Gibbon W, Emery P. Classification of inflammatory arthritis by enthesitis. Lancet. 1998;352(9134):1137–40.
17. Singh JA, Gaffo A. Gout epidemiology and comorbidities. Semin Arthritis Rheum. 2020;50(3S):S11–S6.
18. Agudelo CA, Wise CM. Crystal-associated arthritis. Clin Geriatr Med. 1998;14(3):495–513.
19. Brower AC. Arthritis in black and white. Philadelphia: Saunders; 1988. x, 358 p. p.
20. Parathithasan N, Lee WK, Pianta M, Oon S, Perera W. Gouty arthropathy: review of clinico-pathologic and imaging features. J Med Imaging Radiat Oncol. 2016;60(1):9–20.
21. Abhishek A. Calcium pyrophosphate deposition. Br J Hosp Med (Lond). 2014;75(4):C61–4.
22. Becce F. Diagnosis of calcium pyrophosphate deposition by imaging - current state and challenges remaining. Osteoarthr Cartil. 2019;27(4):545–6.
23. Rosenthal AK, Ryan LM. Calcium pyrophosphate deposition disease. N Engl J Med. 2016;374(26):2575–84.
24. Hayes CW, Conway WF. Calcium hydroxyapatite deposition disease. Radiographics. 1990;10(6):1031–48.
25. Hongsmatip P, Cheng KY, Kim C, Lawrence DA, Rivera R, Smitaman E. Calcium hydroxyapatite deposition disease: imaging features and presentations mimicking other pathologies. Eur J Radiol. 2019;120:108653.
26. Uhthoff HK, Sarkar K, Maynard JA. Calcifying tendinitis: a new concept of its pathogenesis. Clin Orthop Relat Res. 1976;118:164–8.
27. Cuesta-Barriuso R, Gomez-Conesa A, Lopez-Pina JA. Manual and educational therapy in the treatment of hemophilic arthropathy of the elbow: a randomized pilot study. Orphanet J Rare Dis. 2018;13(1):151.
28. Chang CY, Li TY, Cheng SN, Pan RY, Wang HJ, Lin SY, et al. Prevalence and severity by age and other clinical correlates of haemophilic arthropathy of the elbow, knee and ankle among Taiwanese patients with haemophilia. Haemophilia. 2017;23(2):284–91.
29. Malhotra R, Gulati MS, Bhan S. Elbow arthropathy in hemophilia. Arch Orthop Trauma Surg. 2001;121(3):152–7.
30. Dale TM, Saucedo JM, Rodriguez-Merchan EC. Total elbow arthroplasty in haemophilia. Haemophilia. 2018;24(4):548–56.
31. Plut D, Kotnik BF, Zupan IP, Kljucevsek D, Vidmar G, Snoj Z, et al. Diagnostic accuracy of haemophilia early arthropathy detection with ultrasound (HEAD-US): a comparative magnetic resonance imaging (MRI) study. Radiol Oncol. 2019;53(2):178–86.
32. Luo TD, Varacallo M. Diffuse idiopathic skeletal hyperostosis (DISH). Treasure Island (FL): StatPearls; 2020.
33. Beyeler C, Schlapbach P, Gerber NJ, Fahrer H, Hasler F, van der Linden SM, et al. Diffuse idiopathic skeletal hyperostosis (DISH) of the elbow: a cause of elbow pain? A controlled study. Br J Rheumatol. 1992;31(5):319–23.
34. Beyeler C, Thomann SR, Gerber NJ, Kunze C, Aeberli D. Diffuse idiopathic skeletal hyperostosis (DISH) of the elbow: a controlled radiological study. BMC Musculoskelet Disord. 2015;16:119.
35. Shariatzadeh H, Jafari D, Taheri H, Jamshidi K, Pahlevansabagh A. Intra-articular osteochondroma of the elbow: a case report. J Shoulder Elb Surg. 2010;19(3):e1–4.
36. Niu XF, Yi JH, Hu J, Xiao LB. Chronic radial head dislocation caused by a rare solitary osteochondroma of the proximal radius in a child: a case report and review of the literature. BMC Res Notes. 2015;8:131.
37. Murphey MD, Choi JJ, Kransdorf MJ, Flemming DJ, Gannon FH. Imaging of osteochondroma: variants and complications with radiologic-pathologic correlation. Radiographics. 2000;20(5):1407–34.
38. Savvidou OD, Koutsouradis P, Chloros GD, Papanastasiou I, Sarlikiotis T, Kaspiris A, et al. Bone tumours around the elbow: a rare entity. EFORT Open Rev. 2019;4(4):133–42.
39. Douis H, Saifuddin A. The imaging of cartilaginous bone tumours. I. Benign lesions. Skeletal Radiol. 2012;41(10):1195–212.
40. Flemming DJ, Murphey MD. Enchondroma and chondrosarcoma. Semin Musculoskelet Radiol. 2000;4(1):59–71.
41. Murphey MD, Flemming DJ, Boyea SR, Bojescul JA, Sweet DE, Temple HT. Enchondroma versus chondrosarcoma in the appendicular skeleton: differentiating features. Radiographics. 1998;18(5):1213–37; quiz 44–5.
42. Zhu W, Wang W, Mao X, Chen Y. Arthroscopic management of elbow synovial chondromatosis. Medicine (Baltimore). 2018;97(40):e12402.
43. Lu H, Chen Q, Shen H. Pigmented villonodular synovitis of the elbow with rdial, median and ulnar nerve compression. Int J Clin Exp Pathol. 2015;8(11):14045–9.
44. Caruso CA, Leddy TP. Posttraumatic pigmented villonodular synovitis of the elbow after occult fracture: a literature review. J Am Acad Orthop Surg Glob Res Rev. 2017;1(3):e018.
45. Su H, Gould E, Penna J, Meng H. A rare manifestation of pigmented villonodular synovitis of the elbow in a child. Radiol Case Rep. 2008;3(2):156.
46. Cahayadi SD, Antoro A, Swandika B. A giant cell rich osteosarcoma of the proximal ulnar bone treated by elbow arthroplasty: a case report. Int J Surg Case Rep. 2019;58:157–61.
47. Misaghi A, Goldin A, Awad M, Kulidjian AA. Osteosarcoma: a comprehensive review. SICOT J. 2018;4:12.
48. Bansal K, Prasad A, Shahi P, Sehgal A, Kamal S. Extraosseus Ewing's sarcoma of the forearm. Cureus. 2020;12(7):e9051.
49. Puri A, Gulia A, Byregowda S, Ramanujan V. Reconstruction of the elbow and forearm for Ewing

sarcoma of ulna: a new biological technique. Int J Shoulder Surg. 2016;10(2):85–8.
50. Wang C, Lin N. Ewing's sarcoma of the ulna treated with sub-total resection and reconstruction using a non-vascularized, autogenous fibular graft and hernia mesh: a case report. Oncol Lett. 2015;10(4):2067–70.
51. Douis H, Saifuddin A. The imaging of cartilaginous bone tumours. II. Chondrosarcoma. Skeletal Radiol. 2013;42(5):611–26.
52. Rinehart GC, Mustoe TA, Weeks PM. Management of synovial sarcoma of the median nerve at the elbow. Plast Reconstr Surg. 1989;83(3):528–32.
53. Murphey MD, Gibson MS, Jennings BT, Crespo-Rodriguez AM, Fanburg-Smith J, Gajewski DA. From the archives of the AFIP: imaging of synovial sarcoma with radiologic-pathologic correlation. Radiographics. 2006;26(5):1543–65.
54. Kane SF, Lynch JH, Taylor JC. Evaluation of elbow pain in adults. Am Fam Physician. 2014;89(8):649–57.
55. Floemer F, Morrison WB, Bongartz G, Ledermann HP. MRI characteristics of olecranon bursitis. AJR Am J Roentgenol. 2004;183(1):29–34.
56. Skaf AY, Boutin RD, Dantas RW, Hooper AW, Muhle C, Chou DS, et al. Bicipitoradial bursitis: MR imaging findings in eight patients and anatomic data from contrast material opacification of bursae followed by routine radiography and MR imaging in cadavers. Radiology. 1999;212(1):111–6.
57. Yap SH, Griffith JF, Lee RKL. Imaging bicipitoradial bursitis: a pictorial essay. Skelet Radiol. 2019;48(1):5–10.
58. Assuncao JH, Noffs GG, Malavolta EA, Gracitelli MEC, Lima ALM, Ferreira Neto AA. Septic arthritis of the shoulder and elbow: one decade of epidemiological analysis at a tertiary referral hospital. Rev Bras Ortop. 2018;53(6):707–13.
59. Karchevsky M, Schweitzer ME, Morrison WB, Parellada JA. MRI findings of septic arthritis and associated osteomyelitis in adults. AJR Am J Roentgenol. 2004;182(1):119–22.
60. Dong PR, Seeger LL, Yao L, Panosian CB, Johnson BL Jr, Eckardt JJ. Uncomplicated cat-scratch disease: findings at CT, MR imaging, and radiography. Radiology. 1995;195(3):837–9.
61. Kaas L, Struijs PA. Congenital radial head dislocation with a progressive cubitus valgus: a case report. Strategies Trauma Limb Reconstr. 2012;7(1):39–44.
62. Al-Qattan MM, Abou Al-Shaar H, Alkattan WM. The pathogenesis of congenital radial head dislocation/subluxation. Gene. 2016;586(1):69–76.
63. Elliott AM, Kibria L, Reed MH. The developmental spectrum of proximal radioulnar synostosis. Skelet Radiol. 2010;39(1):49–54.
64. Garg G, Gupta SP. Surgical outcome of delayed presentation of congenital proximal radioulnar synostosis. SICOT J. 2015;1:33.
65. Miura T, Nakamura R, Suzuki M, Kanie J. Congenital radio-ulnar synostosis. J Hand Surg Br. 1984;9(2):153–5.
66. Bain G, Gupta P, Phadnis J, Singhi PK. Endoscopic excision of supracondylar humeral spur for decompression of the median nerve and brachial artery. Arthrosc Tech. 2016;5(1):e67–70.
67. Lordan J, Rauh P, Spinner RJ. The clinical anatomy of the supracondylar spur and the ligament of Struthers. Clin Anat. 2005;18(7):548–51.
68. Andreisek G, Crook DW, Burg D, Marincek B, Weishaupt D. Peripheral neuropathies of the median, radial, and ulnar nerves: MR imaging features. Radiographics. 2006;26(5):1267–87.

5 Wrist: Importance and Biomechanics

Bethany U. Casagranda

Wrist

> One really beautiful wrist motion, that is synchronized with your head and heart, and you have it. It looks as if it were born in a minute. Artist: Helen Frankenthaler

Importance and Biomechanics

Wrist mobility not only allows for performance of activities of daily living (ADLs) but also affects our ability to strengthen more proximal muscle groups providing overall stability and proper range of motion of the upper extremity [1].

The wrist is comprised of the distal ends of the radius and ulna, two rows of carpal bones, and the proximal bases of the metacarpal bones. The radiocarpal joint is a synovial joint, condyloid type, and serves as a transition point between the forearm and hand. Facets on the radius allow for true articulations with the scaphoid and lunate. Although the distal radius and ulna are often regarded to as part of the wrist, it is of important note that the ulna does not articulate with the carpus, but articulates with the sigmoid notch of the radius forming the distal radioulnar joint (DRUJ) [2].

B. U. Casagranda (✉)
Department of Radiology, Imaging Institute, Allegheny Health Network, Pittsburgh, PA, USA
e-mail: bethany.casagranda@ahn.org

The articulation between the proximal and distal row is defined as the midcarpal joint. When comparing proximal and distal carpal rows, they possess different kinetic behavior. The proximal carpal row is without true tendon insertions creating an intercalated segment with motion being completely dependent on mechanical forces of the surrounding articulations. The distal carpal row has strong intercarpal ligaments and rigid ligamentous attachments to the metacarpal bases rendering their motion negligible. For this reason, the distal carpal row functions as a part of the fixed hand unit responding to the forces produced from the myotendinous structures of the forearm [3, 4].

Ligaments, classified as extrinsic or intrinsic, help stabilize the wrist and its many articulations. Extrinsic ligaments span from the osseous structures of the distal forearm, retinacula, tendon sheaths, or capsule to the carpal bones [5]. These extrinsic ligaments stabilize the radiocarpal joint with the volar ligaments providing the greatest restraint to excessive motion and contributing to joint stability but allowing coordinated hand and forearm movement during supination [2]. Intrinsic ligaments connect adjacent carpal bones to each other with the scapholunate and lunotriquetral ligaments proving to be most clinically relevant in addition to the triangular fibrocartilage complex which stabilizes the ulnar side of the wrist [2, 5].

Wrist motion is created by three movements of freedom: flexion-extension, radial-ulnar deviation, and supination-pronation. Normal range of

B. U. Casagranda (ed.), *MRI of the Upper Extremity*, https://doi.org/10.1007/978-3-030-81612-4_5

Table 5.1 Normal range of motion for the wrist

Flexion	73°
Extension	71°
Radial deviation	19°
Ulnar deviation	33°
Supination	140°
Pronation	60°

motion has been traditionally studied with universal goniometer and optical motion tracking [6]. Recent studies have reproduced this data utilizing the iPhone gyroscope application [7]. Whether utilizing traditional or advanced technological methods to determine range of motion, testing should be performed with the wrist in near neutral position to allow maximal motion [6]. Normal range of motion for the wrist can be found in Table 5.1 [7, 8].

Biomechanical studies in both men and women have determined the ideal range of motion required to perform common ADLs. Evaluated tasks were achieved with 60° of extension, 54° of flexion, 40° of ulnar deviation, and 17° of radial deviation. Therefore, the majority of ADLs could be accomplished with 70 percent of the maximal range of wrist motion [9].

Radial and ulnar deviation occurs around the anteroposterior axis through the capitate bone. Movements through the transverse axis, again through the capitate bone, create the motions of flexion and extension. Palmar flexion is the most powerful of movements because the flexor muscle groups are considerably stronger than the extensors [10]. Supination and pronation are produced from the rotatory actions of the DRUJ, and therefore, the distal aspects of the radius and ulna are normally regarded as part of the wrist [11].

Simply stated, wrist motion occurs in three planes, but in reality, the movement is more complex with coupling of flexion-extension and radial-ulnar deviation [12]. This movement around the oblique axis has been described as the dart-throwing motion (DTM) of the wrist in orthopedic literature [6] (Fig. 5.1). DTM occurs primarily at the midcarpal joint with less contribution from the radiocarpal joint. More importantly, DTM is found to be the most frequently used motion in ADLs [13, 14] Therefore, midcarpal joint function and understanding of this coupling motion are critical in caring for patients with injuries that may affect their ability to engage in life's activities [15].

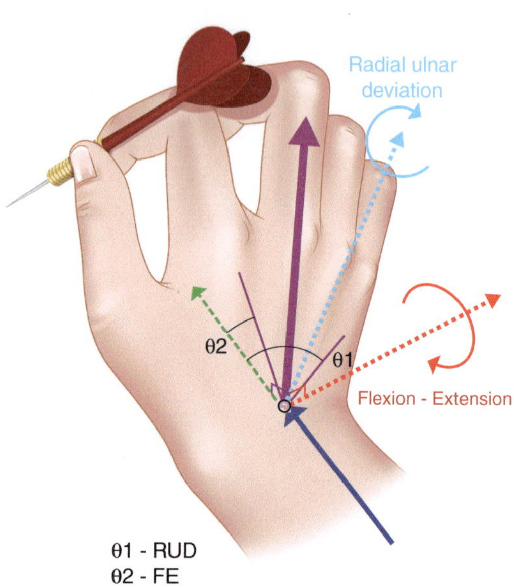

Fig. 5.1 Dart-throwing motion of the wrist

References

1. Cantero-Téllez R, Orza SG, Bishop MD, Berjano P, Villafañe JH. Duration of wrist immobilization is associated with shoulder pain in patients with after wrist immobilization: an observational study. J Exerc Rehabil. 2018;14(4):694–8. https://doi.org/10.12965/jer.36292.146. PMID: 30276195; PMCID: PMC6165988.
2. Erwin J, Varacallo M. Anatomy, shoulder and upper limb, wrist joint. [Updated 2020 Sep 8]. In: StatPearls [Internet]. Treasure Island (FL): StatPearls Publishing; 2020 Jan-. Available from: https://www.ncbi.nlm.nih.gov/books/NBK534779/.
3. Kuo CE, Wolfe SW. Scapholunate instability: current concepts in diagnosis and management. J Hand Surg. 2008;33A:998–1013.
4. Kijima Y, Viegas SF. Wrist anatomy and biomechanics. J Hand Surg Am. 2009;34(8):1555–63. https://doi.org/10.1016/j.jhsa.2009.07.019. PMID: 19801111.
5. Bateni CP, Bartolotta RJ, Richardson ML, Mulcahy H, Allan CH. Imaging key wrist ligaments: what the surgeon needs the radiologist to know. AJR Am J Roentgenol. 2013;200(5):1089–95. https://doi.org/10.2214/AJR.12.9738. PMID: 23617494.
6. Vardakastani V, Bell H, Mee S, Brigstocke G, Kedgley AE. Clinical measurement of the dart throwing

motion of the wrist: variability, accuracy and correction. J Hand Surg Eur. 2018;43(7):723–31. https://doi.org/10.1177/1753193418773329. Epub 2018 May 12. PMID: 29754522; PMCID: PMC6104201.

7. Kim TS, Park D, Lee YB, Han DG, Shim J, Lee YJ, et al. A study on the measurement of wrist motion range using the iPhone 4 gyroscope application. Ann Plast Surg. 2014;73(2):215–21.
8. Braddom RL, Buschbacher RM. Physical medicine & rehabilitation. 3rd ed. Philadelphia: Saunders Elsevier; 2007. p. 21.
9. Ryu JY, Cooney WP 3rd, Askew LJ, An KN, Chao EY. Functional ranges of motion of the wrist joint. J Hand Surg Am. 1991;16(3):409–19. https://doi.org/10.1016/0363-5023(91)90006-w.
10. Platzer W. Color atlas of human anatomy, vol. 1: Locomotor system. 5th ed. Thieme; 2004. ISBN 3-13-533305-1. p. 132 and 172.
11. Kingston B. Understanding joints: a practical guide to their structure and function. Nelson Thornes; 2000. ISBN 0-7487-5399-0. p. 126–7.
12. Li ZM, Kuxhaus L, Fisk JA, Christophel TH. Coupling between wrist flexion-extension and radial-ulnar deviation. Clin Biomech (Bristol, Avon). 2005;20(2):177–83. https://doi.org/10.1016/j.clinbiomech.2004.10.002.
13. Kaufmann R, Pfaeffle J, Blankenhorn B, Stabile K, Robertson D, Goitz R. Kinematics of the midcarpal and radiocarpal joints in radioulnar deviation: an in vitro study. J Hand Surg Am. 2005;30(5):937–42. https://doi.org/10.1016/j.jhsa.2005.05.016. PMID: 16182048.
14. Morimoto H, Murase T, Goto A, Oka K, Sugamoto K, Yoshikawa H. Capitate-based kinematics of the midcarpal joint during wrist radioulnar deviation: an in vivo three-dimensional motion analysis. J Hand Surg. 2004;29A:668–75.
15. Rainbow MJ, Wolff AL, Crisco JJ, Wolfe SW. Functional kinematics of the wrist. J Hand Surg Eur Vol. 2016;41(1):7–21. https://doi.org/10.1177/1753193415616939. Epub 2015 Nov 14.

Wrist: Anatomy and MRI Optimization

6

Asako Yamamoto, Brady K. Huang, and Christine B. Chung

Osseous Anatomy of the Wrist

The wrist joint includes the osseous structures of the distal radius and ulna, carpal bones, and metacarpal bases (Fig. 6.1). The carpal bones form the proximal (scaphoid, lunate, triquetrum) and distal (trapezium, trapezoid, capitate, hamate) carpal rows that are stabilized by intrinsic and extrinsic ligaments to act as a single intercalated segment. The radiocarpal articulation is formed by the distal surface of the radius with the triangular fibrocartilage serving as a soft tissue articular surface extension distal to the ulna. The articular surface of the radius has two shallow fossae that accommodate the scaphoid and lunate. At the dorsum of the distal radius, an osseous prominence is present that serves as an anatomic landmark for the extensor tendons. This is referred to as Lister's tubercle. The midcarpal joint lies between the proximal and distal carpal rows. The articular surfaces of the carpal bones are normally aligned into three arcs (Gilula's arcs) [1]. The proximal (arc I) and distal (arc II) articular surfaces of the proximal row and the opposing joint surface formed by the convexity of the distal row (arc III) comprise the three arcs. Those opposing articular surfaces should be parallel to one another with symmetrical joint spaces [2]. The pisiform is generally considered a sesamoid and not officially housed in either carpal row [3]. Interruption of a uniformly parallel configuration of the joint spaces or a step-off at the articular surface is secondary findings that suggest insufficiency of stabilizing ligamentous structures. When the "ring" of the intercalated segment is broken, the carpal alignment may be affected. Two common anatomical variants can mimic carpal arc step-offs: (1) triquetrum shorter in its proximal-distal dimension than the adjacent lunate (Fig. 6.2a) and (2) proximally prominent hamate articulating with lunate (type II lunate) (Fig. 6.2b). The former variation results in lunotriquetral step-off, whereas the latter affects the third carpal arc. The prevalence of the type 2 lunate was demonstrated to be 50–57% in radiologic studies and up to 73% in cadaveric studies [4–6]. The mean size of the facet was reported as 4.5 mm (range, 2–6 mm) in type II lunate on coronal view [5].

The normal longitudinal axes through the third metacarpal, capitate, lunate, and radius should superimpose, with 0 to 30° (the capitolunate angle) on lateral radiographs [6] (Fig. 6.3a, b). Also, the angle formed between the long axis of the lunate and the scaphoid ranges between 30 and 60° normally (the scapholunate angle). Those

A. Yamamoto · B. K. Huang
Department of Radiology, University of California San Diego, La Jolla, CA, USA

C. B. Chung (✉)
Department of Radiology, University of California San Diego, La Jolla, CA, USA

Department of Radiology, VA San Diego Healthcare System and University of California San Diego, La Jolla, CA, USA
e-mail: cbchung@health.ucsd.edu

B. U. Casagranda (ed.), *MRI of the Upper Extremity*, https://doi.org/10.1007/978-3-030-81612-4_6

parameters are essential for the evaluation of volar intercalated segmental instability (VISI) or dorsal intercalated segment instability (DISI) (Fig. 6.3c–f). Although recognition of a DISI or VISI configuration on MR images can be useful in the assessment of carpal bone alignment, correlation with radiographs is indispensable [7]. The axis of each bone is assessed in the following way: a line parallel to the center of the radial shaft, a line through the midpoints of the lunate proximal and distal articular surfaces, a line through the centers of the capitate head and its distal articular surface, and a line through the midpoints of the scaphoid proximal and distal poles.

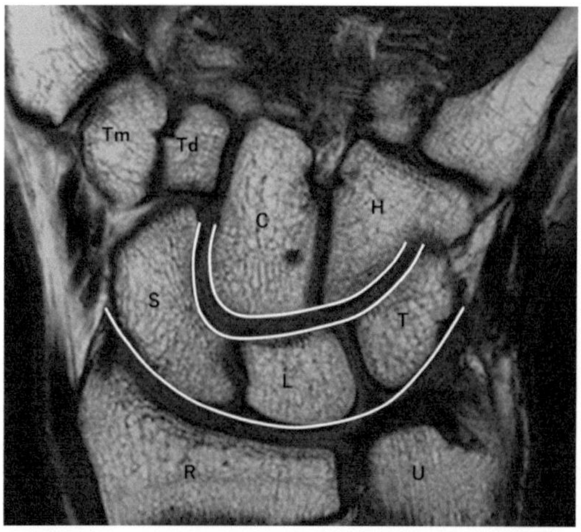

Fig. 6.1 Coronal T1-weighted image of the wrist shows anatomy of carpal bones with lines of Gilula's arc. Abbreviations: Tm Trapezium, Td Trapezoid, C Capitate, H Hamate, S Scaphoid, L Lunate, T Triquetrum, R Radius, U Ulna

To evaluate the anatomical profile of the distal radius, there are three common ways of measurement based on radiographs: radial inclination, radial length, and volar tilt. Radial inclination is measured as the angle between a line drawn from the tip of the radial styloid to the ulnar head articular surface and a second line perpendicular to the longitudinal axis of the radius (Fig. 6.4a). It ranges from 13 to 30° (average 23 degrees) [8, 9]. Radial length can also be measured on PA radiographs or MRI on the coronal plane, normally ranging from 11 to 22 mm (average 12 mm) (Fig. 6.4a). The volar tilt of the radius is measured on the sagittal plane as the angle between a line drawn tangentially across the most distal

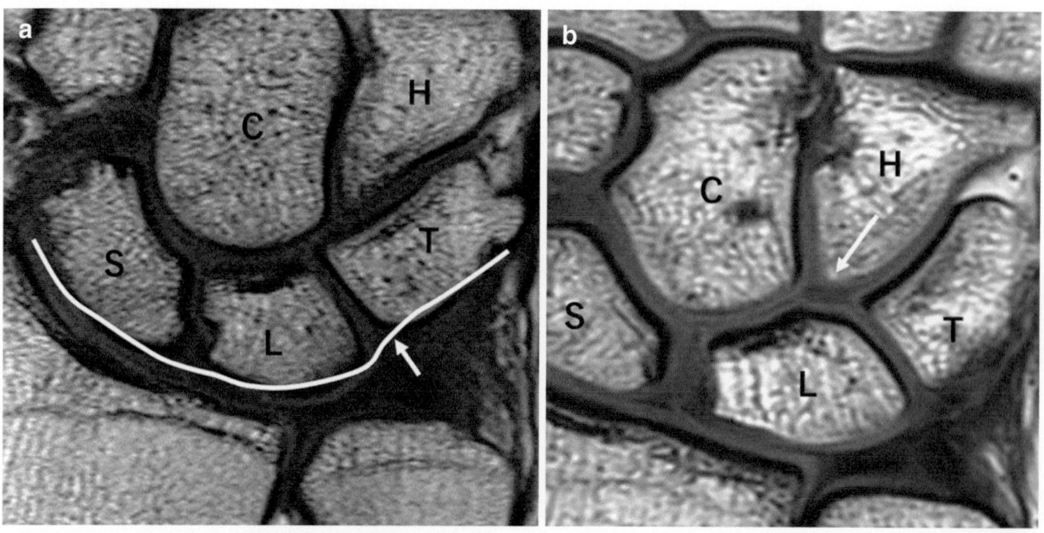

Fig. 6.2 Two common normal variants that mimic carpal arch step-off: (**a**) Short triquetrum. Proximal-distal dimension of triquetrum is shorter than adjacent lunate (L), creating lunotriquetral step-off (arrow) of first carpal arc. Note the proximal configuration of the hamate (H), type I lunate (single distal articular facet for capitate). (**b**) Type II lunate. An additional distal articular facet medially for hamate, affecting the third carpal arc continuity (arrow)

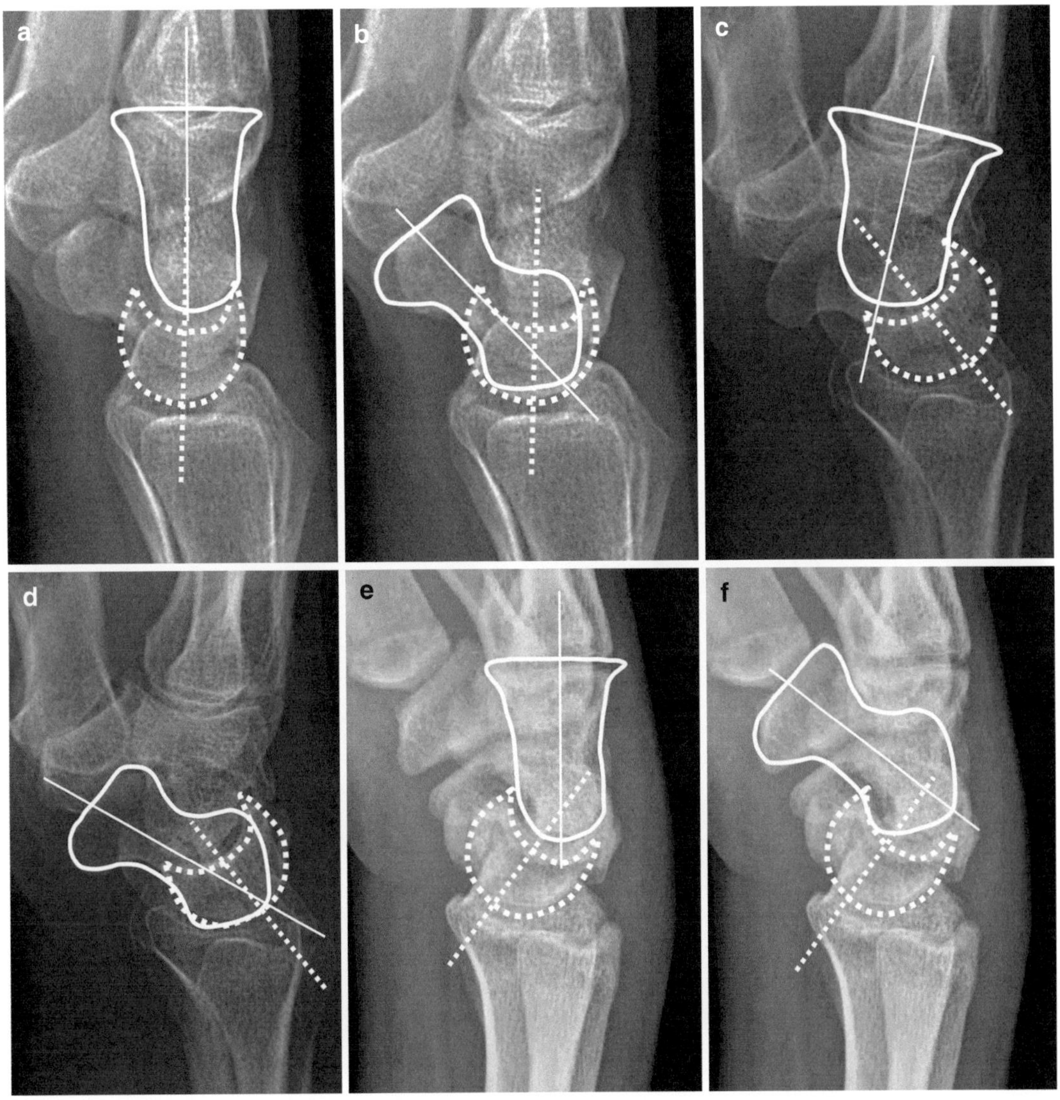

Fig. 6.3 Normal lateral radiograph of the hand with capitolunate angle <30°(**a**) and scapholunate angle between 30 and 60°(**b**). Lateral radiograph with VISI shows capitolunate angle >30°(**c**) and scapholunate angle <30°(**d**). Lateral radiograph with DISI shows capitolunate angle >30°(**e**) and scapholunate angle >60°(**f**)

points of the radial articular surface and a line perpendicular to the midshaft of the radius. Normally this angle ranges from 11° of volar tilt to 4° of dorsal tilt [8] (Fig. 6.4d).

Ulnar variance is the difference in length between the distal radius and ulna. This variance is relevant to the force distribution across the wrist [10]. Ulnar variance is characterized by the differences in apparent lengths of the distal ulna and radius. Ulnar variance is defined as neutral, positive, or negative on the basis of whether the distal articular surface of the ulna is aligned with the distal articular surface of the radius on a neutral posteroanterior imaging (Fig. 6.4a–c) [11]. The ulna is shorter than the radius in negative ulnar variance and longer in positive ulnar variance. Positive variance is defined when the level of the ulna is >2.5 mm beyond the distal articular surface of the radius at the distal radioulnar joint (DRUJ). Negative variance is when the ulnar articular surface is >2.5 mm

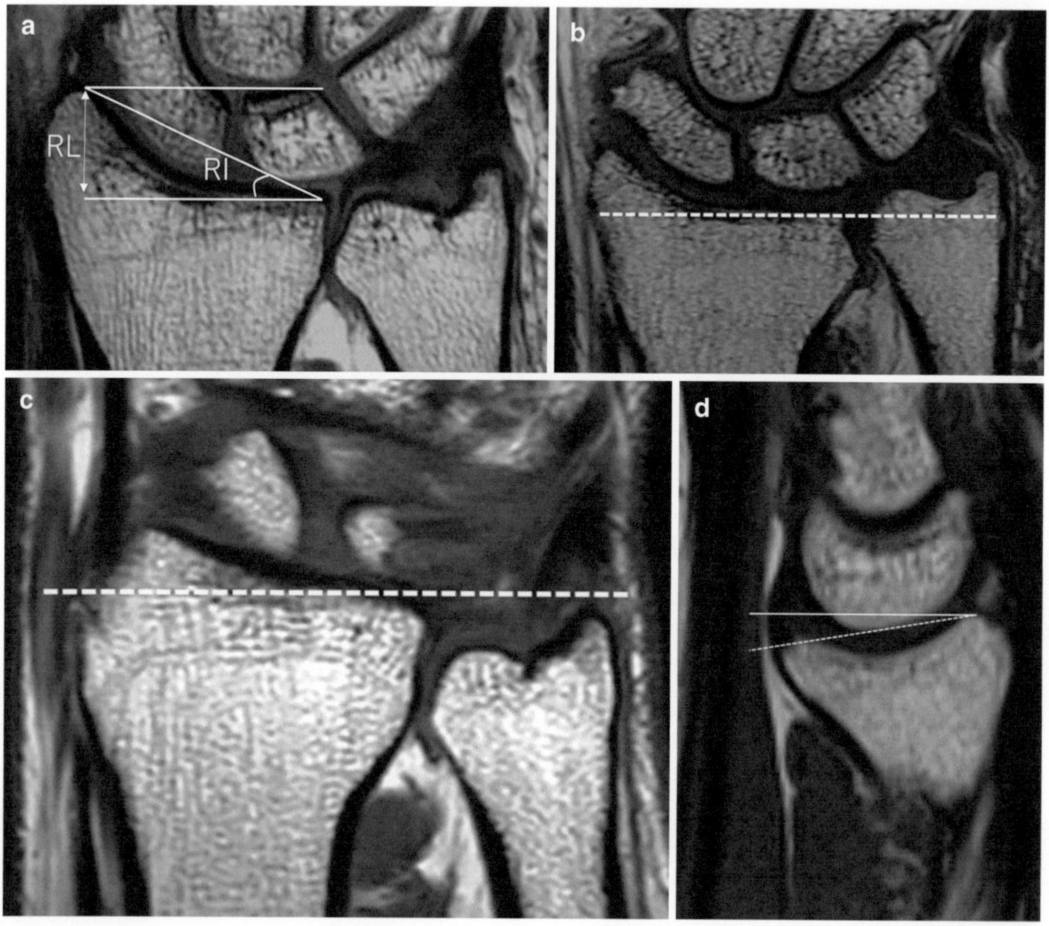

Fig. 6.4 Measurements of the distal radius: RI radial inclination, RL radial length. Ulnar variance is neutral. (**a**) Ulnar variance on coronal T1-weighted images. Positive ulnar (**b**). Negative ulnar variance (**c**). Dotted lines: distal articular surface of the radius. Normal volar tilt on coronal T1-weighted image (**d**)

proximal to the distal articular surface of the radius at the DRUJ [12]. Normally, the radius and ulna are neutral (same length), or there is mild negative ulnar variance. Positive ulnar variance is known to play a key role in ulnar impaction syndrome [12, 13]. Negative ulnar variance has a historic association with Kienbock's disease, but this has been debated in recent orthopedic literature [14, 15].

The DRUJ is formed by the articulation of the sigmoid notch of the radius and ulnar head. This joint is stabilized by the soft tissue and ligamentous components of the triangular fibrocartilage complex (TFCC). It is intimately associated with the sixth extensor compartment, housing the extensor carpi ulnaris.

Guyon's Canal

The ulnar nerve passes through a semirigid longitudinal tunnel known as Guyon's canal or the ulnar tunnel at the palmar aspect of the wrist. It is located superficial to the ulnar aspect of the carpal tunnel and extends from the palmar carpal ligament at the proximal edge of the pisiform to the origin of the hypothenar muscles at the level of the hamulus, approximately 4 cm in distance (Fig. 6.5) [16]. The ulnar nerve, artery, and, occasionally, communicating veins pass through Guyon's canal with accompanying fat tissue. The boundaries are formed by the palmar carpal ligament at the volar aspect, pisiform at the ulnar

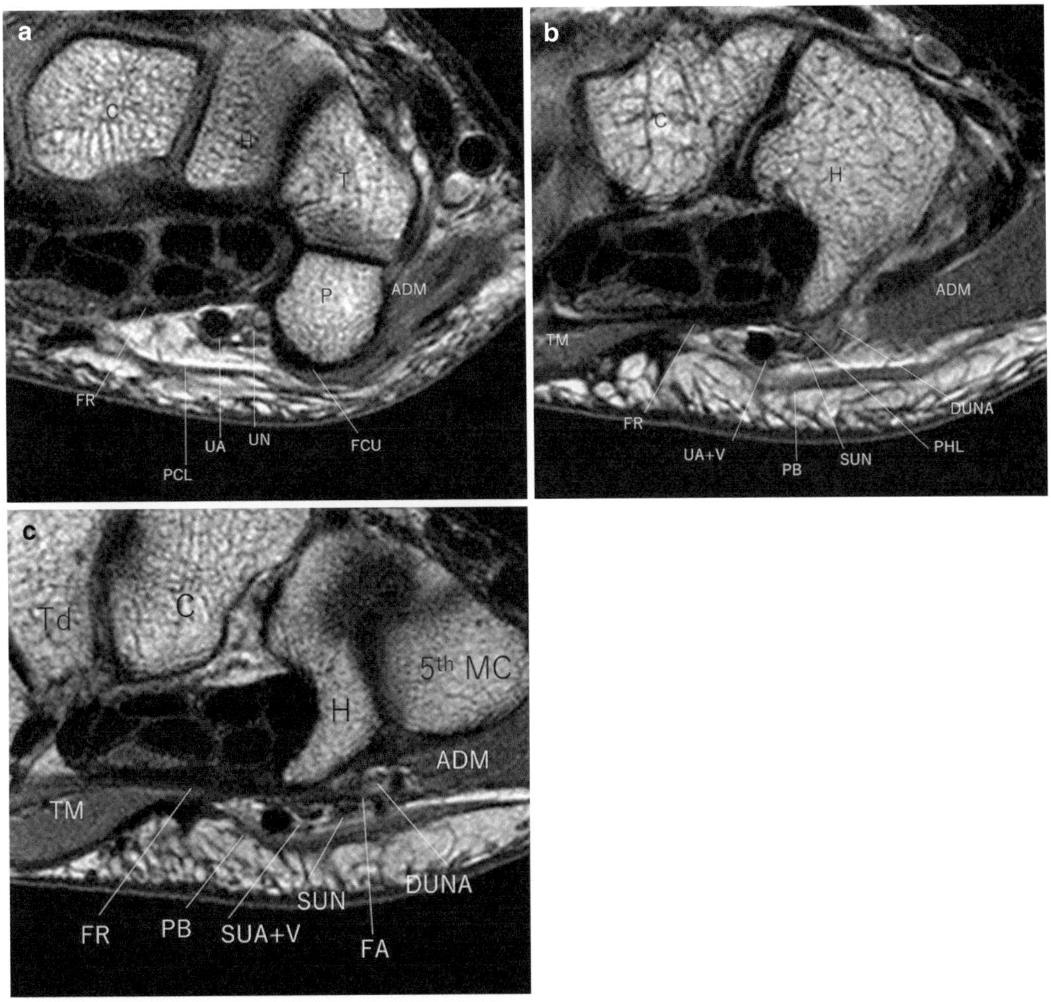

Fig. 6.5 Normal anatomy of Guyon's canal. Axial proton density-weighted MR images of the wrist show anatomy of Guyon's canal in the proximal (**a**), middle-distal (**b**), and distal portion (**c**). Abbreviations: ADM Abductor digiti minimi muscle, DUNA Deep ulnar nerve and artery, FA Fibrous arch of flexor digiti minimi brevis muscle origin, FCU Flexor carpi ulnaris tendon, FR Flexor retinaculum or transverse carpal ligament, H Hamate, P Pisiform, C Capitate, T Triquetrum, Td Trapezoid, MC Metacarpal bone, PB Palmaris brevis muscle, PCL Palmar carpal ligament, SUA Superficial ulnar artery, SUN Superficial ulnar nerve, TM Thenar muscles, UA Ulnar artery, UN Ulnar nerve, V Vein

aspect, and flexor retinaculum of the carpal tunnel at the radial and deep aspect [10]. The ulnar nerve lies between the pisiform bone and the ulnar veins and artery. The transverse carpal ligament, or middle portion of the flexor retinaculum, forms the floor of Guyon's canal as well as the roof of the carpal tunnel; thus, the volumetric changes in one canal can affect the other [17, 18]. The flexor carpi ulnaris (FCU) tendon lies at the ulnar aspect of the ulnar nerve and artery in the forearm and inserts on the pisiform. It partially blends with the palmar carpal ligament and forms the volar boundary of Guyon's canal (Fig. 6.5a) [10].

In the mid-level of Guyon's canal, between the pisiform and hook of hamate, the shape may be triangular or oval (Fig. 6.5b). The boundaries are formed at the volar aspect by the palmar carpal ligament, at the deep aspect by the pisohamate ligament, at the ulnar aspect by the abductor digiti minimi muscle, and at the radial aspect by the flexor retinaculum of the carpal tunnel [19]. Here, the ulnar nerve and artery bifurcate into deep and superficial branches.

At the distal portion of Guyon's canal, the boundaries are formed by the palmaris brevis muscle at the volar and radial aspect, the abductor digiti minimi muscle at the ulnar aspect, and the flexor retinaculum and the hook of hamate dorsally (Fig. 6.5c) [10]. The superficial and deep canals containing the ulnar neurovascular bundles are separated by the fibrous arch of the flexor digiti minimi brevis muscle origin. The deep canal contains the deep motor nerve and artery, whereas the superficial canal contains the superficial sensory nerve and artery [19]. Just distal to the outlet of Guyon's canal, the superficial ulnar artery and the sensory nerve pass volar to the hook of hamate without protective tissues and are vulnerable to mechanical stress or trauma [20].

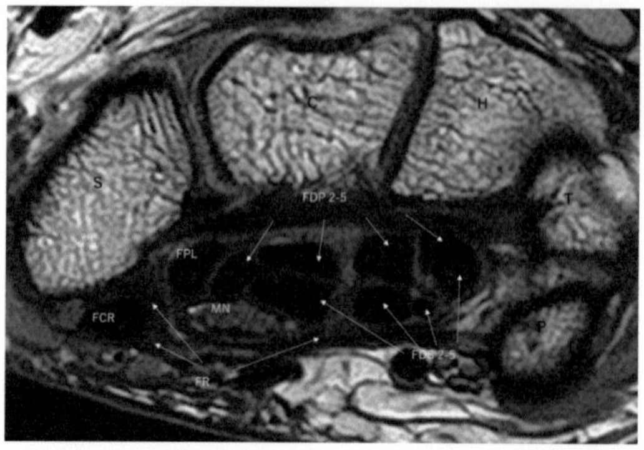

Fig. 6.6 Normal anatomy of carpal tunnel on proton density-weighted axial image. Abbreviations: FCR Flexor carpi radialis, FDP Flexor digitorum profundus, FDS Flexor digitorum superficialis, FPL Flexor pollicis longus, FR Flexor retinaculum, MN Medial nerve, S Scaphoid, C Capitate, H Hamate, T Triquetrum, P Pisiform

Carpal Tunnel

The carpal tunnel is a fibro-osseous tunnel on the palmar side of the wrist. It is bounded by the eight carpal bones and a tough fibrous roof called the transverse carpal ligament (TCL). The carpal tunnel contains eight digital flexor tendons (two for each of the second through fifth rays), flexor pollicis longus (FPL) the radial and ulnar bursae, with the median nerve (Fig. 6.6) [21]. Its dorsal and lateral borders are formed by the scaphoid, triquetrum, lunate, and pisiform proximally and the trapezium, trapezoid, capitate, and hamate distally. This osseous configuration forms a tunnel-like groove called the *sulcus carpi*. The flexor retinaculum forms its palmar boundary and extends from the tuberosities of the scaphoid and the trapezium to the pisiform and the hook of the hamate [22]. In general, the width of the carpal tunnel is narrowest at the level of the hamate hook, located 1 cm beyond the middle of the distal row of the carpal bones about 20 mm [21]. The mean width of the tunnel is 25 mm at its proximal end and 26 mm at its distal border [23]. Variations in the hook of the hamate (hypoplastic, aplastic, or bipartite) in addition to variations in the attachment of the TCL could result in changes in carpal tunnel volume (Fig. 6.7a, b).

The flexor retinaculum is differentiated in three segments: (1) a proximal thin segment called the palmar carpal ligament, (2) the middle tough segment called the TCL, and (3) the distal segment that consists of a thick aponeurosis between the thenar and hypothenar muscles, passing deep to the flexor carpi ulnaris and flexor carpi radialis. The TCL is a thick (2–4 mm) and strong fibrous band. It is attached to the pisiform bone and hook of the hamate medially. Laterally, it splits into two laminae, superficial and deep. The superficial lamina is attached to the tubercle of the scaphoid and trapezium. The deep lamina is attached to the groove on the trapezium. Those two laminae and the osseous groove form a tunnel for flexor carpi radialis (FRC) with its synovial sheath [21]. The volar aspect of the *sulcus carpi* is covered by the extrinsic ligaments, including the palmar lunotriquetral and palmar scaphotriquetral ligaments proximally and the capitate-scaphoid and capitate-trapezium ligaments distally. Usually, a small but variable amount of fatty tissue lies just volar to the capitate-trapezium ligament (Parona's fat pad).

The median nerve is the most volar structure in the carpal tunnel, located just deep to the flexor retinaculum and volar to the flexor digitorum superficialis (FDS) tendons. It is covered by a

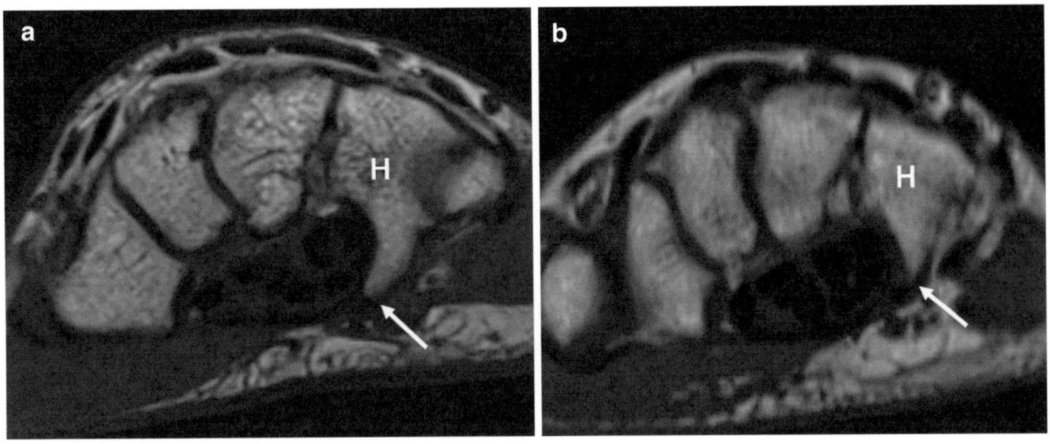

Fig. 6.7 Normal (**a**) and hypoplastic (**b**) hook of hamate on axial T1-weighted images. Note the area of distal carpal tunnel is decreased in (**b**)

layer of cellulo-adipose tissue and adheres to the adjacent ulnar bursa [24]. It changes in position relative to the adjacent tendons on flexion or extension. In extension, the median nerve is usually located anterior to the index finger FDS tendon attached to the flexor retinaculum. In contradistinction, in the flexed position, the median nerve moves dorsally between the FDS of the second finger and flexor pollicis longus tendon. A palmar cutaneous branch arises from median nerve just proximal to the carpal tunnel. Distal to the carpal tunnel, the median nerve divides into medial and lateral branches. The medial branch terminates as two common palmar digital nerves supplying motor innervation to the second lumbrical and sensory innervation to the palm and fingers [25]. The lateral branch gives rise to the proper palmar digital nerves supplying motor innervation to the first lumbrical, sensory innervation to the lateral side of the hand and the thenar motor branch (TMB). The TMB, also referred to as the recurrent motor branch, supplies the abductor pollicis brevis and opponens pollicis muscles, the caput superficiale of the flexor pollicis brevis muscle, and the two radial lumbrical muscles.

Variations of the median nerve are common in the general population including the following four types: type 1 is a single TMB, type 2 has accessory branches of the median nerve at the distal carpal tunnel, type 3 has a high division of the median nerve, and type 4 has the median nerve and its accessory branches proximal to the carpal tunnel [26]. The prevalence of the type 3 variation, a high division of the median nerve resulting in a bifid median nerve, was reported to have a prevalence of 2.6% in a meta-analysis study [27]. In a study performed on 246 carpal tunnel release operations, five of seven patients with the bifid median nerve had an associated persistent median artery [28]. When the median artery persists, it is located on the ulnar aspect of the normal median nerve or between the bifid median nerve components, enveloped by a common perineurium [29]. The presence of hypertrophic muscle within the TCL was reported with a prevalence of 18.2% of hands, with higher prevalence of the TMB variants compared to those without it (23.4% vs 1.7%) [27]. Thus, it is important to recognize a bifid median nerve, persistent median artery, or hypertrophic muscle within the TCL with MRI or US preoperatively.

The four flexor digitorum profundus (FDP) and four FDS tendons arise from muscle bellies proximal to the carpal tunnel. They lie within the ulnar bursa, a sac-like structure lined with a synovial membrane, and are separated from the flexor pollicis longus tendon that resides within the radial bursa [22]. The ulnar bursa extends around the flexor tendons at the level of the carpal tunnel and is composed of three horizontally oriented invaginations of the synovial membrane: (1) a superficial

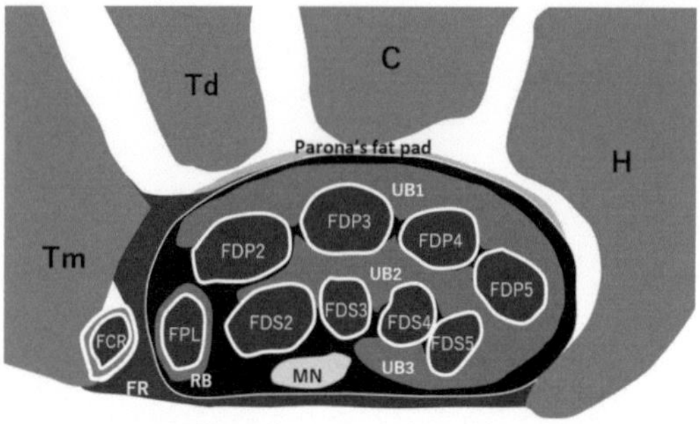

Fig. 6.8 Schematic drawing of the carpal tunnel. Abbreviations: FCR Flexor carpi radialis, FDP Flexor digitorum profundus, FDS Flexor digitorum superficialis, FPL Flexor pollicis longus, FR Flexor retinaculum, MN Medial nerve, RB Radial bursa, UB Ulnar bursa, S Scaphoid, C Capitate, H Hamate, T Triquetrum, P Pisiform

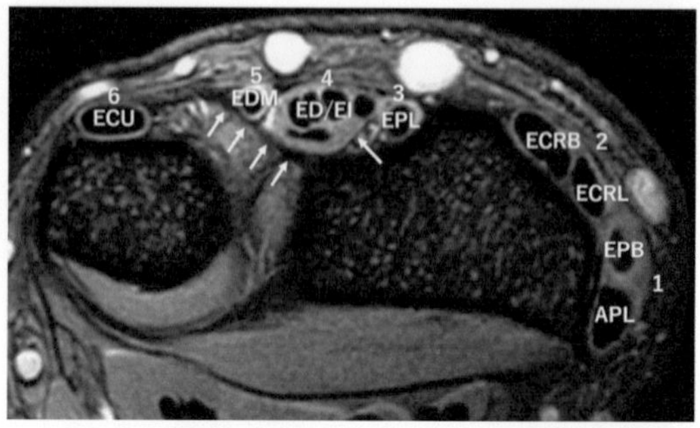

Fig. 6.9 Extensor compartment anatomy. Axial T2*-weighted MR image through the level of the distal radio-ulnar joint showing the six extensor compartments. Arrows show the infratendinous flexor retinaculum. Note the fifth compartment for the extensor digiti minimi tendon (EDM) is purely fibrous

layer situated between the TCL of the flexor retinaculum and the FDS tendons, (2) a middle layer between the FDS tendons and the FDP tendons, and (3) a deep layer situated behind the FDP tendons (Fig. 6.8) [30]. Various patterns of communication between the radial and ulnar bursae, as well as between the bursae and individual tendon sheaths, have been reported. The connection between the ulnar and radial bursae and between the ulnar bursa and flexor digitorum tendon sheath of the fifth digit tendon is typical, with the lack of continuity of the second to fourth flexor tendon sheaths [31]. These communications are of clinical importance in explaining the spread of inflammation, infection, or neoplastic processes.

Extensor Tendons and Extensor Retinaculum

The extensor tendons of the wrist are divided into six compartments along its dorsal aspect. These include the first compartment with the abductor pollicis longus (APL) and extensor pollicis brevis (EPB), the second compartment with the extensor carpi radialis longus (ECRL) and extensor carpi radialis brevis (ECRB), the third compartment with the extensor pollicis longus (EPL), the fourth compartment with the extensor digitorum and extensor indicis, the fifth compartment with the extensor digiti minimi, and the sixth compartment with the extensor carpi ulnaris (ECU). The extensor retinaculum (ER) is a thickening of the distal antebrachial fascia at the level of the inferior radioulnar joint that involves the extensor tendons over the radial, dorsal, and ulnar aspects of the wrist [32]. It consists of two layers, supratendinous and infratendinous (Fig. 6.9) (Table 6.1) [33].

On the radial side of the wrist, the ER attaches at the volar-radial border above the styloid process (Fig. 6.10(I)) blending with the antebrachial fascia, the palmar carpal ligament, and occasionally the fascia overlying the thenar compartment [32]. The ER lies over the tendons to insert into the dorsoradial bony protuberance on the distal radius (Fig. 6.10(II)). Superficial to the first extensor compartment, slips of the ER can form septa that extend between and separate the APL and EPB or even separate individual tendon slips of the APL. The prevalence of supranumerary tendon slips ranged from 74% to 77% for the APL and 2% to 27% for the EPB in cadavers [34–37]. Consistently higher prevalence of supernumerary tendon slips and septation has been reported in patients with De Quervain tenosynovitis. Chang et al. reported multiple tendon slips were also common on MRI, with a prevalence of 74–79% in a control group compared to 91% in a De Quervain tenosynovitis group [38]. In a previous study on CT, the osseous ridge at the floor of the first extensor compartment was found in 23.8% among the general population, with a statistically significant increase in females (19.8%

Table 6.1 Extensor tendons

First compartment (1): Abductor pollicis longus (APL) and extensor pollicis brevis (EPB) tendon
Second compartment (2): Extensor carpi radialis longus and brevis tendons (ECRL, ECRB)
Third compartment (3): Extensor pollicis longus (EPL) tendon
Forth compartment (4): Extensor digitorum (ED) and extensor indicis (EI) tendon
Fifth compartment (5): Extensor digiti minimi (EDM) tendon
Sixth compartment (6): Extensor carpi ulnaris (ECU) tendon

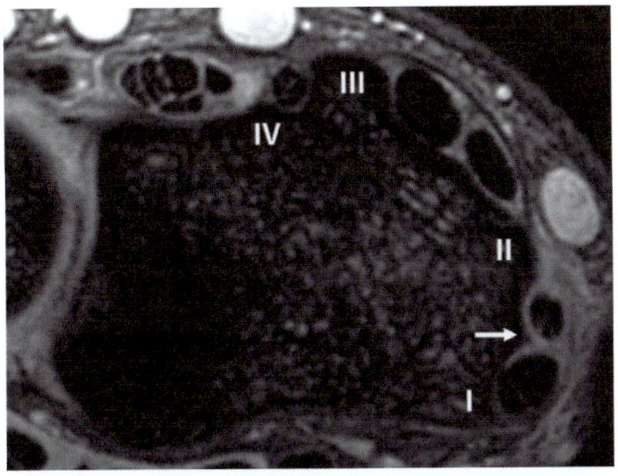

Fig. 6.10 Attachment sites of the extensor retinaculum to the radius on T2*-weighted axial image. Note the osseous protuberance beneath the first extensor compartment (arrow). (I) The volar-radial border above the styloid process, (II) the dorsoradial bony protuberance on the distal radius, (III) Lister's tubercle of the radius, (IV) the osseous prominence on the radius, (I–II) the first compartment containing abductor pollicis longus tendon (APL) and extensor pollicis brevis tendon (EPB), (II–III) the second compartment containing extensor carpi radialis longus and brevis tendons (ECRL, ECRB), (III–IV) the third compartment containing extensor pollicis longus tendon (EPL)

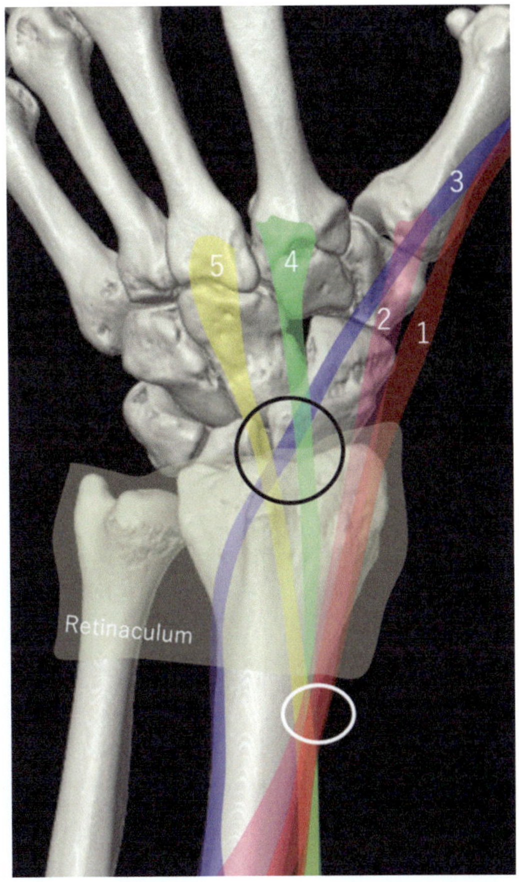

Fig. 6.11 Anatomic diagram shows the distal (black circle) and proximal (white circle) intersections of the extensor tendons. (1) Red, abductor pollicis longus; (2) pink, extensor pollicis brevis; (3) blue, extensor pollicis longus; (4) green, extensor carpi radialis longus; (5) yellow, extensor carpi radialis brevis tendon

in males, 33.3% in females) [39]. An ultrasound anatomical study showed the association between the osseous ridge and the presence of the septation in the first extensor compartment; therefore, it can be an indirect sign of compartmentalization [40]. The bony ridge is observed also on MRI when the slice thickness is appropriate (Fig. 6.10).

The second extensor compartment is formed by the ER located between the dorsoradial bony protuberance (Fig. 6.10(II)) and Lister's tubercle of the radius (Fig. 6.10(III)). As previously noted, this compartment contains the ECRB and ECRL tendons. The insertion of the ER into Lister's tubercle is broad and extends along the entire expanse of the tubercle [32]. Lister's tubercle is an important osseous landmark to separate the second and third extensor compartments. The tendons of the first and second compartments cross each other 4–8 cm proximal to Lister's tubercle (Fig. 6.11) [41]. This intersection creates a vulnerability due to repetitive friction with supination and pronation, flexion, and extension [42]. Routine wrist MRI protocols may not extend proximally to offer full characterization of this region, emphasizing the importance of a detailed clinical history.

The ER crosses the EPL of the third extensor compartment with an attachment from Lister's tubercle (Fig. 6.10(III)) to the osseous prominence on the radius (Fig. 6.10(IV)) [43]. The EPL, ECRB, and ECRL tendons intersect distal to Lister's tubercle with communication of their tendon sheaths at the point of intersection (Fig. 6.11). Lister's tubercle acts as a pulley and therefore creates a vulnerability of the tendons in the setting of intersection syndrome [44].

The supratendinous portion of the ER crosses over the extensor digitorum and extensor indicis to form the fourth and fifth extensor compartments. The ER attaches to an osseous prominence at the dorsoulnar aspect of the radius [32]. The infratendinous portion of the ER is well described on images at the level of the fourth and fifth compartments. The supratendinous and infratendinous portions of the ER coalesce to separate the fourth and fifth extensor compartments [43]. The two portions of the retinaculum continue to surround the extensor digiti minimi tendon and form a purely fibrous fifth compartment.

The ECU tendon of the sixth extensor compartment lies within the subsheath along a groove at the dorsolateral aspect of the ulna. The two portions of the retinaculum meet to form the radial-sided attachment of this compartment [43]. The supratendinous portion of the ER extends over the ECU tendon blending fibers with the volar antebrachial fascia. Ulnarward, it inserts into the sheath of the flexor carpi ulnaris tendon, the pisiform, the pisometacarpal ligament, and the base of the fifth metacarpal [29]. The supratendinous and the infratendinous portions provide blending fibers with the subsheath of the ECU [32]. The ECU tendon centers in its groove in pronation and neutral position (Fig. 6.12) [45]. In supination, the tendon subluxes, and the extensor retinaculum is stretched. The "linea jugata" is the longitudinal fibrous

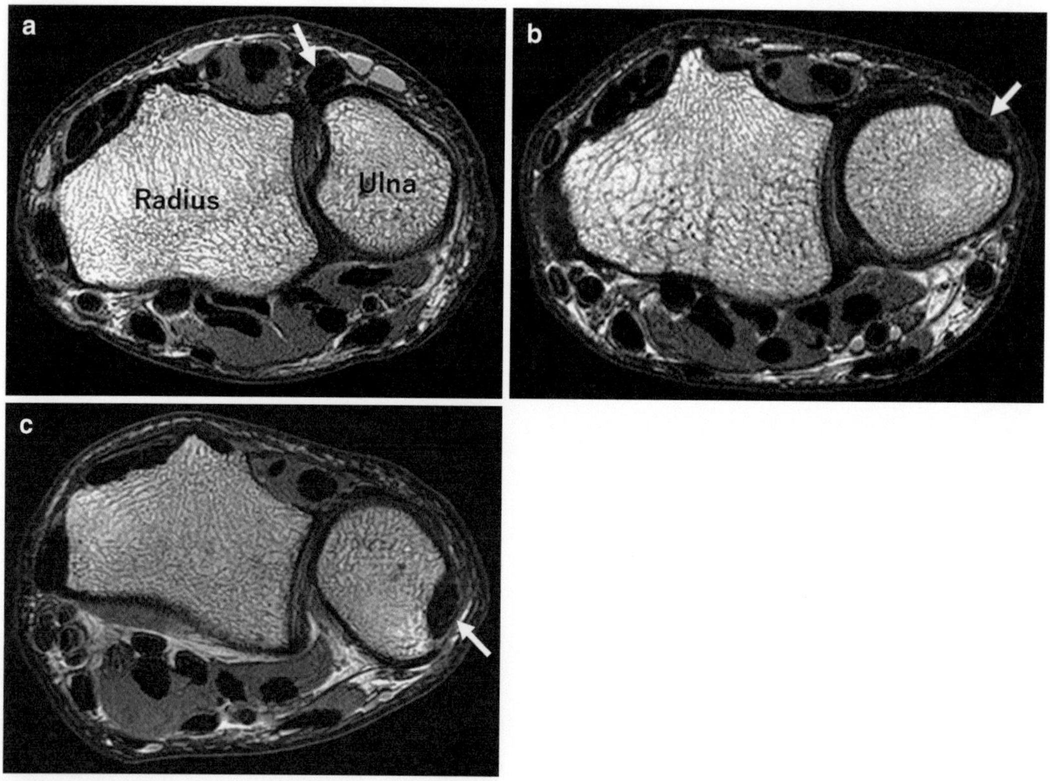

Fig. 6.12 Location of the ECU tendon (arrow) with supination (**a**), neutral (**b**), and pronation (**c**)

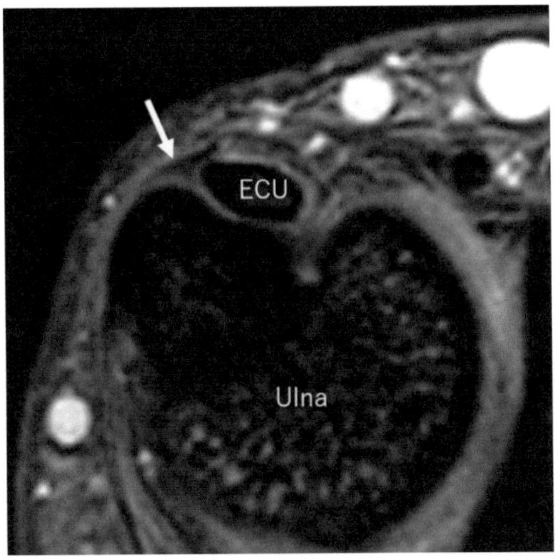

Fig. 6.13 Linea jugata. T2*-weighted axial MR image shows the linea jugata (arrow) stabilizing the ulnar side of the ECU

structure that reinforces the ulnar insertion of the subsheath (Fig. 6.13) [46]. It is an important dynamic stabilizer that helps to prevent ECU tendon luxation during supination [33].

Ligaments of the Wrist

Wrist ligaments are responsible for stability through complex motion about the radiocarpal, ulnocarpal, and DRUJ. The ligaments of the wrist have been classified into two types. Distinction has been made between the extrinsic (radiocarpal and ulnocarpal) and the intrinsic (intercarpal) ligaments (Table 6.2) (Figs. 6.14, 6.15, and 6.16).

Intrinsic Ligaments

Proximal Interosseous Ligaments

There are two proximal intrinsic interosseous wrist ligaments: the scapholunate (SL) ligament and the lunotriquetral (LT) ligament. The proximal intrinsic ligaments cover the dorsal, proximal, and volar aspects of their joints, respectively, leaving the distal aspect open to communicate with the midcarpal joint (Fig. 6.14a, b) [3].

The SL ligament is U-shaped on sagittal section and has three separate zones: dorsal, proximal, and volar components. The dorsal and volar zones are ligamentous, whereas the proximal zone is fibrocartilaginous [10]. The SL ligament is the primary stabilizer of the scapholunate joint. The dorsal zone is the thickest and strongest situated between the proximal pole of the scaphoid and the dorsal portion of the lunate [47]. The volar zone is thin and oriented obliquely from palmar to dorsal progressing from the scaphoid to the lunate; therefore, it is less easily observed on conventional MRI. It combines with the radioscapholunate ligament proximally and inserts on the scaphoid with small connections to the radioscaphocapitate ligament distally [48]. The proximal zone is fibrocartilaginous, similar to the TFCC histologically. DISI can occur due to alteration of SL ligament integrity, with flexion of the scaphoid and extension of the lunate and triquetrum. A recent cadaveric study showed scaphotrapeziotrapezoid ligament or distal intercarpal ligament resection, in association with SL ligament resection, produced DISI [49].

The LT ligament is V-shaped on sagittal section with three separate zones: dorsal, proximal, and volar. The dorsal and volar zones are ligamentous, and the proximal zone is fibrocartilaginous [50]. The volar region is the thickest part and transmits the extension movement of the triquetrum [51]. The dorsal component functions as a restraint to rotation. The dorsal and volar zones of the LT ligament are biomechanically more important than the proximal zone. The proximal zone shows a triangular morphology in >85% of subjects; however, a variety of shapes and MR appearances have been reported [52, 53]. LT ligament instability and the associated capsular damage, typically to the dorsal radiocarpal and dorsal intercarpal ligament, result in VISI. The proximal zone of both SL ligament and LT ligament is best demonstrated on coronal plane (Fig. 6.15b), and the dorsal and volar zones are best identified on axial plane (Fig. 6.16).

Table 6.2 Intrinsic and extrinsic ligaments of the wrist. (Abbreviations in the figures)

Intrinsic ligaments
Proximal interosseous ligaments
Scapholunate ligament (SL)
Lunotriquetral ligament (LT)
Distal interosseous ligaments
Trapeziotrapezoid (TT) ligament
Trapezocapitate (TzC) ligament
Capitohamate (CH) ligament
Palmar midcarpal ligaments
Scaphotrapeziotrapezoid (STT) ligament
Scaphocapitate (SC) ligament
Triquetrocapitate (TC) ligament
Triquetrohamate (TH) ligament
Dorsal intercarpal/intrinsic ligaments (DIC)
Extrinsic ligaments
Radiocarpal
Dorsal radiocarpal (DRC) ligament
Radioscaphocapitate (RSC) ligament
Long radiolunate ligament (LRL)
Short radiolunate ligament (SRL)
Radial collateral ligament (RCL)
Radioscapholunate ligament
Ulnocarpal
Ulnocapitate (UC) ligament
Ulnolunate (UL) ligament
Ulnotriquetral (UT) ligament

Distal Interosseous Ligaments

There are three ligaments connecting the carpal bones of the distal row: trapeziotrapezoid (TT) ligament, trapezocapitate (TzC) ligament, and capitohamate (CH) ligament. Each ligament consists of at least a dorsal and a volar region. The dorsal and volar TT ligaments extend across the entire length of the dorsal and volar joint margin [3]. The TzC ligament includes three zones: the volar, dorsal, and the deep. The deep zone is the strongest crossing the central region of the joint in an angled notch. The CH ligament extends substantially onto the distal half of the volar and the dorsal cortices of the bone [54]. As with the TzC ligament, the deep CH ligament is a thick and square-shaped structure (Fig. 6.14b).

Palmar Midcarpal Ligaments

The four palmar midcarpal ligaments course from the scaphoid or triquetrum to the distal carpal row: the scaphotrapeziotrapezoid (STT) ligament, the scaphocapitate (SC) ligament, the triquetrocapitate (TC) ligament, and the triquetrohamate (TH) ligament (Fig. 6.14a). There is no direct connection between the lunate and the distal carpal row [3]. The STT ligament attaches to the radial and ulnar cortices of the distal pole of the scaphoid proximally. It passes distally to the palmar and radial aspect of the trapezium and the palmar surface of the trapezoid [55, 56]. The SC ligament attaches to the distal pole of the scaphoid proximally and the palmar cortex of the body of the capitate distally. The TC ligament attaches proximally to the distal and radial corner of the triquetrum and the ulnar cortex of the capitate [57]. The triquetrohamate ligament attaches to the distal margin of the palmar cortex of the triquetrum and extends distally to attach to the palmar cortex of the hamate body [54].

Dorsal Intercarpal/Intrinsic Ligaments

The dorsal intercarpal (DIC) ligaments attach the dorsal tubercle of the triquetrum proximally to the dorsal ridge and radial surface of the scaphoid and in half of individuals the dorsal cortex of the trapezoid (Figs. 6.14d and 6.15c) [3, 58]. The DIC ligaments play the role of a secondary stabilizer associated with the dorsal radiocarpal ligament; however, the SL ligament is the primary stabilizer of the scapholunate joint [48]. They form a lateral V-shaped structure with an apex in the triquetrum that stabilizes the dorsal scapholunate interval [58].

Extrinsic Ligaments

Radiocarpal Ligaments

On the volar side, the radioscaphocapitate (RSC) ligament and the long radiolunate (LRL) liga-

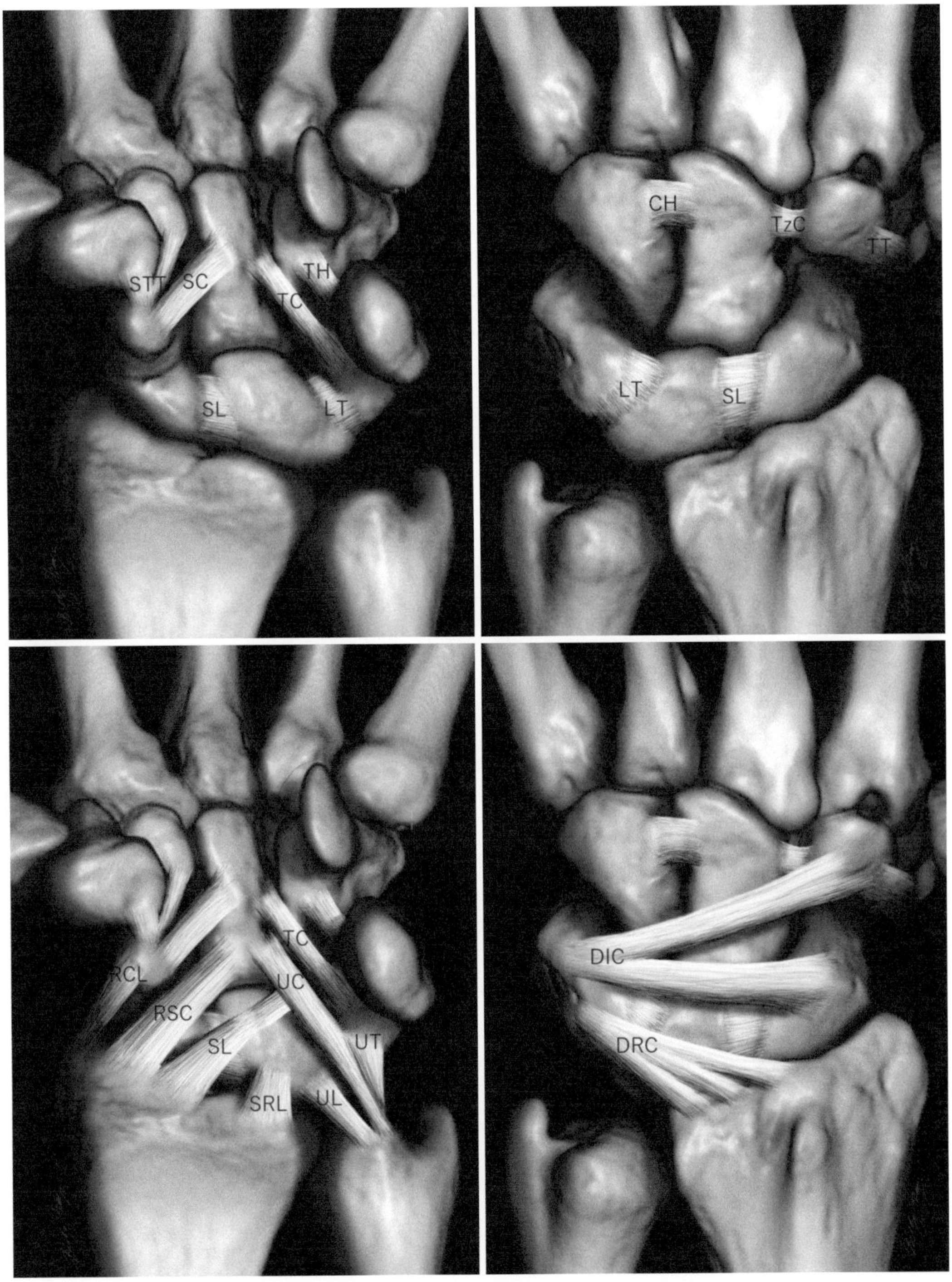

Fig. 6.14 Schematic drawing of the intrinsic and extrinsic ligaments. Volar intrinsic ligaments (**a**), dorsal deep intrinsic ligaments (**b**), volar extrinsic ligaments (**c**), and dorsal intercarpal/intrinsic and extrinsic ligaments (**d**). Abbreviations: see Table 6.2 for ligaments

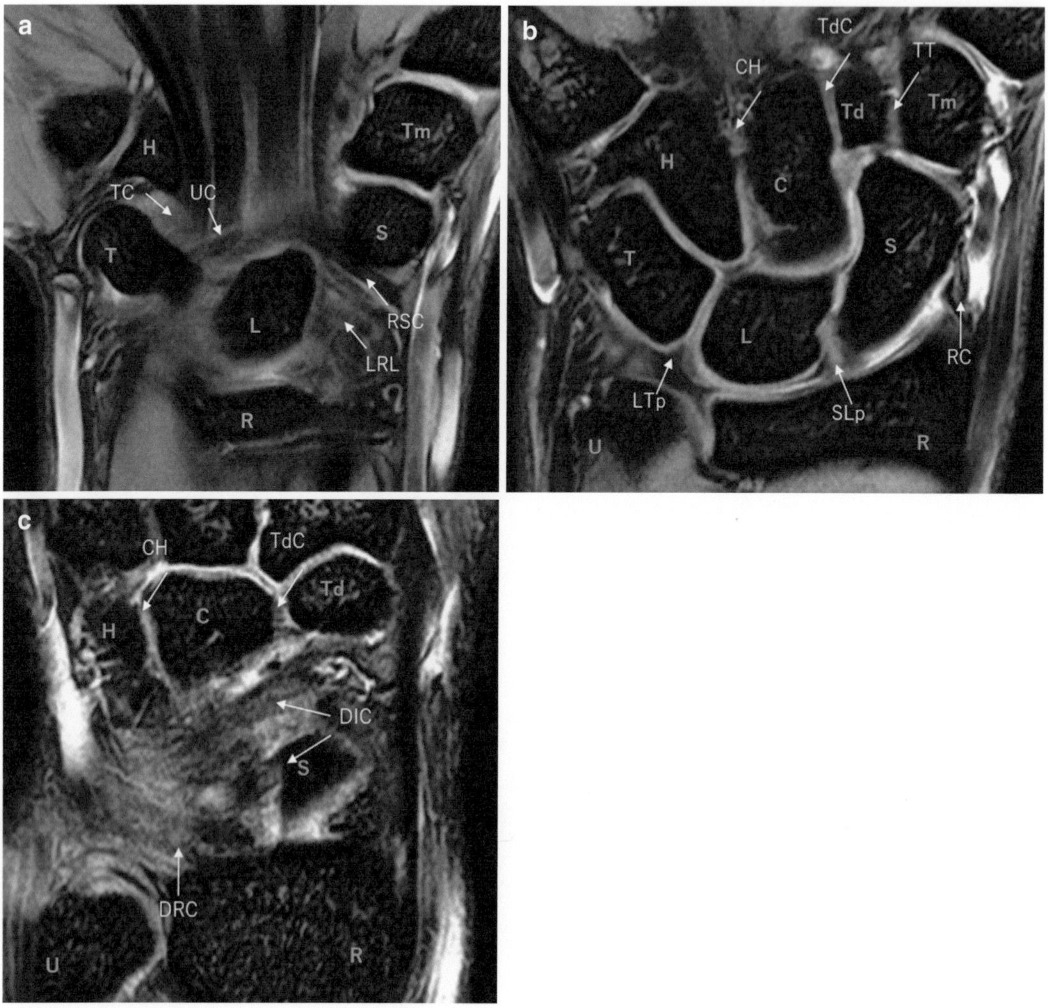

Fig. 6.15 Anatomical images of the wrist ligaments on T2*-weighted coronal images. The proximal zone of both SL ligament and LT ligament are best demonstrated on this plane. Abbreviations: see Table 6.2 for ligaments. d dorsal zone, v volar zone, p proximal zone, R radius, L ulna, S scaphoid, L lunate, T triquetrum, Tm trapezium, Td trapezoid, C capitate, H hamate

ment are the two main ligamentous stabilizers of the scapholunate joint (Figs. 6.13c and 6.14a) [48]. The RSC ligament is the most radial extrinsic ligament and forms the entire radial radiocarpal and a part of the palmar radiocarpal joint capsule [55]. It extends diagonally from the radial styloid process to the region of the middle of the scaphoid fossa with connection to the fibers from the ulnocapitate (UC) ligament [57]. This structure is also referred to as the palmar arcuate ligament [59]. The LRL ligament, or volar radiolunotriquetral ligament, extends from the distal palmar rim of the radius to terminate in the lunate at the radial aspect of its palmar cortex over the lunate [60]. It plays a role in stabilization of the lunate in extension [49]. The short radiolunate (SRL) ligament originates proximally from the entire width of the lunate fossa of the distal radius and attaches to the radial half of the palmar cortex of the lunate [61]. The radial collateral ligament (RCL) extends from the tip of the styloid process of the radius and inserts on the distal pole and waist of the scaphoid and the palmar surface of the trapezium [62]. Another volar-sided extrinsic ligament, the radioscapholunate ligament is found just ulnar to the long radiolunate ligament. There is some question as to whether this is a true ligament [63].

The dorsal radiocarpal (DRC) ligament (Figs. 6.14d and 6.15c), also called as the dorsal radiolunotriquetral ligament, is comprised of oblique fibers of approximately 1.5 mm thickness and attaches to the dorsal rim of the distal radius proximally and the dorsal cortex of the triquetrum, giving a firm attachment to the dorsoulnar corner of the lunate [64]. It is the most important dorsal extrinsic ligament to stabilize the lunate and scaphoid [65].

There are three identified ulnocarpal ligaments: the ulnocapitate (UC) ligament, the ulnolunate (UL) ligament, and the ulnotriquetral (UT) ligament (Figs. 6.14c and 6.15a). The UC ligament is the only ulnocarpal ligament that attaches directly to the ulnar head [66]. It attaches to the fovea region of the ulnar head proximally and interdigitates with the fibers of the RSC ligament distally as mentioned above.

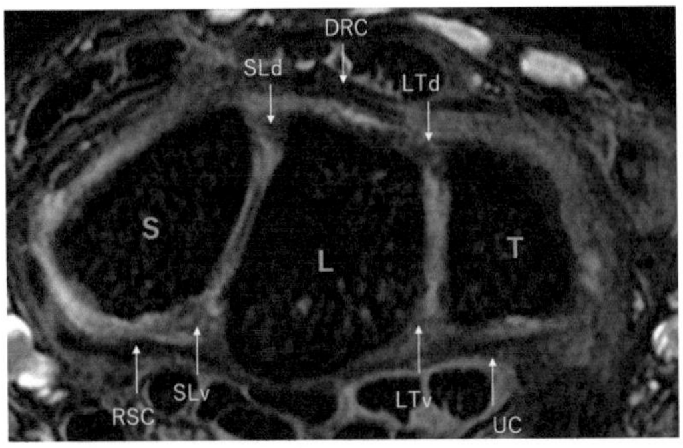

Fig. 6.16 Anatomical image of the ligaments on T2*-weighted axial image at the level of the proximal carpal row. The dorsal and volar zones are best identified on this plane. Abbreviations: S Scaphoid, L Lunate, T Triquetrum, SL Scapholunate ligament, LT Lunotriquetral ligament, RSC Radioscaphocapitate ligament, DRC Dorsal radiocarpal ligament, UC Ulnocapitate ligament, d Dorsal zone, v Volar zone

The Triangular Fibrocartilage Complex

The triangular fibrocartilage complex (TFCC) comprises the following structures: (1) triangular fibrocartilage disc, (2) radioulnar ligaments, (3) triangular ligament, (4) meniscal homologue, (5) ulnar collateral ligament (UCL), (6) volar ulnocarpal ligaments (ulnolunate and ulnotriquetral), and (7) extensor carpi ulnaris (ECU) tendon sheath (Figs. 6.17 and 6.18). The TFCC plays a role as the main stabilizer of the ulnar-sided wrist and the DRUJ. The TFCC articulates between the proximal carpal row and the distal ulna, facilitating smooth motion of the wrist, transmitting axial loads between the ulna and carpal bones, and serving as an extension of the proximal radial articular surface.

1. Triangular Fibrocartilage Disc

The triangular fibrocartilage disc appears as an asymmetric biconcave rectangular shape in the coronal plane (Fig. 6.17b, c). In contradistinction to the attachment of the dorsal and volar radioulnar ligaments mentioned later, there is a continuous transition from the central fibrocartilaginous disc to the hyaline cartilage of the sigmoid notch [67]. The shape of the disk remains constant throughout wrist motion when the ulnocarpal joint is stable. The morphology of the disc varies with ulnar variance [10]. The disc with the ulnar plus variance is thin and, therefore, more vulnerable to biomechanical stress.

2. Dorsal and Volar Radioulnar Ligaments

The dorsal and volar radioulnar ligaments form the main components of dorsal and volar marginal portion of the triangular fibrocartilage disc. The ligaments attach to the dorsal and volar rim of the distal radius directly at the level of the sigmoid notch and the middle and distal thirds of the styloid process via chondral-apophyseal entheses (Fig. 6.17a, b, d) [68]. The dorsal and volar radioulnar ligaments are well recognized in axial MR images (Fig. 6.18). The most superficial fibers of the dorsal radioulnar ligament contribute to the formation of the ECU tendon sheath ulnarly [22].

3. Triangular Ligament

The triangular ligament, a synonym of the ulnar side of the triangular fibrocartilage, anchors the

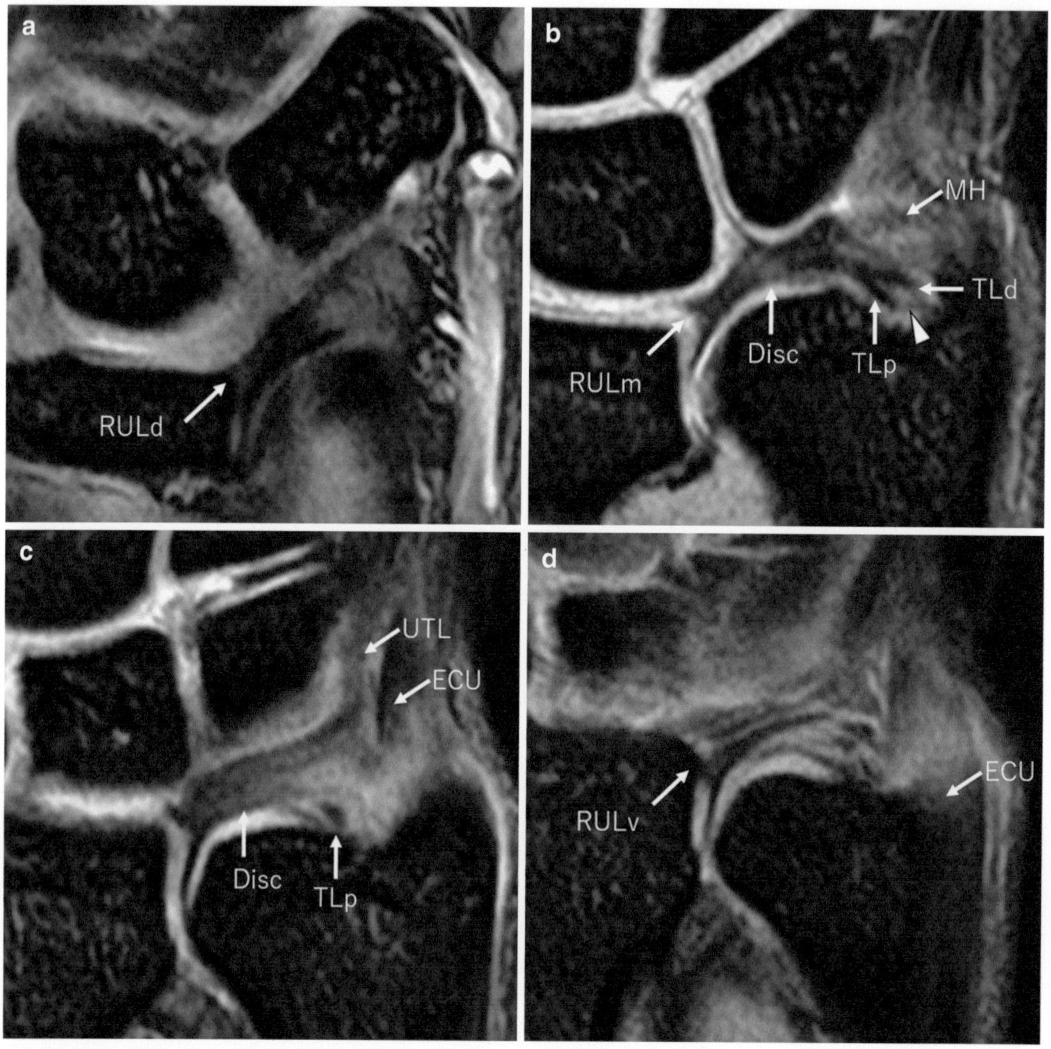

Fig. 6.17 Coronal anatomical images of the TFCC. Abbreviations: RULd distal radioulnar ligament dorsal attachment, RULm distal radioulnar ligament middle attachment, RULv distal radioulnar ligament volar attachment, TLp triangular ligament proximal lamina, TLd triangular ligament distal lamina, MH meniscus homologue, UTL ulnotriquetral ligament, ECU extensor carpi ulnaris tendon

disc of triangular fibrocartilage to the ulnar styloid process. It extends along the entire surface to the most proximal aspect of the fovea of the styloid process and the tip [67]. The triangular ligament usually bifurcates into two laminae (proximal and distal) as the ligament extends toward the ulna (Fig. 6.17b, c) [69]. The distal lamina inserts into the fibro- or hyaline-like cartilage of the tip of the ulnar styloid [70]. The normal MRI appearance of the triangular ligament is a band with striated pattern (arrowhead). The internal signal is higher compared with the disc, due to its histological structure as a combination of collagen fibers and vascular-rich connective tissue [71].

4. Meniscal Homologue

The meniscal homologue is an inconsistent structure formed by a thickening of the ulnar side of the joint capsule. The meniscal homologue extends from the ulnar styloid to the dorsal edge of the triquetrum, the hamate, and the base of the fifth metacarpal [72]. It is best depicted in the coronal plane as a triangle-shaped structure with hypointense signal (Fig. 6.17b). The prestyloid recess is a synovium-lined saccular space bordered by the meniscal homologue distally, the TFCC attachments to the ulnar styloid process proximally, and the central TFCC disk radially [73]. Commonly there is a direct connection to the rest of the radiocarpal compartment.

5. Ulnar Collateral Ligament

The concept of the UCL is nebulous but considered as the loose connective tissue that extends from the horizontal portion of the TFCC to join the subsheath of the ECU [74].

6. Volar Ulnocarpal Ligaments (ulnotriquetral and ulnolunate ligaments)

The UT and UL ligaments both originate proximally from the volar radioulnar ligament.

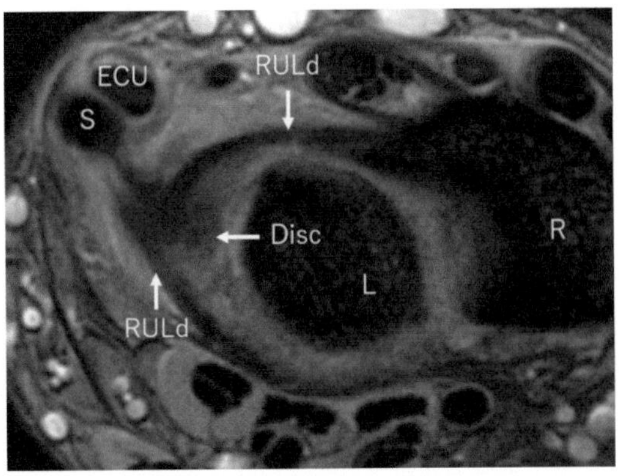

Fig. 6.18 Axial image of the TFCC. Abbreviations: RULd distal radioulnar ligament dorsal attachment, RULv distal radioulnar ligament volar attachment, ECU extensor carpi ulnaris tendon, R radius, S styloid process

(3) They stabilize the lunate and, therefore, the proximal row of the carpal bones [61]. The UT ligament is intimately associated with the meniscal homologue. There is no direct attachment to the ulna. Assessment of their proximal attachment on MRI can be difficult because of the heterogeneous appearance due to the interspersed vascular loose connective tissue [75, 76]. Also, there is no clear demarcation between the UL and the UT ligaments proximally, but there are distinct attachment sites distally (Fig. 6.17c) [3].

7. Extensor Carpi Ulnaris (ECU) Subsheath

The ECU courses along the dorsolateral aspect of the ulnocarpal joint, is situated within the ulnar notch, and covered by fibrous tissue referred to as the ECU subsheath (Fig. 6.17c, d) [72]. As described above, a part of the dorsal radioulnar ligament and the dorsal radial metaphyseal arcuate ligament merge and reinforce the ECU subsheath [55]. They are further reinforced by the extensor retinaculum and ulnar collateral ligament which blends with the ECU subsheath. The ECU subsheath is an important stabilizer of the ulnar side of the TFCC.

Imaging Protocols for the Wrist

Thin and contiguous slices with high signal-to-noise ratio are essential to evaluate the structures in the wrist joint as above discussed. Our routine noncontrast 3T wrist MR protocol is included in Table 6.3. Higher magnetic field such as 3T, with adequate coil selection such as wrist coil or microcoils for small field of view, is required. For

Table 6.3 Routine wrist MR protocol

Sequence	FOV	TR/TE	ST	SG	Matrix
Coronal T2FS	10 cm	3500–4000/60–90	3 mm	0.3 mm	320
Coronal T1	10 cm	450–500/13–15	3 mm	0.3 mm	320
Coronal PD 3D	10 cm	2000–2500/18–30	1.4 mm	0	288
3D reconstructed in axial and sagittal					
Sagittal T1	10 cm	450–500/13–15	3 mm	0.3 mm	384
Axial T2FS	10 cm	3500–4000/60–90	2.5 mm	0.5 mm	320
Axial T1	10 cm	600–850/10–15	2.5 mm	0.5 mm	384

Abbreviations: *FOV* field of view, *TR* repetition time, *TE* echo time, *ST* slice thickness, *SG* slice gap the SLL injury evaluation, higher specificity at 3T compared with 1.5T is demonstrated in the recent meta-analysis study; however, that of MR arthrography with 3T was still superior. MRA may be considered when higher diagnostic performance is demanded to avoid invasive arthroscopy [77].

Acknowledgments All healthy wrist images were acquired on a Vantage Galan 3T, Canon Medical Systems.

Authors thank Ms. Christine Duxbury and Mr. Yurian Falls of Canon Medical for their supports in parameter optimizations and acquisitions.

References

1. Metz VM, Wunderbaldinger P, Gilula LA. Update on imaging techniques of the wrist and hand. Clin Plast Surg. 1996;23(3):369–84.
2. Resnik CS. Wrist and hand injuries. Semin Musculoskelet Radiol. 2000;4(2):193–204.
3. Berger RA. The anatomy of the ligaments of the wrist and distal radioulnar joints. Clin Orthop Relat Res. 2001;383:32–40.
4. Viegas SF, Patterson RM, Hokanson JA, Davis J. Wrist anatomy: incidence, distribution, and correlation of anatomic variations, tears, and arthrosis. J Hand Surg Am. 1993;18(3):463–75.
5. Pfirrmann CW, Theumann NH, Chung CB, Trudell DJ, Resnick D. The hamatolunate facet: characterization and association with cartilage lesions--magnetic resonance arthrography and anatomic correlation in cadaveric wrists. Skeletal Radiol. 2002;31(8):451–6.
6. Goldfarb CA, Yin Y, Gilula LA, Fisher AJ, Boyer MI. Wrist fractures: what the clinician wants to know. Radiology. 2001;219(1):11–28.
7. Zanetti M, Hodler J, Gilula LA. Assessment of dorsal or ventral intercalated segmental instability configurations of the wrist: reliability of sagittal MR images. Radiology. 1998;206(2):339–45.
8. Weissman BNW, Sledge C. Orthopedic radiology. Philadelphia: Saunders; 1986. p. 111–67.
9. Solgaard S. Angle of inclination of the articular surface of the distal radius. Radiologe. 1984;24(7):346–8.
10. Vezeridis PS, Yoshioka H, Han R, Blazar P. Ulnar-sided wrist pain. Part I: anatomy and physical examination. Skeletal Radiol. 2010;39(8):733–45.
11. Mann FA, Wilson AJ, Gilula LA. Radiographic evaluation of the wrist: what does the hand surgeon want to know? Radiology. 1992;184(1):15–24.
12. Cerezal L, del Pinal F, Abascal F, Garcia-Valtuille R, Pereda T, Canga A. Imaging findings in ulnar-sided wrist impaction syndromes. Radiographics. 2002;22(1):105–21.
13. Imaeda T, Nakamura R, Shionoya K, Makino N. Ulnar impaction syndrome: MR imaging findings. Radiology. 1996;201(2):495–500.
14. van Leeuwen WF, Oflazoglu K, Menendez ME, Ring D. Negative ulnar variance and Kienböck disease. J Hand Surg Am. 2016;41(2):214–8.
15. Stahl S, Stahl AS, Meisner C, Hentschel PJH, Valina S, Luz O, Schaller HE, Lotter O. Critical analysis of causality between negative ulnar variance and Kienböck disease. Plast Reconstr Surg. 2013;132(4):899–909.
16. Gross MS, Gelberman RH. The anatomy of the distal ulnar tunnel. Clin Orthop Relat Res. 1985;196:238–47.
17. Brooks JJ, Schiller JR, Allen SD, Akelman E. Biomechanical and anatomical consequences of carpal tunnel release. Clin Biomech (Bristol, Avon). 2003;18(8):685–93.
18. Goitz RJ, Fowler JR, Li ZM. The transverse carpal ligament: anatomy and clinical implications. J Wrist Surg. 2014;3(4):233–4.
19. Zeiss J, Jakab E, Khimji T, Imbriglia J. The ulnar tunnel at the wrist (Guyon's canal): normal MR anatomy and variants. AJR Am J Roentgenol. 1992;158(5):1081–5.
20. Blum AG, Zabel JP, Kohlmann R, Batch T, Barbara K, Zhu X, et al. Pathologic conditions of the hypothenar eminence: evaluation with multidetector CT and MR imaging. Radiographics. 2006;26(4):1021–44.
21. Ghasemi-Rad M, Nosair E, Vegh A, Mohammadi A, Akkad A, Lesha E, et al. A handy review of carpal tunnel syndrome: from anatomy to diagnosis and treatment. World J Radiol. 2014;6(6):284–300.
22. Lewis OJ, Hamshere RJ, Bucknill TM. The anatomy of the wrist joint. J Anat. 1970;106(Pt 3):539–52.
23. Cobb TK, Dalley BK, Posteraro RH, Lewis RC. Anatomy of the flexor retinaculum. J Hand Surg Am. 1993;18(1):91–9.
24. Robbins H. Anatomical study of the median nerve in the carpal tunnel and etiologies of the carpal-tunnel syndrome. J Bone Joint Surg Am. 1963;45:953–66.
25. Demircay E, Civelek E, Cansever T, Kabatas S, Yilmaz C. Anatomic variations of the median nerve in the carpal tunnel: a brief review of the literature. Turk Neurosurg. 2011;21(3):388–96.
26. Lanz U. Anatomical variations of the median nerve in the carpal tunnel. J Hand Surg Am. 1977;2(1):44–53.
27. Henry BM, Zwinczewska H, Roy J, Vikse J, Ramakrishnan PK, Walocha JA, et al. The prevalence of anatomical variations of the median nerve in the carpal tunnel: a systematic review and meta-analysis. PLoS One. 2015;10(8):e0136477.
28. Beris AE, Lykissas MG, Kontogeorgakos VA, Vekris MD, Korompilias AV. Anatomic variations of the median nerve in carpal tunnel release. Clin Anat. 2008;21(6):514–8.
29. Gassner EM, Schocke M, Peer S, Schwabegger A, Jaschke W, Bodner G. Persistent median artery in the carpal tunnel: color Doppler ultrasonographic findings. J Ultrasound Med. 2002;21(4):455–61.

30. Resnick D. Roentgenographic anatomy of the tendon sheaths of the hand and wrist: tenography. Am J Roentgenol Radium Ther Nucl Med. 1975;124(1):44–51.
31. Aguiar RO, Gasparetto EL, Escuissato DL, Marchiori E, Trudell DJ, Haghighi P, et al. Radial and ulnar bursae of the wrist: cadaveric investigation of regional anatomy with ultrasonographic-guided tenography and MR imaging. Skeletal Radiol. 2006;35(11):828–32.
32. Palmer AK, Skahen JR, Werner FW, Glisson RR. The extensor retinaculum of the wrist: an anatomical and biomechanical study. J Hand Surg Br. 1985;10(1):11–6.
33. Taleisnik J, Gelberman RH, Miller BW, Szabo RM. The extensor retinaculum of the wrist. J Hand Surg Am. 1984;9(4):495–501.
34. Motoura H, Shiozaki K, Kawasaki K. Anatomical variations in the tendon sheath of the first compartment. Anat Sci Int. 2010;85(3):145–51.
35. Roy AJ, Roy AN, De C, Banerji D, Das S, Chatterjee B, et al. A cadaveric study of the first dorsal compartment of the wrist and its content tendons: anatomical variations in the Indian population. J Hand Microsurg. 2012;4(2):55–9.
36. Leao L. De Quervain's disease; a clinical and anatomical study. J Bone Joint Surg Am. 1958;40-A(5):1063–70.
37. Choi SJ, Ahn JH, Lee YJ, Ryu DS, Lee JH, Jung SM, et al. de Quervain disease: US identification of anatomic variations in the first extensor compartment with an emphasis on subcompartmentalization. Radiology. 2011;260(2):480–6.
38. Chang CY, Kheterpal AB, Vicentini JRT, Huang AJ. Variations of anatomy on MRI of the first extensor compartment of the wrist and association with DeQuervain tenosynovitis. Skeletal Radiol. 2017;46(8):1047–56.
39. Gurses IA, Turkay R, Inci E, Ors S, Onal Y, Ozel S, et al. Sex differences in the radial grooves in the first extensor compartment. Skeletal Radiol. 2016;45(7):955–8.
40. Rousset P, Vuillemin-Bodaghi V, Laredo JD, Parlier-Cuau C. Anatomic variations in the first extensor compartment of the wrist: accuracy of US. Radiology. 2010;257(2):427–33.
41. de Lima JE, Kim HJ, Albertotti F, Resnick D. Intersection syndrome: MR imaging with anatomic comparison of the distal forearm. Skeletal Radiol. 2004;33(11):627–31.
42. Lee RP, Hatem SF, Recht MP. Extended MRI findings of intersection syndrome. Skeletal Radiol. 2009;38(2):157–63.
43. Massaki AN, Tan J, Huang BK, Chang EY, Trudell DJ, Resnick DL. Extensor retinaculum of the wrist: gross anatomical correlation with MR imaging after ultrasound-guided tenography with emphasis on anatomical features in wrist dorsiflexion responsible for tendon impingement. Skeletal Radiol. 2013;42(12):1727–37.
44. Parellada AJ, Gopez AG, Morrison WB, Sweet S, Leinberry CF, Reiter SB, et al. Distal intersection tenosynovitis of the wrist: a lesser-known extensor tendinopathy with characteristic MR imaging features. Skeletal Radiol. 2007;36(3):203–8.
45. Pfirrmann CW, Theumann NH, Chung CB, Botte MJ, Trudell DJ, Resnick D. What happens to the triangular fibrocartilage complex during pronation and supination of the forearm? Analysis of its morphology and diagnostic assessment with MR arthrography. Skeletal Radiol. 2001;30(12):677–85.
46. Carneiro RS, Fontana R, Mazzer N. Ulnar wrist pain in athletes caused by erosion of the floor of the sixth dorsal compartment: a case series. Am J Sports Med. 2005;33(12):1910–3.
47. Berger RA. The gross and histologic anatomy of the scapholunate interosseous ligament. J Hand Surg Am. 1996;21(2):170–8.
48. Rajan PV, Day CS. Scapholunate interosseous ligament anatomy and biomechanics. J Hand Surg Am. 2015;40(8):1692–702.
49. Perez AJ, Jethanandani RG, Vutescu ES, Meyers KN, Lee SK, Wolfe SW. Role of ligament stabilizers of the proximal carpal row in preventing dorsal intercalated segment instability: a cadaveric study. J Bone Joint Surg Am. 2019;101(15):1388–96.
50. Johnstone DJ, Thorogood S, Smith WH, Scott TD. A comparison of magnetic resonance imaging and arthroscopy in the investigation of chronic wrist pain. J Hand Surg Br. 1997;22(6):714–8.
51. Zlatkin MB, Chao PC, Osterman AL, Schnall MD, Dalinka MK, Kressel HY. Chronic wrist pain: evaluation with high-resolution MR imaging. Radiology. 1989;173(3):723–9.
52. Smith DK, Snearly WN. Lunotriquetral interosseous ligament of the wrist: MR appearances in asymptomatic volunteers and arthrographically normal wrists. Radiology. 1994;191(1):199–202.
53. Yoshioka H, Tanaka T, Ueno T, Shindo M, Carrino JA, Lang P, et al. High-resolution MR imaging of the proximal zone of the lunotriquetral ligament with a microscopy coil. Skeletal Radiol. 2006;35(5):288–94.
54. Ritt MJ, Bishop AT, Berger RA, Linscheid RL, Berglund LJ, An KN. Lunotriquetral ligament properties: a comparison of three anatomic subregions. J Hand Surg Am. 1998;23(3):425–31.
55. Berger RA. The ligaments of the wrist. A current overview of anatomy with considerations of their potential functions. Hand Clin. 1997;13(1):63–82.
56. Drewniany JJ, Palmer AK, Flatt AE. The scaphotrapezial ligament complex: an anatomic and biomechanical study. J Hand Surg Am. 1985;10(4):492–8.
57. Taleisnik J. The ligaments of the wrist. J Hand Surg Am. 1976;1(2):110–8.
58. Viegas SF, Yamaguchi S, Boyd NL, Patterson RM. The dorsal ligaments of the wrist: anatomy, mechanical properties, and function. J Hand Surg Am. 1999;24(3):456–68.

59. Chang W, Peduto AJ, Aguiar RO, Trudell DJ, Resnick DL. Arcuate ligament of the wrist: normal MR appearance and its relationship to palmar midcarpal instability: a cadaveric study. Skeletal Radiol. 2007;36(7):641–5.
60. Mak WH, Szabo RM, Myo GK. Assessment of volar radiocarpal ligaments: MR arthrographic and arthroscopic correlation. AJR Am J Roentgenol. 2012;198(2):423–7.
61. Shahabpour M, De Maeseneer M, Pouders C, Van Overstraeten L, Ceuterick P, Fierens Y, et al. MR imaging of normal extrinsic wrist ligaments using thin slices with clinical and surgical correlation. Eur J Radiol. 2011;77(2):196–201.
62. Siegel DB, Gelberman RH. Radial styloidectomy: an anatomical study with special reference to radiocarpal intracapsular ligamentous morphology. J Hand Surg Am. 1991;16(1):40–4.
63. Berger RA. Arthroscopic anatomy of the wrist and distal radioulnar joint. Hand Clin. 1999;15(3):393–413, vii.
64. Mizuseki T, Ikuta Y. The dorsal carpal ligaments: their anatomy and function. J Hand Surg Br. 1989;14(1):91–8.
65. Mitsuyasu H, Patterson RM, Shah MA, Buford WL, Iwamoto Y, Viegas SF. The role of the dorsal intercarpal ligament in dynamic and static scapholunate instability. J Hand Surg Am. 2004;29(2):279–88.
66. Garcia-Elias M. Soft-tissue anatomy and relationships about the distal ulna. Hand Clin. 1998;14(2):165–76.
67. Benjamin M, Evans EJ, Pemberton DJ. Histological studies on the triangular fibrocartilage complex of the wrist. J Anat. 1990;172:59–67.
68. Horiuchi S, Nimura A, Tsutsumi M, Suzuki S, Fujita K, Nozaki T, et al. Anatomical relationship between the morphology of the styloid process of the ulna and the attachment of the radioulnar ligaments. J Anat. 2020;237:1032–9.
69. Yoshioka H, Tanaka T, Ueno T, Carrino JA, Winalski CS, Aliabadi P, et al. Study of ulnar variance with high-resolution MRI: correlation with triangular fibrocartilage complex and cartilage of ulnar side of wrist. J Magn Reson Imaging. 2007;26(3):714–9.
70. Nakamura T, Takayama S, Horiuchi Y, Yabe Y. Origins and insertions of the triangular fibrocartilage complex: a histological study. J Hand Surg Br. 2001;26(5):446–54.
71. Cody ME, Nakamura DT, Small KM, Yoshioka H. MR imaging of the triangular fibrocartilage complex. Magn Reson Imaging Clin N Am. 2015;23(3):393–403.
72. Zhan HL, Li WT, Bai RJ, Wang NL, Qian ZH, Ye W, et al. High-resolution 3T magnetic resonance imaging of the triangular fibrocartilage complex in Chinese wrists: correlation with cross-sectional anatomy. Chin Med J (Engl). 2017;130(7):817–22.
73. Milz S, Sicking B, Sprecher CM, Putz R, Benjamin M. An immunohistochemical study of the triangular fibrocartilage complex of the wrist: regional variations in cartilage phenotype. J Anat. 2007;211(1):1–7.
74. Daunt N. Magnetic resonance imaging of the wrist: anatomy and pathology of interosseous ligaments and the triangular fibrocartilage complex. Curr Probl Diagn Radiol. 2002;31(4):158–76.
75. Chidgey LK, Dell PC, Bittar ES, Spanier SS. Histologic anatomy of the triangular fibrocartilage. J Hand Surg Am. 1991;16(6):1084–100.
76. Kauer JM. The articular disc of the hand. Acta Anat (Basel). 1975;93(4):590–605.
77. Hafezi-Nejad N, Carrino JA, Eng J, Blackmore C, Shores J, Lifchez SD, et al. Scapholunate interosseous ligament tears: diagnostic performance of 1.5 T, 3 T MRI, and MR arthrography-A systematic review and meta-analysis. Acad Radiol. 2016;23(9):1091–103.

Wrist Pathology – Traumatic

7

Teresa T. Martin-Carreras and Jenny T. Bencardino

Background

The wrist has frequently been regarded as the most complex joint in the human body [1, 2]. Composed of multiple small carpal joints, it allows for substantial motion in the sagittal and coronal planes. Coupled with the radioulnar joints, it also facilitates three-dimensional rotational movements about the longitudinal axis of the forearm [2]. Additionally, it also serves as one of the main functional joints of daily activities, making it especially susceptible to traumatic injuries [3]. In the last two decades, magnetic resonance (MR) imaging of the wrist has seen remarkable advancements and has greatly benefitted from the use of dedicated surface coils and increasing magnetic field strength. Today's MR imaging capabilities allow us to noninvasively finely depict smaller and more subtle osseous, soft tissue, and cartilaginous pathology [4]. As a result, MR imaging of the wrist has become an instrumental asset in rendering accurate diagnoses and facilitating subsequent treatment.

Excellent anatomic detail can be elucidated using T1-weighted and high-resolution proton density images. T2-weighted images are useful in demonstrating alterations in water content seen in many pathologic conditions. In addition, fluid-sensitive sequences such as T2-weighted fat-suppressed sequences and short tau inversion recovery (STIR) can serve to highlight the differences between low-signal ligaments, tendons, triangular fibrocartilage complex (TFCC), and abnormal free water content in the setting of pathology. A 3T system is preferable, as it can provide nearly twofold in signal-to-noise (SNR) ratio, and dedicated multichannel phase-array surface coils should be used when imaging the wrist. Sequences should be obtained in the axial, oblique sagittal, and oblique coronal planes. Magnetic resonance arthrography (MRA) can also provide additional benefits including joint distention, increased contrast-to-noise ratio, and assessment of abnormal patterns of compartmental communication [4, 5].

Osseous Injuries

Scaphoid Fractures

The scaphoid is the most commonly injured carpal bone, accounting for 60% of all carpal fractures. The most common mechanism of

T. T. Martin-Carreras (✉)
Department of Radiology, Division of Musculoskeletal Imaging and Intervention, University of Wisconsin Hospital and Clinics, Madison, WI, USA
e-mail: TMartin-Carreras@uwhealth.org

J. T. Bencardino
Department of Radiology, Division of Musculoskeletal Imaging, Hospital of the University of Pennsylvania, Philadelphia, PA, USA

B. U. Casagranda (ed.), *MRI of the Upper Extremity*, https://doi.org/10.1007/978-3-030-81612-4_7

injury is a fall on an outstretched hand (FOOSH), typically with the wrist in greater than 90-degree dorsiflexion. Injury may also occur from a direct blow or excess axial loading with the wrist in flexion and extension [6, 7]. Patients may present with minimal swelling, mildly decreased range of motion, snuffbox tenderness, and/or radial-sided wrist pain [6]. Fractures of the waist account for two-thirds of all scaphoid fractures, and the majority are non-displaced (Fig. 7.1). Fractures of the distal third/pole of the scaphoid represent 25% of scaphoid fractures, and fractures of the proximal third/pole of the scaphoid occur in 5–10% of cases [7]. The Herbert classification system is most commonly used because it's primarily based on the distinction between stable (type A) and unstable (type B) (Fig. 7.2) acute scaphoid fractures, a difference which guides clinical and operative management. Scaphoid tubercle fractures and incomplete waist fractures are considered stable in the Herbert classification system, whereas comminuted fractures, fracture dislocations, oblique distal pole fractures, proximal pole fractures, and complete/displaced waist fractures are considered unstable. Delayed unions (type C) and established nonunion (type D) are also included in the classification system [6].

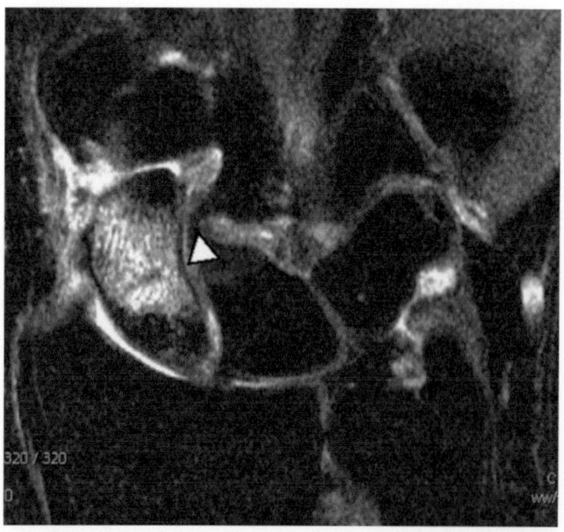

Fig. 7.1 *Stable scaphoid fracture*. Coronal fat-suppressed T2-weighted image demonstrates an incomplete stable scaphoid waist fracture line (arrowhead) outlined by bone marrow edema representing contusions of the distal pole and scaphoid waist

If a scaphoid fracture is suspected, initial imaging typically begins with wrist radiography. However, a large meta-analysis revealed that scaphoid fractures are not identified on initial radiographs in 16% of cases [8]. If initial radiographs are negative for fracture but there remains clinical concern for scaphoid fracture, one of two options may then be enacted. One option is to place the patient in a thumb spica short arm cast and repeat wrist radiographs in 10–14 days. Alternatively, the second option is to obtain MR imaging of the wrist [9]. MR imaging has been shown to have sensitivity and specificity nearing 100% for scaphoid fracture detection. It also avoids radiation and prevents unnecessary immobilization and lost productivity in negative cases, an important consideration in the athletic population [6].

On MR images, fractures are seen as a low signal intensity line on all MR sequences. Bone contusions describe an occult injury of the trabecular bone without an obvious fracture line and may be referred to as a "microfracture." MR is also very sensitive at detecting bone contusions which appear as high signal intensity on STIR and T2-weighted fat-suppressed images [10].

Missed scaphoid fractures can result in serious consequences including fracture nonunion (Fig. 7.3). Eventually, nonunion can progress to posttraumatic osteoarthritis and carpal collapse secondary to carpal instability, an entity known as scaphoid nonunion advanced collapse (SNAC) wrist.

Fractures of the scaphoid distal pole have a better prognosis than fractures of the proximal pole related to the retrograde blood supply to the scaphoid. Blood vessels originating from the dorsal carpal branch of the radial artery enter the scaphoid through a capsular insertion on the dorsal ridge. They account for 70–80% of the scaphoid's intra-osseous blood supply, and they represent the only vascular supply to the proximal pole. On the palmar side, superficial palmar branch vessels from the radial artery enter at the palmar lateral aspect of the scaphoid tubercle accounting for 20–30% of the blood supply to the scaphoid, but only to the distal pole [11].

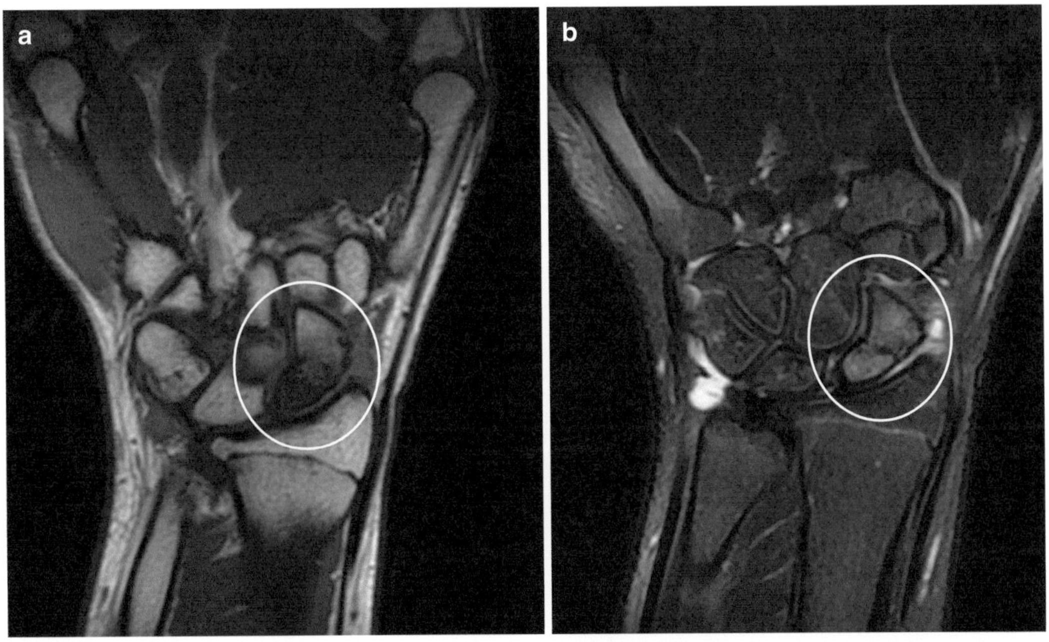

Fig. 7.2 *Unstable scaphoid fracture.* Coronal T1-weighted image (**a**) and coronal T2-weighted fat-suppressed image (**b**) demonstrate an unstable obliquely oriented fracture of the scaphoid extending from the waist to the proximal pole with diffuse bone marrow edema throughout the scaphoid

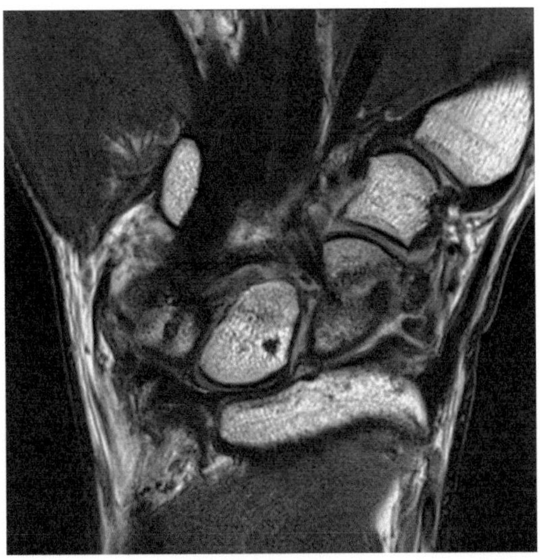

Fig. 7.3 *Scaphoid nonunion advanced collapse (SNAC).* Coronal T1-weighted image demonstrates SNAC wrist posttraumatic osteoarthritis at the articulation of the distal scaphoid fragment and radial scaphoid fossa

Scaphoid Nonunion

Nonunion is typically defined as being present when there are imaging signs consistent with the lack of fracture healing (i.e., sclerosis/neocortex, cyst formation, collapse, and bone resorption) or when osseous bridging has not occurred over a period of 6 months from the time of fracture. Causes of nonunion are multifactorial and include a delay in beginning treatment, displacement of fracture fragments, inadequate immobilization, instability due to ligamentous injury, and inadequate blood supply of the proximal fragment [12]. Scaphoid nonunion can lead to avascular necrosis, also known as osteonecrosis (Fig. 7.4). When fracture nonunion involves the middle third of the scaphoid, the incidence of osteonecrosis is 30%. However, when fracture nonunion involves the proximal one-fifth of the scaphoid, the incidence increases to 100%. The

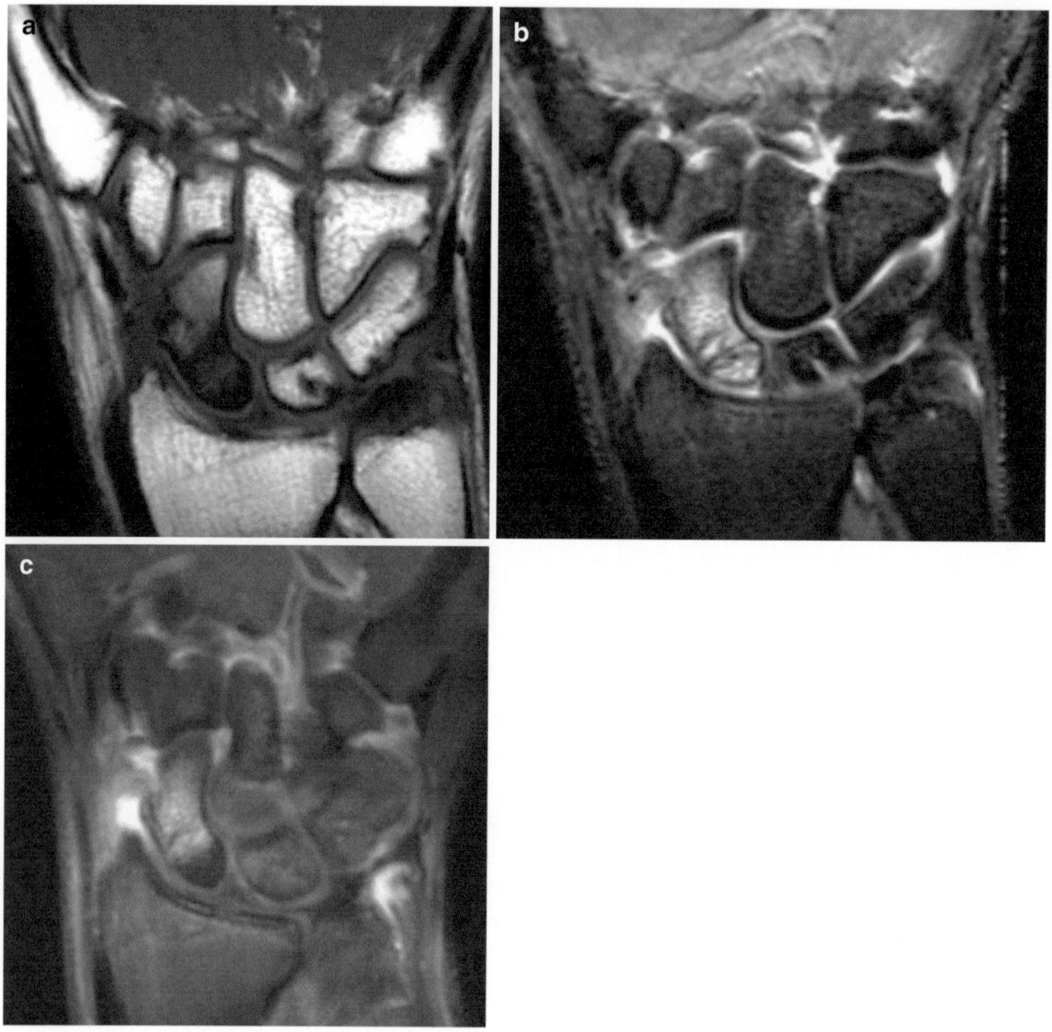

Fig. 7.4 *Avascular necrosis in the setting of scaphoid nonunion*. A 30-year-old male presents with persistent wrist pain 9 months after trauma. Coronal T1-weighted (**a**) and coronal T2-weighted fat-suppressed (**b**) images reveal scaphoid fracture nonunion with loss of normal fat marrow signal and diffuse bone marrow edema throughout the bone. Postcontrast coronal T1-weighted fat-suppressed imaging (**c**) shows increased enhancement in region of bone marrow edema distal to the fracture. However, the edematous bone proximal to the fracture is hypointense even when compared to the normally enhancing adjacent carpal bones. Findings are concerning for avascular necrosis. (Case is courtesy of Dr. Bethany Casagranda)

viability of the proximal fragment determines whether a nonvascularized or vascularized bone graft is used. MR imaging is the modality of choice to assess the viability of the proximal fracture fragment in cases of scaphoid nonunion. However, the most reliable MR imaging protocol for this purpose is not universally agreed upon [13]. Several studies have shown that delayed contrast enhancement MR images can predict the viability of the proximal fracture fragment better than non-contrast images when surgical punctate bleeding points of the proximal pole are used as a reference standard [14, 15]. A separate study compared delayed contrast-enhanced MR imaging with dynamic contrast-enhanced MR imaging and found that delayed contrast-enhanced imaging was superior [16]. However, Anderson et al. found a poor correlation between delayed contrast enhancement when compared to intraoperative findings of osteonecrosis (54% sensitivity). Meanwhile, their study found that confluent decreased T1 signal in the proximal fragment on non-contrast images had a sensitivity of 100% for detection of osteonecrosis when compared to intraoperative findings [17].

Ulnocarpal Abutment Syndrome

Ulnocarpal abutment syndrome is a condition which results from distinct ulnar-sided pathology resulting from abutment of the distal end of the ulna against the ulnar-sided carpus. This syndrome is often seen in patients with ulnar positive variance, malunion of the distal radius, Madelung deformity, trauma that impacts the growth of the distal radius relative to the ulna, and elbow or forearm trauma, such as radial head or Essex-Lopresti injury patterns [18]. While more commonly seen in patients with ulnar positive variance, it can also be seen in patients with neutral or ulnar negative variance. Prolonged impaction leads to degenerative changes of the triangular fibrocartilage complex (discussed later in the chapter); chondromalacia of the lunate, triquetrum, and distal ulnar head; resultant instability of the lunotriquetral joint; and ultimately degenerative arthrosis of the ulnocarpal and distal radioulnar joint (DRUJ) [19]. MR findings include focal abnormal signal intensity of the ulnar aspect of the lunate, of the radial aspect of the triquetrum, or less commonly of the radial aspect of the ulnar head. Subchondral bone marrow edema which can be seen on fat-suppressed T2-weighted and STIR images is often an indirect sign of chondromalacia and an early finding of ulnocarpal abutment syndrome (Fig. 7.5). With syndrome progression, subchondral sclerosis may be seen as areas of low signal intensity on T1-weighted images and high signal intensity on T2-weighted images. Subchondral cysts can also be seen as well-defined areas of low signal intensity on T1 and high signal intensity on T2-weighted images [18].

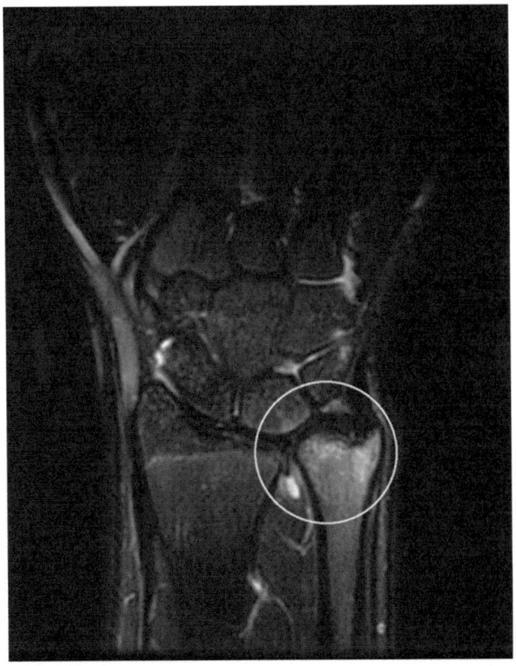

Fig. 7.5 *Ulnocarpal abutment.* Coronal fat-suppressed T2-weighted image demonstrates early signs of ulnocarpal abutment including bone marrow edema of the distal ulna and ulnar aspect of the lunate (white circle). Positive ulnar variance is also present

Kienböck's Disease

Kienböck's disease is a progressive and debilitating process characterized by avascular necrosis of the lunate. Patients most commonly present with pain in the dorsal aspect of the wrist at the radiolunate facet, decreased range of motion, swelling, and weakness of the affected hand. Many patients endorse a history of trauma; however, this history may not always be present. The cause of Kienböck's disease remains in debate; however, it is likely multifactorial and results from varying degrees of anatomic factors (e.g., negative ulnar variance, oblong or square lunate geometry), disrupted vascularity, and traumatic insults to the lunate [20, 21]. A number of staging systems exist for Kienböck's disease classification, with the Lichtman staging system often regarded as having the most clinical relevance. The classification consists of four stages with two subclassifications for stage 3. In stage 1, radiographs are normal, and MR imaging is particu-

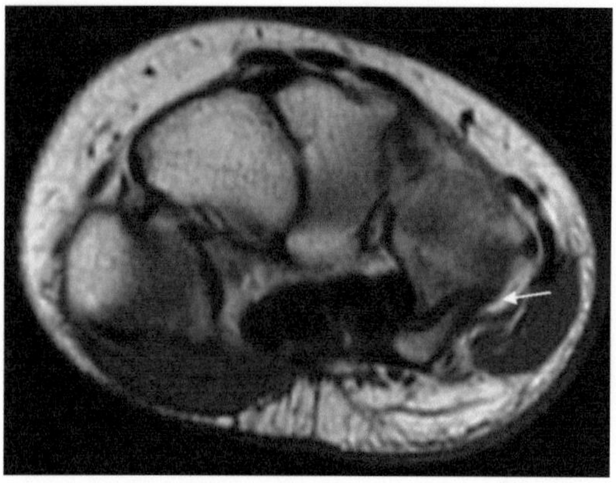

Fig. 7.7 *Hook of hamate fracture*. Axial T1-weighted image demonstrates an acute hook of the hamate fracture (arrow)

larly useful as it can detect bone marrow edema and subtle trabecular microfractures (Fig. 7.6) that may be radiographically occult. Stage 2 is characterized by lunate sclerosis which can be architecturally normal or demonstrate early collapse on the radial side. In stage 3, there is collapse of the entire lunate. This is the most common stage at initial presentation. This stage is subdivided into stage 3A without carpal collapse and 3B with diminished carpal height and fixed palmar flexion of the scaphoid. Finally, stage 4 is characterized by the presence of generalized arthritic change in the carpus, in addition to the findings of stage 3 [20–22].

Ulnar Styloid Fractures

Fractures of the ulnar styloid may occur as an isolated injury from a direct blow to the dorsal or ulnar wrist, or they may occur in conjunction with other wrist fractures in traumatic settings such as a fall. Patients often present with a weakened grip, ulnar-sided wrist pain worsened by ulnar deviation and twisting of the wrist, and limited range of motion. While these fractures are easily diagnosed at radiography, approximately 65% result in nonunion and ulnar-sided wrist disorders [23]. The extensor carpi ulnaris tendon sheath, ulnocarpal ligaments, and TFCC all originate from the distal ulna and serve to preserve the congruency of the

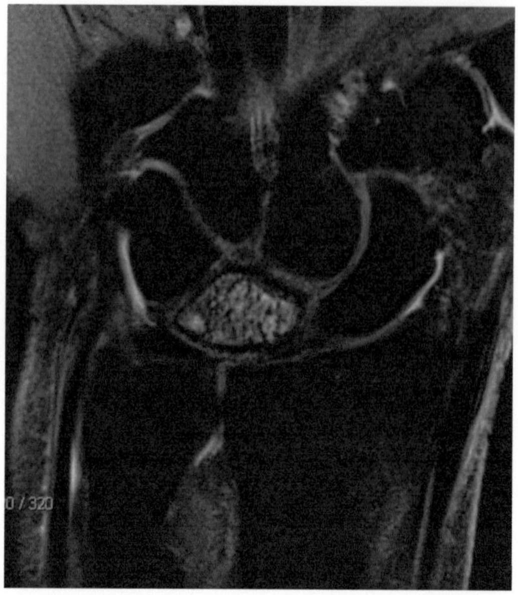

Fig. 7.6 *Kienböck's disease*. Coronal fat-suppressed T2-weighted image demonstrates negative ulnar variance and bone marrow edema and microfractures of the lunate

DRUJ. If only the tip of the ulnar styloid is fractured, the TFCC will remain intact since its attachments are near the base of the styloid, and the DRUJ will accordingly remain stable. However, more complex ulnar styloid fractures may result in avulsion of the ulnar attachments of the TFCC (a palmer grade 1B TFCC injury discussed later in the chapter) and a pattern of injury which may ultimately lead to DRUJ instability [24].

Hamate Fractures

Hamate fractures may involve the body or the hook, with the hook being the most common. The hook of the hamate fractures (Fig. 7.7) is commonly seen in swinging sports including baseball, golf, and tennis. Fractures typically result from direct compression and repetitive microtrauma. Early diagnosis and treatment are important to decrease the risk of complications which include nonunion, flexor digitorum profundus tendon ruptures, ulnar neuropathy (Fig. 7.8), and ulnar artery injury. MR imaging is the best imaging modality to diagnose a hamate fracture and simultaneously evaluate all of its potential complications [13].

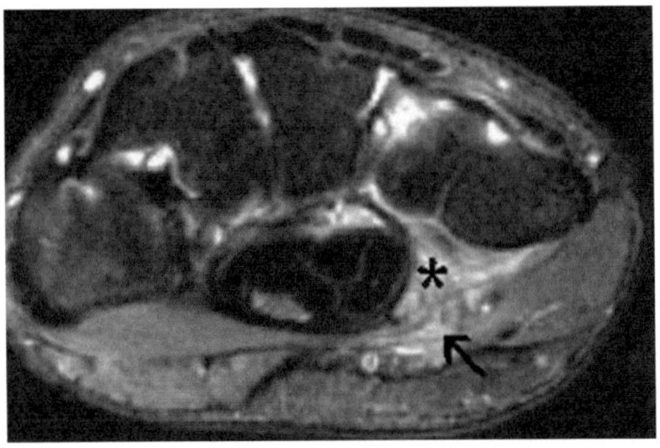

Fig. 7.8 *Ulnar neuropathy in the setting of hook of the hamate fracture.* Axial T2-weighted fat-suppressed image one slice distal to the expected location of the hook of the hamate (asterisk) demonstrates the associated extensive perineural edema at the level of Guyon's canal (arrow)

Triquetrum Fractures

Triquetrum fractures account for up to 3.5% of all wrist injuries and represent the second most common carpal bone fracture after scaphoid fractures. Three types of triquetral fractures have been described: cortical dorsal (most common), body, and cortical palmar fractures. Most triquetral fractures are seen after FOOSH injuries. However, the mechanism of injury resulting in triquetral fractures remains controversial. To date, two major theories have been proposed. The first theory suggests the fracture results from avulsion of the dorsal capsular ligaments, whereas the second theory suggests that the fracture is the result of ulnocarpal impaction caused by an elongated styloid process [25]. The main dorsal carpal ligaments insert on the dorsum of the triquetrum, including extrinsic (dorsal radiocarpal and dorsal ulnotriquetral) and intrinsic (dorsal intercarpal) ligaments, each with separate attachment sites. While dorsal triquetral fractures rarely lead to nonunion, they are frequently associated with ligamentous injuries which can result in early arthritis and instability. While radiography is the recommended initial modality for acute wrist injuries, in the setting of negative radiographs with a confounding clinical exam, early MR imaging would be a suitable choice. In the case of triquetral fractures, MR imaging can provide the diagnosis, and it can also serve to assess for concomitant ligamentous injury [13].

Ligament Injuries

Interosseous Ligaments of the Wrist

The intrinsic or interosseous ligaments are intracapsular structures, and they originate and insert on carpal bones. The two most important interosseous ligaments are the scapholunate and lunotriquetral ligaments. These intrinsic ligaments connect the proximal carpal row and preclude communication between the radiocarpal and midcarpal joints. These ligaments are U-shaped and have dorsal and volar ligamentous components, with a thinner membranous/cartilaginous central component [1]. MR sequences in the coronal and axial planes allow for direct assessment of the scapholunate and lunotriquetral ligaments. However, MR arthrography has been shown to be more sensitive than standard MR for detecting abnormalities of these intrinsic wrist ligaments [26].

Scapholunate Ligament Injury

Schapholunate dissociation which results from injury to the scapholunate ligament (SLL) is the most common form of carpal instability. Patients often present with weakness and pain about the dorsal radial aspect of the wrist. The SLL is composed of thick, dorsal collagen bundles, a feature which renders its dorsal component the most important for carpal stability. Volarly, the ligament is less thick and less taut in order to accommodate the articulating surfaces of the lunate and scaphoid rendering it weaker than the dorsal component [5]. Scapholunate ligament tears typically occur in the setting of axial overload injuries or hyperextension with supination as can be seen in the context of a fall [27]. Understanding the anatomy of each SLL component is important, since the site and extent of ligament disruption may be used to differentiate between a traumatic tear and degenerative changes. For example, a complete ligamentous tear or involvement of the dorsal or volar portions of the ligament indicates a traumatic origin, whereas central perforations are more compatible with sequela of physiological degeneration [28]. Complete tears of the SLL

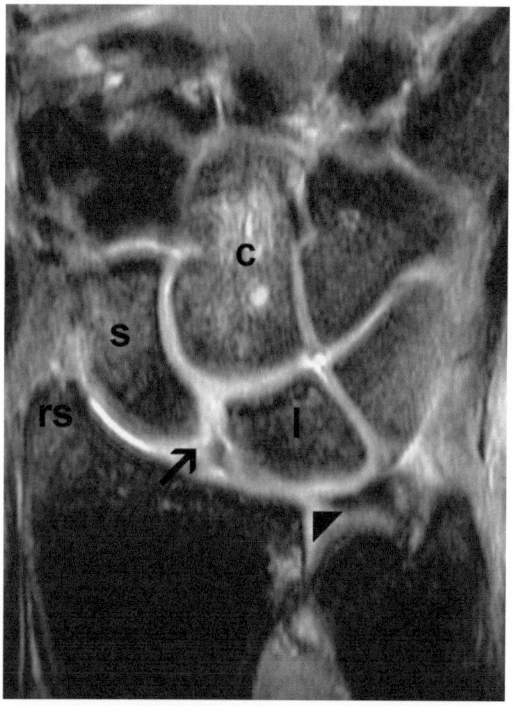

Fig. 7.9 *Complete SLL tear.* Coronal fat-suppressed T2-weighted image demonstrates full-thickness tear of the scapholunate ligament at its scaphoid insertion (arrow) with resultant widening of the scapholunate interval. Also seen is radial avulsion of the triangular fibrocartilage (arrowhead) and bone marrow contusions of nearly all carpal bones as well as the radial styloid. L lunate, c capitate, s scaphoid, rs radial styloid

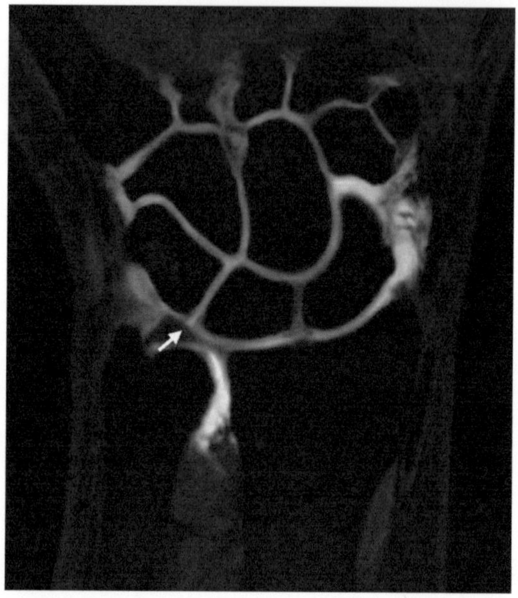

Fig. 7.10 *Complete LTL tear.* Coronal fat-suppressed 3D spoiled gradient image demonstrates a full-thickness tear of the lunotriquetral ligament (white arrow) with intra-articular contrast extending to the midcarpal row. Intra-articular contrast injections of the radiocarpal and distal radioulnar joints were performed for this MR arthrogram examination

(Fig. 7.9) are seen as absence of the ligament or as distinct areas of discontinuity within the ligament with corresponding fluid-like T2 hyperintensity [5]. Partial tearing is typically characterized by focal thinning or irregularity in a portion of the ligament, and they more commonly affect the weaker volar ligamentous attachment. When there is accompanying injury to the secondary wrist stabilizers, dorsal intercalated segment instability (DISI) develops, and over time, subsequent wrist osteoarthritis and scapholunate advanced collapse (SLAC) wrist may result [23]. These complications will be discussed later in the chapter.

Lunotriquetral Ligament Injury

Lunotriquetral ligament (LTL) tears are reportedly only one-sixth as common as SLL tears. Isolated lunotriquetral ligament (LTL) tears may result from a FOOSH or a direct blow. Patients often present with tenderness and swelling to the ulnar side of the wrist over the LTL articulation which can be palpated between the fourth and fifth wrist extensor compartments, and they may also present with a weakened grip [29, 30]. In contradistinction to the SLL, the volar component is the most stout and considered the major constraint to lunotriquetral motion [30]. Similar to SLL tears, LTL complete tears are diagnosed when there is a distinct area of discontinuity with increased signal on fluid-sensitive sequences (Fig. 7.10) or complete absence of the ligament. Fraying, thinning, distorted morphology, or abnormal ligament course may also indicate the presence of a tear [4]. As with the SLL, degenerative tears of the LTL generally involve the membranous portion with intact dorsal and volar components. When there is accompanying injury to the radiocarpal extrinsic ligamentous stabilizers, volar intercalated segment instability

(VISI) will often result (discussed later in the chapter) [1].

Capsular Ligaments of the Wrist

The capsular ligaments of the wrist are so named because they derive part or all of their substance from the capsule of the wrist. In this chapter, we will cover the most clinically relevant capsular ligaments. The extrinsic capsular ligaments are ligaments that originate from the distal forearm and insert on the carpus. Of the extrinsic capsular ligaments, the volar ligaments are strongest and provide the most contribution to carpal stability. The radioscaphocapitate is considered the primary volar capsular ligament. It originates from the lateral aspect of the radial styloid and courses underneath the waist of the scaphoid and is an important contributor to scaphoid stability. On MR imaging, it is seen as a low-signal structure with striations.

Deep to the extensor tendons and extensor retinaculum lie the dorsal capsular ligaments which are not considered as important as the volar capsular ligaments. The dorsal radiocarpal ligament is the primary dorsal extrinsic capsular ligament. It originates from Lister's tubercle and inserts on the dorsal aspect of the triquetrum. As it courses, it sends a few fibers to the lunate and is sometimes also referred to as the dorsal radiolunotriquetral ligament. It serves to provide stability to the proximal carpal row. The dorsal radiocarpal ligament is typically the culprit that causes dorsal avulsion of the triquetrum. These ligaments can be seen on coronal images but are better assessed on axial and sagittal images. Similar to the volar ligaments, the dorsal extrinsic ligaments may demonstrate a striated appearance which should not be mistaken for ligament tears [1, 4, 31].

Another important dorsal capsular ligament is the dorsal intercarpal ligament (DICL) which always attaches to the dorsal aspect of the triquetrum; however, there is some variation in its attachment on the radial side of the carpus. Generally, however, the DICL attaches to the scaphoid and trapezium on the radial aspect of the wrist.

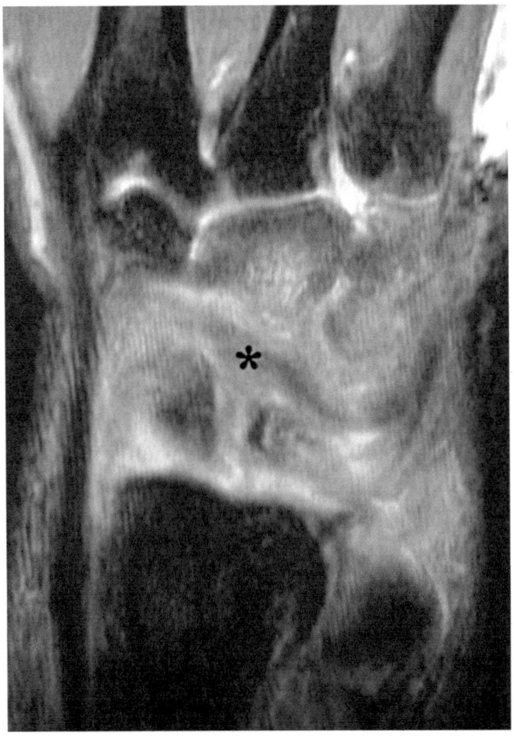

Fig. 7.11 *Dorsal intercarpal ligament (DICL) injury.* Coronal fat-suppressed T2-weighted images demonstrate partial thickness rupture of the DICL (asterisk) with associated surrounding high T2 signal likely reflecting a combination of edema, hemorrhage, and inflammation

While injury to the dorsal ligaments is not uncommon, complete disruption of the ligaments is rare. Injury to the dorsal wrist ligaments more commonly manifests as sprains or partial tears. On MR imaging, there is associated distortion of the ligament morphology and surrounding high T2 signal from edema, hemorrhage, and/or inflammation. When a partial tear is present, the ligament will be distorted, and fluid will be seen between ligament fibers (Fig. 7.11) [32].

Carpal Instability

Generally speaking, carpal instability can be defined as a disturbance of the static and dynamic balance of forces within the wrist which exist under normal conditions, leading to loss of the normal anatomic alignment. The most important ligaments for carpal stability are the scapholunate and lunotriquetral ligaments. The SLL counteracts the inherent tendency of the lunate to dorsiflex, and the LTL serves the same function for the triquetrum. As previously noted, the most common type of carpal instability is schapholunate dissociation [1, 33]. When there is disruption of the SLL, MRI will show a dorsal tilt of the lunate, hyperflexion of the scaphoid, and incongruity of Gilula's arcs known as DISI deformity. MR arthrography may be helpful to assess for tears or excessive stretching of the secondary ligamentous stabilizers of the scaphoid [27]. In the case of volar intercalated segment instability (VISI) deformity, a complete tear of the LTL is typically seen in combination with disruption of one of the secondary stabilizers of the lunotriquetral joint such as the dorsal radiocarpal ligament. On imaging, palmar tilt of the lunate will often be seen [33]. However, it's worth nothing that these carpal relationships are best evaluated on radiographs, as studies have shown that sagittal MRI exaggerates these relationships [1].

Triangular Fibrocartilage Complex

The triangular fibrocartilage complex (TFCC) stabilizes the distal radioulnar joint (DRUJ) by behaving as a cushion for the ulnar head and lunate during axial loading and ulnar deviation of the wrist. TFCC tears often result from a FOOSH or a hyperpronation injury to the forearm [34]. The clinical presentation of TFCC injuries typically include ulnar-sided wrist pain and an audible or palpable click upon rotation of the forearm [20]. Anatomic factors such as positive ulnar variance can also predispose patients to both acute and chronic degenerative injuries [35]. The TFCC is composed of tendon, ligaments, and cartilage. Components include the triangular fibrocartilage articular disc, volar and dorsal radioulnar ligaments, volar ulnotriquetral and ulnolunate ligaments, ulnar collateral ligament, extensor carpi ulnaris (ECU) tendon sheath, and meniscal homologue [34].

MR imaging is the modality of choice to evaluate TFCC injuries. A tear or defect of the TFCC will typically appear as a linear band of increased signal intensity on T1-weighted images, which further increases on PD- and T2-weighted sequences. A communicating defect (full-thickness) tear can be suspected when the abnormal signal extends to both articular surfaces. A non-communicating defect is suspected when the abnormal signal involves only one articular surface, either the distal radioulnar joint or the radiocarpal joint surface [4]. The Palmer classification divides TFCC tears into traumatic (Class 1) and degenerative (Class 2) categories. While knowledge of this classification system is useful, it is important to recognize that this system is not exhaustive, and it does not cover all of the components of the TFCC. With regard to traumatic injury of the TFCC, Palmer Class 1 tears are subclassified according to the location of injury. Class 1A tears are the most common traumatic subtype of tear, and they involve the central fibrocartilage disk. They are most frequently localized at the radial side and frequently show a complex configuration. Class 1B tears are peripheral tears of the TFCC near or at its insertion on the distal ulna. These tears may be purely ligamentous involving avulsions from the ulnar attachments of the TFCC, or they can be associated with a fracture through the base of the ulnar styloid process and DRUJ instability (Fig. 7.12). Class 1C tears are distal avulsions and involve the volar ligaments, namely, the ulnolunate and ulnotriquetral ligaments. These ligaments are robust making this injury pattern uncommon. When it does occur, however, this injury can result in ulnocarpal instability with palmar migration of the ulnar carpus. Class 1D tears are characterized by avulsion of the TFCC from its radial attachment at the sigmoid notch of the radius. They can also be associated with avulsion fractures of the sigmoid notch [35].

Nerve Injuries

Carpal Tunnel Syndrome

Peripheral nerve compression syndromes refer to irritation and pressure injuries of nerves where they pass through anatomical bottlenecks and

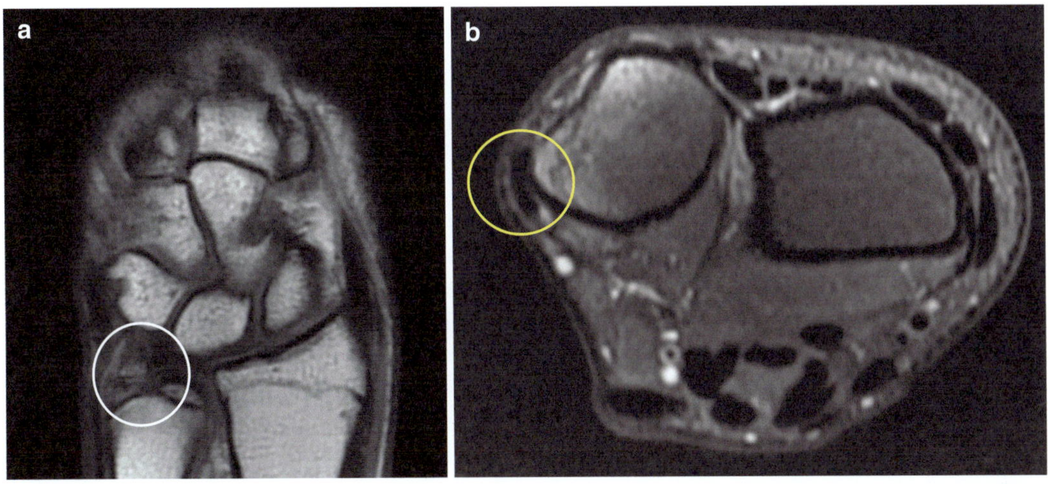

Fig. 7.12 *Palmer 1B traumatic TFCC injury*. Coronal T1-weighted image of the wrist (**a**) in the setting of acute traumatic avulsion the triangular fibrocartilage articular disc from its ulnar styloid and foveal attachments with associated ulnar styloid avulsion fracture (white circle). Axial T2 fat-suppressed sequence (**b**) reveals bone marrow edema and dorsal subluxation of the distal ulna at the level of the distal radioulnar joint. Extensor carpi ulnaris tendon is dislocated (yellow circle)

fibro-osseous canals. Carpal tunnel syndrome is by far the most common peripheral nerve compression syndrome and results from compression of the median nerve beneath the transverse carpal ligament [36]. The carpal tunnel floor is formed by the carpal bones, the roof is formed by the transverse carpal ligament, the scaphoid and the trapezium are on the radial side, and the pisiform and hook of the hamate are on the ulnar side. Patients with carpal tunnel syndrome may present with wrist pain, paresthesias and numbness involving the first through third fingers, and radial aspect of the fourth finger [37]. The carpal tunnel encompasses nine tendons, the four flexor digitorum superficialis tendons, the four flexor digitorum profundus tendons, and the flexor pollicis longus tendon in addition to the median nerve which lies along the volar superficial aspect of the tunnel [38].

Carpal tunnel syndrome can result from repetitive microtrauma, and increased incidence has been associated with repetitive flexion and extension of the wrist. These repetitive motion activities may result in flexor tenosynovitis, a predisposing factor to carpal tunnel syndrome [23]. Many other pathologic processes, traumatic and nontraumatic in etiology, may compress the median nerve within the carpal tunnel including anomalous muscles, ganglion cysts, fracture fragments, bone spurs, inflammatory synovial pannus, rice bodies, and amyloid deposits [5].

A confirmatory clinical evaluation for carpal tunnel syndrome includes a positive Phalen's test, which elicits worsened paresthesias after 30–60 seconds of maximal passive wrist flexion, and a positive Tinel's sign, which demonstrates paresthesias in a median nerve distribution elicited by gentle tapping over the carpal tunnel [38]. Median nerve conduction testing may demonstrate a decreased conduction testing at the level of the wrist, and needle-electrode electromyography may assist in detecting denervation of the intrinsic hand muscles [39].

MRI findings of carpal tunnel syndrome can be divided into four major categories: (1) increased nerve size (Fig. 7.13), (2) flattening of the nerve, (3) bowing of the flexor retinaculum, and (4) increased T2 signal within the median nerve. Axial MR images are best to compare the cross-sectional area of the nerve at the radiocarpal joint and at the pisiform bone level. In patients with carpal tunnel syndrome, the nerve size is approximately two to three times larger at the level of the pisiform compared to the size of the nerve at the radiocarpal

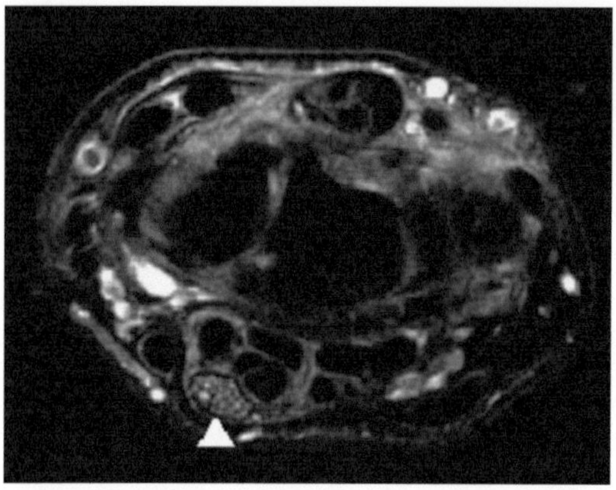

Fig. 7.13 *Carpal tunnel syndrome at the level of the proximal tunnel.* Axial fat-suppressed T2-weighted image demonstrates high signal intensity and enlargement of the median nerve (arrowhead)

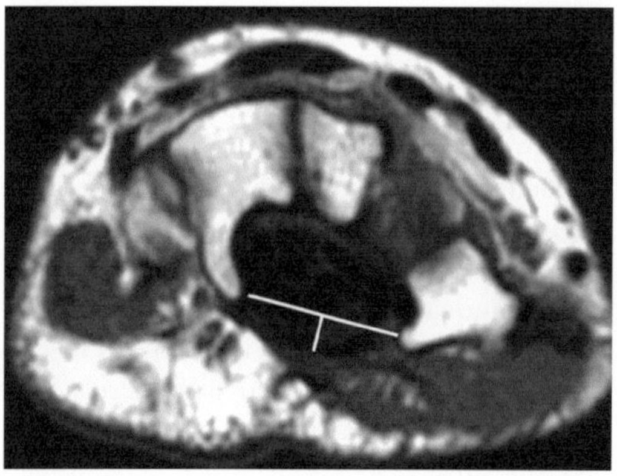

Fig. 7.14 *Carpal tunnel syndrome's retinacular bowing.* At the level of the transverse carpal ligament, axial PD-weighted image shows increased bowing ratio determined by dividing the palmar displacement of the retinaculum (short line) by the distance between the hamate hook to the trapezium tubercle (long line)

joint [39]. The ratio between the major and minor axis of the nerve at the level of the DRUJ and at the level of the hook of the hamate can be used to assess for nerve flattening with a ratio of three being indicative of disease. Normally, the flexor retinaculum at the level of the hook of the hamate should be flat or slightly convex. The degree of bowing is determined by dividing the distance of palmar displacement of the retinaculum by the distance between the hook of the hamate and the tubercle of the trapezium (Fig. 7.14). In normal patients, this ratio varies from 0 to 0.15; however, in patients with carpal tunnel syndrome, the ratio varies from 0.14 to 0.26 [5]. Most nerves in the body demonstrate a slightly increased T2 signal on fat-suppressed T2-weighted images, and as such, it can be difficult to assess for disease. However, intense increase in signal within the nerve is fairly diagnostic of disease. Lesions causing mass effect on the carpal tunnel such as ganglia, bursae, fracture fragments, proliferative synovitis, and aberrant muscles can also be easily depicted with MR imaging. Aberrant muscles demonstrate signal isointense to muscle on all pulse sequences. MR imaging is also useful in identifying persistent median arteries or veins within the carpal tunnel, an important finding to recognize and report in order to avoid inadvertent injury to these vessels during surgery [5].

Ulnar Tunnel Syndrome

Guyon's canal, or the ulnar tunnel, originates at the proximal edge of the palmar carpal ligament and extends distally to the fibrous arch of the hypothenar muscles at the level of the hamate hook. The ulnar nerve, ulnar artery, concomitant veins, and connective fatty tissue lie within the ulnar tunnel. Compression of the ulnar nerve, while seen most commonly at the elbow, can occasionally occur at the wrist in Guyon's canal. The loss of sensation along the dorsal ulnar-sided aspect of the hand seen in ulnar tunnel syndrome (UTS) can aid in distinguishing elbow and forearm ulnar neuropathy [40].

The ulnar nerve can undergo compression at three potential sites within Guyon's canal: (a) zone I which extends from the proximal edge of the palmar carpal ligament to the bifurcation of the ulnar nerve into the deep motor and superficial sensory branches, (b) zone II which extends from the bifurcation of the ulnar nerve just distal to the fibrous arch of the hypothenar muscles and which contains the deep motor branch of the ulnar nerve, and (c) zone III which is parallel to zone II and contains the superficial sensory branch of the ulnar nerve. The clinical presentation can provide clues regarding the site of ulnar nerve compression. Combined sensory and motor deficits are seen in zone I lesions, zone II lesions demonstrate pure motor deficits, and isolated sensory deficits are noted with zone III compression. Most patients undergo ulnar nerve compression at either zone I or zone III. In greater than 50% of patients, the compression can occur in more than one zone [40, 41].

Ulnar nerve compression within Guyon's canal can either be idiopathic or secondary to trauma [41]. A displaced hook of the hamate fracture or an enlarged hook of the hamate are recognized offending causes. Isolated compressive neuropathy of the deep terminal motor branch of the ulnar nerve in cyclists has been termed handlebar palsy. This palsy is related to prolonged riding with the hands pressed against the handle bars. As no sensory fibers are affected, the patients often do not become aware of an ongoing nerve compression until a severe nerve compression develops [42]. Other causes for UTS include tumors, musculotendinous variants, aberrant fibrous bands, vascular lesions such as ulnar artery pseudoaneurysm, and thrombosis [38].

MR imaging findings of UTS include increased size and increased signal in the nerve and its branches, a finding best seen on axial MR sequences. Space-occupying lesions such as ganglions, lipomas, hemangiomas, vascular lesions, posttraumatic scarring, and obliteration of the fat around the nerves are other causes of UTS. Evaluation for the presence of aberrant muscles should be made, as this is a common cause of UTS that is easily overlooked. The hook of hamate fractures is often associated with edema and scarring in the adjacent Guyon's' canal (Fig. 7.8). Assessment for muscle denervation edema and atrophy in the hypothenar and intrinsic muscles should be made, although this is a less common finding [38, 41].

Wartenberg Syndrome

Wartenberg syndrome, also known as cheiralgia paresthetica, results from entrapment of the superficial branch of the radial nerve. Other descriptive terms used to refer to the syndrome include handcuff neuropathy or neuropraxia, wristlet watch neuritis, or watch-strap nerve compression. The superficial branch of the radial nerve can be compressed at any point along its course, but it is believed to be at greatest risk along the posterior aspect of the brachioradialis as the nerve transitions from a deep to a subcutaneous structure. The entrapment results from scissoring or traction on the superficial branch of the radial nerve in the fascia joining the tendons of the extensor carpi radialis longus and the brachioradialis and is aggravated by pronation of the forearm or ulnar deviation of the wrist. Many different causes for compression of the superficial branch of the radial nerve have been described including trauma, diabetes, de Quervain' s disease, anatomic variants, and tight fascial bands [43, 44]. Additionally, traumatic compression can also result from direct compression by handcuffs or tight watchbands or due to distal radius fractures or closed reduction. Patients often report pain and paresthesias along the dorsum of the distal forearm, thumb, and index finger, symptoms which can mimic de Quervain stenosing tenosynovitis. While both of these syndromes may demonstrate pain with ulnar deviation of the wrist, Wartenberg syndrome pain is typically present at rest and may have an associated positive Tinel sign. While electrodiagnostic testing is often negative in cases of Wartenberg syndrome, it should be performed as part of a thorough workup and may be helpful if positive [45].

Muscle, Tendon, and Soft Tissue Injuries

Flexor Tendons

Digital flexor tendon injuries in the wrist include lacerations (Fig. 7.15) and less commonly closed ruptures [46]. Closed ruptures are usually the result of a series of chronic conditions that result in weakening of the tendons such as rheumatoid arthritis, osteoarthritis, scaphoid nonunion, Kienböck's disease, hamate hook fractures, nonhealed distal radial fractures, carpal dislocations,

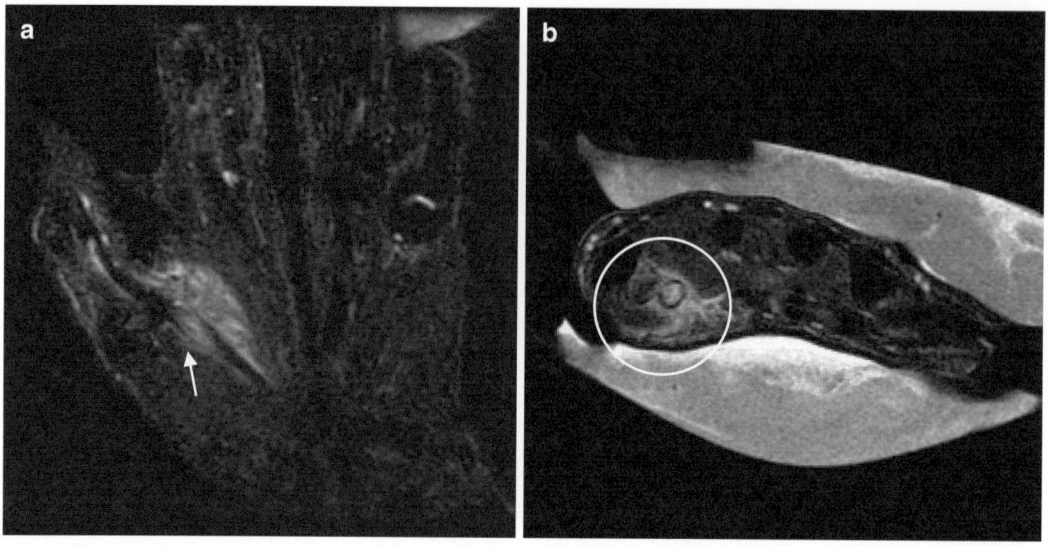

Fig. 7.15 *Flexor tendon laceration*. Coronal T2 (**a**) and axial T2-weighted fat-suppressed (**b**) images demonstrate a traumatic laceration of the flexor pollicis longus tendon with surrounding peritendinous edema in a patient who suffered a penetrating injury

and certain medications including corticosteroids, quinolone antibiotics, and aromatase inhibitors [47–49]. Rapid hyperextension of a flexed finger, most frequently seen in football or rugby players or less commonly following an electrical injury, can also lead to acute closed ruptures [5].

Drape et al. found MR imaging to be useful in displaying the zone of rupture, assessing the tendon edges, and accurately measuring the gap between retracted tendon ends [46]. Additionally, MR imaging can evaluate the integrity of the adjacent tendons prior to tendon grafting and aid in locating the retracted tendon edges [50, 51].

Flexor Carpi Radialis

Flexor carpi radialis (FCR) tenosynovitis is often the result of trauma from either direct injury or chronic repetitive microtrauma. On clinical evaluation, patients often present with pain and crepitus over the FCR tendon just proximal to the flexor creases of the wrist. MR imaging findings include thickening of the tendon sheath with associated hyperintensity on fluid-sensitive images (Fig. 7.16). As a result of its close proximity to the FCR tendon, median nerve irritation may also occur. MR imaging is useful in diagnosing FCR tenosynovitis as the clinical diagnosis can be difficult, often mistaken for scaphotrapezial joint arthritis, soft tissue ganglion, scaphoid and radial fractures, and lastly Linburg syndrome which is often asymptomatic [52, 53].

Flexor Carpi Ulnaris

Flexor carpi ulnaris (FCU) tendinopathy is quite common and typically results from repetitive ulnar deviation, such as from repetitive hammering. It can also result from repetitive high-speed impact with a ball as seen in racquet sports and golf. On MR imaging, signs of tendinopathy are increased signal on T1- and T2-weighted images. In cases with associated calcific tendinopathy, calcific deposits will produce "blooming" or susceptibility artifact on gradient-echo sequences [54].

Extensor Tendons

The abductor pollicis longus (APL) and extensor pollicis brevis (EPB) tendons comprise the contents of the first extensor compartment which sits

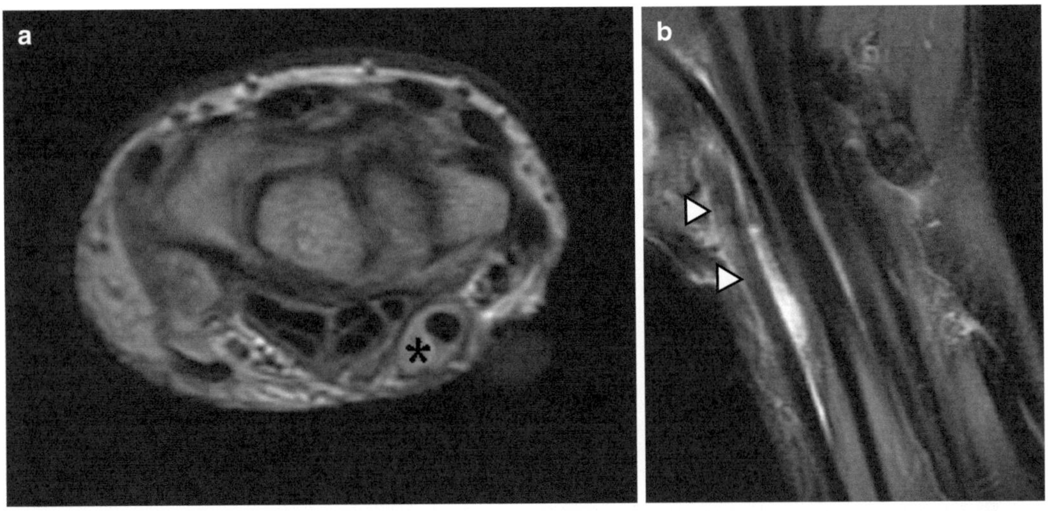

Fig. 7.16 *Tenosynovitis of the FCR with partial tendon rupture*. Axial proton density (**a**) and coronal fat-suppressed T2-weighted (**b**) images show fluid distending the FCR tendon sheath (asterisk) with associated tendon intrasubstance tearing (arrowheads) at the level of the scaphoid-trapezium joint

along the dorsolateral aspect of the wrist. These tendons overlie the radial styloid, are variably separated by a septum, and are held in place by the overlying extensor retinaculum. The intervening septum may range from partial to complete, and it can predispose to the development of de Quervain tenosynovitis [55]. In one cadaveric study, up to 40% of studied wrists demonstrated some degree of septation within the first extensor compartment [56].

de Quervain tenosynovitis is most commonly idiopathic; however, other predisposing etiologies include rheumatoid arthritis, acute traumatic injuries, and chronic repetitive microtrauma from radial and ulnar deviation of the wrist. It is related to shear microtrauma and repetitive gliding of the abductor pollicis longus and extensor pollicis brevis tendons over the radial styloid [57].

Most commonly, de Quervain's tenosynovitis occurs at the level of or slightly proximal to the radial styloid. Patients often present with pain and swelling along the radial aspect of the wrist which can be reproduced by provocative maneuvers such as the Finkelstein test [55]. While the diagnosis is often made clinically, MR imaging characteristics typically include first extensor compartment tendinopathy (ranging from tendon thickening to split tearing), tenosynovitis, and peritendinous edema (Fig. 7.17). MR imaging can also assess the course of the superficial radial nerve prior to surgical intervention [58].

Intersection Syndrome

Intersection syndrome is an overuse syndrome which occurs approximately 4–8 cm proximal to Lister's tubercle of the radius where the first extensor compartment tendons (abductor pollicis longus and extensor pollicis brevis) cross over the second extensor compartment tendons (extensor carpi radialis longus and extensor carpi radialis brevis) [59]. Patient's often present with radial-sided wrist pain, swelling, tenderness, and crepitus at the site of crossover [60]. This inflammatory process of the second extensor compartment tendons occurs in the setting of chronic overuse and friction and is commonly associated with sports-related activities, such as rowing, canoeing, tennis, horseback riding, and skiing [61, 62]. Occupations which require repeated extension and flexion of the wrist can result in intersection syndrome as seen in individuals who perform extensive typing [63].

However, intersection syndrome can sometimes be overlooked clinically, and as a result,

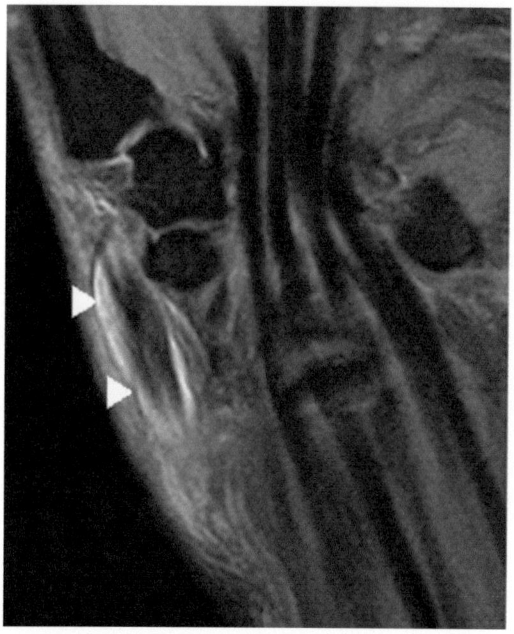

Fig. 7.17 *de Quervain's tenosynovitis*. Coronal fat-suppressed T2-weighted image demonstrates first extensor compartment peritendinous edema, tendon sheath effusion, and tendon thickening (arrowheads)

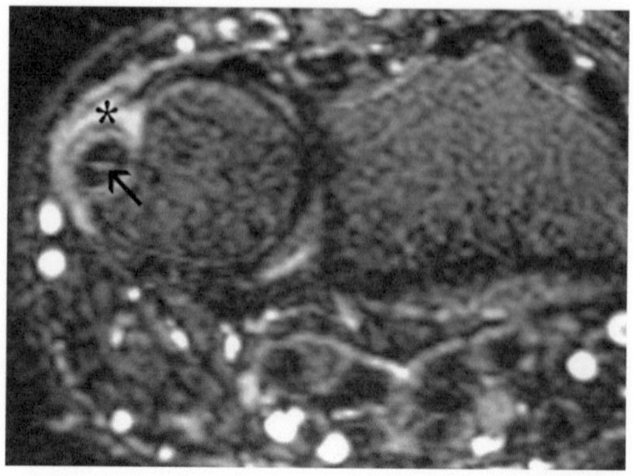

Fig. 7.18 *ECU tendon partial tear*. Axial fat-suppressed T2-weighted image shows intrasubstance longitudinal split tear of the ECU tendon (arrow) with associated peritendinous edema (asterisk) at the level of the ulnar styloid

MR imaging can significantly aid in making the correct diagnosis. MR findings include thickening and interstitial fluid concentrically surrounding the first and second extensor compartment tendons and their tendon sheaths, beginning at the point of crossover and extending proximally. These findings are best seen on fluid-sensitive sequences [64].

Extensor Carpi Ulnaris

The extensor carpi ulnaris (ECU) tendon courses through the sixth extensor compartment and is held within the groove of the head of the ulna by a deep retinaculum. Abnormalities include tendinopathy, tenosynovitis, rupture, subluxation, or dislocation. The mechanism of injury is believed to be forced wrist supination and flexion with ulnar deviation. Tenosynovitis of the ECU is very common, and this can lead to tendon instability [65].

ECU subluxation or dislocation typically results from injury to the ECU tendon subsheath in the setting of trauma or rheumatic disease and may cause ulnar-sided wrist pain. The ECU tendon subsheath is an independent layer of connective tissue underneath the extensor retinaculum which stabilizes the ECU tendon as discussed in detail in Chap. 6. ECU tendon dislocation may result from numerous etiologies including recurrent instability, distal forearm fractures with extensor retinaculum disruption, and posttraumatic alteration of biomechanics involving the DRUJ [66].

MR imaging appearance of tenosynovitis of the ECU tendon includes circumferential hyperintense T2 signal within the tendon sheath, thickening of the tendon sheath, and peritendinous edema. With continued stress, the tendon may degenerate with resultant tendinopathy, tearing, or a combination of both (Fig. 7.18). Closed, nonrheumatoid ruptures of the ECU tendon are rare but have been previously described in tennis and hockey players [58]

References

1. Davis KW, Blankenbaker DG. Imaging the ligaments and tendons of the wrist. Semin Roentgenol. 2010;45(3):194–217.
2. Schmitt R, Froehner S, Coblenz G, Christopoulos G. Carpal instability. Eur Radiol. 2006;16(10):2161–78.

3. Bruno F, Arrigoni F, Palumbo P, Natella R, Maggialetti N, Reginelli A, et al. The acutely injured wrist. Radiol Clin North Am. 2019;57(5):943–55.
4. Ringler MD. MRI of wrist ligaments. J Hand Surg. 2013;38(10):2034–46.
5. Bencardino JT, Rosenberg ZS. Sports-related injuries of the wrist: an approach to MRI interpretation. Clin Sports Med. 2006;25(3):409–32.
6. Fowler JR, Hughes TB. Scaphoid fractures. Clin Sports Med. 2015;34(1):37–50.
7. Clementson M, Björkman A, Thomsen NOB. Acute scaphoid fractures: guidelines for diagnosis and treatment. EFORT Open Rev. 2020;5(2):96–103.
8. Hunter JC, Escobedo EM, Wilson AJ, Hanel DP, Zink-Brody GC, Mann FA. MR imaging of clinically suspected scaphoid fractures. Am J Roentgenol. 1997;168(5):1287–93.
9. Murthy NS. The role of magnetic resonance imaging in scaphoid fractures. J Hand Surg. 2013;38(10):2047–54.
10. Karantanas A, Dailiana Z, Malizos K. The role of MR imaging in scaphoid disorders. Eur Radiol. 2007;17(11):2860–71.
11. Ko JH, Pet MA, Khouri JS, Hammert WC. Management of scaphoid fractures. Plast Reconstr Surg. 2017;140(2):333e–46e.
12. Smith M, Bain GI, Turner PC, Watts AC. Review of imaging of scaphoid fractures. ANZ J Surg. 2010;80(1–2):82–90.
13. Murthy NS, Ringler MD. MR imaging of carpal fractures. Magn Reson Imaging Clin N Am. 2015;23(3):405–16.
14. Schmitt R, Christopoulos G, Wagner M, Krimmer H, Fodor S, van Schoonhoven J, et al. Avascular necrosis (AVN) of the proximal fragment in scaphoid nonunion: Is intravenous contrast agent necessary in MRI? Eur J Radiol. 2011;77(2):222–7.
15. Cerezal L, Abascal F, Canga A, García-Valtuille R, Bustamante M, del Piñal F. Usefulness of gadolinium-enhanced MR imaging in the evaluation of the vascularity of scaphoid nonunions. Am J Roentgenol. 2000;174(1):141–9.
16. Donati OF, Zanetti M, Nagy L, Bode B, Schweizer A, Pfirrmann CWA. Is dynamic gadolinium enhancement needed in MR imaging for the preoperative assessment of scaphoidal viability in patients with scaphoid nonunion? Radiology. 2011;260(3):808–16.
17. Anderson SE, Steinbach LS, Tschering-Vogel D, Martin M, Nagy L. MR imaging of avascular scaphoid nonunion before and after vascularized bone grafting. Skeletal Radiol. 2005;34(6):314–20.
18. Sachar K. Ulnar-sided wrist pain: evaluation and treatment of triangular fibrocartilage complex tears, ulnocarpal impaction syndrome, and lunotriquetral ligament tears. J Hand Surg. 2012;37(7):1489–500.
19. Acott TR, Greenberg JA. Ulnar abutment syndrome in the athlete. Orthop Clin North Am. 2020;51(2):227–33.
20. Porteous R, Harish S, Parasu N. Imaging of ulnar-sided wrist pain. Can Assoc Radiol J. 2012;63(1):18–29.
21. Cross D, Matullo KS. Kienböck disease. Orthop Clin North Am. 2014;45(1):141–52.
22. Ansari MT, Chouhan D, Gupta V, Jawed A. Kienböck's disease: where do we stand? J Clin Orthop Trauma. 2020;11(4):606–13.
23. Cockenpot E, Lefebvre G, Demondion X, Chantelot C, Cotten A. Imaging of sports-related hand and wrist injuries: sports imaging series. Radiology. 2016;279(3):674–92.
24. Hauck RM, Skahen J, Palmer AK. Classification and treatment of ulnar styloid nonunion. J Hand Surg. 1996;21(3):418–22.
25. Becce F, Theumann N, Bollmann C, Omoumi P, Richarme D, Guerini H, et al. Dorsal fractures of the triquetrum: MRI findings with an emphasis on dorsal carpal ligament injuries. Am J Roentgenol. 2013;200(3):608–17.
26. Lee YH, Choi YR, Kim S, Song H-T, Suh J-S. Intrinsic ligament and triangular fibrocartilage complex (TFCC) tears of the wrist: comparison of isovolumetric 3D-THRIVE sequence MR arthrography and conventional MR image at 3 T. Magn Reson Imaging. 2013;31(2):221–6.
27. LiMarzi GM, O'Dell MC, Scherer K, Pettis C, Wasyliw CW, Bancroft LW. Magnetic resonance arthrography of the wrist and elbow. Magn Reson Imaging Clin N Am. 2015;23(3):441–55.
28. Zanetti M, Saupe N, Nagy L. Role of MR imaging in chronic wrist pain. Eur Radiol. 2007;17(4):927–38.
29. Henderson CJ, Kobayashi KM. Ulnar-sided wrist pain in the athlete. Orthop Clin North Am. 2016;47(4):789–98.
30. Nicoson MC, Moran SL. Diagnosis and treatment of acute lunotriquetral ligament injuries. Hand Clin. 2015;31(3):467–76.
31. Ringler MD, Murthy NS. MR imaging of wrist ligaments. Magn Reson Imaging Clin N Am. 2015;23(3):367–91.
32. Steinbach LS, Smith DK. MRI of the wrist. J Clin Imag. 2000;24:298–32.
33. Timins E. MR imaging of the major carpal stabilizing ligaments: normal anatomy and clinical. Radiographics. 1995;15(3):575–87.
34. Ng AWH, Griffith JF, Fung CSY, Lee RKL, Tong CSL, Wong CWY, et al. MR imaging of the traumatic triangular fibrocartilaginous complex tear. Quant Imaging Med Surg. 2017;7(4):443–60.
35. Cody ME, Nakamura DT, Small KM, Yoshioka H. MR imaging of the triangular fibrocartilage complex. Magn Reson Imaging Clin N Am. 2015;23(3):393–403.
36. Assmus H, Antoniadis G, Bischoff C. Carpal and cubital tunnel and other, rarer nerve compression syndromes. Dtsch Aerzteblatt Online [Internet]. 2015 Jan 5 [cited 2020 Sep 19]. Available from: https://www.aerzteblatt.de/10.3238/arztebl.2015.0014.
37. Dong Q, Jacobson JA, Jamadar DA, Gandikota G, Brandon C, Morag Y, et al. Entrapment neuropathies in the upper and lower limbs: anatomy and MRI features. Radiol Res Pract. 2012;2012:1–12.

38. Miller TT, Reinus WR. Nerve entrapment syndromes of the elbow, forearm, and wrist. Am J Roentgenol. 2010;195(3):585–94.
39. Andreisek G, Crook DW, Burg D, Marincek B, Weishaupt D. Peripheral neuropathies of the median, radial, and ulnar nerves: MR imaging features. Radiographics. 2006;26(5):1267–87.
40. Chen S-H, Tsai T-M. Ulnar tunnel syndrome. J Hand Surg. 2014;39(3):571–9.
41. Murata K, Shih J-T, Tsai T-M. Causes of ulnar tunnel syndrome: a retrospective study of 31 subjects. J Hand Surg. 2003;28(4):647–51.
42. Capitani D, Beer S. Handlebar palsy - a compression syndrome of the deep terminal (motor) branch of the ulnar nerve in biking. J Neurol. 2002;249(10):1441–5.
43. Lanzetta M, Foucher G. Entrapment of the superficial branch of the radial nerve (Wartenberg's syndrome): A report of 52 cases. Int Orthop [Internet]. 1993 Dec [cited 2020 Sep 20];17(6). Available from: http://link.springer.com/10.1007/BF00180450.
44. Tosun N, Tuncay I, Akpinar F. Entrapment of the sensory branch of the radial nerve (Wartenberg's Syndrome): an unusual cause. Tohoku J Exp Med. 2001;193(3):251–4.
45. Dang AC, Rodner CM. Unusual compression neuropathies of the forearm, part I: radial nerve. J Hand Surg. 2009;34(10):1906–14.
46. Drapé J-L, Tardif-Chastenet de Gery S, Silbermann-Hoffman O, Chevrot A, Houvet P, Alnot J-Y, et al. Closed ruptures of the flexor digitorum tendons: MRI evaluation. Skeletal Radiol. 1998;27(11):617–24.
47. Saitoh S, Hata Y, Murakami N, Nakatsuchi Y, Seki H, Takaoka K. Scaphoid nonunion and flexor pollicis longus tendon rupture. J Hand Surg. 1999;24(6):1211–9.
48. Kato N, Nemoto K, Arino H, Ichikawa T, Fujikawa K. Ruptures of flexor tendons at the wrist as a complication of fracture of the distal radius. Scand J Plast Reconstr Surg Hand Surg. 2002;36(4):245–8.
49. Knobloch K. Drug-induced tendon disorders. In: Ackermann PW, Hart DA, editors. Metabolic influences on risk for tendon disorders [Internet]. Cham: Springer International Publishing; 2016. [cited 2021 Mar 20]. p. 229–38. (Advances in Experimental Medicine and Biology; vol. 920). Available from: http://link.springer.com/10.1007/978-3-319-33943-6_22.
50. Kumar BA, Tolat AR, Threepuraneni G, Jones B. The role of magnetic resonance imaging in late presentation of isolated injuries of the flexor digitorum profundus tendon in the finger. J Hand Surg. 2000;25(1):95–7.
51. Rubin DA, Kneeland JB, Kitay GS, Naranja RJ. Flexor tendon tears in the hand: use of MR imaging to diagnose degree of injury in a cadaver model. Am J Roentgenol. 1996;166(3):615–20.
52. Irwin LR, Outhwaite J, Burge PD. Rupture of the flexor carpi radialis tendon associated with scapho-trapezial osteoarthritis. J Hand Surg. 1992;17(3):343–5.
53. Rennie WR, Muller H. Linburg syndrome. Can J Surg. 1998; 41(4):306–8.
54. Yamabe E, Nakamura T, Pham P, Yoshioka H. The athlete's wrist: ulnar-sided pain. Semin Musculoskelet Radiol. 2012;16(04):331–7.
55. Plotkin B, Sampath SC, Sampath SC, Motamedi K. MR imaging and US of the wrist tendons. Radiographics. 2016;36(6):1688–700.
56. Jackson WT, Viegas SF, Coon TM, Stimpsom KD, Frogameni AD, Simpson JM. Anatomical variations in the first extensor compartment of the wrist. J Bone Jt Surg. 1986;68-A(6):923–6.
57. Rettig AC. Athletic injuries of the wrist and hand: part II: overuse injuries of the wrist and traumatic injuries to the hand. Am J Sports Med. 2004;32(1):262–73.
58. Meraj S, Gyftopoulos S, Nellans K, Walz D, Brown MS. MRI of the extensor tendons of the wrist. Am J Roentgenol. 2017;209(5):1093–102.
59. Adams JE, Habbu R. Tendinopathies of the hand and wrist. J Am Acad Orthop Surg. 2015;23(12):741–50.
60. Patrick NC, Hammert WC. Hand and wrist tendinopathies. Clin Sports Med. 2020;39(2):247–58.
61. Hanlon DP, Luellen JR. Intersection syndrome: a case report and review of the literature. J Emerg Med. 1999;17(6):969–71.
62. de Lima JE, Kim H-J, Albertotti F, Resnick D. Intersection syndrome: MR imaging with anatomic comparison of the distal forearm. Skeletal Radiol. 2004;33(11):627–31.
63. Chatterjee R, Vyas J. Diagnosis and management of intersection syndrome as a cause of overuse wrist pain. BMJ Case Rep. 2016;2016:bcr2016216988.
64. Costa CR, Morrison WB, Carrino JA. MRI features of intersection syndrome of the forearm. Am J Roentgenol. 2003;181(5):1245–9.
65. Chauhan A, Jacobs B, Andoga A, Baratz ME. Extensor tendon injuries in athletes. Sports Med Arthrosc Rev. 2014;22(1):45–55.
66. Kaiser P, Kellermann F, Arora R, Henninger B, Rudisch A. Diagnosing extensor carpi ulnaris tendon dislocation with dynamic rotation MRI of the wrist. Clin Imaging. 2018;51:323–6.

8 Wrist Pathology: Non-traumatic

Amanda M. Crawford, Maryam Soltanolkotabi, and Nancy Major

Congenital

Carpal Coalitions

Epidemiology

Individual carpal bones can be fused either by osseous, cartilaginous, or fibrous fusion, resulting in carpal coalition. Carpal coalitions are relatively common, estimated to occur in 0.1% of the population [1]. Coalitions involving the same carpal row are more commonly idiopathic in etiology, while coalitions spanning the proximal and distal carpal rows are seen in the postinfectious, metabolic, or syndrome-related setting [1, 2]. Idiopathic coalitions are more common in people of West African descent [1]. Intercarpal fusion can also be inherited in a dominant pattern. The most common coalition is lunotriquetral (Fig. 8.1). Other described coalitions include capitate-hamate, capitate-trapezoid, scaphotrapezial (Fig. 8.2), and scaphoid-lunate. While osseous fusions are typically asymptomatic, cartilaginous and fibrous coalitions can be painful [2]. Biomechanical stresses at the site of fusion may also become symptomatic [1].

Imaging Features

Several classification systems have been used to describe carpal coalition. In 1952, Minnaar characterized coalitions as either incomplete with pseudarthrosis (type I), coalition with a notch of incomplete division of the two bones (type II), complete lunotriquetral coalition in isolation (type III), or complete lunate-triquetral fusion with other carpal bone coalitions (type 4) [3]. Singh et al. classified intercarpal fusions based more on morphology, focusing on the shape of the coalesced bones, the specific site of fusion, and whether the fusion is non-osseous [4]. The Burnett classification is simpler, suggesting a dichotomy of either osseous fusion and non-osseous fusion to include both synchondrosis (united by cartilage) and syndesmosis (united by fibrous tissue) [5]. While the Minnaar classification system has been widely used, the Burnett classification, with its emphasis on osseous versus non-osseous fusion, likely has more clinical significance.

Another goal of imaging is to evaluate for other causes of fusion: postinfectious and post-inflammatory states can result in ankylosis. Radiologic studies can be used to evaluate for such inflammatory arthropathies such as rheumatoid arthritis, juvenile idiopathic arthritis, psoriatic arthritis, and Reiter's syndrome.

A. M. Crawford (✉) · M. Soltanolkotabi
Department of Radiology, University of Utah, Salt Lake City, UT, USA
e-mail: Amanda.Crawford@utah.edu

N. Major
Department of Radiology, University of Colorado, Aurora, CO, USA

B. U. Casagranda (ed.), *MRI of the Upper Extremity*, https://doi.org/10.1007/978-3-030-81612-4_8

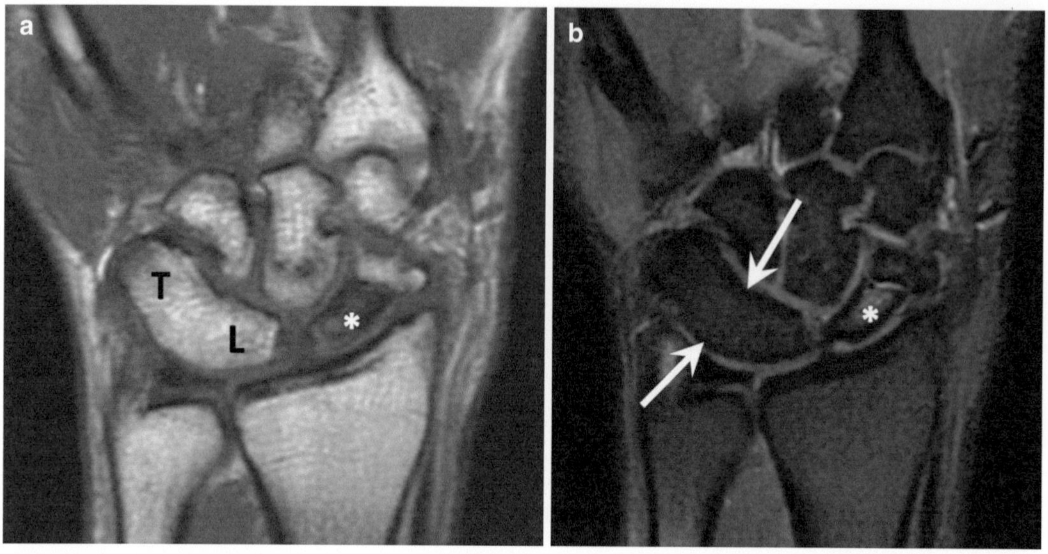

Fig. 8.1 Lunotriquetral coalition. Coronal T1 (**a**) and PD fat-suppressed (**b**) images show coalition of the lunate (L) and triquetrum (T). No cleft (white arrows) present making this a Minnaar type III coalition. Coalition was incidentally noted during the evaluation of a scaphoid fracture with nonunion and avascular necrosis of the proximal pole (*)

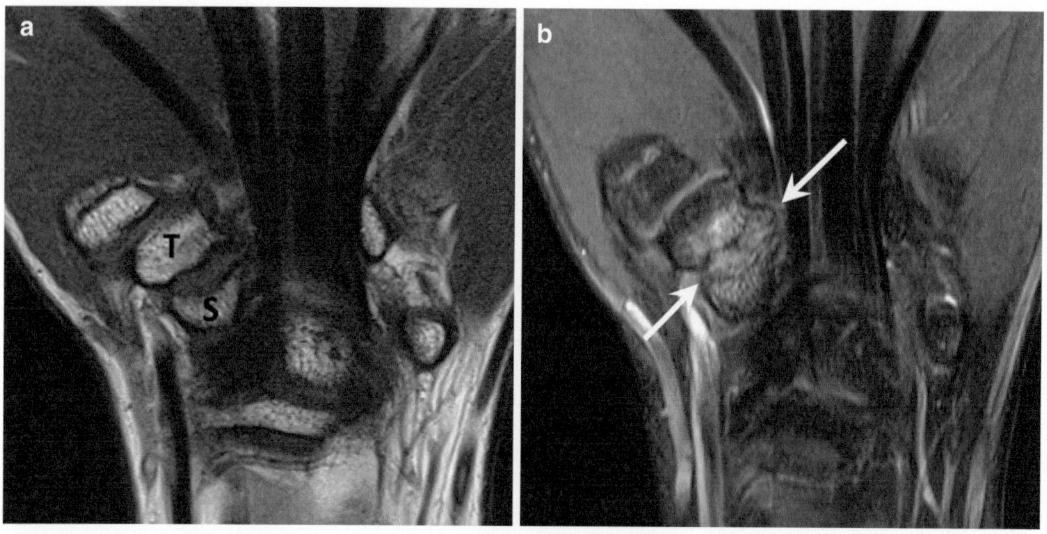

Fig. 8.2 Symptomatic scaphotrapezial coalition. Coronal T1 image (**a**) shows irregular articulation between the scaphoid (S) and trapezium (T). Coronal PD fat-suppressed image (**b**) reveals the non-osseous fusion of the scaphoid and trapezium (white arrows). Bone marrow edema is present along the margins of the coalition

Special MRI Considerations

Magnetic resonance imaging (MRI) is helpful in the evaluation of intercarpal coalitions by detecting non-osseous fusions including the synchondroses and syndesmoses. Osseous fusions will exhibit uniform or near-uniform marrow signal across the coalition site. While many coalitions are asymptomatic, it is proposed that altered biomechanics of the wrist related to increased motion of the unfused carpal joints may result in pain from increased stress or sprains [1]. MRI can also identify features related to symptoms, which may manifest as edema-like signal on fluid bright sequences and subchondral cystic changes.

Variant Lunate Morphology

Epidemiology

Two lunate morphologies are typically described and are similar in prevalence, with studies citing frequency of variant morphology as 50–57.5% [6, 7]. Type I lunate has only one facet at the midcarpal joint, while type II lunate has two facets, with the additional facet articulating with the hamate (Fig. 8.3) [6]. The associated reactive changes can be identified in the proximal pole of the hamate or articulating aspect of the lunate in the setting of type II lunate morphology [2, 6].

Imaging Features

Radiographs clearly depict the variant osseous relationships between the lunate and hamate but will only depict more advanced stages of cartilage degeneration with subchondral sclerosis and osteophyte formation. Variable rates of cartilage damage have been reported as it relates to type II lunate morphology. Many studies report higher rates of chondromalacia and hamate marrow edema associated with the presence of a hamatolunate facet. Pfirrmann et al. found that cartilage lesions in the proximal pole of the hamate reached up to 63.6–81.8% with the additional facet and only 18.2–27.3% with type I morphology [7].

Special MRI Considerations

The thin hyaline layers and multiple articulating surfaces make the articular cartilage of the wrist particularly difficult to assess on MRI. Past studies of cartilage defects of the wrist have proven inadequately sensitive when compared to arthroscopy [8]. With the increased availability of 3T magnets as well as the tailoring of sequences and dedicated wrist coils, evaluation of the wrist cartilage is improving. More recent literature describes good image quality and high performance in the evaluation of wrist cartilage on 3T 3D TrueFISP sequences [9]. Results from research in biochemical and 7T MRI are promising for the future of wrist cartilage evaluation [10, 11].

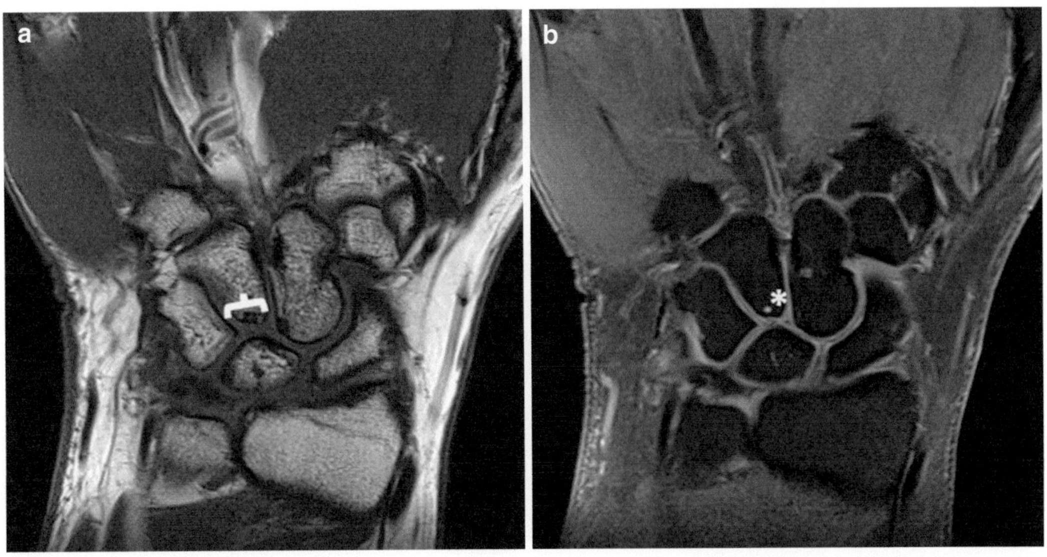

Fig. 8.3 Type II lunate. Coronal T1 (**a**) and coronal T2 fat-suppressed (**b**) images depict type II lunate with a hamatolunate facet (bracket). Hyperintensity across the articulation as well as subchondral sclerosis and subchondral cystic change of the hamate (*) suggests articular cartilage damage

Accessory Ossicles

Epidemiology

At least 20 accessory ossicles have been described in the wrist [2]. These congenital secondary ossification centers are separate from the traditional bones of the wrist and should not be mistaken for fracture fragments or ossific bodies in the absence of trauma or degeneration. The true incidence of these ossicles is unclear as they are often mistaken for un-united fractures or attributed to post-traumatic change. The most frequently identified ossicles of the wrist are seen at a rate of about 1–2% of the population and are discussed in general decreasing frequency below (Fig. 8.4).

The *lunula* can be fused with the distal portion of the ulnar styloid process or be positioned just distal to it within the meniscal homologue [2].

The *os styloideum, or carpal boss*, is located at the dorsal base of the second or third metacarpal and may or may not be fused. In some cases, this anatomic variant can become symptomatic due to limitation in hand motion and friction producing inflammation of overlying soft tissue structures. This ossicle can be palpable and may simulate a dorsal ganglion [2].

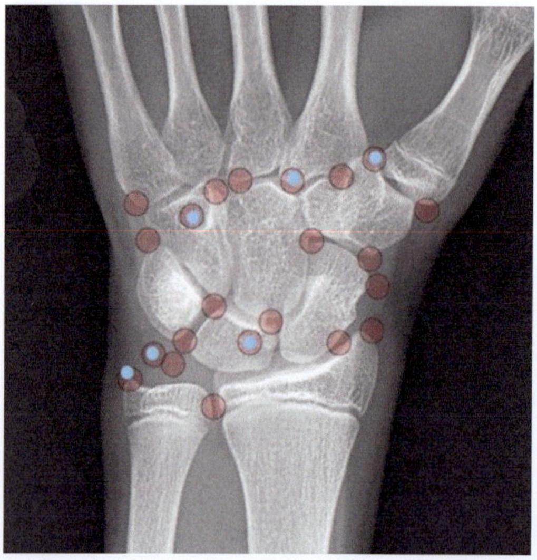

Fig. 8.4 Accessory ossicles of the wrist. The wrist has many accessory ossicles illustrated as red dots by Dr. Jeremy Jones, Radiopaedia.org, rID: 24102. More common ossicles specifically discussed in this chapter have been additionally annotated with superimposed blue dots

Additional common ossicles include *os epilunate* which is dorsal to the lunate (Fig. 8.5), *os triangulare* which is positioned distal to the ulnar fovea, and *trapezium secondarium* which lies superomedially to the palmar aspect of the trapezium [2].

The *os hamuli proprium, or bipartite hamate*, is an ossicle at the site of the hook of the hamate. This os has been associated with ulnar tunnel syndrome, and patients with this accessory ossicle have high rates of carpal tunnel syndrome (CTS), reported as high as 95.2% [12]. It has been proposed that variations in the hook of the hamate may decrease the volume of the carpal tunnel and thus predispose to CTS [12].

Imaging Features

Accessory ossicles will appear well-corticated on radiographs: distinct from adjacent carpal bones. Ossicles will appear the same as bone on all MRI sequences. Although often asymptomatic, accessory ossicles demonstrating edema-like signal on T2-weighted sequences may be indicative of a problematic ossicle. Edema-like signal of the surrounding soft tissues or adjacent bones should increase this suspicion.

Madelung Deformity

Epidemiology

Madelung deformity of the wrist is a rare condition affecting the distal forearms of individuals in the first and second decades of life with up to 80% of cases occurring between 11 and 15 years of age [13]. The deformity can occur in isolation but is common in Leri-Weill dyschondrosteosis and has a 4:1 female predominance [14]. Madelung variant deformities can occur in the setting of Turner syndrome, multiple hereditary exostoses, and Ollier's disease or may be post-traumatic in etiology. Premature closure of the medial volar distal radial physis results in increased volar tilt and inclination of the radial articular surface. In turn, the lunate migrates proximally, and the relatively longer ulna displaces dorsally relative to the carpus producing a "bayonet" deformity [13, 14]. An injury to the

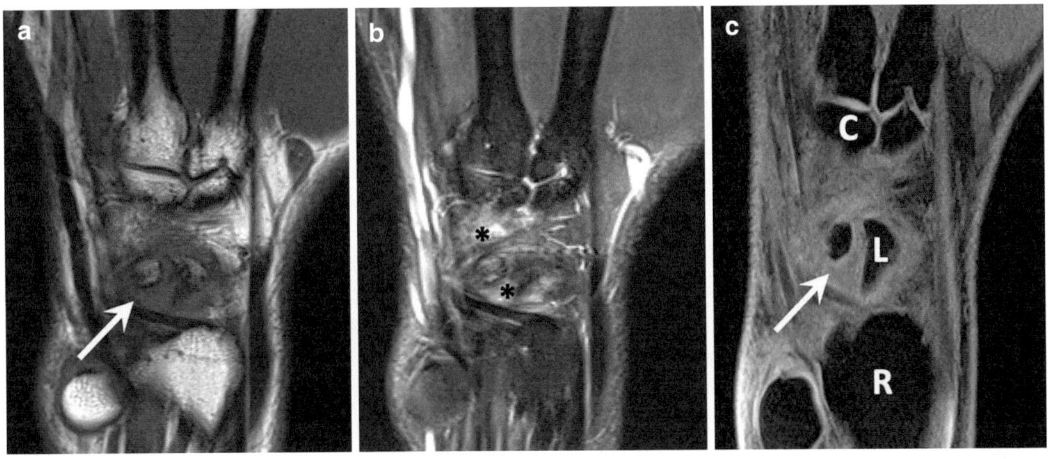

Fig. 8.5 Os epilunatum. Coronal T1 image (**a**) demonstrating an os epilunatum (white arrow) at the dorsal aspect of the lunate and capitate articulation. Coronal T2 fat-suppressed image (**b**) depicts edema-like signal of the ossicle and surrounding soft tissues (*) consistent with site of dorsal wrist pain. Coronal T1 VIBE (**c**) depicts the ossicle (white arrow) as it relates to the distal radius (R), lunate (L), and capitate (c)

dorsal physis can result in "reverse" Madelung deformity: causing dorsal tilt of the distal radius.

Imaging Features

Anatomic changes of Madelung deformity are best seen in their entirety on radiographs of the wrist and forearm. True congenital Madelung deformity (Fig. 8.6) and variants including the "distal radius" variant, "entire radius" variant, and "reverse" Madelung deformities can be differentiated by the presence of Vickers ligament, an anomalous radiolunate ligament [14]. Those with Vickers ligament will have a corresponding notch at the origin of the ligament at the distal medial radius. The hypertrophic ligament tethers the proximal carpal row to the radius, more commonly at the lunate but occasionally at the triquetrum. Entire radius Madelung deformity has similar but more pronounced features of distal radius Madelung deformity including more pronounced radial bowing and increased radiocapitellar distance. An injury to the dorsal physis can result in "reverse" Madelung deformity, causing dorsal tilt of the distal radius.

Special MRI Considerations

MRI is the modality of choice for identifying Vickers ligament and distinguishing true Madelung deformity from variants. MRI can also detect the physeal bridge of the medial volar physis. Additionally, MRI is the most sensitive modality for identifying associated injuries to ligaments and triangulofibrocartilage (TFCC) injuries which can occur because of the altered biomechanics of the deformed wrist. The assessment for posttraumatic etiologies is also aided by MRI which may show paraphyseal edema from repetitive microtrauma as would be seen in "gymnast wrist."

Inflammatory/Infection

Carpal Tunnel Syndrome

Epidemiology

Carpal tunnel syndrome (CTS) is a compressive neuropathy of the median nerve at the level of the carpal tunnel which affects 0.1–1% of the general population [15]. It most commonly affects patients between 30 and 60 years of age and can be bilateral in up to half of cases. CTS can have both intrinsic and extrinsic causes including space-occupying pathologies within the carpal tunnel, trauma, or abnormalities involving the median nerve itself.

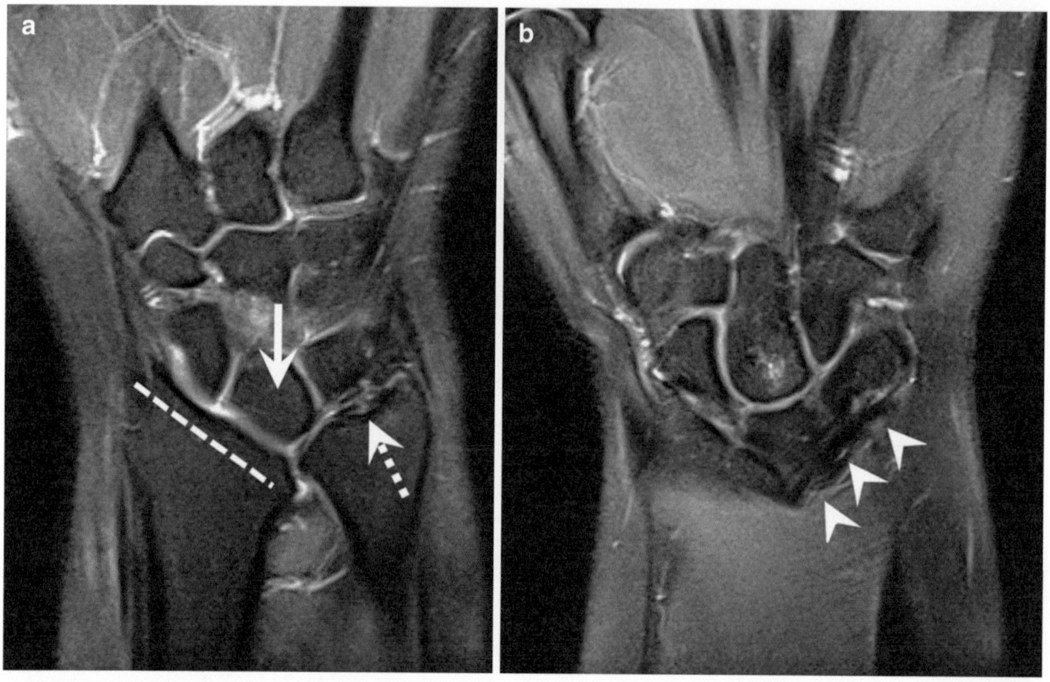

Fig. 8.6 Madelung deformity. Coronal PD fat-suppressed image (**a**) shows increased radial inclination (dashed line) and proximal migration of the lunate (white arrow). The TFCC is also torn (dashed arrow). Coronal PD fat-suppressed image (**b**) shows Vickers ligament (arrowheads)

Imaging Features

Normal MRI appearance of the median nerve in the axial plane is round at the level of the distal radius and elliptical at the level of the pisiform. The nerve should be T1 isointense to muscle and mildly T2 hyperintense. The nerve is surrounded by perineural fat and consists of a fascicular pattern on T1- and T2-weighted sequences. Imaging features of CTS include palmar bowing of the flexor retinaculum, increase of the cross-sectional area of the median nerve by more than 2 mm^2 between the level of the hamate and pisiform, increased T2 signal hyperintensity, and fascicular swelling. Secondary signs of denervation injury of the thenar muscles may also be present (Fig. 8.7) [15].

Special MRI Considerations

In addition to detecting changes to the compressed median nerve, MRI is helpful in determining the cause of neuropathy. CTS is common in patients with rheumatoid arthritis, estimated to occur at a rate of 23% [15]. Most often, symptoms develop insidiously as a result of flexor tenosynovitis but may also be a consequence of severe destructive changes of the carpus. MRI can be used to characterize synovial hyperplasia and evaluate for tenosynovitis and early destructive change.

Infectious tenosynovitis can result in compression of the median nerve by inflammatory exudates. MRI will exhibit T1-hypointense and T2-hyperintense fluid distending the tendon sheath with enhancement of a thickened synovium following the administration of gadolinium-based contrast.

In the posttraumatic setting, MRI can help identify neuromas which may develop as a result of complete transection or partial injury. Neuromas are disorganized fibroneuronal tissue whose bulbous enlargement and T2 heterogeneous hyperintensity are attributed to a combination of fascicles, intralesional hemorrhage, and fibrosis. Post-contrast enhancement of posttraumatic neuromas will also be heterogeneous. They can be differentiated from peripheral nerve sheath

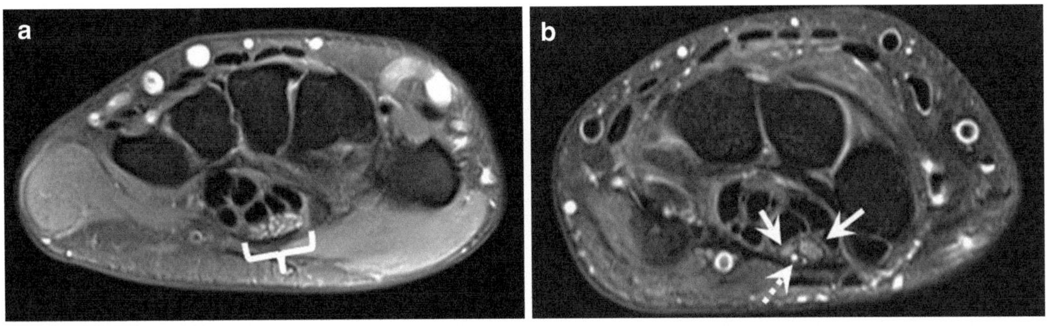

Fig. 8.7 Carpal tunnel syndrome. Axial PD fat-suppressed image (**a**) through the level of the distal carpal tunnel depicts enlarged median nerve with increased fluid signal and fascicular swelling (bracket). Axial PD fat-suppressed image (**b**) through the level of the carpal tunnel in another patient presenting with CTS details a bifid median nerve (arrows) and persistent median artery (dashed arrow)

tumor (PNST) by clinical history and absence of "target sign" often seen in PNST.

It is important to evaluate for the bifid median nerve, a normal median nerve variant which bifurcates within or proximal to the carpal tunnel rather than distal to it. Due to its higher cross-sectional area, bifid median nerves are more susceptible to CTS. The bifid nerve is often associated with a persistent median artery of the forearm which is easily detected on ultrasound and MRI and positioned between the two nerve bundles (Fig. 8.7). Noting this anatomy is important before surgical release of the flexor retinaculum to avoid inadvertent injury to the nerve.

Tenosynovitis

de Quervain Tenosynovitis

Epidemiology

de Quervain tenosynovitis (Fig. 8.8) is a chronic overuse injury of the first compartment of the wrist resulting in stenosing tenosynovitis of the extensor pollicis brevis (EPB) and abductor pollicis longus (APL). Racquet sports, fishing, golf, early motherhood, and frequent text messaging have been associated with this condition characterized by radial-sided wrist pain [16].

Imaging Features

Radiographic features of de Quervain tenosynovitis are nonspecific but include soft tissue swelling over the radial styloid and reactive changes of the subjacent radial styloid seen as periosteal reaction and erosion. MRI fluid-sensitive sequences delineate hyperintensity of the first compartment tendon sheaths with distension by fluid and inflammatory cells. Tendinopathy of the EPB and APL tendons may be present, including tendon thickening or longitudinal split tearing. Inflammation may extend into the adjacent soft tissue and osseous structures as edema-like signal.

Special MRI Considerations

Aside from inflammatory findings, MRI can aid in the characterization of variant anatomy which can predispose to de Quervain tenosynovitis as well as provide prognostic and clinical decision-making information. The presence of multiple tendon slips may create increased friction and predispose to tenosynovitis. More common in the APL than the EPB, the normal appearance is that of multiple tendon slips. Knowing this helps distinguish normal anatomy from longitudinal tears and guides the appropriateness of surgical intervention [17].

The first extensor compartment can be split into partial or complete subcompartments by the presence of a septum. In these cases, the EPB is typically more severely affected, and failure to treat both subcompartments may lead to worse clinical outcomes. The septum is easier to visualize on ultrasound, but indirect features of a septum can be seen on MRI, including

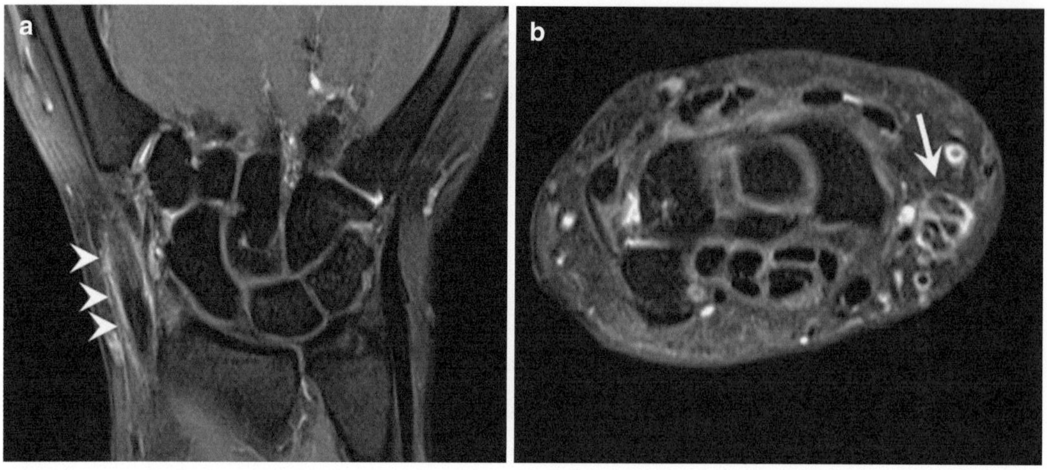

Fig. 8.8 de Quervain tenosynovitis. Coronal (**a**) and axial PD fat-suppressed images (**b**) demonstrating hyperintensity of the first compartment tendon sheaths (arrowheads). Increased signal within the APL and EPB tendons (white arrow)

asymmetric tendon involvement, presence of a bony ridge, and a double groove on the radial floor [17].

Distal Intersection Syndrome

Epidemiology

Distal intersection syndrome (Fig. 8.9) is a less common extensor compartment inflammatory condition affecting the second and third dorsal compartments where the extensor pollicis longus (EPL) crosses over the extensor carpi radialis longus (ECRL) and extensor carpi radialis brevis (ECRB) tendons. Intrinsic stenosing tenosynovitis or compression from the extensor retinaculum may contribute to this inflammatory process. Many cases are attributed to overuse or blunt trauma to the EPL tendon. A foramen communicates between the tendon sheaths of these compartments which may propagate findings of tenosynovitis from one compartment to the other. This syndrome should not be confused with intersection syndrome or proximal intersection syndrome involving the first and second extensor compartments where their myotendinous junctions cross in the distal forearm producing radial and dorsal sided pain 4–6 cm proximal to the wrist joint.

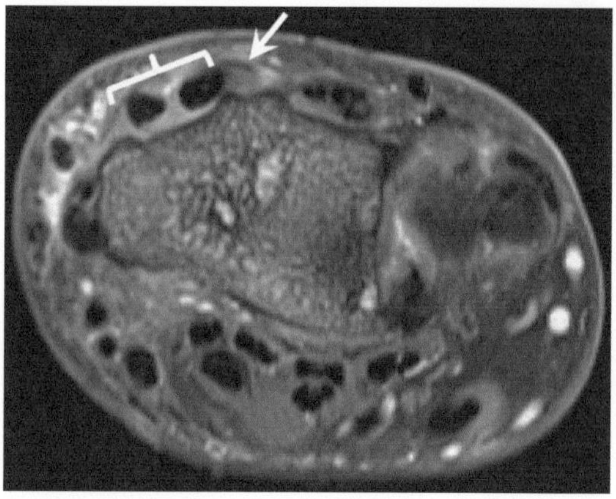

Fig. 8.9 Distal intersection syndrome. The EPL (white arrow) begins to cross over the second compartment (bracket) in the axial PD fat-suppressed image. Hyperintensity surrounds the tendons of the second compartment with increased signal in the EPL

Imaging Features

This entity can clinically present as a mass in the distal forearm or wrist. Knowledge of the anatomy aids in MRI diagnosis. MRI features of distal intersection syndrome include thickening of the EPL, ECRL, and ECRB tendons with or without intrasubstance signal changes. Fluid signal surrounds the tendons at the level of the intersection and adjacent soft tissues, and osseous structures may also show increased T2 signal and edema-like signal.

Infectious Tenosynovitis

Epidemiology

Most infections of the hand are related to minor trauma with overlooked or neglected wounds. Patients who are immunocompromised are more susceptible, and additional predisposing factors include diabetes mellitus, peripheral vascular disease, renal failure, intravenous drug use, alcohol consumption, steroids, and arthritis [18]. Infections of the hand and wrist are capable of spreading easily via flexor and extensor tendon sheaths. Common organisms affecting the flexor and extensor tendons are *Mycobacterium tuberculosis*, atypical mycobacterium or nontuberculous mycobacteria (NTM), and pyogenic bacteria (*Staphylococcus* and *Streptococcus*) [15]. Timely diagnosis of infectious flexor tenosynovitis is imperative to prevent significant spread related to the common tendon sheath. Neurovascular compromise can also occur.

Imaging Features

Fluid-sensitive sequences show high-signal-intensity fluid and inflammatory cell distension of tendon sheaths (Figs. 8.10 and 8.11). Flexor tendon tenosynovitis can spread from tendon sheaths of the thumb into the radial bursa or from small finger tendon sheaths into the ulnar bursa. Infection can also spread into the space of Parona, a potential space deep to the flexor tendons described in Chap. 6 and from one bursa to the other resulting in a "horseshoe" abscess.

Special MRI Considerations

Although there are a variety of pathogens that can cause infectious tenosynovitis, many of the imaging features are similar.

MRI features of tuberculous tenosynovitis will often be nonspecific for the pathogen and may mimic inflammatory arthropathies, pigmented villonodular synovitis, gout, or tumor. However, some imaging findings may point toward tuberculous infection. In contrast to more common tenosynovial infections, tuberculous tenosynovitis demonstrates hypointense synovium on T2-weighted images in 40% of cases suggestive of granuloma [19]. Foci of hypointense T2 and T2* signal may also be present within the synovial fluid and may indicate debris or rice bodies [19]. These foci will also not enhance following gadolinium contrast administration.

Septic Arthritis

Epidemiology

Septic arthritis (Fig. 8.12) is most commonly caused by penetrating injury but may also result

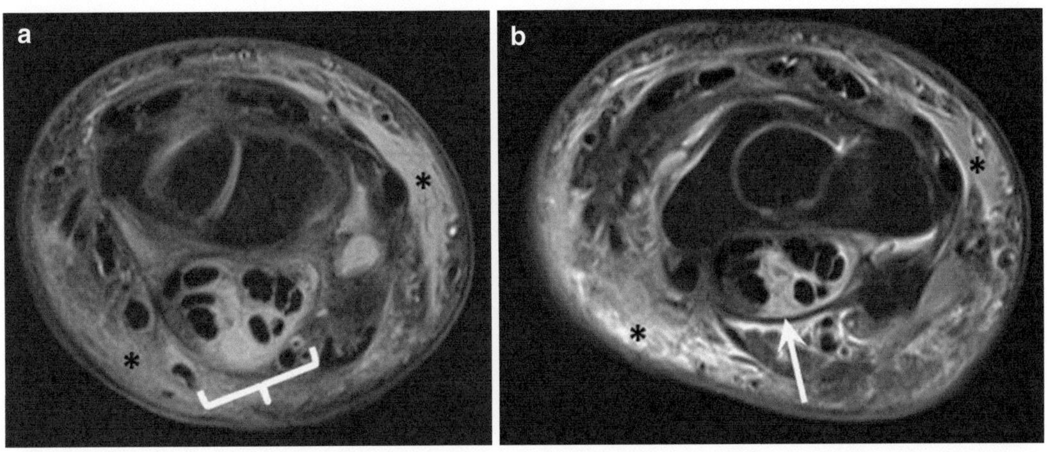

Fig. 8.10 Infectious tenosynovitis in intravenous drug use. Axial PD fat-suppressed image (**a**) shows hyperintense distension of multiple flexor tendon sheaths (bracket). Axial T1 fat-suppressed and contrast-enhanced image (**b**) demonstrates enhancing synovium (white arrow) and enhancing subcutaneous edema (*), a feature of cellulitis

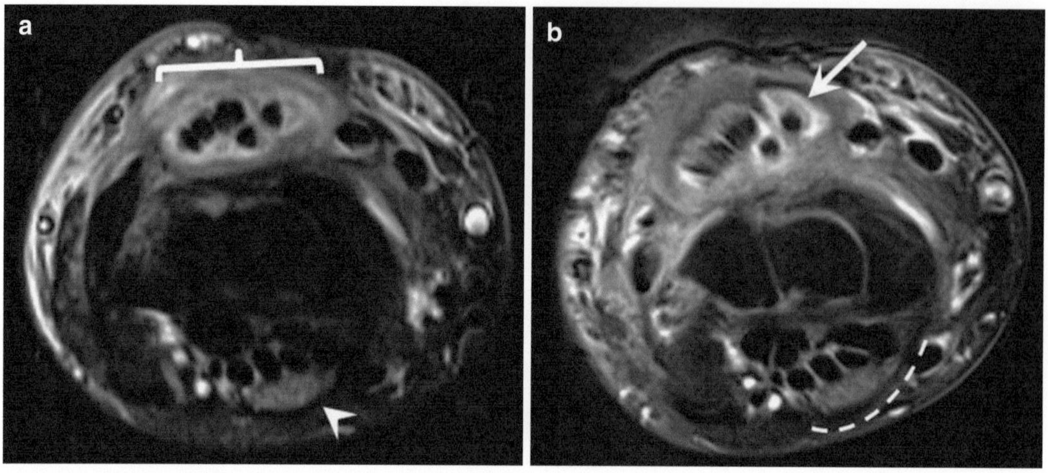

Fig. 8.11 Sporotrichosis tenosynovitis. Axial STIR image (**a**) depicts hyperintense distension of the extensor tendon sheaths (bracket) and compressive neuropathy of the median nerve with increased nerve caliber (arrowhead). Contrast-enhanced T1 fat-suppressed image (**b**) shows bowing of the flexor retinaculum (dashed line) and enhancement of the synovium (white arrow)

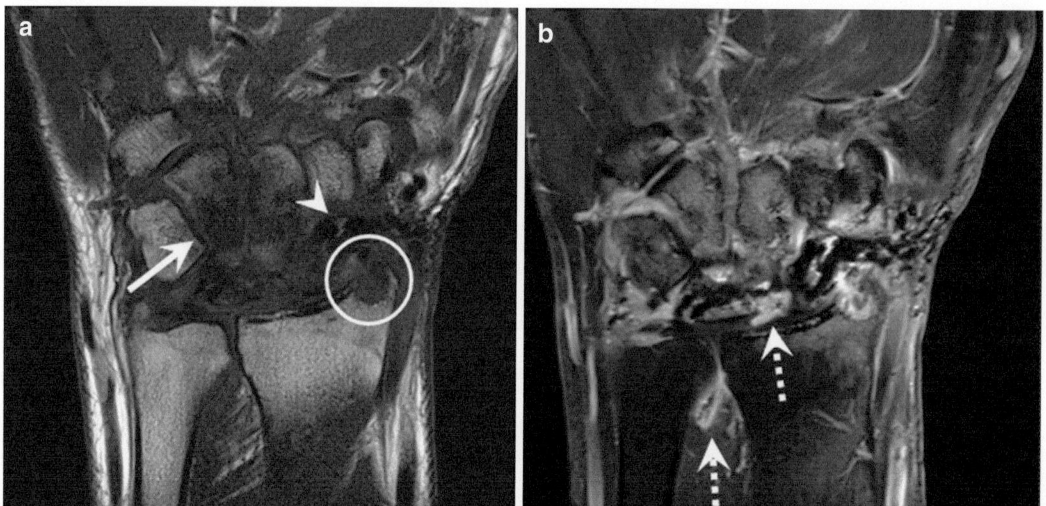

Fig. 8.12 Septic arthritis in the postoperative wrist. Coronal T1 image (**a**) shows osseous erosion (circle) and T1 marrow hypointensity of the capitate and hamate (arrow) consistent with osteomyelitis. Foci of signal loss are consistent with prior surgical intervention (scapholunate ligament reconstruction) and/or with the presence of gas-forming organism. The scaphoid and lunate are fragmented and sclerotic from prior avascular necrosis and advanced osteoarthritis. Post-contrast-enhanced coronal T1 image (**b**) highlights joint effusion with synovial enhancement (dashed arrows)

from contiguous spread of infection from an adjacent structure. The prompt and accurate diagnosis of septic arthritis is important to prevent cartilage damage and joint destruction.

Imaging Features

Radiographs of the septic joint will reveal joint effusion, bone erosions, periostitis, and periarticular soft tissue swelling. Joint space narrowing may also be present but occurs later in the disease process. On MRI, fluid-sensitive sequences will reveal hyperintense joint distension. Following the administration of gadolinium contrast, post-contrast image will show synovial enhancement and may help differentiate rim-enhancing soft tissue abscesses from adjacent cellulitis.

Special MRI Considerations

MRI is the most sensitive modality for the early detection of osteomyelitis. If soft tissue infection or abscess contacts the bone, careful scrutiny of the cortex may reveal periosteal thickening as would be seen in reactive periostitis. Cortical changes and erosions in conjunction with subjacent loss of normal T1 marrow signal are concerning for osteomyelitis.

Arthritis

Rheumatoid Arthritis

Epidemiology

Rheumatoid arthritis (RA) (Fig. 8.13) is a systemic rheumatologic disease estimated to affect 1% of the population [20]. Inflammatory changes typically affect the hands first with the peak incidence in the fourth and fifth decades.

Imaging Features

Classic radiographic features of rheumatoid arthritis include symmetric joint involvement, "bare area" erosions, periarticular osteopenia, and concentric joint space narrowing. RA has a predilection for the ulnar styloid. MRI is the most sensitive modality for detecting early erosive changes of rheumatoid arthritis. It also clearly depicts other features of rheumatoid arthritis including joint effusions, early erosions, synovial pannus, and soft tissue and osseous edema-like signal. Not only is MRI sensitive in detection, but also it aids in assessing disease activity which is necessary for disease management.

Synovitis is the earliest abnormality to appear in RA and has intermediate to low T1 signal, high T2 signal, enhancement, and increased synovial volume. Joint effusion can be differentiated from synovitis by using heavily T2-weighted sequences or T1 post-contrast images. Fibrotic pannus appears in later stage RA and will be hypointense on T2-weighted sequences.

Although nonspecific, bone marrow edema is considered to be an early marker of inflammation and is commonly reported in RA.

Erosions are defined as sharply marginated juxtaarticular bone lesions with associated cortical loss. Erosions will demonstrate loss of normal T1 marrow hyperintensity and hyperintensity of T2-weighted and STIR images. Erosions will also enhance following administration of gadolinium contrast – a feature which helps differentiate them from fluid-filled cystic lesions.

As discussed earlier, distinguishing etiologies for tenosynovitis can be difficult. RA typically affects the dorsal compartments, most

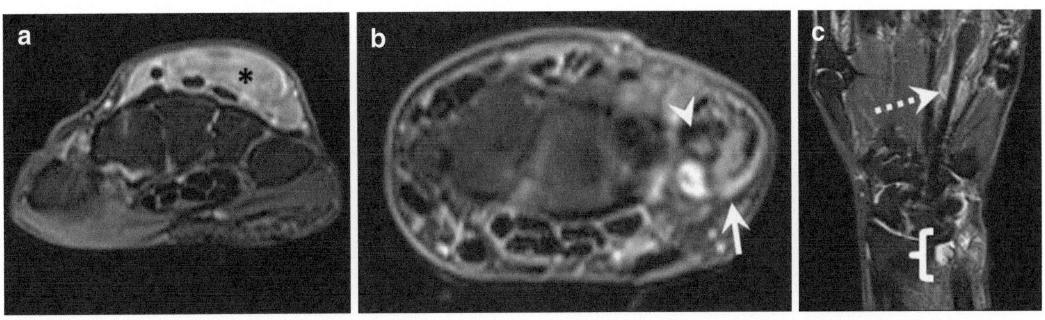

Fig. 8.13 Rheumatoid arthritis. Axial T2 fat-suppressed image (**a**) shows large volume of tenosynovium in the dorsal compartments (*). Axial T2 fat-suppressed image (**b**) demonstrates ECU tendinosis (white arrow) and erosion of the ulnar styloid (arrowhead). Coronal STIR image (**c**) depicts flexor tenosynovitis (dashed arrow) and distal radioulnar joint effusion (bracket)

frequently involving the extensor carpi ulnaris (ECU).

Special MRI Considerations

Although RA typically affects both hands, it is recommended to image the more symptomatic side not only to be more sensitive but also to save time. The Outcomes Measures in Rheumatoid Arthritis Clinical Trials (OMERACT) MR imaging study group recommends imaging in at least two planes (preferably coronal and axial), T1-weighted imaging before and after gadolinium contrast (fat suppression preferred following contrast), and a fat-suppressed T2-weighted or STIR sequence [21]. Contrast may be withheld if osseous changes alone are important.

Psoriatic Arthritis

Epidemiology

Psoriatic arthritis (Fig. 8.14) is a seronegative spondyloarthropathy that has a prevalence of approximately 0.5% but affects approximately 25% of those with psoriasis. Psoriatic arthritis most commonly affects the hand. In contrast to RA, psoriatic arthritis can affect any small hand joint as a monoarthritis or oligoarthritis.

Imaging Features

Isolated tenosynovitis with synovitis or soft tissue inflammation results in dactylitis or "sausage digit" which may be the first clinical findings. Flexor tendon involvement is more common than extensor, and several fingers can be involved simultaneously. Although the synovitis of RA and psoriatic arthritis are difficult to distinguish from one another, psoriatic arthritis causes an inflammation of the periosteum which creates a characteristic periostitis. More advanced psoriatic arthritis can present with more aggressive disruption of the cortex, "pencil-in-cup" deformities to the distal interphalangeal joints, and inflammatory changes of underlying cancellous bone.

Special MRI Considerations

Dynamic contrast-enhanced studies have been shown to highlight active versus chronic inactive inflammation in psoriatic arthritis [22]. The hyperemia of active inflammation will enhance earlier, while delayed enhancement is more likely in fibrotic synovial thickening. Dynamic contrast evaluation may also help in differentiating RA from psoriatic arthritis with more abrupt washout described in psoriatic arthritis. A dynamic contrast-enhanced protocol described

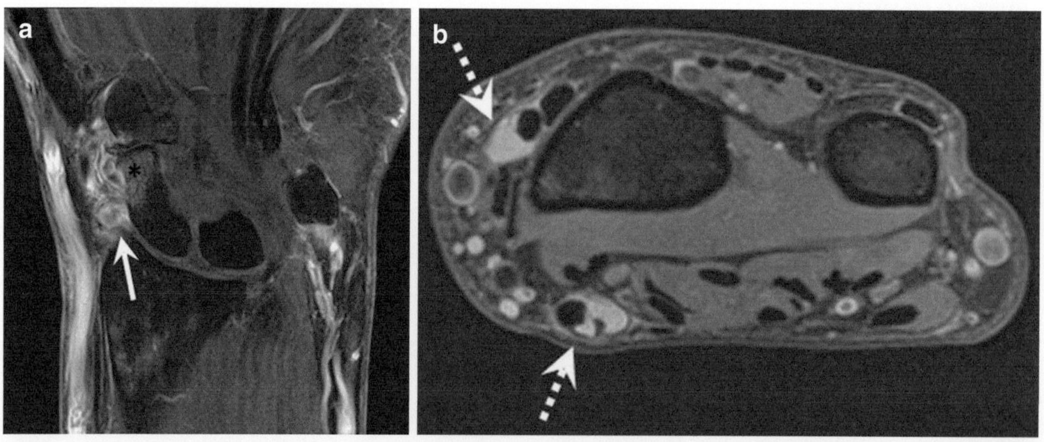

Fig. 8.14 Oligoarticular psoriatic arthritis. Coronal T1 fat-suppressed and contrast-enhanced image (**a**) depicts enhancing synovitis (white arrow). There is cortical disruption of the scaphoid with edema-like signal of the bone (*). Axial PD fat-suppressed image (**b**) reveals tenosynovitis of both the FCR and ECRL (dashed arrows)

by Schwenzer et al. [23] utilizes a 3D encoded spoiled gradient-echo sequence to measure contrast medium uptake in the synovial tissue to calculate relative enhancement rates at 35 seconds, 52 seconds, 3 minutes, and 15 minutes. Observations at 15 minutes are statistically significant for decreased relative enhancement in psoriatic arthritis relative to rheumatoid arthritis.

Gout

Epidemiology

The incidence of gout (Fig. 8.15) has increased in recent history with a prevalence of approximately 4% in the United States. Deposition of monosodium urate (MSU) crystals in the joints and soft tissues triggers an inflammatory response causing soft tissue and bone changes.

Imaging Features

Features of gouty arthropathy include joint effusion, eccentric "punched-out" erosions with sclerotic margins, and overhanging edges. Surrounding soft tissues may contain tophi, mass-like deposits of MSU. Although MRI is sensitive for early soft tissue and osseous abnormalities, it is less specific than dual-energy computed tomography (DECT). In addition to detecting osseous erosions, newer CT technologic advances have allowed for the specific detection of uric acid by exploiting the photon energy-dependent attenuation. DECT software can directly quantify the MSU volume and demonstrate responses to therapy on follow-up scans [24].

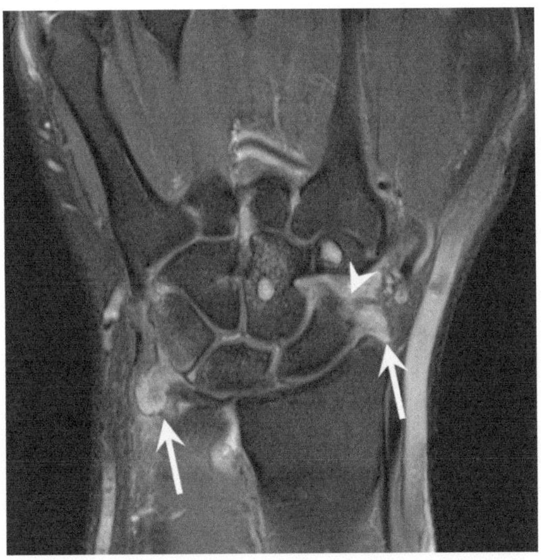

Fig. 8.15 Gout. Coronal PD fat-suppressed image illustrates heterogeneously intense joint effusion (white arrows) and small cortical erosions (arrowheads). Incidental note is made of type II lunate morphology and associated cartilage loss

Special MRI Considerations

Features of gout on MRI can be variable. Tophi are hypointense on T1-weighted images and have heterogeneous hyperintensity with T2-weighted and fluid-sensitive sequences. Following the administration of gadolinium contrast, tophi can uniformly enhance or be centrally non-enhancing. The erosions of infection can mimic gout; however, the presence of associated soft tissue ulceration supports infection.

Calcium Pyrophosphate Dihydrate Deposition Disease (CPPD)

Epidemiology

The prevalence of CPPD is high and increases with age reaching up to 25% of patients aged 85 and older [25]. CPPD can progress to a destructive arthropathy with many features in common with osteoarthritis (Fig. 8.16).

Imaging Features

CPPD and osteoarthritis can have a similar appearance. In distinction to osteoarthritis, CPPD tends to be more symmetric and is more likely to involve non-weight-bearing joints. CPPD is also notable for prominent subchondral cystic changes. On radiographs, chondrocalcinosis will commonly be present at the triangular fibrocartilage complex and lunotriquetral ligaments.

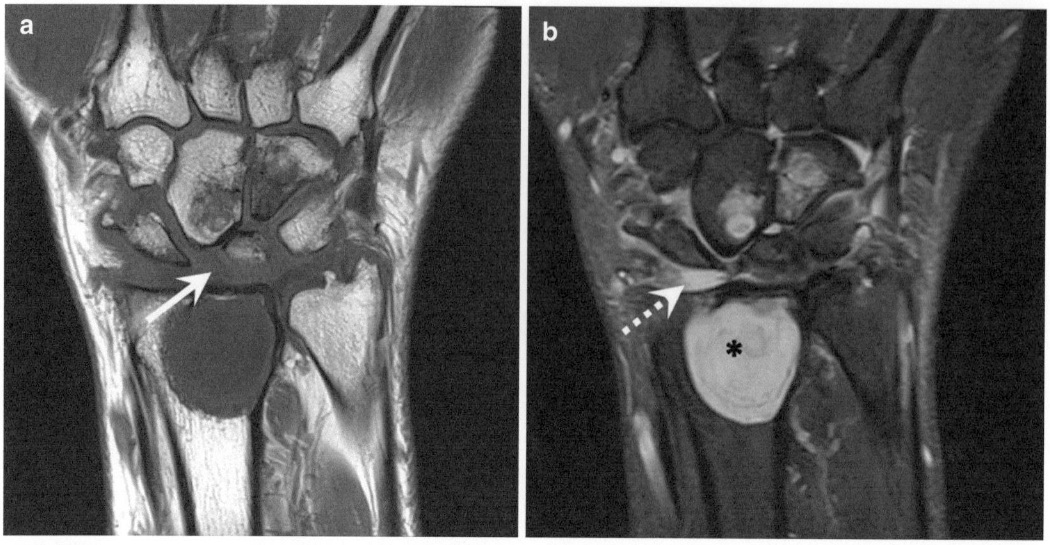

Fig. 8.16 CPPD with SLAC wrist. Coronal T1 images (**a**) reveals widened scapholunate interval seen with scapholunate tear (white arrow) as well as proximal migration of the capitate. Coronal PD fat-suppressed image (**b**) demonstrates cartilage damage of the radioscaphoid articulation (dashed arrow) as well as large subchondral cysts of the distal radius (*) and capitate

Special MRI Considerations

An interesting feature of CPPD is the frequently comorbid SLAC (scapholunate advanced collapse) wrist. Pyrophosphate deposition in the scapholunate ligament leads to ligamentous laxity and eventual disruption. As the capitate migrates proximally, osteoarthritis develops first at the radioscaphoid articulation and then the capitolunate articulation. Other features of CPPD, such as subchondral cysts, are also well characterized on MRI. The TFCC and lunotriquetral mineralization may also be detected on MRI.

Hemophilia

Epidemiology

Hemophilia (Fig. 8.17) is a rare inherited bleeding disorder in which approximately half of patients suffer from hemophilic arthropathy. Recurrent intra-articular hemorrhage results in iron deposition stimulating synovitis and causing progressive cartilage and subchondral bone damage.

Imaging Features

As joints will often be affected at an early age, radiographs may demonstrate epiphyseal enlargement related to hyperemia. Additional radiographic features reflect secondary degenerative changes including osteophytes, subchondral sclerosis, and subchondral cysts. MRI is the most sensitive modality for assessing articular and periarticular structural damage related to hemophilic arthropathy. MR depicts synovial hypertrophy as well as signs of occult bleeding and hemosiderin deposits. In earlier stages of the disease, with only few episodes of intra-articular hemorrhage, changes may be difficult to detect. As the disease recurs, periarticular erosions and subchondral cysts will form.

Special MRI Considerations

MRI specific to assessing hemophilic arthropathy may be tailored to detect small foci of hemosiderin deposition. One may consider adding gradient-echo (GRE) sequences to highlight susceptibility artifact from these deposits. The same deposits will similarly degrade evaluation of the synovium and cartilage, and standard pulse sequences such

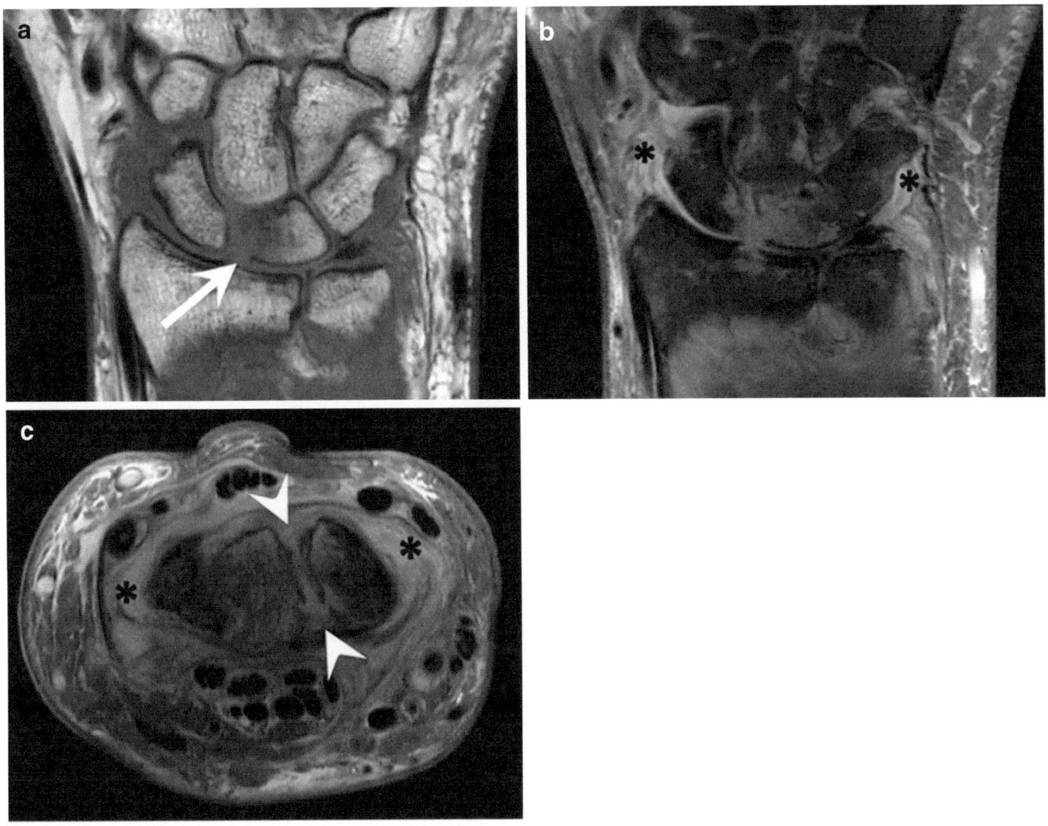

Fig. 8.17 Hemophilic arthropathy. Coronal T1 (**a**) shows focal areas of cortical erosion and cartilage destruction involving the radial aspect of the lunate and central articular surface of the radius (white arrow). Coronal T2 fat-suppressed image (**b**) depicts heterogeneous joint effusion and extensive synovitis (*). Axial PD fat-suppressed image (**c**) illustrates complete disruption of the scapholunate ligament (arrowheads)

as T1, T2, and PD are recommended as they do not depend on T2* relaxation time and can overcome blooming artifact seen on GRE sequences.

Benign Osseous Lesions

Intraosseous Ganglion Cysts

Epidemiology

Intraosseous ganglion cysts are benign bone processes with similar internal mucoid viscous contents to synovial cysts and lack a synovial or epithelial lining in contrast to synovial cysts Peak incidence is in the fourth and fifth decades of life with a small male predominance. These lesions have a tendency for the long bones of the lower extremity and proximal carpal bones. An intraosseous ganglion is distinct from subchondral cystic changes seen with degenerative joint disease. Subchondral cystic changes are often due to overlying high-grade articular cartilage loss and are frequently seen in conjunction with joint space narrowing and osteophyte formation. Intraosseous ganglion cysts are not seen in association with degenerative joint disease. However, the majority of literature on the pathophysiology of this entity suggests a potential fine articular communication.

Imaging Features

On radiography, intraosseous ganglion cysts appear as a well-defined lucent lesion near a joint, mostly small (1–2 cm), and without aggressive features.

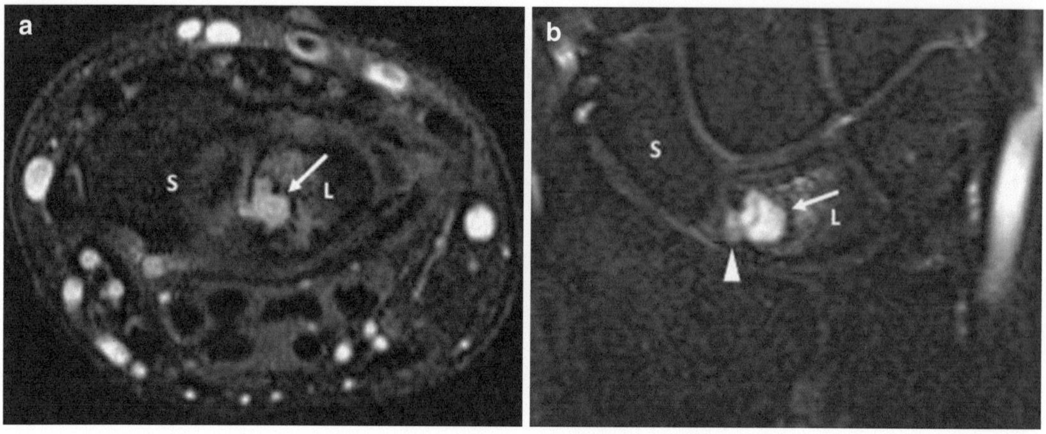

Fig. 8.18 Intraosseous ganglion cyst. Axial PD fat-suppressed image (**a**) of the wrist shows a well-circumscribed fluid intensity structure (white arrow) within the radial aspect of the lunate (L). Coronal T2 fat-suppressed image of the wrist (**b**) depicts the lunate intraosseous ganglion cyst, communicating with the scapholunate interval (arrowhead). The scaphoid bone (S) is annotated for orientation. Note the lack of osteophytes and joint space narrowing that would be seen with a subchondral cyst

Special MRI Considerations

Intraosseous ganglion cysts are often seen as unilocular T1-hypointense and T2-hyperintense structures within the carpal bones. These structures often demonstrate a thin sclerotic rim and do not enhance on gadolinium-enhanced sequences. When enhancement is present, it is in the form of thin and peripheral without nodular or mass-like enhancement. Intraosseous ganglion cysts are often away from the articular surface. When these structures are subchondral, overlying degenerative changes are absent (Fig. 8.18).

Enchondroma

Epidemiology

Enchondromas are most common within the hands and feet (phalanges, metacarpals, and metatarsals). These benign neoplasms are less frequently found in the carpus [26]. Of the 110 cases of hand enchondromas reported by Takigawa et al., only two cases involved the carpal bones – the scaphoid and the lunate [27]. Emecheta et al. reported only 3 enchondromas in a series of 86 treated carpal lesions [28]. The scaphoid is the most common location for carpal enchondromas and is often asymptomatic unless a pathologic fracture occurs [29, 30]. Malignant transformation of carpal enchondromas has not been reported.

Imaging Features

Enchondromas of the carpus are similar in appearance on radiography to enchondromas of the metacarpals and phalanges. These lesions are intramedullary, mildly expansile, and do not reveal significant matrix mineralization unlike enchondromas within larger tubular bones. They may have mild endosteal scalloping but have no aggressive features.

Special MRI Considerations

On MRI, enchondromas are well-circumscribed and somewhat lobulated intramedullary lesions. Carpal enchondromas demonstrate low to intermediate T1 and high T2 signal. Aggressive features such as periosteal reaction and associated soft tissue mass are not seen. These lesions have variable enhancement patterns but predominantly exhibit peripheral thin enhancement.

Osteoid Osteoma

Epidemiology

Carpal bones are involved in only 2% of cases of osteoid osteoma. The scaphoid and capitate are the most frequent sites of involvement in the carpus. There is a male predominance and patients are often in their second and third decades of life [31]. Clinical presentation is very typical with pain, worse at night.

Imaging Features

Radiography can reveal a lucent nidus, occasionally with a central sclerotic focus of mineralized osteoid. The nidus is surrounded by reactive sclerosis. These findings are exceptionally hard to see on wrist radiography due to superimposition of structures and small bone size. Thin-slice CT utilizing bone algorithm best reveals the lucent central nidus with associated osseous sclerosis and benign periosteal reaction to better advantage than radiography or MRI. Bone scan imaging will reveal a central focus of marked increased uptake (nidus) in a background of increased activity [32].

Special MRI Considerations

MRI findings of osteoid osteoma can be confounding due to the degree of marrow edema that often accompanies these lesions; however, it is the most *sensitive* modality in detecting osteoid osteomas [33]. Commonly, a demarcated nidus of hypointense signal surrounded by edema is seen on fluid-sensitive sequences. Dynamic gadolinium-enhanced sequences show peak enhancement in arterial phase with early partial washout in the majority of cases. Liu et al. concluded that osteoid osteomas can be imaged with greater conspicuity by using dynamic gadolinium-enhanced sequences compared to non-contrast-enhanced MRI and with equal to improved conspicuity compared to thin-section CT [34]. Rarely is this technique necessary for evaluation.

Aggressive Osseous Lesions

Giant Cell Tumor of Bone

Epidemiology

Giant cell tumor of bone (GCTOB) is a benign, locally aggressive primary bone tumor. The distal radius accounts for 10–12% of cases with the remainder of the wrist bones rarely affected. GCTOB most often occurs in skeletally mature patients between the ages of 20 and 40 years old with a slight female predominance [35].

Imaging Features

When GCTOB occurs in the wrist, it is often centrally located, in contradistinction to elsewhere in the skeleton where it is eccentric in location. GCTOB occurs near an articular surface and exhibits a geographic lucent appearance with a narrow zone of transition but lacks a sclerotic margin. This absence of a sclerotic border distinguishes GCTOB from intraosseous ganglion. Thinning of the cortex and expansile remodeling of bone are also common radiographic features.

The utility of CT in evaluation of these lesions is limited to evaluation of matrix. GCTOB will not have a mineralized matrix. While CT improves delineation of cortical thinning, periosteal reaction, and pathologic fractures, these findings are well shown with MRI [35–38].

Special MRI Considerations

MRI demonstrates a hypointense rim and T1/T2 predominantly isointense-hypointense solid components. Giant cell tumors are characteristic on MRI because of the low T1 and T2 signal due to the presence of hemosiderin. This imaging characteristic distinguishes GCTOB from other pathologic lesions. Fluid-fluid levels as can be seen in aneurysmal bone cysts may also occur within GCTOB. Often, when ABC components predominate, the solid part of the tumor is located peripherally [38]. Solid versus cystic component detection is aided by the use of contrast and is important to avoid misdiagnosis and to direct biopsy. While the cystic components may have thin, wispy peripheral enhancement, the solid sections diffusely enhance, reflecting hypervascularity seen on pathology (Fig. 8.19).

Soft Tissue Lesions

Soft tissue sarcomas predominantly occur in the extremities; however, these tumors comprise only 1% of all cancers [39]. It is estimated that

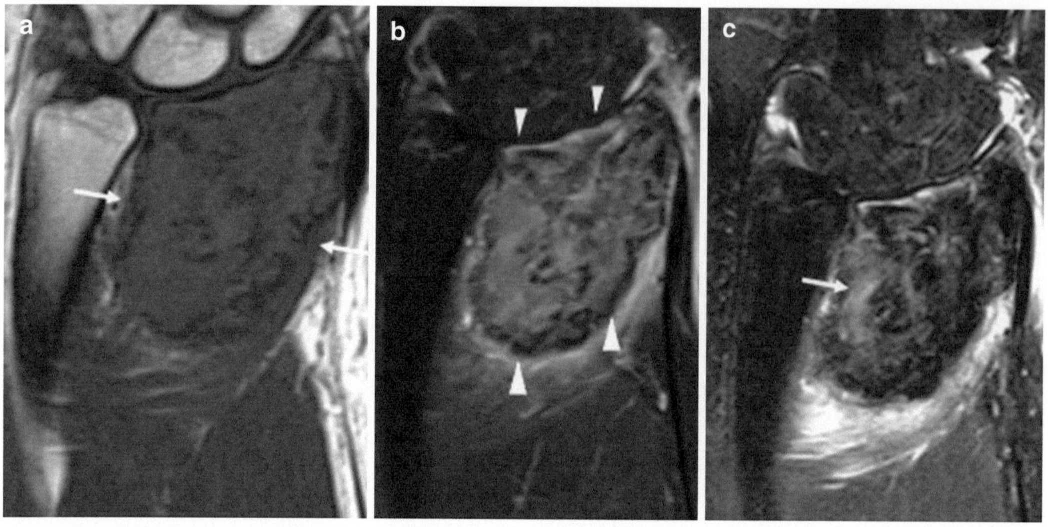

Fig. 8.19 Giant cell tumor of bone. Coronal T1 image (**a**) shows cortical thinning both medially and laterally (arrows). Note low signal elements on T1-weighted imaging. Coronal T2 fat-suppressed image (**b**) shows a subarticular, expansile, heterogeneously isointense to predominantly low signal intramedullary lesion within the distal radius (arrowheads). Coronal T1 fat-suppressed post-contrast image (**c**) illustrates heterogeneous enhancement (arrow)

less than 1% of upper limb tumors occur in the wrist and hand [39]. Rarity of these tumors results in scarce literature describing their imaging findings. Additionally, it has been demonstrated that approximately 41% of soft tissue sarcomas of the hand/wrist were initially excised under the assumption that they were not malignant [40]. This disappointing statistic stresses that most atypical hand/wrist tumors do not undergo appropriate investigation via imaging and pathologic sampling prior to excision. More accurate identification can result in proper treatment and surgical excision when appropriate.

Benign Soft Tissue Lesions

Synovial Cysts

Synovial cysts are the most common benign soft tissue lesions encountered in the wrist [41]. Although the exact mechanism of cyst formation is unknown, it is widely speculated that extra-articular mucin droplets coalesce to form the main body of the cyst. Thereafter, the "cyst wall" and stalk connecting the cyst to a nearby synovial joint are formed [42]. In the majority of cases, these cysts occur spontaneously and gradually over time increase in size; however, 15% of patients describe a chronological relationship between the appearance of the cyst and an injury [41, 43, 44]. The clinical course of these cysts is unpredictable and variable as they can appear and disappear spontaneously. Synovial cysts are lined with synovium as extensions of the joint. Ganglion cysts do not have a synovial lining. Clinicians, including radiologists, often use the terms interchangeably. Ganglion cysts are typically located along tendon sheaths, whereas the synovial cysts often arise from a joint.

Epidemiology

Wrist synovial cysts are commonly encountered in young adults between the ages of 20 and 40 years. There is a 2:1 female to male ratio and both wrists are equally affected. 60–70% of wrist synovial cysts are dorsally located. Dorsal wrist cysts often communicated with the scapholunate joint and communicate with a region of dorsal scapholunate ligament degeneration [41, 45, 46]. Less commonly, these cysts may arise from the pisotriquetral articulation or be seen within the floor of the carpal tunnel. Carpal tunnel floor cysts often originate from the scaphotrapeziotrapezoid joint, but any carpometacarpal joint may give rise to these cysts.

Imaging Features

Palpable cysts are best evaluated with ultrasound initially. Radiographs can be helpful in depiction of foci of mineralization, alluding to internal calcification or phleboliths. On ultrasound, a cyst is well-circumscribed and anechoic with posterior acoustic enhancement and possible thin internal septations or fine internal echoes. Cysts can be multi-loculated and their stalk may be seen extending to a synovial joint. On color Doppler imaging, simple cyst walls usually do not contain low. Thick-walled cysts may appear as solid lesions when excessively applied pressure with the ultrasound probe results in cyst collapse, especially because these cysts' walls often demonstrate flow on color Doppler evaluation. Care must be taken to apply the least amount of pressure when evaluating cysts with ultrasound.

Occult dorsal cysts of the hand and wrist often present with pain. These cysts are best evaluated with ultrasound or MRI. When ulnar or median nerve symptoms are encountered, MRI may be superior in evaluation of neuropathy. Carpal floor cysts may be harder to evaluate by ultrasound due to shadowing caused by multiple osseous prominences in the carpus.

Special MRI Considerations

MRI is utilized in the radiologic evaluation of synovial cysts when atypical imaging features are expected or encountered on ultrasound or radiographic imaging. On MRI, a typical synovial cyst shows low T1 signal compared to skeletal muscle and fluid-like T2 signal intensity. It can contain thin septations and its wall should be barely perceptible on T2 imaging. Due to the ability to image with thin-slice thickness, cyst walls are often better visualized on 3D steady-state free precession (SSFP) or fast imaging employing steady-state acquisition (FIESTA) with thin, 1 mm, slice thickness. Additionally, these thin-slice sequences can depict the cyst stalk well. On gadolinium-enhanced sequences, thin peripheral enhancement is often visualized except in small cysts where global enhancement is often encountered due to difficulty in separating the internal fluid component (Fig. 8.20).

Synovial cysts that are not dorsal in the hand and wrist tend to have a more variable course and origin and thus may benefit from further radiologic evaluation with MR imaging. Additionally, when there is doubt as to whether a cyst is simple, MRI with IV contrast can be obtained. Hemorrhagic cysts can have a variable MR appearance on T1- (possibly with intrinsic T1 hyperintense signal) and T2 (often heterogeneously hyperintense)-weighted imaging. In some cases, hemorrhagic cysts contain a fluid-fluid level. Gradient-echo (GRE) T2-weighted imaging can aid in the depiction of hemosiderin deposits by taking advantage of magnetic susceptibility. Contrast-enhanced T1 nonfat-suppressed sequences to allow for subtraction postprocessing are invaluable in evaluation of hemorrhagic cysts as these cysts may contain intrinsic T1 hyperintense signal. Ruptured cysts can also pose a diagnostic dilemma on initial radiologic evaluation. MRI will more readily show pericapsular infiltration of non-enhancing fluid. The partially collapsed cyst may exhibit thin enhancement due to the apposition of its walls. Thick-walled cysts were found in 27% of cases in an ultrasound study by Teefey et al. [47]. These cysts are often painful and may benefit from therapeutic injection.

According to Freire et al., the majority of dorsal wrist cysts are not associated with scapholunate ligament tears and even when the ligament is abnormal intraligamentous cysts are rarely found [48]. Opinions in this regard vary, and some authors have found correlation between these cysts and scapholunate ligament instability. The presence of a cyst warrants close inspection of the scapholunate ligament.

Lipomas

Epidemiology

Lipomas account for approximately one-half of all soft tissue tumors and are the most common subcutaneous neoplasm [49]. The vast majority

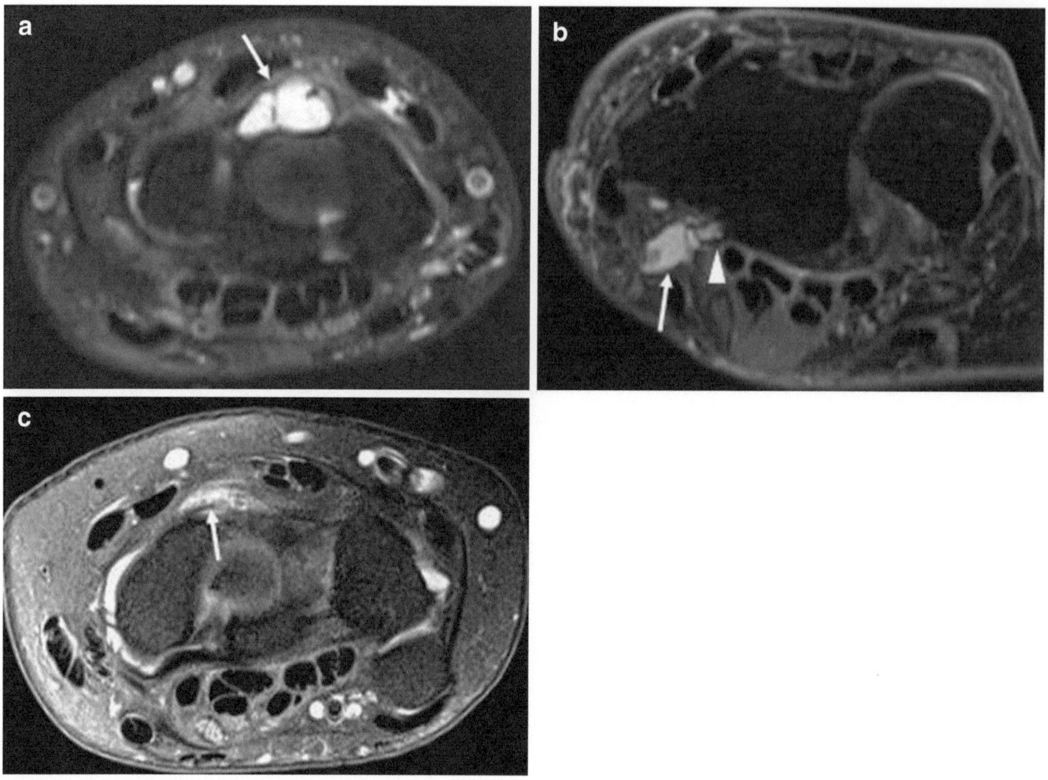

Fig. 8.20 Synovial cysts of the wrist. Axial PD fat-suppressed image (**a**) shows a dorsal synovial cyst (arrow). Axial PD fat-suppressed image (**b**) demonstrates a volar synovial cyst (arrow) in communication with the radiocarpal joint (arrowhead). Axial PD fat-suppressed image (**c**) depicts a ruptured dorsal carpal synovial cyst with ill-defined fluid signal (arrow)

of lipomas are benign. These lesions most commonly occur in the fifth to seventh decades of life and are more common in obese patients [49]. Lipomas are broadly categorized as superficial versus deep with superficial lipomas being subcutaneous in location and often less than 5 cm in size. Deep lipomas are located beneath the superficial fascia and are intramuscular or, less often, intermuscular [50, 51]. Deep lipomas of the extremities are larger than their superficial counterparts; thus, the term *infiltrating* lipoma has been applied to these lesions [52].

Imaging Features

Small lipomas may not be easily identifiable on radiography, but large lipomas can be seen as well-defined, uniformly radiolucent mass-like structures within the soft tissues without subjacent osseous abnormalities. On sonography, lipomas are well-circumscribed, hyperechoic structures that may or may not have internal septae. Lipomas are without posterior acoustic enhancement and may have slight heterogeneity. The thin capsule may be difficult to identify on sonography. CT demonstrates well-defined homogenous adipose tissue with Hounsfield unit measurements reflecting fat content (−65 to −120) [53]. Lipomas commonly contain thin, <2 mm, septae on CT and MR imaging (37–49% of cases) [53–57]. When areas of mineralization within a lipomatous lesion are encountered, a well-differentiated liposarcoma/atypical lipomatous tumor should be considered [49].

Special MRI Considerations

On MR imaging, lipomas show isointense signal relative to subcutaneous fat, regardless of pulse sequence. The thin fibrous capsule often exhibits

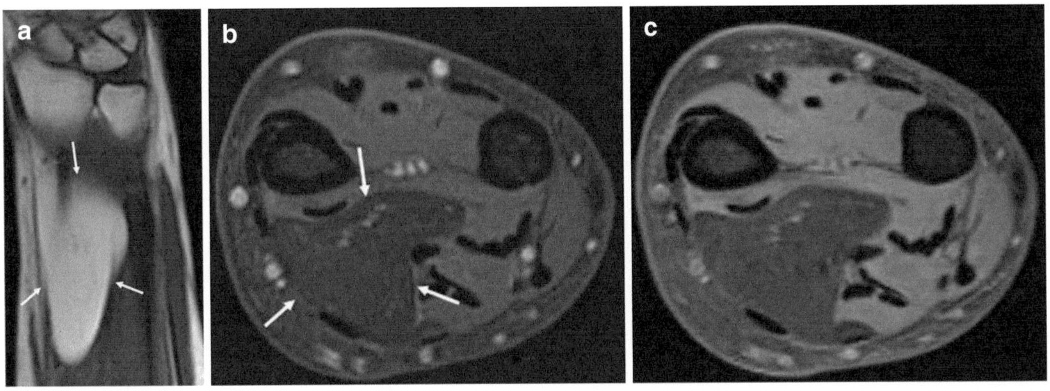

Fig. 8.21 Deep lipoma. Coronal T1 nonfat-suppressed image (**a**) depicts intrinsic T1 hyperintense signal within the mass without nodular or septal hypointense regions (arrows). Axial PD fat-suppressed image (**b**) shows a PD hypointense to skeletal muscle mass in the volar distal forearm, insinuating between musculature (arrows). Axial T1 fat-suppressed image (**c**) exhibits no thick septal or nodular enhancement

hypointense signal on all pulse sequences and thin enhancement after contrast. It is important to note contrast is not necessary to make this diagnosis. Thin septae within lipomas often do not enhance. The capsule is not seen in intramuscular lesions. Additionally, intramuscular lesions may demonstrate irregular margins due to interdigitation with surrounding muscle (Fig. 8.21). Subcutaneous lesions without a distinct capsule are termed *nonencapsulated lipomas* and are difficult to detect on MR imaging [58]. Skin markers placed on the margins of the palpable abnormality may aid diagnosis in these cases.

Pigmented Villonodular Synovitis

Epidemiology

Pigmented villonodular synovitis (PVNS) is an uncommon metaplastic process involving the synovium characterized by hemosiderin deposition [59, 60]. The World Health Organization nomenclature designates *localized* giant cell tumor of the tendon sheath (L-GCTTS) for pigmented villonodular bursitis and pigmented villonodular tenosynovitis [59, 60]. L-GCTTS primarily occurs in the tendon sheaths of the hand and foot and demonstrates more delineated margins, whereas *diffuse* giant cell tumor of the tendon sheath (D-GCTTS) commonly occurs in the larger joints, has a more irregular multinodular growth pattern, and may recur. It is important to be sure the entire joint has been evaluated as small foci of D-PVNS will lead to persistence of pathology.

PVNS has an estimated annual occurrence of 9.2 and 1.8 cases per one million population for the extra-articular and intra-articular forms, respectively. L-GCTTS is the most common form (Fig. 8.22). Patients are commonly in the third to fifth decades of life at diagnosis. L-GCTTS has a mild female predilection, while D-GCTTS has an equal occurrence in both sexes (Fig. 8.23) [61–63]. Lesions are almost always monoarticular and solitary without association with other disorders [64]. GCTTS most commonly involves the hand or wrist (65–89% of cases) and is second only to synovial cysts in incidence of masses presenting in the hand/wrist. The volar hand/wrist is affected twice as often as dorsal, in contrast to synovial cysts in this location [61, 64].

Imaging Features

Radiography has a limited role in the diagnosis of PVNS in the wrist. If mineralization is present on X-ray, GCTTS is not a clinical consideration. Calcifications may be present in the setting of recurrence. Periosteal reaction may occur and is reported in less than 10% of cases. In the upper extremity, pressure erosions of the osseous structures are uncommon.

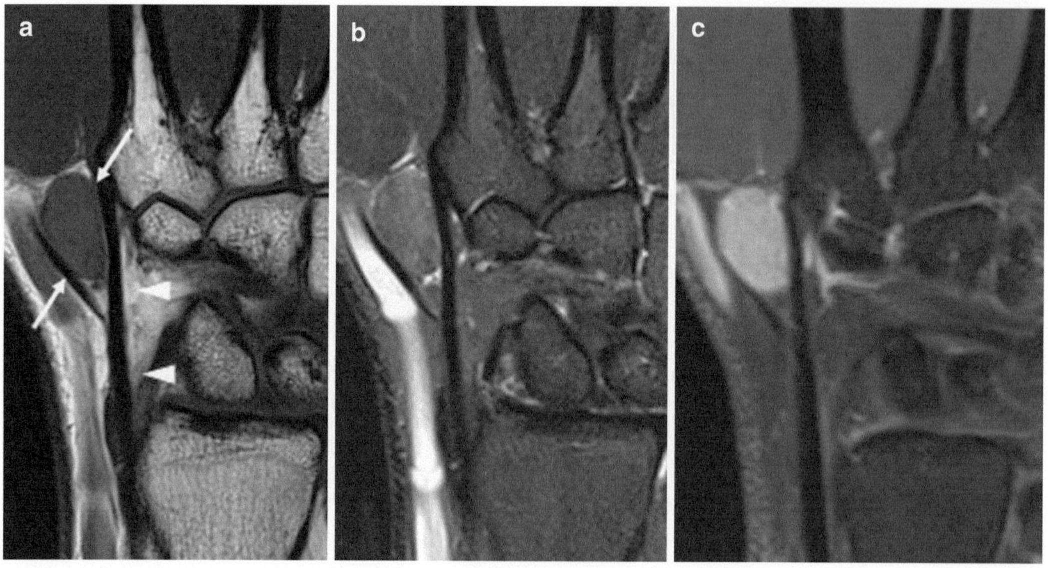

Fig. 8.22 L-GCTTS. Coronal T1 nonfat-suppressed image (**a**) shows T1 isointense mass (arrows) arising from the second extensor compartment of the wrist and abutting the extensor carpi radialis longus tendon (arrowheads). Coronal T2 fat-suppressed image (**b**) shows homogeneous iso-slightly hyperintense signal relative to skeletal muscle. Note the punctate low signal elements within the mass representing the presence of hemosiderin. Coronal T1 fat-suppressed post-contrast image (**c**) depicts homogeneous mild enhancement of the mass

Special MRI Considerations

Almost all focal forms of PVNS are well-circumscribed and have isointense T1 and hypointense T2 signal. Small scattered foci and/or capsules of hypointensity are extremely common both on T1- and T2-weighted sequences due to the presence of hemosiderin deposits. Similar findings are seen with the more diffuse forms of PVNS; however, these entities are often not well-circumscribed. Hemosiderin deposits within these lesions result on blooming on GRE sequence which can be a helpful addition to the protocol in suspected cases. Contrast is not required for the diagnosis as the presence of hemosiderin and the imaging appearance are pathognomonic for this lesion. Should contrast be given, these lesions predominantly demonstrate homogeneous enhancement; however, a minority can have heterogeneous enhancement patterns.

Benign Neurogenic Tumors

Benign neurogenic tumors of the wrist include traumatic neuroma, neural fibrolipoma, nerve sheath ganglion, and benign peripheral nerve sheath tumors (PNSTs) which include schwannomas and neurofibromas. Nerve sheath ganglions will not be discussed given their relative rarity in the upper extremity.

Traumatic Neuromas

Traumatic neuromas are a result of nonneoplastic proliferation of the proximal end of a severed or injured nerve. This entity essentially consists of a tangled, multidirectional, regenerating axonal mass and can arise 1–12 months after transection or injury and have no malignant potential [65]. Although the most frequent site is the lower extremity, traumatic neuromas can occur along the course of any injured nerve. In the wrist, this phenomenon is most commonly seen with the radial nerve [66, 67]. These lesions are best depicted on MRI and typically have T1 isointense and T2 hyperintense signal to skeletal muscle. Heterogeneous signal is thought to be related to histologic morphology of nerve fascicles, often termed “fascicular sign” [64, 65].

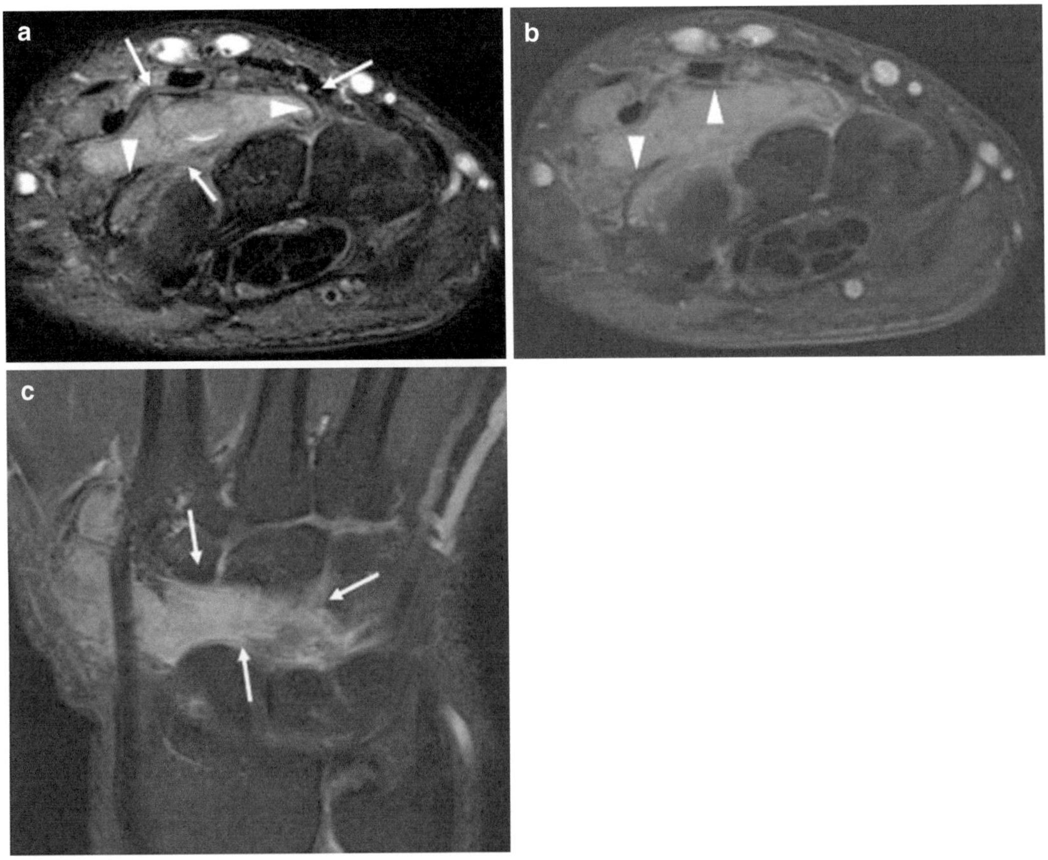

Fig. 8.23 D-GCTTS. Axial T2 fat-suppressed (**a**), axial T1 fat-suppressed post-contrast (**b**), and coronal T1 fat-suppressed post-contrast (**c**) images demonstrate large slightly heterogeneous T2 signal intra-articular mass within the distal carpal row (arrows). Thin linear hypointense signal within the mass (arrowheads) suggestive of hemosiderin deposition

Neural Fibrolipoma

Epidemiology

Also known as fibrolipomatous hamartoma of the nerve, the exact cause of these lesions is unknown, but hypertrophy of mature fat and fibroblasts in the epineurium has been postulated. Patients are usually younger than 30 years of age without sex preference or familial predilection [68]. The upper extremity and particularly the median nerve are most commonly affected with 78–96% of neural fibrolipoma cases located in the upper extremity, and 85% of those cases studied by Silverman and Enzinger involved the median nerve [68]. In 27–67% of patients, macrodactyly is seen in association with neural fibrolipoma, and the second and third digits are most often affected [68, 69].

Imaging Features

Radiographs are often normal in patients with neural fibrolipoma without macrodactyly. In patients with macrodactyly, soft tissue and osseous overgrowth is commonly seen. The digits have broad and long bones with splaying of the distal ends. This overgrowth is more prominent volarly and results in bowing [70].

On ultrasound evaluation, neural fibrolipoma mirrors its histology demonstrating alternating bands of hyperechoic (lipomatous elements) and hypoechoic structures (nerves) resulting in a "cable-like" appearance.

Special MRI Considerations

The MR appearance of these lesions is pathognomonic due to the perineural fat proliferation around the nerve roots resulting in the appearance of a coaxial cable (Fig. 8.24).

Benign PNSTs

Epidemiology and Histology

Benign PNSTs are often classified into schwannomas and neurofibromas. Furthermore, three types of neurofibromas have been described: focal, diffuse, and plexiform. All of these lesions have cellular elements that are closely related to normal Schwann cells [71, 72]. Both schwannomas and neurofibromas occur most commonly in 20- to 30-year-old patients without sex predilection. Neurofibromas have a higher incidence than schwannomas.

Schwannomas are often solitary, not associated with neurofibromatosis-1 (NF-1), with non-aggressive features, slow growth, and small size (<5 cm) [72]. Schwannomas most often occur along the flexor surfaces of the extremities, especially the ulnar nerve. The hallmark of schwannomas on histologic examination are regions of Antoni A and B elements [72]. Antoni A predominant lesions are more cellular, whereas Antoni B predominant lesions have more myxoid material and will contain more T2 hyperintense signal. Larger schwannomas can degenerate resulting in cystic changes, internal calcifications, hemorrhage, and fibrosis [72]. Schwannomas have a true capsule and are separable from the nerve on surgical excision [73].

Focal neurofibromas are the most common subtype and constitute 90% of all neurofibromas. They are slow growing and are often small (<5 cm). Histologically, neurofibromas contain an abundance of collagen and do not often undergo degeneration or exhibit myxoid regions [71, 72]. Deep-seated focal neurofibromas of large nerves have true capsules; however, lesions affecting small nerves although well-circumscribed often extend beyond the epineurium. On the contrary, diffuse neurofibromas are usually ill-defined and infiltrative. Neurofibromas are intermixed and inseparable from the normal nerve tissue on surgical exploration [71, 72].

Theoretically, schwannomas and neurofibromas can be differentiated on the basis of their location relative to the nerve. Schwannomas are eccentric to the nerve, while neurofibromas demonstrate an intimate and intermixed relationship with the underlying nerve. In practice, however, this distinction is impossible to delineate on imaging due to almost identical signal intensity of these lesions and the underlying nerves.

Imaging Features

Radiography is often normal in patients with benign PNSTs as osseous involvement and mineralization are rare. Occasionally, large

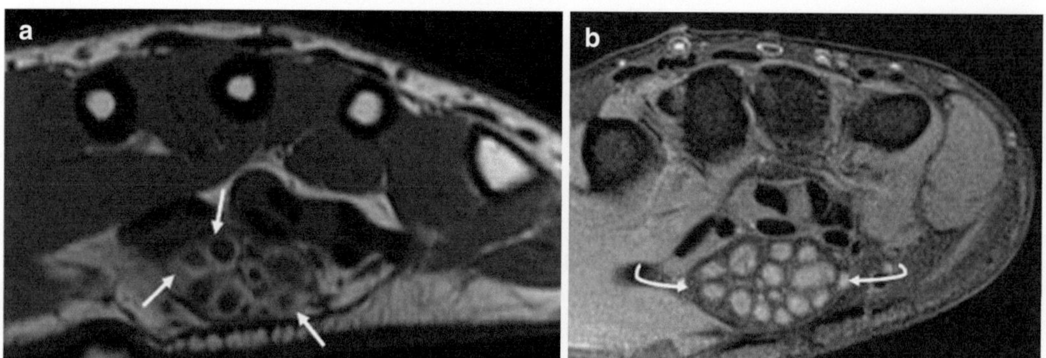

Fig. 8.24 Median nerve fibrolipoma. Axial T1 nonfat-suppressed (**a**) and PD fat-suppressed (**b**) images demonstrate hypertrophy of epineural fat exhibiting intrinsic T1 hyperintense signal (arrows) with enlarged median nerve fascicles (curved arrows)

fusiform soft tissue masses with surrounding fat density may be seen. As with all soft tissue tumors, these lesions are more readily characterized by MRI. PNSTs are always in the distribution of a nerve and characteristically fusiform with the affected nerve entering and exiting them [74].

Special MRI Considerations

MRI is superior in the characterization of benign PNSTs. Signal intensity of these lesions is often nonspecific with isointense T1 and hyperintense T2 signal (occasionally mimicking fluid signal). The "fluid-like" signal on T2WI is rather characteristic of PNSTs and can aid in distinguishing this pathologic process from other lesions mentioned in this chapter. Diffuse plexiform neurofibromas can demonstrate predominantly hypointense T1 signal related to their high collagen content. Signal heterogeneity is less common in benign PNSTs unless large and undergoing degeneration.

Benign PNST's capsule is thin, hypointense on all pulse sequences, and surrounds the PNST. PNSTs frequently have well-circumscribed margins with the exception of diffuse and plexiform neurofibromas. A rim of fat often surrounds neurogenic neoplasms and is termed the *split-fat sign* and is particularly easy to identify on T1-weighted sequences (Fig. 8.25) [74]. Simply, it alludes to the preservation of perineural fat, and while nonspecific, it suggests tumor origin within the intermuscular space where the neurovascular bundles often course.

The *target sign* has been used in the description of these lesions on T2-weighted MR images and consists of low-intermediate central signal (collagenous tissue) with peripherally high signal intensity (myxoid tissue) and is pathognomonic for these lesions [75–77] (Fig. 8.26). The *fascicular sign* is another characteristic appearance of these lesions with multiple small ring-like structures with peripheral higher signal intensity on T2- or PD-weighted sequences [70]. Not unexpectedly, the fascicular sign is more often seen with benign PNSTs.

Variable enhancement is seen with PNSTs, but in lesions with a target sign, more prominent central enhancement is detected. Increased degree of contrast enhancement, nodular enhancement, and heterogeneous enhancement patterns is more commonly seen with malignant PNSTs [78]. It is worth noting that plexiform neurofibromas do not typically enhance after contrast administration.

Subtle fatty infiltration and atrophy of the muscles innervated by the nerve associated with the PNST have been reported but are infrequent [79]. This finding is not common with other soft tissue masses and may be helpful in arriving at the diagnosis. Comparison with unaffected normal extremity on nonfat-suppressed T1 sequences may be beneficial in such cases.

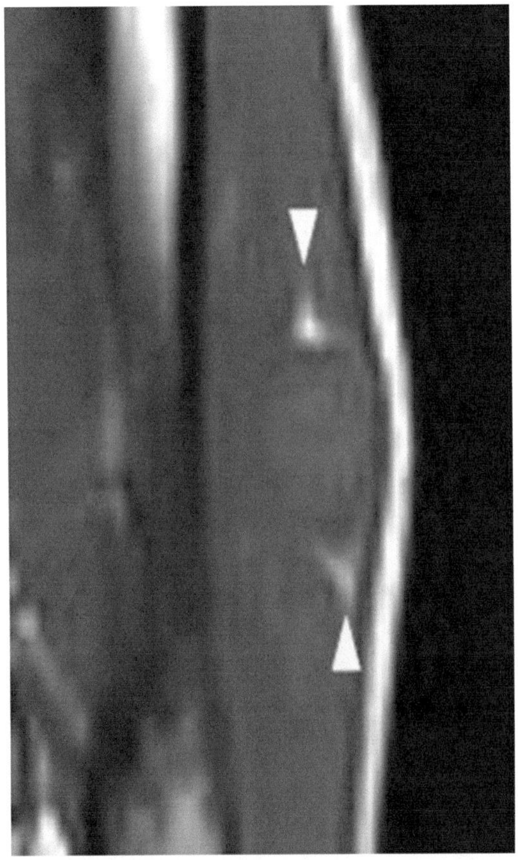

Fig. 8.25 Split-fat sign. Coronal T1 nonfat-suppressed image exhibit split-fat sign as T1 hyperintense signal (arrow heads) at the superior and inferior margins of the mass, alluding to preservation of perineural fat and intermuscular location of the tumor

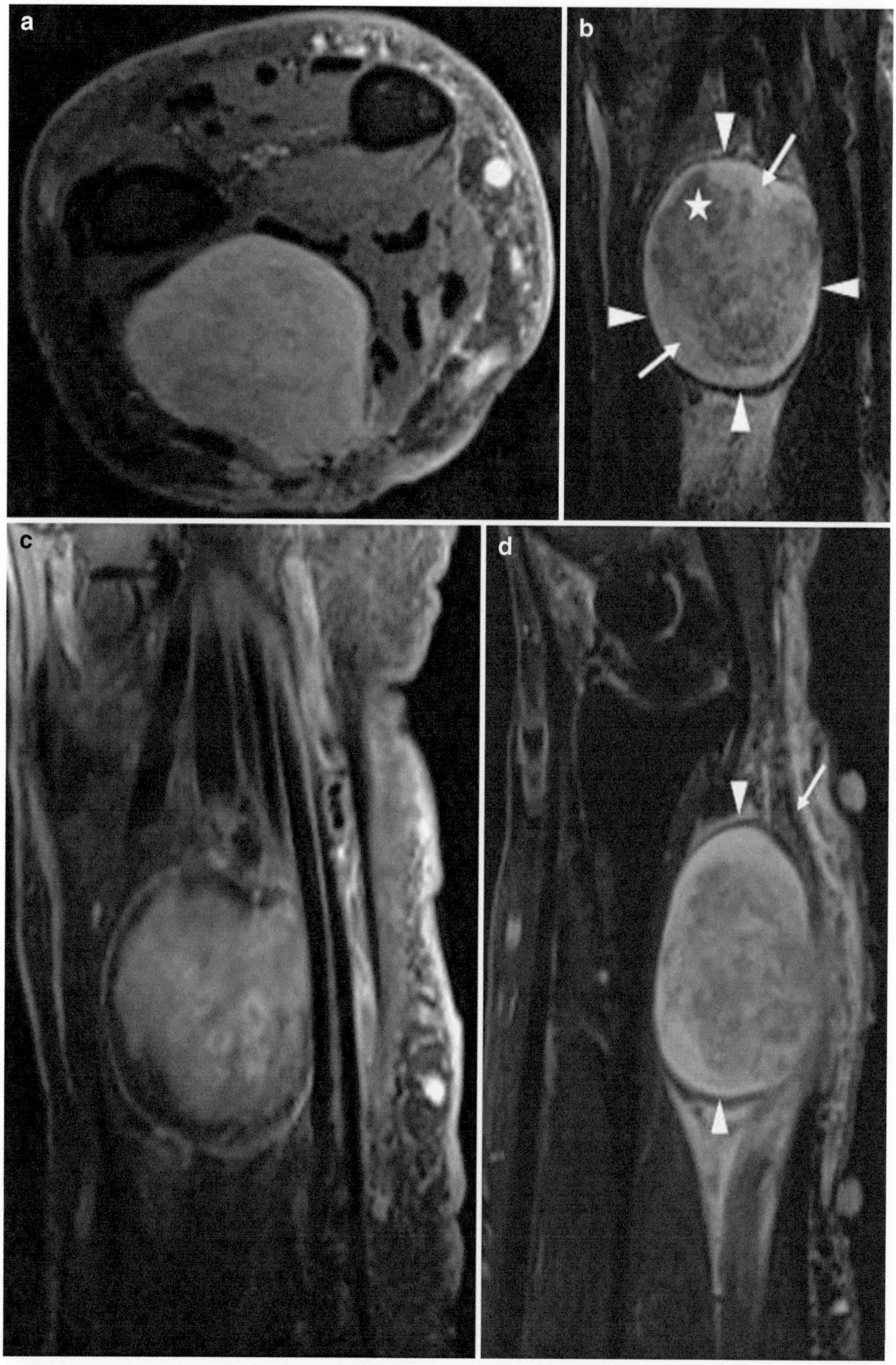

Fig. 8.26 Median nerve schwannoma. Axial PD fat-suppressed image (**a**) shows a heterogeneous, hyperintense mass within the volar wrist. Coronal STIR (**b**) demonstrating the target sign with a large "bullseye," low central signal (asterisk), and high peripheral signal (arrows). The thin hypointense capsule is also well seen (arrowheads). Coronal T1 fat-suppressed post-contrast image (**c**) shows target pattern of enhancement in this mass. Sagittal T2 fat-suppressed image (**d**) shows eccentric location of this mass in relation to the median nerve (arrow). Thin hypointense capsule (arrowheads) and target sign can also be seen

Extra-Skeletal Chondroma

Epidemiology and Histology

Extra-skeletal chondroma is also known as chondroma of soft parts and is almost entirely composed of hyaline cartilage without connection to bone or periosteum [80]. It is histologically very similar to juxtacortical chondroma [81]. It is usually smaller than 3 cm and found in the hands and feet [82]. This tumor occurs predominantly in the adult population between 30 and 60 years with slight male predominance [80]. It is thought to arise from soft tissue fibrous stroma rather than mature cartilaginous or osseous tissue [83].

Imaging Features

The literature on radiographic features of extra-skeletal chondroma of the wrist and hand is sparse, in part due to small size and uncommon mineralization. These tumors may be seen as soft tissue masses which may have mineralization if large (33–70% of cases) [84]. Mineralization is often in rings and arcs pattern, as expected due to the chondroid nature of the lesion. Osseous pressure erosions may be seen in rare cases [84–86].

Special MRI Considerations

Extra-skeletal chondromas are similar to juxtacortical chondromas in MRI features meaning they often exhibit intermediate T1 signal and high T2 signal with thin peripheral enhancement. When internal mineralization is present, hypointense signal may be seen.

Malignant Soft Tissue Lesions

The most common aggressive soft tissue sarcomas of the upper extremity include alveolar rhabdomyosarcoma, synovial sarcoma, and myxofibrosarcoma [40].

Alveolar Rhabdomyosarcoma

Epidemiology and Histology

Rhabdomyosarcoma is the most common soft tissue sarcoma in children and accounts for 4.5% of childhood malignancies. Alveolar rhabdomyosarcoma is a histologic subtype of rhabdomyosarcoma, accounts for 20% of cases of rhabdomyosarcoma, and has the worst prognosis. It is more common in older children and young adults between the ages of 10 and 25 years. It most commonly arises from the deep soft tissues of the extremities and has an indolent growth pattern [87]. Alveolar rhabdomyosarcoma is a highly cellular tumor with fibrous stroma and fibrovascular septae that tend to exhibit peripheral discohesion and areas of necrosis resulting in an alveoli-like appearance [88].

Imaging Features

Radiographic, sonographic, and CT appearance of alveolar rhabdomyosarcoma is similar to other soft tissue sarcomas and is nonspecific.

Special MRI Considerations

On MR imaging, alveolar rhabdomyosarcoma has nonspecific signal characteristics often seen with other soft tissue sarcomas including T1 isointense to slightly hyperintense to skeletal muscle and T2 heterogeneously hyperintense signal. Twenty-five percent of cases exhibit involvement of adjacent bone in the form of cortical erosions or subperiosteal new bone formation. Involvement of surrounding muscles and fascia is common [89].

Synovial Sarcoma

Epidemiology and Histology

Synovial sarcomas are rare soft tissue masses that comprise approximately 18% of upper extremity soft tissue sarcomas [40]. They predominantly affect young adults, presenting as slowly growing masses within the deep soft tissues adjacent to the large joints of the lower extremity and less commonly in the wrist [90]. Synovial sarcomas get their name because on microscopic examination they resemble synovium, but these tumors stain for epithelial markers (keratin), whereas synovium does not.

Imaging Features

Radiographic features of these tumors are highly nonspecific. Thirty percent of synovial sarcomas reveal peripheral dystrophic calcification that does not resemble ossified or chondroid matrix described as psammomatous (or sand-like) [90]. As with all soft tissue sarcomas adjacent to bone, smooth pressure erosions of the cortex may be seen. Osseous invasion can occur [91]. Ultrasound and CT findings are also nonspecific with heterogeneous, predominantly hypoechoic mass with internal flow on sonographic and color Doppler evaluation and heterogeneously enhancing mass on CT images. CT is superior in depiction of internal calcifications compared to other modalities.

Special MRI Considerations

On MR imaging, synovial sarcomas are usually multilobulated, well-circumscribed lesions, measuring less than 5 cm, and are T1 isointense to slightly hyperintense to skeletal muscle and T2 heterogeneously hyperintense masses (sometimes very intensely high in signal). *Triple sign* has been used to describe synovial sarcomas' signal characteristics on MR imaging and alludes to hypointense (calcification or fibrosis), intermediate (cellular component), and hyperintense (hemorrhage or necrosis) signal within these lesions [92]. Other soft tissue sarcomas may have a triple sign (particularly malignant fibrous histiocytoma); therefore, this sign alone lacks specificity [90]. Synovial sarcomas often reveal heterogeneous enhancement owing to their varied internal histology. Multilobulated appearance with large intervening septae was described in larger lesions and is especially well depicted on T2-weighted images [93, 94]. Osseous involvement, be it pressure erosions or marrow invasion, is seen in up to 21% of cases [92, 95]. Neurovascular encasement is not uncommon and must be assessed to aid in appropriate surgical planning and is believed to be due to the intermuscular origin of these tumors where the neurovascular bundle is also often seen [90]. Intermuscular location often results in a *split-fat sign* (Fig. 8.25).

The importance of a high degree of suspicion for synovial sarcoma in cyst-like-appearing lesions in the wrist cannot be overemphasized. When in doubt, administration of gadolinium contrast can prove exceedingly helpful as synovial sarcoma will demonstrate contrast enhancement, and, as stated previously, fluid-filled structures will show thin, peripheral enhancement [90].

References

1. Defazio MV, et al. Carpal coalition: a review of current knowledge and report of a single institution's experience with asymptomatic intercarpal fusion. Hand (N Y). 2013;8(2):157–63.
2. Timins ME. Osseous anatomic variants of the wrist: findings on MR imaging. Am J Roentgenol. 1999;173(2):339–44.
3. Devilliers Minnaar AB. Congenital fusion of the lunate and triquetral bones in the South African Bantu. J Bone Joint Surg Br. 1952;34-b(1):45–8.
4. Singh P, Tuli A, Choudhry R, Mangal A. Intercarpal fusion- a review. J Anat Soc India. 2003;52(2):2003-7–2003-12.
5. Burnett SE. Hamate-pisiform coalition: morphology, clinical significance, and a simplified classification scheme for carpal coalition. Clin Anat. 2011;24(2):188–96.
6. Malik AM, et al. MR imaging of the type II lunate bone: frequency, extent, and associated findings. AJR Am J Roentgenol. 1999;173(2):335–8.
7. Pfirrmann C, et al. The hamatolunate facet: characterization and association with cartilage lesions – magnetic resonance arthrography and anatomic correlation in cadaveric wrists. Skelet Radiol. 2002;31(8):451–6.
8. Haims AH, et al. MRI in the diagnosis of cartilage injury in the wrist. Am J Roentgenol. 2004;182(5):1267–70.
9. Rehnitz C, et al. Comparison of modern 3D and 2D MR imaging sequences of the wrist at 3 tesla. Rofo. 2016;188(8):753–62.
10. Mori V, et al. Differences of radiocarpal cartilage alterations in arthritis and osteoarthritis using morphological and biochemical magnetic resonance imaging without gadolinium-based contrast agent administration. Eur Radiol. 2019;29(5):2581–8.
11. Chang G, et al. MRI of the wrist at 7 tesla using an eight-channel array coil combined with parallel imaging: preliminary results. J Magn Reson Imag: JMRI. 2010;31(3):740–6.
12. Vaz A, Trippia CR. Small but troublesome: accessory ossicles with clinical significance. Radiol Bras. 2018;51(4):248–56.

13. Claiborne EM, Kautz FG. Madelung's deformity of the wrist: with report of a case. Radiology. 1936;27(5):594–9.
14. Ali S, et al. Madelung deformity and Madelung-type deformities: a review of the clinical and radiological characteristics. Pediatr Radiol. 2015;45(12):1856–63.
15. Kumari A, et al. Tingling hand: magnetic resonance imaging of median nerve pathologies within the carpal tunnel. Pol J Radiol. 2019;84:e484–90.
16. Meraj S, et al. MRI of the extensor tendons of the wrist. Am J Roentgenol. 2017;209(5):1093–102.
17. Goyal A, Srivastava DN, Ansari T. MRI in De Quervain tenosynovitis: is making the diagnosis sufficient? Am J Roentgenol. 2018;210(3):W133–4.
18. Patel DB, et al. Hand infections: anatomy, types and spread of infection, imaging findings, and treatment options. Radiographics. 2014;34(7):1968–86.
19. Hsu C-Y, Lu H-C, Shih TT-F. Tuberculous infection of the wrist: MRI features. Am J Roentgenol. 2004;183(3):623–8.
20. Taouli B, et al. Rheumatoid arthritis of the hand and wrist: comparison of three imaging techniques. Am J Roentgenol. 2004;182(4):937–43.
21. Narvaez JA, et al. MR imaging of early rheumatoid arthritis. Radiographics. 2010;30(1):143–63.
22. Spira D, et al. MRI findings in psoriatic arthritis of the hands. AJR Am J Roentgenol. 2010;195(5):1187–93.
23. Schwenzer NF, et al. The role of dynamic contrast-enhanced MRI in the differential diagnosis of psoriatic and rheumatoid arthritis. Am J Roentgenol. 2010;194(3):715–20.
24. Girish G, Glazebrook KN, Jacobson JA. Advanced imaging in gout. Am J Roentgenol. 2013;201(3):515–25.
25. Omoumi P, et al. Imaging in gout and other crystal-related arthropathies. Rheum Dis Clin N Am. 2016;42(4):621–44.
26. Forthman CL, Segalman KA. Lesions and tumors of the carpus. Hand Clin. 2006;22(4):435–46; abstract vi.
27. Takigawa K. Chondroma of the bones of the hand. A review of 110 cases. J Bone Joint Surg Am. 1971;53(8):1591–600.
28. Emecheta IE, Bernhards J, Berger A. Carpal enchondroma. J Hand Surg Br. 1997;22(6):817–9.
29. Masada K, et al. Chondroma of the scaphoid. J Bone Joint Surg Br. 1989;71(4):705.
30. Takka S, Poyraz A. Enchondroma of the scaphoid bone. Arch Orthop Trauma Surg. 2002;122(6):369–70.
31. Murray PM, Berger RA, Inwards CY. Primary neoplasms of the carpal bones. J Hand Surg Am. 1999;24(5):1008–13.
32. Greenspan A, et al. Differential diagnosis in orthopaedic oncology. 2nd ed. Philadelphia: Lippincott Williams & Wilkins. xi; 2007. 529 p.
33. Assoun J, et al. Osteoid osteoma: MR imaging versus CT. Radiology. 1994;191(1):217–23.
34. Liu PT, et al. Imaging of osteoid osteoma with dynamic gadolinium-enhanced MR imaging. Radiology. 2003;227(3):691–700.
35. Larsson SE, Lorentzon R, Boquist L. Giant-cell tumor of bone. A demographic, clinical, and histopathological study of all cases recorded in the Swedish Cancer Registry for the years 1958 through 1968. J Bone Joint Surg Am. 1975;57(2):167–73.
36. Kricun ME. Imaging of bone tumors. Philadelphia: W.B. Saunders. xv; 1993. 677 p.
37. Greenspan A, Borys D. Radiology and pathology correlation of bone tumors: a quick reference and review. Philadelphia: Wolters Kluwer; 2016. p. xiv, 440 pages.
38. Moser RP Jr, et al. From the archives of the AFIP. Giant cell tumor of the upper extremity. Radiographics. 1990;10(1):83–102.
39. Muramatsu K, et al. Musculoskeletal sarcomas in the forearm and hand: standard treatment and microsurgical reconstruction for limb salvage. Anticancer Res. 2013;33(10):4175–82.
40. Nicholson S, Milner RH, Ragbir M. Soft tissue sarcoma of the hand and wrist: epidemiology and management challenges. J Hand Microsurg. 2018;10(2):86–92.
41. Angelides AC, Wallace PF. The dorsal ganglion of the wrist: its pathogenesis, gross and microscopic anatomy, and surgical treatment. J Hand Surg Am. 1976;1(3):228–35.
42. Gude WM. V, Ganglion cysts of the wrist; pathophysiology, clinical picture, and management. Curr Rev Musculoskelet Med. 2008;1:205–11.
43. Barnes WE, Larsen RD, Posch JL. Review of ganglia of the hand and wrist with analysis of surgical treatment. Plast Reconstr Surg. 1964;34:570–8.
44. Nelson CL, Sawmiller S, Phalen GS. Ganglions of the wrist and hand. J Bone Joint Surg Am. 1972;54(7):1459–64.
45. Kuhlmann JN, et al. [Ganglions of the wrist: proposals for topographical systematization and natural history]. Rev Chir Orthop Reparatrice Appar Mot. 2003;89(4):310–9.
46. Cardinal E, et al. Occult dorsal carpal ganglion: comparison of US and MR imaging. Radiology. 1994;193(1):259–62.
47. Teefey SA, et al. Ganglia of the hand and wrist: a sonographic analysis. AJR Am J Roentgenol. 2008;191(3):716–20.
48. Freire V, et al. Imaging of hand and wrist cysts: a clinical approach. AJR Am J Roentgenol. 2012;199(5):W618–28.
49. Murphey MD, et al. From the archives of the AFIP: benign musculoskeletal lipomatous lesions. Radiographics. 2004;24(5):1433–66.
50. Rydholm A, Berg NO. Size, site and clinical incidence of lipoma. Factors in the differential diagnosis of lipoma and sarcoma. Acta Orthop Scand. 1983;54(6):929–34.

51. Myhre-Jensen O. A consecutive 7-year series of 1331 benign soft tissue tumours. Clinicopathologic data. Comparison with sarcomas. Acta Orthop Scand. 1981;52(3):287–93.
52. Regan JM, Bickel WH, Broders AC. Infiltrating benign lipomas of the extremities; report of two cases. Proc Staff Meet Mayo Clin. 1946;21:175.
53. Ohguri T, et al. Differential diagnosis of benign peripheral lipoma from well-differentiated liposarcoma on MR imaging: is comparison of margins and internal characteristics useful? AJR Am J Roentgenol. 2003;180(6):1689–94.
54. Kransdorf MJ, et al. Imaging of fatty tumors: distinction of lipoma and well-differentiated liposarcoma. Radiology. 2002;224(1):99–104.
55. Kransdorf MJ, et al. Fat-containing soft-tissue masses of the extremities. Radiographics. 1991;11(1):81–106.
56. Ha TV, et al. MR imaging of benign fatty tumors in children: report of four cases and review of the literature. Skelet Radiol. 1994;23(5):361–7.
57. Gaskin CM, Helms CA. Lipomas, lipoma variants, and well-differentiated liposarcomas (atypical lipomas): results of MRI evaluations of 126 consecutive fatty masses. AJR Am J Roentgenol. 2004;182(3):733–9.
58. Roberts CC, Liu PT, Colby TV. Encapsulated versus nonencapsulated superficial fatty masses: a proposed MR imaging classification. AJR Am J Roentgenol. 2003;180(5):1419–22.
59. Murphey MD, et al. Pigmented villonodular synovitis: radiologic-pathologic correlation. Radiographics. 2008;28(5):1493–518.
60. Wang C, et al. Giant cell tumor of the tendon sheath: magnetic resonance imaging findings in 38 patients. Oncol Lett. 2017;13(6):4459–62.
61. Hughes TH, et al. Pigmented villonodular synovitis: MRI characteristics. Skelet Radiol. 1995;24(1):7–12.
62. Flandry F, Hughston JC. Pigmented villonodular synovitis. J Bone Joint Surg Am. 1987;69(6):942–9.
63. Goldblum JR, et al. Enzinger and Weiss's soft tissue tumors. 6th ed. Philadelphia: Saunders/Elsevier; 2014. p. xiv, 1155 p.
64. Kransdorf MJ, Murphey MD. Soft tissue tumors: post-treatment imaging. Radiol Clin N Am. 2006;44(3):463–72.
65. Boutin RD, Pathria MN, Resnick D. Disorders in the stumps of amputee patients: MR imaging. AJR Am J Roentgenol. 1998;171(2):497–501.
66. Attarian DE. Neuromas of the superficial radial nerve. Mil Med. 1988;153(8):393–4.
67. Stahl S, Kaufman T, Ben-David B. Neuroma of the superficial branch of the radial nerve after intravenous cannulation. Anesth Analg. 1996;83(1):180–2.
68. Silverman TA, Enzinger FM. Fibrolipomatous hamartoma of nerve. A clinicopathologic analysis of 26 cases. Am J Surg Pathol. 1985;9(1):7–14.
69. Amadio PC, Reiman HM, Dobyns JH. Lipofibromatous hamartoma of nerve. J Hand Surg Am. 1988;13(1):67–75.
70. Murphey MD, et al. From the archives of the AFIP. Imaging of musculoskeletal neurogenic tumors: radiologic-pathologic correlation. Radiographics. 1999;19(5):1253–80.
71. Kransdorf MJ. Malignant soft-tissue tumors in a large referral population: distribution of diagnoses by age, sex, and location. AJR Am J Roentgenol. 1995;164(1):129–34.
72. Harkin JC, Reed RJ. Tumors of the peripheral nervous system, Atlas of tumor pathology. Washington: Armed Forces Institute of Pathology; 1969. 174 p
73. Kransdorf MJ, Murphey MD. The use of gadolinium in the MR evaluation of soft tissue tumors. Semin Ultrasound CT MR. 1997;18(4):251–68.
74. Cohen LM, Schwartz AM, Rockoff SD. Benign schwannomas: pathologic basis for CT inhomogeneities. AJR Am J Roentgenol. 1986;147(1):141–3.
75. Suh JS, et al. Peripheral (extracranial) nerve tumors: correlation of MR imaging and histologic findings. Radiology. 1992;183(2):341–6.
76. Burk DL Jr, et al. Spinal and paraspinal neurofibromatosis: surface coil MR imaging at 1.5 T1. Radiology. 1987;162(3):797–801.
77. Lewis TT, Kingsley DP. Magnetic resonance imaging of multiple spinal neurofibromata-neurofibromatosis. Neuroradiology. 1987;29(6):562–4.
78. Moon WK, Im JG, Han MC. Malignant schwannomas of the thorax: CT findings. J Comput Assist Tomogr. 1993;17(2):274–6.
79. Stull MA, et al. Magnetic resonance appearance of peripheral nerve sheath tumors. Skelet Radiol. 1991;20(1):9–14.
80. Kransdorf MJ, Meis JM. From the archives of the AFIP. Extraskeletal osseous and cartilaginous tumors of the extremities. Radiographics. 1993;13(4):853–84.
81. Le Corroller T, Bouvier-Labit C, Champsaur P. Diffuse mineralization of forearm extraskeletal chondroma. Joint Bone Spine. 2008;75(4):479–81.
82. Papagelopoulos PJ, et al. Extraskeletal chondroma of the foot. Joint Bone Spine. 2007;74(3):285–8.
83. De Riu G, et al. Soft-tissue chondroma of the masticatory space. Int J Oral Maxillofac Surg. 2007;36(2):174–6.
84. Chung EB, Enzinger FM. Chondroma of soft parts. Cancer. 1978;41(4):1414–24.
85. Zlatkin MB, et al. Soft-tissue chondromas. AJR Am J Roentgenol. 1985;144(6):1263–7.
86. Dahlin DC, Salvador AH. Cartilaginous tumors of the soft tissues of the hands and feet. Mayo Clin Proc. 1974;49(10):721–6.
87. Weiss AR, et al. Histologic and clinical characteristics can guide staging evaluations for children and adolescents with rhabdomyosarcoma: a report from the Children's Oncology Group Soft Tissue Sarcoma Committee. J Clin Oncol. 2013;31(26):3226–32.
88. Morotti RA, et al. An immunohistochemical algorithm to facilitate diagnosis and subtyping of rhabdomyosarcoma: the Children's Oncology Group experience. Am J Surg Pathol. 2006;30(8):962–8.
89. Stein-Wexler R. Pediatric soft tissue sarcomas. Semin Ultrasound CT MR. 2011;32(5):470–88.

90. Murphey MD, et al. From the archives of the AFIP: imaging of synovial sarcoma with radiologic-pathologic correlation. Radiographics. 2006;26(5):1543–65.
91. Meyers SP. MRI of bone and soft tissue tumors and tumorlike lesions: differential diagnosis and atlas. Stuttgart; New York: Thieme; 2008. p. xv, 798 p.
92. Jones BC, Sundaram M, Kransdorf MJ. Synovial sarcoma: MR imaging findings in 34 patients. AJR Am J Roentgenol. 1993;161(4):827–30.
93. Tateishi U, et al. Synovial sarcoma of the soft tissues: prognostic significance of imaging features. J Comput Assist Tomogr. 2004;28(1):140–8.
94. Blacksin MF, et al. Synovial sarcoma: frequency of nonaggressive MR characteristics. J Comput Assist Tomogr. 1997;21(5):785–9.
95. Morton MJ, et al. MR imaging of synovial sarcoma. AJR Am J Roentgenol. 1991;156(2):337–40.

9 Hand: Importance and Biomechanics

Bethany U. Casagranda

Hand

> Man is the metre of all things, the hand is the instrument of instruments, and the mind is the form of forms. —Greek Philosopher: Aristotle

Importance and Biomechanics

According to Aristotle, the hand is the "tool of tools." It can convey strength, power, and protection in one venue while providing generosity, hospitality, and support in another. Hand gestures are used to express a statement or display an emotion. People lay hands upon an object in order to bless or heal. Raising one's hand is an appropriate gesture when asking a question among a group [1]. Hands can provide sight for the blind or a voice for the deaf. It is a tool, a symbol, and a weapon. Science, philosophy, art, religion, and many cultures have been influenced by the importance of the hand and handedness. But in the end, not to dispute its importance, the human hand is simply a product of excellence in primate evolution [2].

Man alone has a hand.

B. U. Casagranda (✉)
Department of Radiology, Imaging Institute, Allegheny Health Network, Pittsburgh, PA, USA
e-mail: bethany.casagranda@ahn.org

The hand is defined as the terminal, grasping or prehensile, aspect of the upper extremity in humans consisting of the wrist, palm, digits, and opposable thumb [3]. Although both humans and primates have four digits and an opposable thumb, the human thumb is well-developed with sharp divergence of approximately 80° with respect to the other metacarpals [4]. The human thumb is comparatively stronger and longer than the primate thumb. Human hands have greater mobility with movements of rotation, flexion, and extension at the level of the wrist and the digits. Humans capitalize on this difference by not only using the hand to grasp but to produce limitless fine motor movements. Therefore, the hand acts as an instrument with innumerable uses supporting the concept of the hand as being a uniquely human characteristic [2, 5].

In addition to structural advancements, humans have evolved extensive cerebral cortical systems for controlling the hand. The cerebral cortex possesses monosynaptic control over motor neurons whose axons connect with the hand muscles. In effect, these direct connections have moved the hand "closer" to the cerebral cortex. Furthermore, the corticospinal tracts provide rapid access to the hand from other cortical areas and subcortical structures, including the cerebellum and basal ganglia, known to be intimately involved in motor control. Haptic perception and sophisticated sensory information from the mechanoreceptive sensors of the skin, densest at

B. U. Casagranda (ed.), *MRI of the Upper Extremity*, https://doi.org/10.1007/978-3-030-81612-4_9

the level of the fingertips, allow feedback to further advance hand movements [6].

Multiple muscle groups are recruited to perform functional opposition of the thumb which is a necessity to pinch, grip, or grasp objects. These include abductor pollicis brevis, opponens pollicis, and superficial head of the flexor pollicis brevis. They work together on the trapeziometacarpal joint (basal joint) and the metacarpophalangeal (MCP) joint. Antagonistic forces to this group include extensor pollicis longus and adductor pollicis which contribute to supination, extension, and adduction forces of the thumb [4].

Digits of the hand are identified as 1 through 5 with the thumb being 1 (Fig. 9.1). Finger length from longest to shortest is 3 > 4 > 2 > 5 > 1 [2].

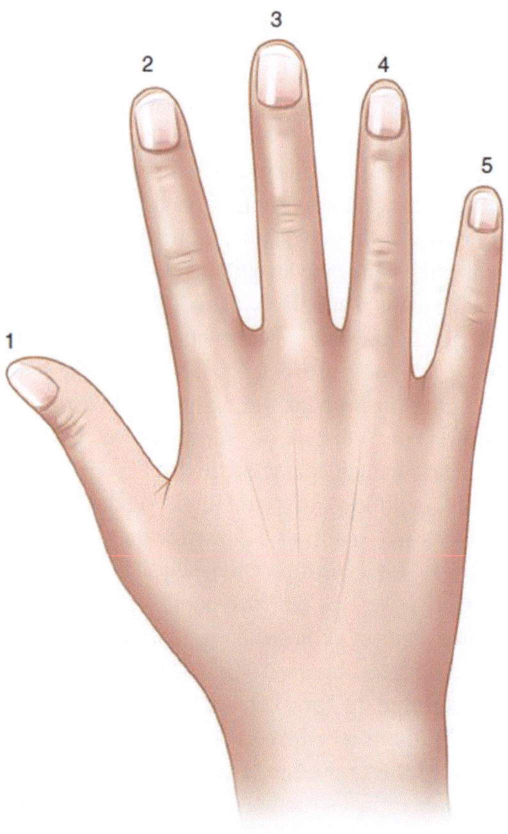

Fig. 9.1 Conventional method of identifying the digits of the hand

Therefore, other identifiers for the third digit include middle finger or the long finger. The third digit provides the most flexion force and participates in power grip and precision movements as expected given its central location. The fourth digit, or ring finger, is felt to cause the least amount of impairment to hand function if lost. Although the fifth digit, small finger, has the least flexion strength, it was only second to the thumb in importance of hand function. This is thought to be related to the fifth carpal metacarpal joint which is highly mobile yet strengthen by the hypothenar musculature [4].

In addition to the strength and agility of the digits, other joints of the upper extremity must have the correct balance of stability and mobility to create effective hand motion. The hand relies on the wrist and forearm's ability to rotate with the elbow in varying degrees of flexion. Forearm rotation involves the proximal radioulnar joint (PRUJ), distal radioulnar joint (DRUJ), and humeroradial joint also known as the radiocapitellar joint. The PRUJ and DRUJ are uniaxial pivot joints, and the radiocapitellar joint is a limited ball and socket joint. A common clinical mistake is to focus on the wrist or elbow in a patient with upper extremity pain or dysfunction without proper assessment of forearm biomechanics [7].

Although rotation of the forearm occurs at the level of the aforementioned joints, the curvature of the forearm bones contribute to rotation as well. Both the radius and the ulna are curved anteriorly in both the sagittal and frontal planes. The two curvatures of the radius are the "supinator" and "pronator" curvatures named after its muscle attachments. The ulna's two curvatures resemble an elongated "s" in the sagittal plane with anterior concavity. These curvatures allow greater rotation of the bones in relation to each other than if the bones were perfectly straight (Fig. 9.2) [7]. With the addition of upper arm rotation at the level of the shoulder, these movement combinations allow for proper placement of the more distal joints in space (Fig. 9.3) [7, 8].

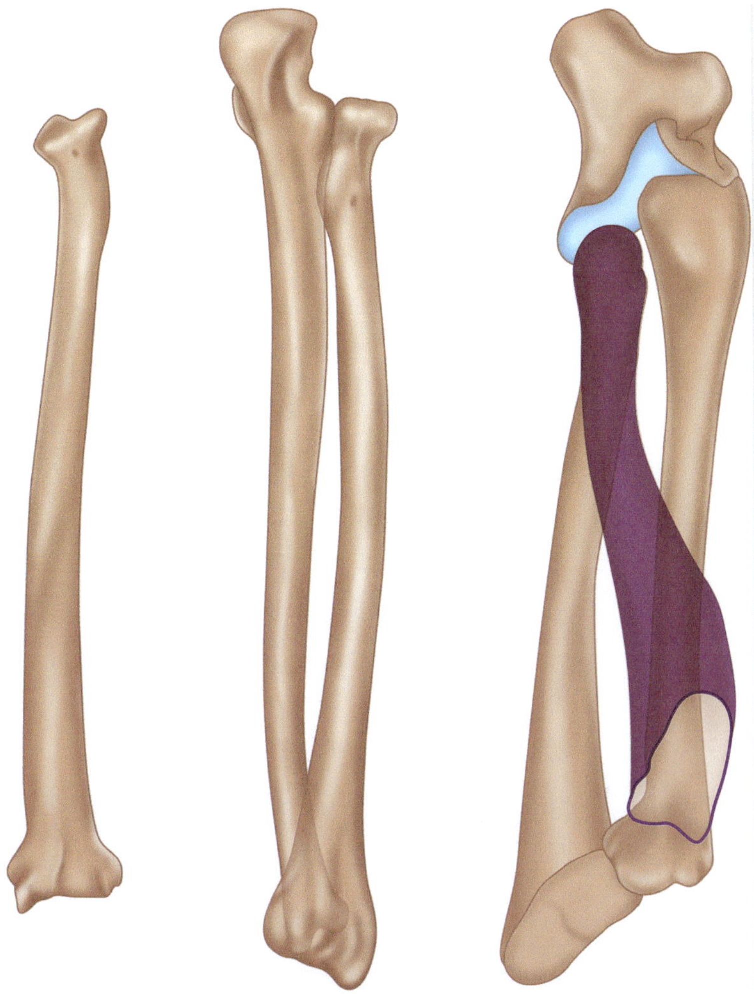

Fig. 9.2 Curvatures of the radius and ulna are essential to rotation of the forearm

Once the shoulder, elbow, and wrist place the hand in position, the complex biomechanical system of arches support the work the hand must perform. The scaffolding or osseous arches of the hand on which the myotendinous structures pull are either transverse or longitudinal in direction. Arches are created by the bony segments of the hand. Two transverse arches are formed by the carpal bones proximally and the metacarpal heads distally. Longitudinal arches are created by the bones comprising each of the five digits. Arches resist greater forces than other structures so the hands were built to work. However, it is important to note that arches are only as strong as its base, and therefore, a stable wrist is necessary to perform standard hand movements [4].

Most hand movements are made up of seven maneuvers: precision pinch (Fig. 9.4), oppositional pinch (Fig. 9.5), key pinch (Fig. 9.6), directional grip (Fig. 9.7), hook grip (Fig. 9.8), power grasp (Fig. 9.9), and span grasp (Fig. 9.10).

Although hand maneuvers are predefined, studies focused on natural hand movements have confirmed similar findings when comparing real-life patterns of digit independence, movement times, and relationships between fingers to previously published laboratory data [9]. From its basic use to its remarkable ability to evolve, the hand is largely responsible for the creative manifestations that characterize the human species [2].

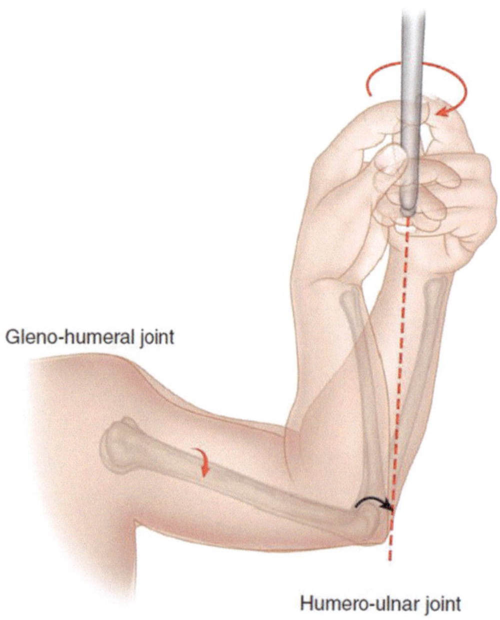

Fig. 9.3 All joints of the upper extremity contribute motion that properly places the hand in space

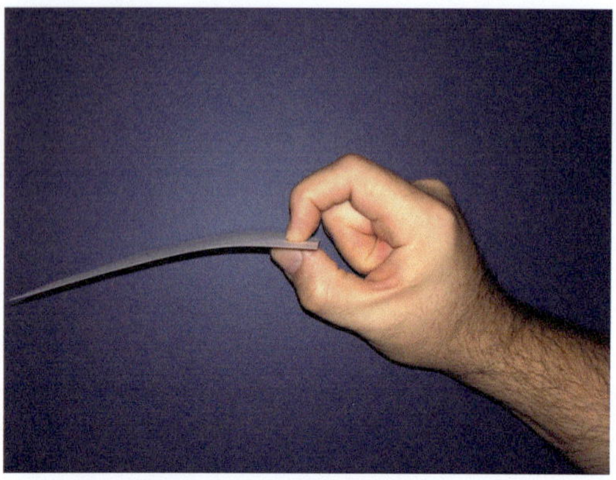

Fig. 9.4 Precision pinch maneuver

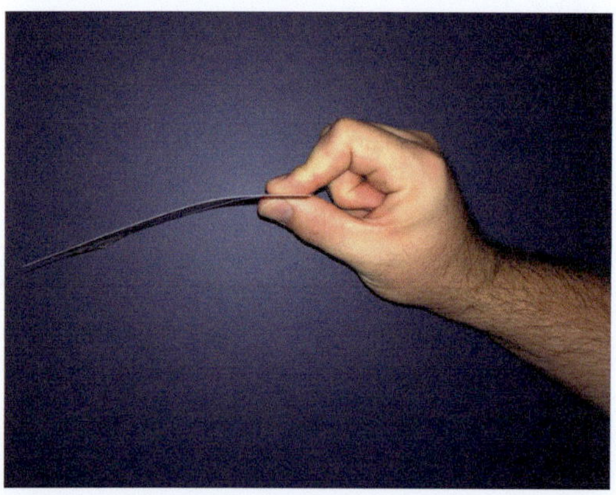

Fig. 9.5 Oppositional pinch maneuver

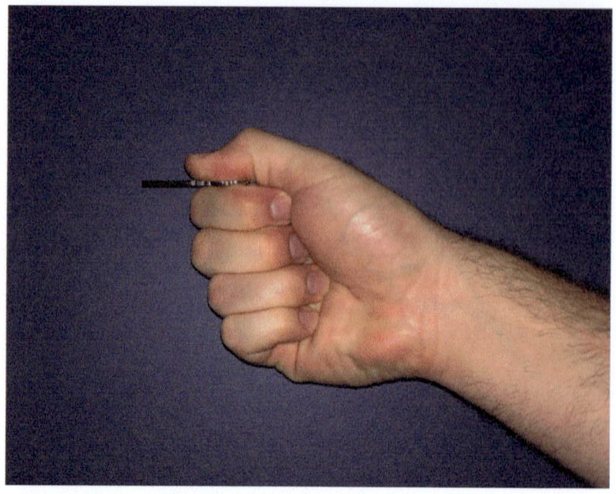

Fig. 9.6 Key pinch maneuver

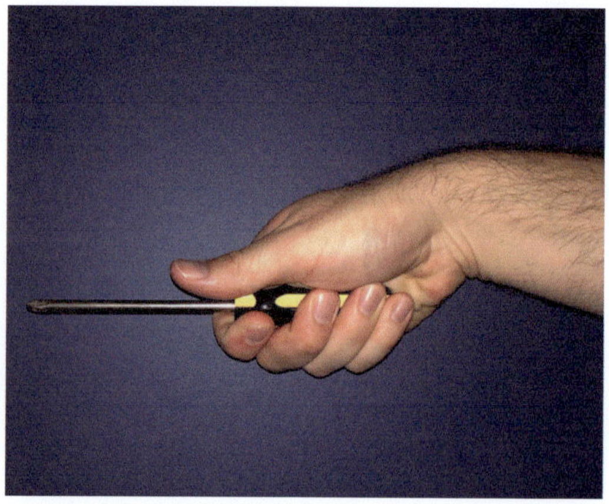

Fig. 9.7 Directional grip maneuver

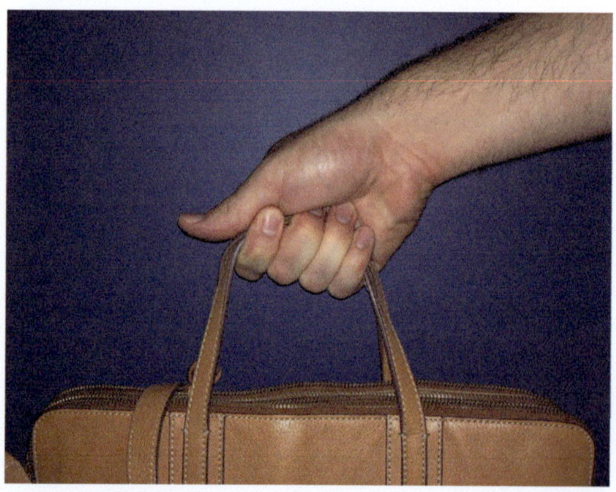

Fig. 9.8 Hook grip maneuver

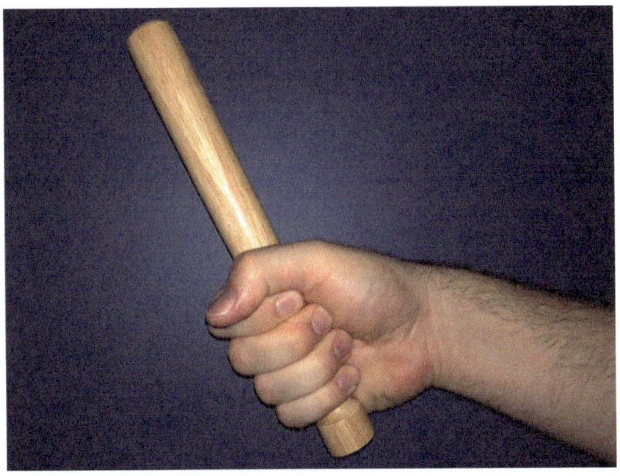

Fig. 9.9 Power grasp maneuver

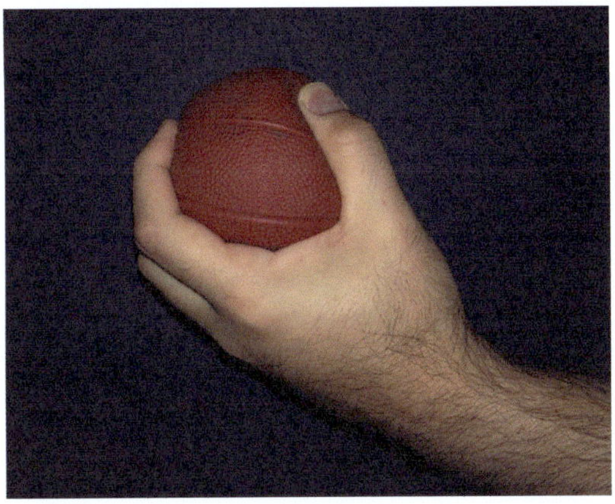

Fig. 9.10 Span grasp maneuver

References

1. http://umich.edu/~umfandsf/symbolismproject/symbolism.html/H/hand.html#:~:text=According%20to%20Aristotle%2C%20the%20hand,and%20friendship%20(shake%20hands).
2. Alpenfels EJ. The anthropology and social significance of the human hand. Artif Limbs. 1955;2(2):4–21.
3. https://definition.org/define/hand/American.Heritage(R) Dictionary of the English Language, Fifth Edition. Copyright (c) 2011 by Houghton Mifflin Harcourt Publishing Company. Published by Houghton Mifflin Harcourt Publishing Company.
4. Duncan SF, Saracevic CE, Kakinoki R. Biomechanics of the hand. Hand Clin. 2013;29(4):483–92. https://doi.org/10.1016/j.hcl.2013.08.003. Epub 2013 Oct 15. PMID: 24209947.
5. Gargulinski R. Human vs. primate hands. 2018. Updated 2020 Oct 28. Available from: https://sciencing.com/human-vs-primate-hands-6137415.html.
6. Flanagan JR, Johansson RS. Encyclopedia of the human brain. Academic Press; 2002. Hand movements:399–414.
7. Soubeyrand M, Assabah B, Bégin M, Laemmel E, Dos Santos A, Crézé M. Pronation and supination of the hand: anatomy and biomechanics. Hand Surg Rehabil. 2017;36(1):2–11. https://doi.org/10.1016/j.hansur.2016.09.012. Epub 2016 Oct 27. PMID: 28137437.
8. Dimon T. The body of motion: its evolution and design. Berkeley: North Atlantic Books; 2011. p. 39–42.
9. Ingram JN, Körding KP, Howard IS, Wolpert DM. The statistics of natural hand movements. Exp Brain Res. 2008;188(2):223–36. https://doi.org/10.1007/s00221-008-1355-3. Epub 2008 Mar 28. PMID: 18369608; PMCID: PMC2636901.

10 Hand – Anatomy and MRI Optimization

Tetyana Gorbachova, Angela Atinga, and Linda Probyn

Normal MRI Anatomy of the Hand

Capsular Anatomy

Overview

The capsular anatomy of the metacarpophalangeal (MCP) joint, proximal interphalangeal (PIP) joint, and distal interphalangeal (DIP) joints is organized in a similar fashion; lateral capsular reinforcements are provided by the proper and accessory collateral ligaments on the radial and ulnar sides of the joint, and the volar capsule is comprised of a thick fibrocartilaginous structure, referred to as the volar or palmar plate (Fig. 10.1). The proper and accessory collateral ligaments share their proximal site of attachment at the proximal osseous aspect of the joint, whereas distally the proper collateral ligaments insert on the distal osseous margin of the joint and accessory collateral ligaments fan out in palmar direction to broadly insert on the volar plate [1, 2] (Fig. 10.2). The volar plates of the lesser MCP joints are connected by the deep transverse metacarpal ligament (DTML) [3]. On MRI, the coronal plane provides best visualization of the proper collateral ligaments, the sagittal plane best depicts the volar plate, and the axial images add visualization of both structures and accessory collateral ligaments. In addition to capsuloligamentous structures, the extensor and flexor system of the finger is essential to the stability to the MCP, DIP, and PIP joints.

The lesser carpometacarpal (CMC) joints can be divided into two groups separated by the ligamentous attachments between hamate and fourth metacarpal and occasionally enclosed in separate synovial cavities: second and third CMC joints and fourth and fifth CMC joints. Functionally, the first and second CMC joints are nearly immobile. There is a short range of gliding at the fourth and fifth CMC joints with a small degree of flexion and rotation. The CMC joints are stabilized by dorsal, volar, and interosseous ligaments [4].

T. Gorbachova (✉)
Department of Radiology, Einstein Healthcare Network, Sidney Kimmel Medical College at Thomas Jefferson University, Philadelphia, PA, USA
e-mail: GorbachT@einstein.edu

A. Atinga · L. Probyn
Department of Medical Imaging, University of Toronto, Sunnybrook Health Sciences Centre, Toronto, ON, Canada
e-mail: Angela.atinga@sunnybrook.ca; Linda.probyn@sunnybrook.ca

B. U. Casagranda (ed.), *MRI of the Upper Extremity*, https://doi.org/10.1007/978-3-030-81612-4_10

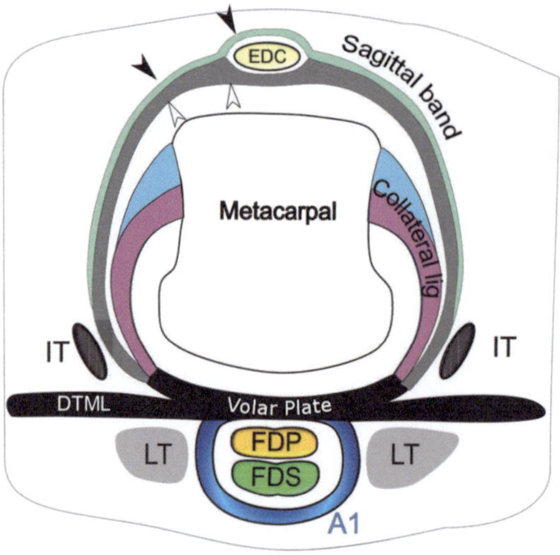

Fig. 10.1 *Supporting structures of the MCP joint at the level of the metacarpal head.* Schematic drawing of the capsuloligamentous structures as well as the flexor and extensor apparatuses of the finger. The dorsal and volar structures connect, forming a cylindrical fibrous envelope around the MCP joint. Proximally, proper and accessory collateral ligaments attach to the metacarpal, while distally, the proper collateral ligament (blue) attaches to the base of the proximal phalanx (not illustrated), and accessory collateral ligament (purple) extends to the volar plate. The digital flexor tendons (FDP and FDS) are anchored to the volar plate by A1 pulley. The volar plates of the fingers are interconnected by the deep transverse metacarpal ligament (DTML). The lumbrical muscles and tendons (LT) are located superficial to the DTML, while interosseous tendons (IT) are located deep to the DTML. The extensor hood at the level of the MCP joint is represented by a sagittal band with superficial (black arrowheads) and deep (white arrowheads) layers that envelope extensor digitorum communis (EDC) tendon. (Modified from Ref. [2])

Hand Musculature

Extrinsic muscles acting on the hand originate in the forearm and elbow, and their tendons pass through the wrist to insert on the hand. Intrinsic hand muscles are located within the hand itself. The intrinsic muscles are subdivided into three groups: thenar muscles (discussed separately), hypothenar muscles, and central group. The hypothenar group includes palmaris brevis, abductor digiti minimi, flexor digiti minimi brevis, and opponens digiti minimi muscles. The central group, sometimes referred to as deep or metacarpal muscles, is comprised of lumbrical, palmar interossei, and dorsal interossei muscles. The interosseous muscles arise from the metacarpal bones and insert directly on to the proximal phalanx and to the dorsal aponeurosis of each finger. Three palmar interosseous muscles adduct the fingers at the MCP joints to the long axis of the middle finger. Four dorsal interosseous muscles function to abduct fingers at the MCP joints in relation to the long axis of the middle finger, resulting in spreading of the fingers. The dorsal interossei are bipennate muscles, with each muscle arising from the two adjacent metacarpal bones. The four lumbrical muscles are unique in that they have both a tendinous origin and insertion, originating from the flexor digitorum profundus tendons and inserting on the dorsal aponeurosis.

On an axial image obtained at the level of the mid hand, the lumbrical muscle bellies are recognized along the radial and slightly volar aspect of the flexor digitorum profundus tendons. The interosseous muscles are further dorsal in location with their muscle bellies filling the intermetacarpal spaces. At the level of the MCP joint, the tendons of the intrinsic hand muscles can be identified by their relationship to the DTML: the lumbrical tendons are located superficial to the DTML, while the interosseous tendons are deep to the DTML [3, 5] (Fig. 10.3).

Extensor Apparatus

The complex anatomy of the flexor and extensor tendons of the hand is better understood by considering their different biomechanical requirements. The organization of the extensor apparatus is dictated by the functional demands for stability and integrated functioning [6]. Therefore, compared to the flexors, the extensor apparatus has a much more delicate aponeurotic character [2, 5]. The extensor tendons and retinacular structures form a plexiform construct around the finger that has been likened to a Chinese finger trap or a functional homolog of an exoskeleton [7] (Fig. 10.4). Dorsal aponeurotic sheets of tissue

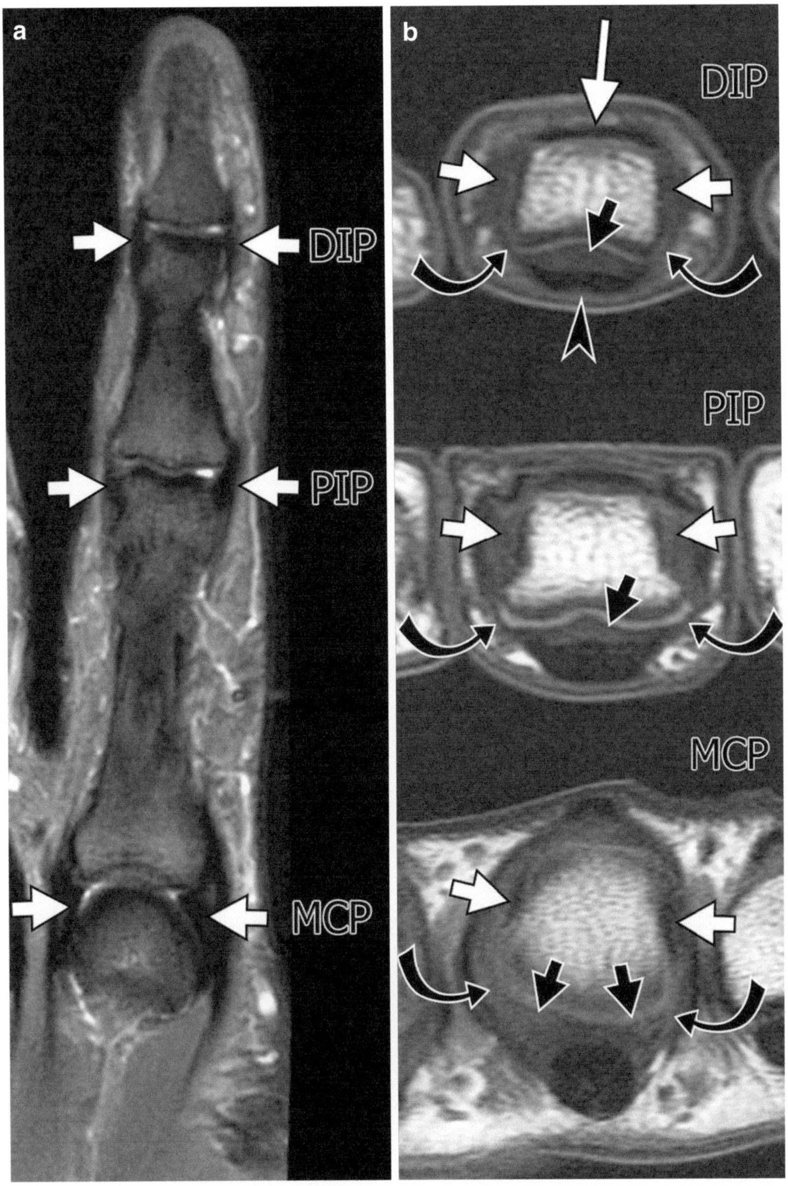

Fig. 10.2 *Capsuloligamentous anatomy of the finger.* Coronal STIR MR image (**a**) demonstrates proper collateral ligaments (arrows) on the radial and ulnar sides of the MCP, PIP, and DIP joints. Axial T1-weighted MR images (**b**) obtained through the proximal margin of each joint depict proper collateral ligaments (short white arrows), accessory collateral ligaments (curved arrows), and the volar plates (short black arrows). The terminal extensor tendon (long white arrow) and flexor digitorum profundus tendon (black arrowhead) are intimately related to the joint capsule

represent the meeting point of tendons associated with different muscles and allow coordination between the extrinsic (extensor digitorum communis (EDC), extensor indicis, extensor digiti minimi) and intrinsic (lumbrical and interosseous) muscles [1, 8, 9]. The EDC trifurcates at proximal phalanx to form a central slip, which inserts on the base of the middle phalanx, and

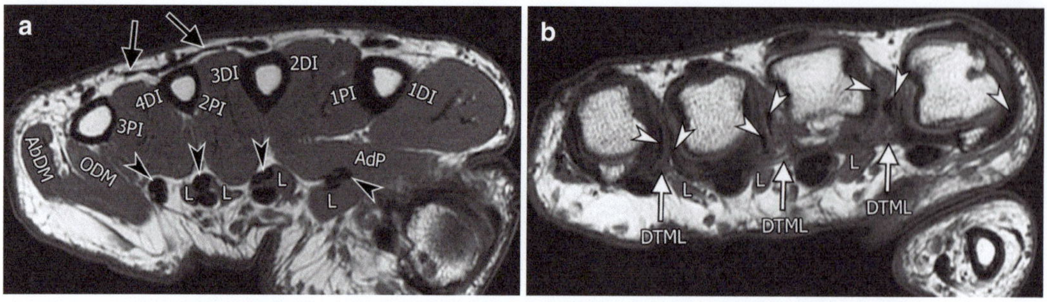

Fig. 10.3 *Intrinsic muscles of the hand.* Axial T1-weighted fat-suppressed images through the mid hand (**a**) and MCP joints (**b**) demonstrate the lumbrical muscles (L) along the radial and slightly volar side of the flexor digitorum profundus tendons (black arrowheads). The dorsal interosseous (1–4 DI) and palmar interosseous (1–3 PI) muscles bellies fill in the intermetacarpal spaces. Note the position of the lumbrical muscles (L) and interosseous tendons (white arrowheads) relative to the DTML (white arrows). Juncturae tendinum (black arrows) interconnect the extrinsic extensor tendons. AdP adductor pollicis, AbDM abductor digiti minimi, ODM opponens digiti minimi

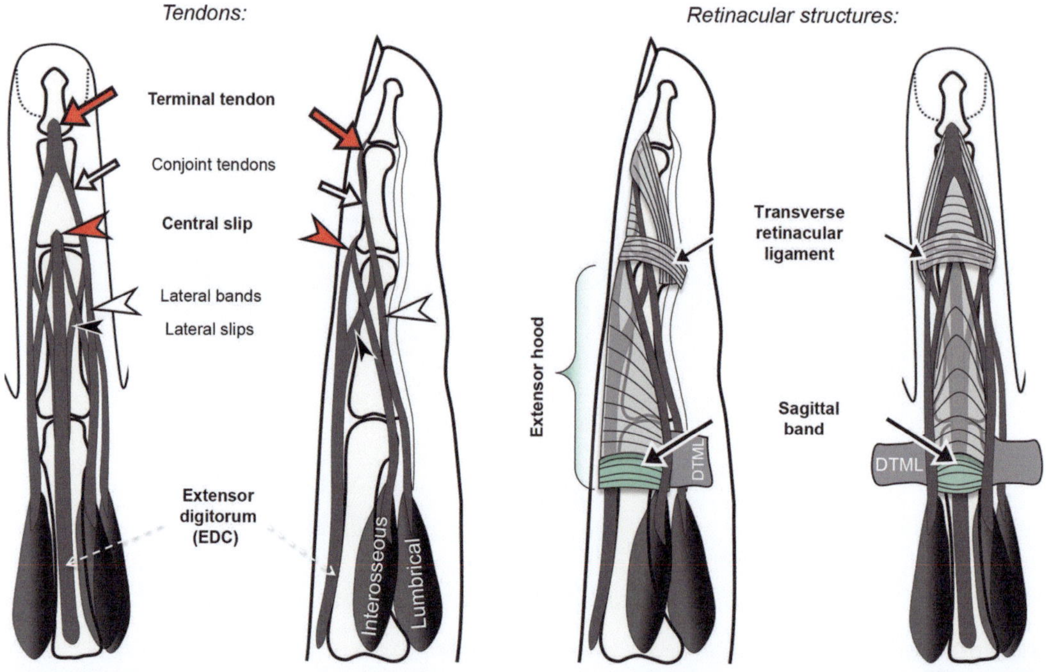

Fig. 10.4 *Extensor apparatus of the finger*. The central slip of the extensor digitorum communis (EDC) tendon inserts on the base of the middle phalanx (red arrowheads), and the two lateral slips (black arrowheads) join the lateral bands from the interossei and lumbrical tendons (white arrowheads) to form the conjoint tendons (white arrows). The conjoint tendons merge to form the terminal extensor tendon (red arrows) which inserts on the base of the distal phalanx. The sagittal band (long black arrow) is a part of the extensor hood at the level of MCP joint. The transverse retinacular ligament (short black arrow) is located at the level of PIP joint. DTML deep transverse metacarpal ligament. (Modified from Ref. [2])

two flanking lateral slips. The lateral slips join the two lateral bands, formed by interossei and lumbrical tendons, to form conjoint tendons. The interossei and lumbrical tendons also give off the medial bands that connect with the central slip distally near its insertion. Conjoint tendons merge distally to form a terminal extensor tendon which inserts on the base of distal phalanx (Fig. 10.4).

At the dorsum of the hand, stabilizing retinacular structures are represented by juncturae tendinum, fibrous bands that connect the slips of the extensor digitorum [10] (Fig. 10.3). There is considerable anatomic variability of the extensor apparatus that includes variations in extensor tendons and juncturae, more common toward the ulnar side of the hand [10].The index finger is more independent as it is critical for a delicate precision grip, so it has the least variable extensor tendon anatomy and the least prominent juncturae [6].

In the finger, the principal stabilizing retinacular structure is referred to as the extensor hood or dorsal aponeurotic expansion [8]. The sagittal band is an important part of the extensor hood at the level of the MCP joint (Figs. 10.1 and 10.5). A thicker deep layer and very thin superficial layer of the sagittal band envelope the extensor tendon and continue around either side of the joint to connect to the volar plate, stabilizing the extensor tendon over the MCP joint [1, 11]

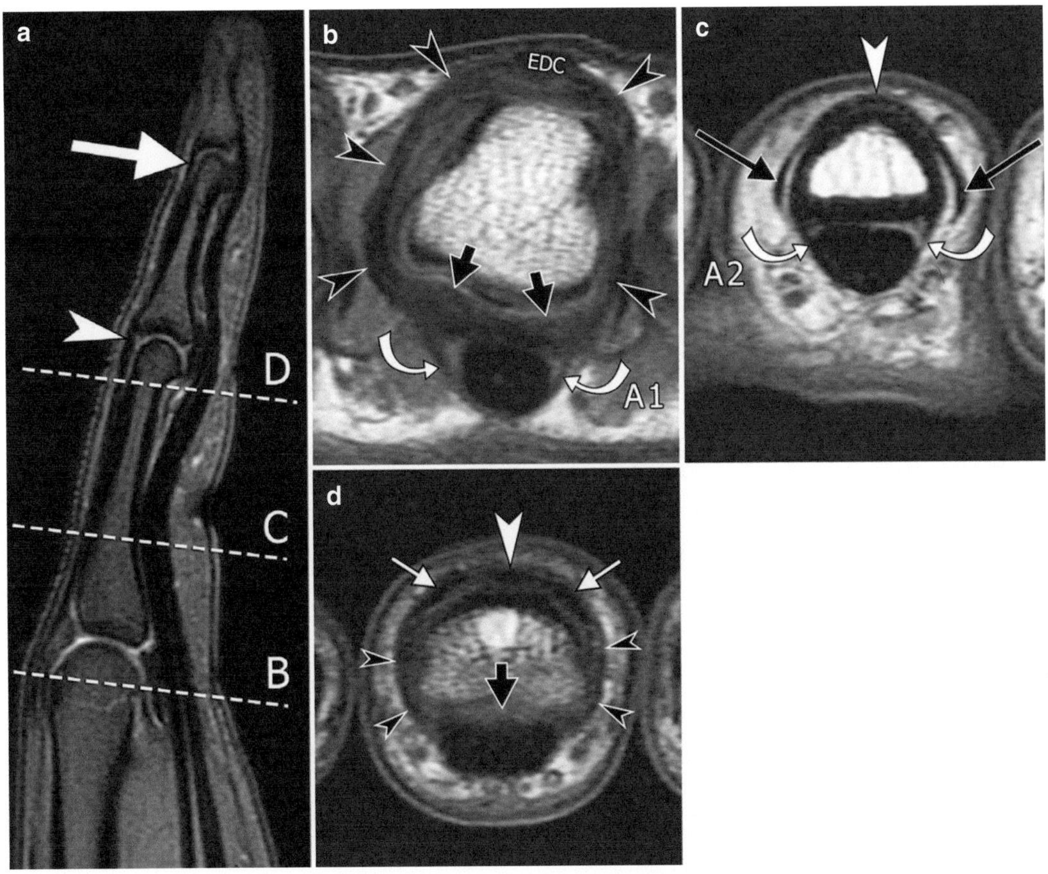

Fig. 10.5 *Extensor apparatus of the finger*. Sagittal proton density-weighted fat-suppressed MR image (**a**) shows insertions of the central slip of the extensor tendon (white arrowhead) and the terminal extensor tendon (large white arrow). Axial T1-weighted MR images at the level of the MCP joint (**b**) and proximal (**c**) and distal (**d**) aspect of the proximal phalanx demonstrate the sagittal band (black arrowheads) as it encircles the EDC tendon and wraps around the MCP joint to connect to the volar plate (short black arrows, **b**). Further distally the extensor hood is formed by the central slip (white arrowhead) and lateral bands (long black arrows, **c**) connected by transverse fibers. At the level of the proximal aspect of the PIP volar plate (short black arrow, **d**), the transverse retinacular ligament (small black arrowheads, **d**) connects the conjoint tendons (small white arrows) to the flexor sheath. A1 and A2 flexor pulleys are shown (curved arrows, **b**, **c**)

(Figs. 10.1 and 10.5). Distal to the sagittal bands, the extensor hood is formed by transverse and oblique fibers which arise from the interossei and lumbricals tendons. At the proximal interphalangeal (PIP) joint, a structure analogous to the sagittal band is referred to as the transverse retinacular ligament and connects the conjoint lateral bands to the flexor sheath. Further distally, a "mini hood" is formed by oblique retinacular ligaments and a triangular ligament that bridges the conjoint tendons.

Flexor Apparatus

Morphologic features of the flexor apparatus are dictated by their functional demands of power and precision. Flexion of the fingers can be carried further than extension as fingers can generally be flexed toward the palm at three neighboring joints. In extension, however, fingers are merely returned to a straight position. Greater excursion of the flexor tendons necessitates additional anatomic structures to prevent tendons bowstringing and facilitate gliding of the tendons [6, 12]. The flexor tendons run through fibro-osseous tunnels that are lined by synovium. The floor or dorsal aspect of each tunnel is composed of palmar surfaces of the proximal and middle phalanges, DTML, and volar plates of the MCP, PIP, and DIP joints. The palmar aspect is formed by fibrous sheets attached to the periosteum of the phalanges and to the volar plates. Local thickenings of these fibrous sheaths are referred to as pulleys [13, 14].

The flexor tendons of the second through fifth fingers include the flexor digitorum profundus (FDP) tendon that inserts at the volar base of the distal phalanx and flexor digitorum superficialis (FDS) that inserts on the midportion of the middle phalanx. At the level of the metacarpal head and proximally FDS lies superficial to the FDP. Distal to the metacarpal, the FDS tendon splits forming a ring aperture to allow passage of the FDP which subsequently becomes the more superficially located tendon. The two portions of the FDS reunite at Camper's chiasm located deep to the FDP [3]. The advantage of this anatomic arrangement is that in addition to pulleys, the tendons themselves contribute to maintaining their position close to the bone as one tendon forms a sling for the other (Fig. 10.6).

Pulleys maintain close apposition of the tendon to the bone and help flexor tendon tracking. The finger pulley system is composed of annular and cruciform pulleys (Fig. 10.7). Annular pulleys serve to stabilize the tendon during motion, while cruciate pulleys facilitate deformation of the tendon sheath during flexion. Annular pulleys are identified on MR imaging as transversely oriented well-defined areas of tendon sheath thickening [15]. The odd-numbered pulleys, A1, A3, and A5, are located at the level of the MCP, PIP, and DIP joints, respectively. Cruciform pulleys are delicate crisscrossing web-like fibers interposed between annular pulleys and not typically visualized on clinical MR imaging. The most biomechanically important and most frequently injured pulleys are the A2 and A4 pulleys. The A2 is the longest pulley, covering the proximal two thirds of the proximal phalanx. The A4 pulley covers the midportion of the middle phalanx [15]. Annular pulleys are best depicted on axial MR images as thin low signal intensity struts anchoring the flexor tendons to the volar plates at the level of the joints or to the volar surface of the bone along the phalangeal osseous attachments. On sagittal images, the annular pulleys can be observed as local thickenings of low signal intensity along the palmar aspect of the tendon sheaths. The locations of cruciform pulleys can be indirectly demonstrated as areas of pleating of the synovial sheaths near the PIP and DIP joints in the presence of tenosynovitis (Fig. 10.7).

On MRI, the interplay between the FDS and FDP is best followed on sequential axial images. Additional longitudinal assessment of the tendons and their insertions is performed in the sagittal plane (Figs. 10.6 and 10.7). When following the course of the flexor tendons on axial images, it is important to remember that they are true to their names within the wrist and hand. Distal to the A1 pulley, the FDS divides into radial and

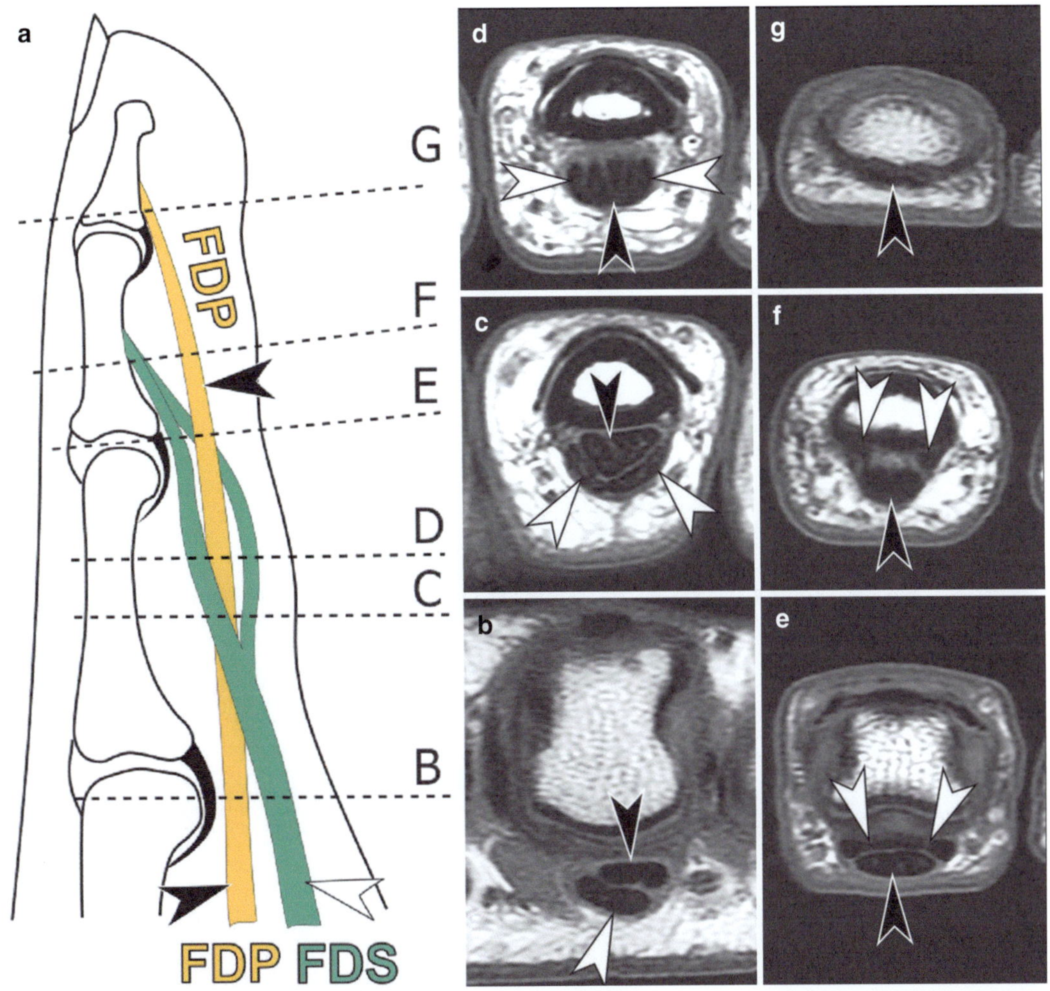

Fig. 10.6 *Flexor tendon anatomy of the finger*. Diagram (**a**) and sequential axial T1-weighted MR images (**b–g**, proximal to distal) depict the course of the FDP (black arrowheads) and FDS (white arrowheads). At the level of the metacarpal head (**b**) and proximally, FDS lies superficial to the FDP. Distal to the metacarpal, FDS tendon splits (**c**, **d**) forming an aperture to allow passage of the FDP. Distal to this point FDP becomes the more superficially located tendon. The two portions of the FDS reunite at Camper's chiasm located deep to the FDP (**e**). FDS inserts on the midportion of the middle phalanx (**f**), and FDP inserts at the volar base of the distal phalanx (**g**). (6A modified from Ref. [2])

ulnar slips, and along the course of the A2 pulley, the superficialis and profundus tendons swap their locations so that further distally FDS is located deep to FDP [15]. The FDP tendon may display a median longitudinal groove or two separate slips [16] (Fig. 10.8).

Synovial sheaths provide nutrition and lubrication to the tendons. To enable greater longitudinal excursion of the flexor tendons in the wrist and hand, the flexor synovial sheaths extend beyond the boundaries of the corresponding retinacular structures. Because the metacarpal bones of the thumb and little finger have the greatest mobility compared to other fingers, their flexor tendon synovial sheaths pass without interruption from fingers to the wrist [12]. The synovial sheaths of the thumb and little finger often communicate with the radial and ulnar bursae at the wrist, respectively. The flexor tendon sheaths of the index, long, and ring fingers typically do not

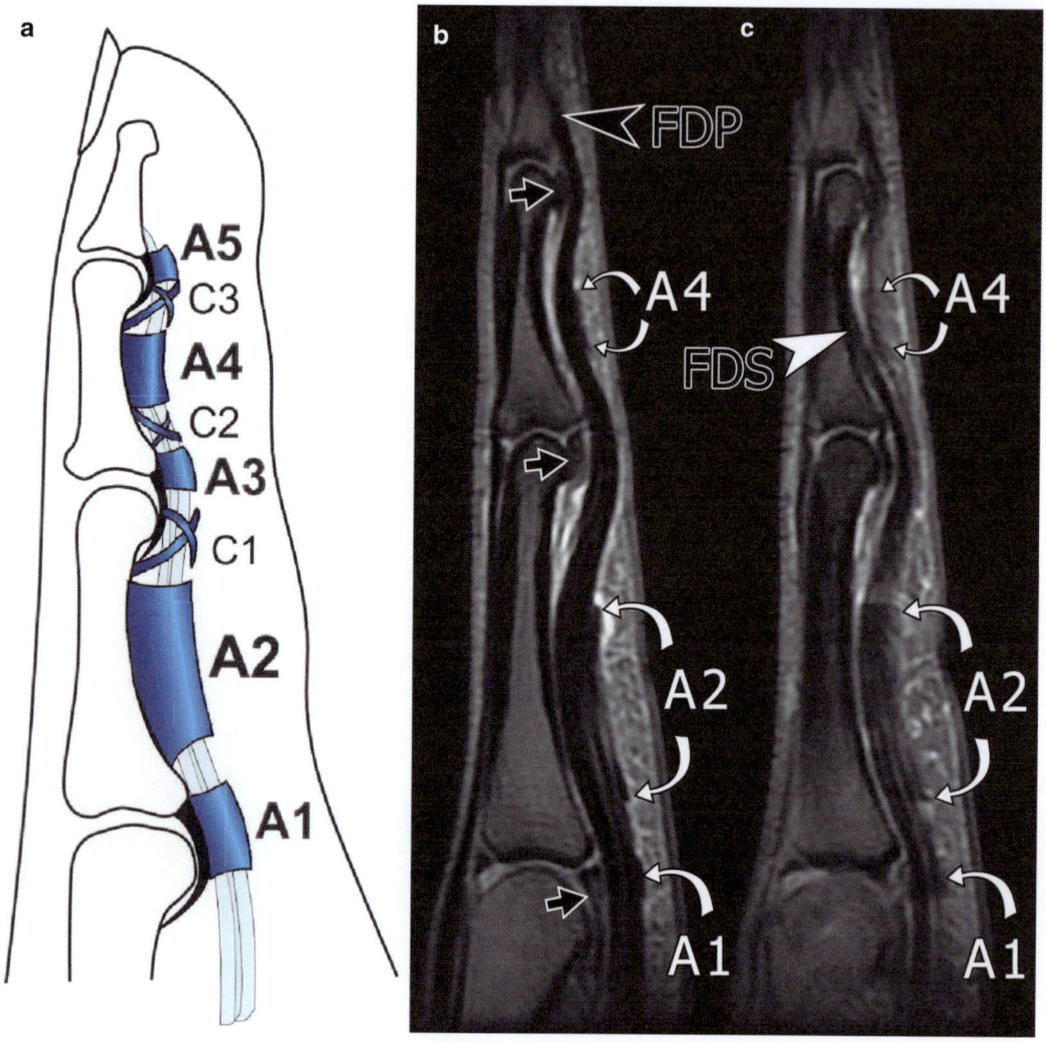

Fig. 10.7 *Flexor tendon pulley system of the fingers.* The pulley systems are composed of five transversely oriented annular pulleys (A1–A5) and three cruciform pulleys (C1–C3) (**a**). Midline sagittal (**b**) and parasagittal (**c**) proton density-weighted fat-suppressed MR images of the long finger depict annular pulleys (curved arrows) as local thickening of low signal intensity along the palmar aspect of the flexor tendon sheaths. Note the relationship of the pulleys to the volar plates (black arrows) and to the insertions of the FDS (white arrowhead) and FDP (black arrowhead). (7A modified from Ref. [2])

have as great a proximal extent; these sheaths begin at the level of the metacarpal necks proximal to the DTML and terminate distally at the insertion of the FDP. The multiple anatomic variations in communications of the palmar bursae and finger tendon sheaths may necessitate imaging of the entire hand and wrist when evaluating pathology affecting the synovial sheaths, in particular infection [17, 18].

Vascular and Digital Nerve Anatomy

Overview

Arterial blood supply to the hand is provided by a superficial palmar arch, formed by anastomosis between the continuation of the ulnar artery and superficial volar branch of the radial artery, and the more proximal deep palmar arch, formed by the deep branch of the radial artery as it passes

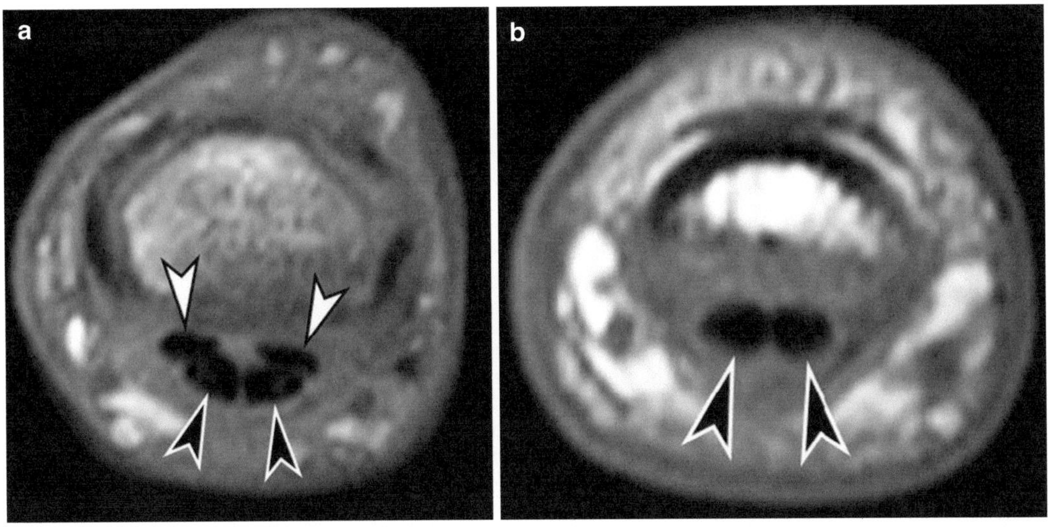

Fig. 10.8 *Flexor tendons of the finger*. Axial T1-weighted MR images at the level of the PIP joint distal to the chiasm (**a**) and just proximal to the DIP joint (**b**) demonstrate the relationship of the FDS (white arrowheads) and FDP (black arrowheads). Note the presence of two distinct slips of the FDP tendon, a normal anatomic variation

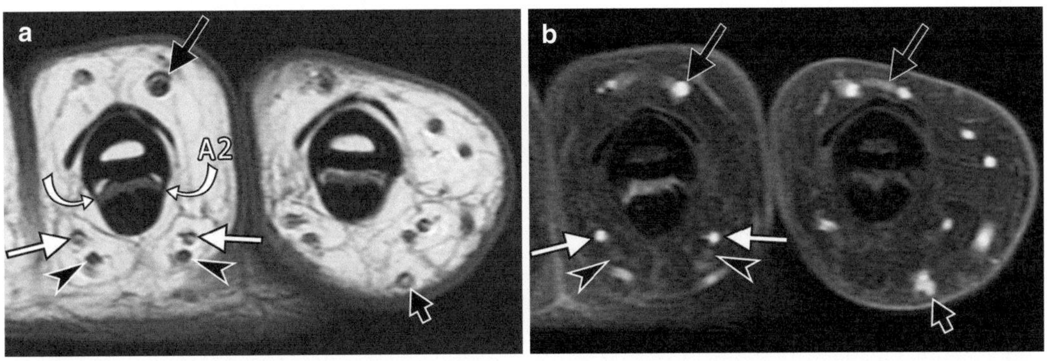

Fig. 10.9 *Vascular and digital nerve anatomy of the finger*. Axial T1-weighted (**a**) and T1-weighted fat-suppressed gadolinium-enhanced images (**b**) of the index and long fingers at the mid diaphysis of the proximal phalanx demonstrate radial and ulnar palmar digital arteries (white arrows) and proper digital nerves (black arrowheads). The venous system is represented by the proximal venous arch (long black arrow) and palmar veins (short black arrows). A2 pulleys (curved arrows)

from dorsal to the deep volar hand and anastomoses with one or both deep volar branches of the ulnar artery. The superficial palmar arch has greater anatomic variability with several patterns of complete or incomplete arch described in the literature [19]. Common digital arteries originate from the superficial arch. Each finger has two palmar digital arteries that originate from the bifurcation of the common digital artery at the level of the base of the proximal phalanx and course along the radial and ulnar side of the flexor tendon sheath dorsal to the proper digital nerves [20] (Fig. 10.9). Communicating branches of the digital arteries form three transfers of palmar arches in the finger: proximal, middle, and distal. The pulp of the finger and nail matrix are nourished by the matrix arches and longitudinal arteries.

In the regions where tendons are surrounded by true synovial sheaths, the vessels enter the

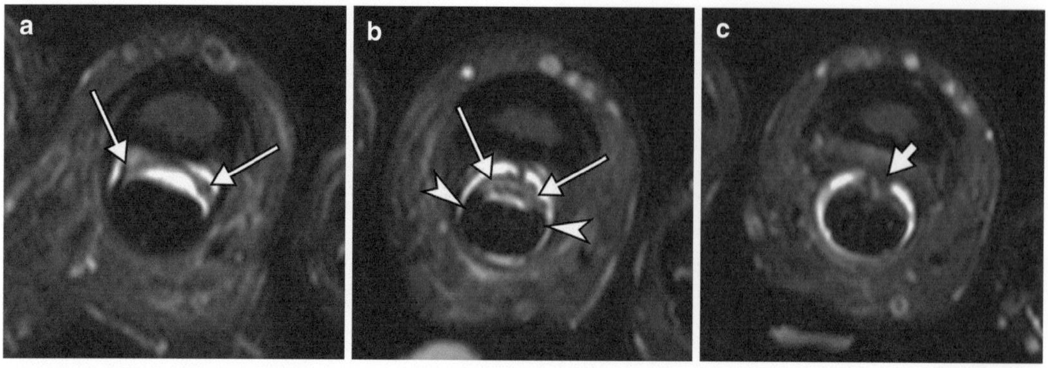

Fig. 10.10 *Vincular system of the flexor tendons.* Axial T2-weighted fat-suppressed MR images (**a**–**c**) of the ring finger in a 44-year-old man with subacute A2 pulley injury with increased conspicuity of the vincula due to flexor tenosynovitis and tendon bowstringing. The radial and ulnar vincula longa superficialis (long white arrows, **a** and **b**) arise from the radial and ulnar side of the base of the proximal phalanx and attach to FDS (arrowheads) just proximal to the Camper's chiasm. Vinculum breve superficialis (short white arrow, **c**) arises from the membranous part of the volar plate of the PIP joint and attaches to the chiasm

tendon via mesotenon that, along with synovial fluid, provides a nutritional pathway to the tendon. In digital flexor tendons, the blood supply is delivered via thin strands of synovium called the vincula tendinum. The vincula carry minute vessels and connect to the dorsal part of the tendons (Fig. 10.10). In the digital canal, each flexor tendon typically has two kinds of vincula, the short and the long. The short vincula of FDS and FDP (vinculum breve superficialis and vinculum breve profundus) are found consistently in all fingers. The long vincula (vinculum longum superficialis and vinculum longum profundus) may vary in type and differ in each finger [21].

The motor and sensory innervation of the hand is provided by three nerves: median, ulnar, and radial nerves [20, 22]. Variations from the classical nerve distribution are extremely common in the hand. Distal to the transverse carpal ligament, the *median nerve* gives off a short recurrent motor branch for the thenar musculature and continues as three common digital nerves. The first common digital nerve divides into three proper volar digital nerves supplying the thumb and radial side of the index finger. The second and third common digital nerves each divide into two proper digital nerves that supply the ulnar side of the index finger, both sides of the third finger, and radial side of the fourth finger. Each proper digital nerve gives off a dorsal branch that joins the dorsal digital nerve from the superficial branch of the radial nerve and supplies the dorsal aspect of the distal phalanx. At Guyon's canal, the *ulnar nerve* divides into the deep motor and superficial sensory branches. The superficial sensory branch of the ulnar nerve continues in a straight course and divides into the fourth common digital nerve that supplies the ulnar side of the fourth ray and radial side of the little finger and a proper palmar digital nerve that supplies the ulnar side of the little finger. The deep motor branch of the ulnar nerve crosses the palm and innervates intrinsic hand muscles including all the interossei muscles and third and fourth lumbrical muscles. The innervation of the thenar musculature is provided by the median nerve and deep branch of the ulnar nerve, while hypothenar musculature is entirely supplied by the deep ulnar nerve. The superficial branch of the *radial nerve* divides into dorsal digital nerves that provide sensation to the radial aspect of the dorsum of the hand, dorsum of the thumb and index and long fingers, and dorsal radial side of the ring finger.

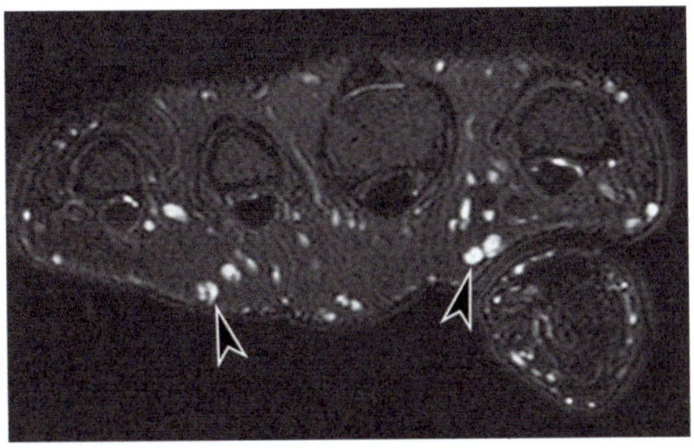

Fig. 10.11 *Pacinian corpuscles.* Axial T2-weighted fat-suppressed images of the hand distal to the MCP joints in a 53-year-old man demonstrate multiple round and oval hyperintense nodules (arrowheads) in the subcutaneous fat of the palm representing prominent Pacinian corpuscles. Following intravenous administration of gadolinium contrast, there is no enhancement of these nodules

Recent studies have demonstrated that hyperintense palmar subcutaneous nodules in the hands and proximal fingers frequently observed on clinical MRI examinations represent normal Pacinian corpuscles and should not be mistaken for pathological conditions [23, 24]. The corpuscles are sensory receptors for vibration and deep pressure. On MRI, they appear as round or oval, 1–5 mm in diameter, non-enhancing, T2-hyperintense subcutaneous nodules, separate from the vessels, concentrated in subcutaneous fat of palms around the MCP joints (Fig. 10.11).

Anatomic Zones of the Extensor and Flexor Hand Tendons

To provide an organized approach to the anatomic structures and lesion localization, a topographic classification of zones has been developed for the flexor and extensor tendons. According to the Kleinert and Verdan classification, the hand and wrist encompass five flexor and eight extensor zones that are numbered distal to proximal [25].

The extensor zones alternate between the joint lines (odd-numbered zones) and the areas in between the joints (even-numbered zones)

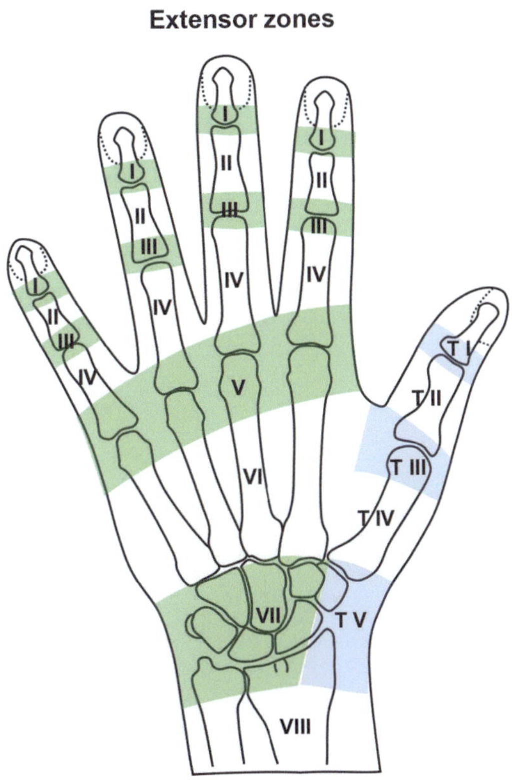

Fig. 10.12 *Extensor tendon zones of the fingers and thumb.* These topographic zones are labeled distal to proximal with odd-numbered zones (green and blue) located over the joints and the even-numbered located in between the joints. Zone VII of the hand and Zone V of the thumb include wrist extensor compartments

(Fig. 10.12). The topographic division of the flexor tendons into the zones takes into account the interplay between the FDP and FDS, presence of the pulleys and synovial sheaths, and vascular supply delivered via vincula (Fig. 10.13). Of particular importance is flexor Zone II that spans a relatively large area at the palmar aspect of the finger (Fig. 10.14). Zone II starts distal to the insertion of the FDS at the volar base of the middle phalanx and stops proximally at the distal palmar fold, which corresponds to the proximal margin of A1 pulley on MRI. Due to the complexity of this region, injuries to flexor Zone II carry worst prognosis and used to be called "no man's land."

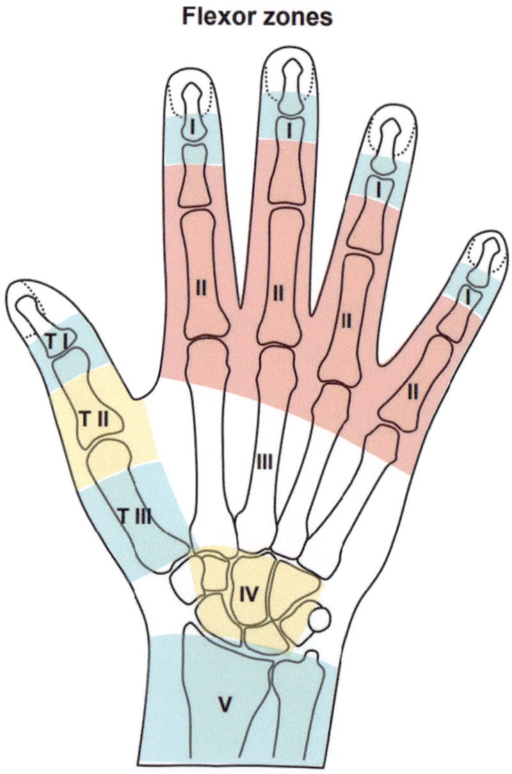

Fig. 10.13 *Flexor tendon zones of the fingers and thumb.* In the finger, Zone I extends from the distal phalanx to the middle phalanx, Zone II extends from the middle phalanx to the distal palmar fold, Zone III extends from the level proximal to the MCP joint to the distal part of the flexor retinaculum of the carpal tunnel, Zone IV consists of the carpal tunnel, and Zone V includes structures proximal to the carpal tunnel. In the thumb, Zone I (T I) includes the region of the interphalangeal joint, Zone II (T II) is the region of the MCP joint, and Zone III (T III) includes the first metacarpal

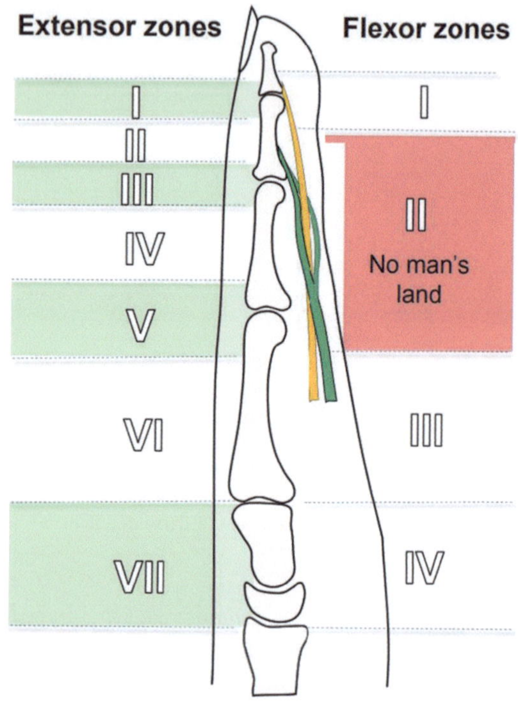

Fig. 10.14 *Extensor and flexor zones of the fingers.* Lateral view of the finger demonstrates designation of the extensor and flexor tendon zones. Flexor Zone II (red) spans area that includes FDS insertion (green tendon) distally and distal palmar fold and proximal edge of A1 pulley proximally, "no man's land"

Normal MR Imaging Anatomy of the Thumb

Osseous and Capsuloligamentous Anatomy of the Thumb

Thumb CMC Joint

The first CMC joint is a unique semi-constrained biconcave saddle joint between the base of the first metacarpal and distal surface of the trapezium [26, 27]. The joint has a wide range of movement and is inherently unstable, requiring many ligaments for support [28, 29]. Although up to 16 ligaments have been described in cadaveric hands, only some of these ligaments provide most of the stability at the CMC joint and are visible on MRI (Fig. 10.15). For a dedicated thumb CMC joint MRI, the imaging planes are prescribed to the thumb, as described later under MRI optimization [27].

The dorsal ligament complex, also referred to as the dorsal deltoid ligament, is best seen on sagittal MR images of the thumb. The dorsal deltoid ligament is comprised of three ligaments: the dorsal radial ligament (DRL), dorsal central ligament (DCL), and posterior oblique ligament (POL). The DRL attaches to the dorsal radial tubercle of the trapezium and the dorsal edge of the first metacarpal base, adjacent to the abductor pollicis longus (AbPL) tendon. This is the thickest ligament and most easily seen on MR images [30]. The DCL is adjacent to the DRL, being more dorsal and ulnar [31]. The POL attaches to the dorsal trapezium and dorsal base of the first

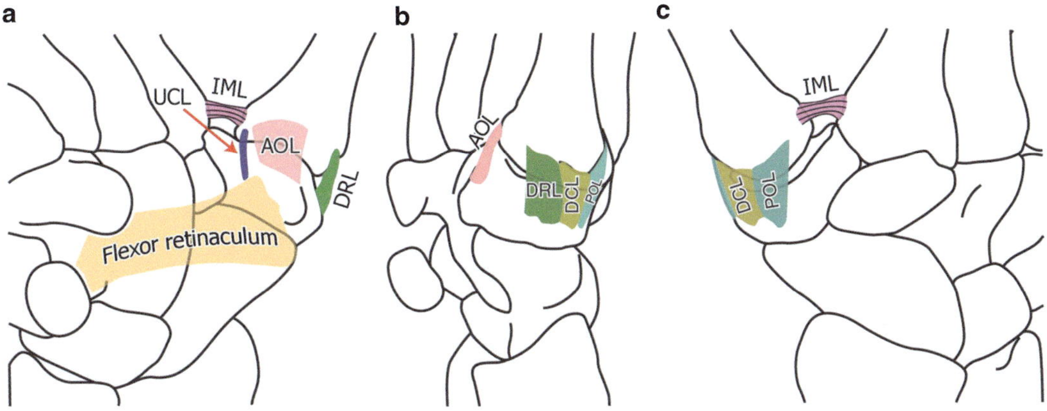

Fig. 10.15 *Supporting ligaments of the first CMC joint.* The ulnar collateral ligament (UCL, red arrow, **a**) originates from the distal ulnar margin of the flexor retinaculum (yellow band) and trapezial ridge and courses ulnar to the anterior oblique ligament (AOL), also known as the beak ligament, attaching to the volar ulnar tubercle of the base of the thumb metacarpal. The dorsal deltoid ligament consists of three ligaments, the dorsal radial ligament (DRL), dorsal central ligament (DCL), and posterior oblique ligament (POL), traverse from the trapezium to the first metacarpal base. The intermetacarpal ligament (IML) (**a**, **c**) traverses from the bases of the first and second metacarpals. (Modified from Ref. [31])

metacarpal. These dorsal ligaments act as a primary restraint to dorsal radial metacarpal dislocation [27, 32]. Given their broad range of attachment and support provided, the dorsal ligaments have been likened to a deltoid-type structure [28]. The intermetacarpal ligament (IML) attaches to the dorsal aspect of the first and second metacarpal bases and restrains thumb movements, particularly abduction. It can be difficult to see on MR imaging but is most visible on coronal images [30] (Figs. 10.15 and 10.16).

The volar ligament complex is thinner than the dorsal ligaments but still functionally important and is best seen on sagittal MR images (Fig. 10.16e, f) [30]. The most important volar ligament is the anterior oblique ligament (AOL), also called the beak ligament, which attaches to the volar tubercle of the trapezium and to the volar tubercle, or a "beak," of the thumb metacarpal. AOL has superficial and deep components [30] (Fig. 10.16f).This ligament resists volar or dorsal stress [26, 27, 32]. The ulnar collateral ligament (UCL) attaches proximally to the trapezium along the distal and ulnar margins of the flexor retinaculum and distally to the volar ulnar base of the first metacarpal [30]. The UCL of the first CMC joint can be difficult to visualize on MR imaging.

Thumb MCP Joint

The thumb MCP joint is a condyloid joint which allows flexion, extension, adduction, abduction, and circumduction. The most common location of sesamoid bones in the hand is at the first MCP joint [33]. Sesamoid bones act as a pulley system that provides tendons with a smooth surface over which to glide [33]. The flexor pollicis brevis (FPB) tendon inserts onto the radial sesamoid bone and the radial base of the proximal phalanx of the thumb, whereas the adductor pollicis (AdP) tendon inserts onto the ulnar sesamoid bone and ulnar base of the proximal phalanx [30]. The volar plate is a wedge-shaped fibrocartilage plate that reinforces the volar joint capsule and extends between the two first MCP sesamoid bones [30, 33] (Fig. 10.17).

The radial collateral ligament (RCL) and ulnar collateral ligament (UCL) are the primary stabilizers to varus and valgus stresses of the MCP joint, respectively [30]. The proper RCL and UCL originate at the dorsal aspect of the first metacarpal head and insert at the volar aspect of the first proximal phalangeal base. The accessory RCL and UCL are adjacent to the volar aspect of the proper collateral ligaments and extend from the metacarpal heads to the volar plate and sesamoid bones. The proper and accessory collateral

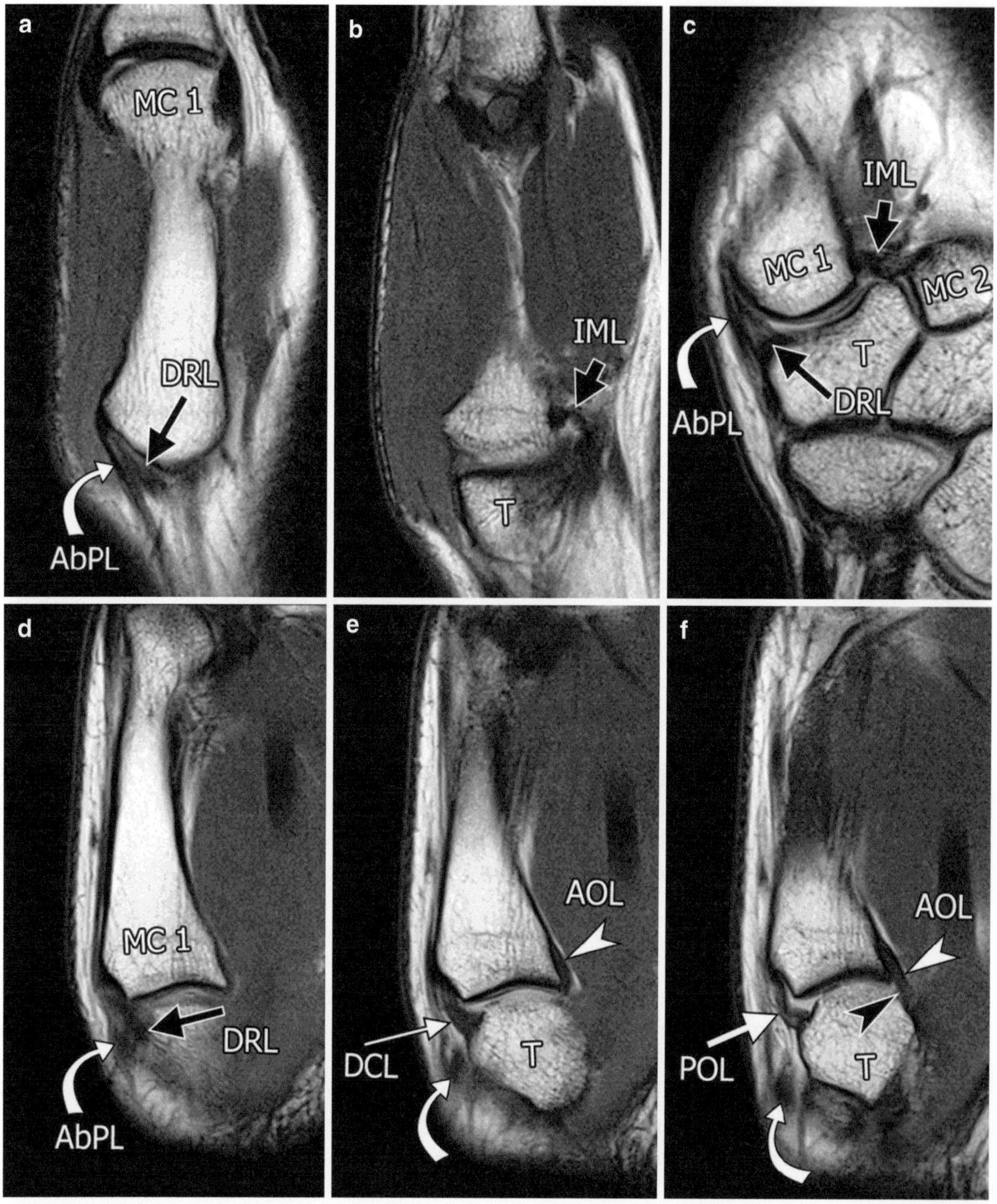

Fig. 10.16 *MR imaging of the supporting ligaments of the first CMC joint.* The image planes described are relative to the thumb CMC joint and metacarpal, the latter of which is pronated compared to the remainder of the hand and wrist through a range of between 45 and 60 degrees. Coronal (**a**, **b**) and coronal oblique (**c**) proton density-weighted MR images depict the DRL (long black arrow) coursing between the dorsal radial tubercle of the trapezium (T) and the dorsal radial edge of the first metacarpal (MC1) base, deep to the AbPL insertion (curved arrow). IML (short black arrow) traverses between the bases of the first (MC1) and second metacarpals. Sequential sagittal proton density-weighted MR images (radial to ulnar with respect to wrist, **d–f**) demonstrate DRL deep to AbPL and the more dorsally located DCL (thin white arrow) and POL (thick white arrow). The AOL courses at the volar and ulnar aspect of the joint. Note the superficial (white arrowhead) and deep (black arrowhead) components of the AOL

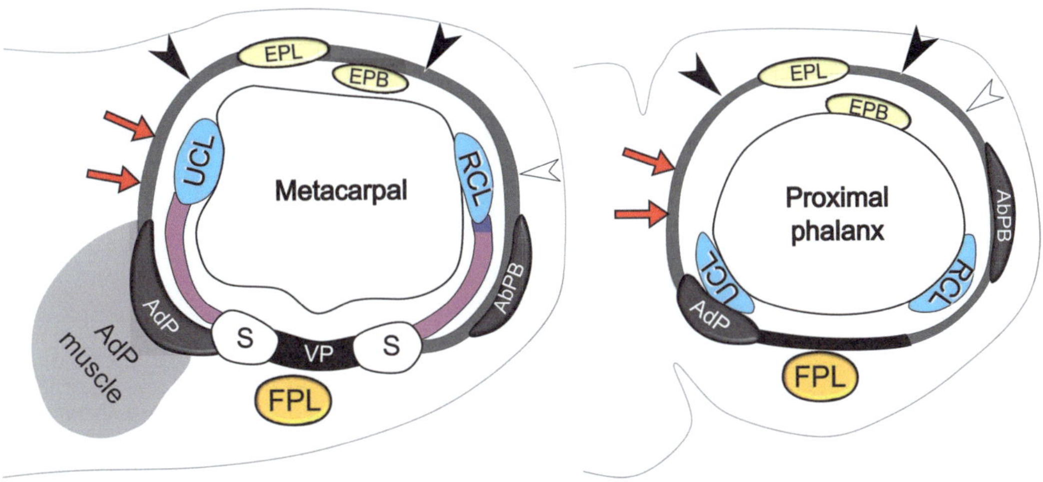

Fig. 10.17 *Anatomy of the first MCP joint*. Axial schematic images at the level of the first metacarpal (MC) head and proximal phalanx. The sagittal band (black arrowheads at the level of the MC head) and extensor hood (black arrowheads at the level of the proximal phalanx) encircle the extensor pollicis longus (EPL) tendon. The adductor pollicis muscle (AdP) and tendon are located at the ulnar and volar aspect of the joint. The adductor aponeurosis (red arrows) is continuous with the sagittal band and extensor hood on the ulnar side. The abductor pollicis brevis (AbPB) tendon and abductor aponeurosis (white arrowhead) blend with the radial side of the sagittal band and extensor hood. The extensor pollicis brevis (EPB) tendon is at the radial aspect of the EPL and deep to the radial sagittal band and extensor hood. The ulnar collateral ligament (UCL) and radial collateral ligament (RCL) are seen at the ulnar and radial aspect of the MC head, respectively, and traverse toward the volar aspect at the level of the proximal phalanx. The volar plate (VP) traverses between the sesamoids (S), deep to the flexor pollicis longus (FPL) tendon. The accessory collateral ligaments are shown in purple

ligaments are taught reciprocally during flexion and extension [34]. Palmar ligaments extend from the metacarpal head to the sesamoid (metacarpal sesamoid ligament) and from the sesamoid to the proximal phalanx (sesamoid phalangeal ligament) (Fig. 10.18).

Thumb IP Joint

The interphalangeal joint of the thumb shares the same anatomy as the interphalangeal joints of the lesser digits, discussed earlier in this chapter.

Muscle and Tendon Anatomy of the Thumb

The intrinsic muscles at the thumb form the thenar eminence, the palmar muscular bulge on the radial side of the hand at the base of the thumb. It comprises the opponens pollicis (OP), abductor pollicis brevis (AbPB), and flexor pollicis brevis (FPB) muscles, all originating at the flexor retinaculum (Fig. 10.19). The OP originates from the tubercle of the trapezium and the flexor retinaculum and inserts into the lateral margin of the first metacarpal. It medially rotates the thumb with flexion at the first CMC joint permitting opposition. The AbPB arises from the scaphoid and trapezium tubercles and the flexor retinaculum. It is superficial to the OP and inserts at the lateral base of the proximal phalanx of the thumb and abducts the thumb. The superficial head of the FPB arises from the tubercle of the trapezium and flexor retinaculum, passing along the radial margin of the flexor pollicis longus (FPL) tendon. The deep head, if present, arises from the trapezoid and capitate and the transverse carpal ligaments of the distal carpal row. It lies just radial to the abductor pollicis muscle and permits flexion at the MCP joint. Both heads of the FPB insert on the radial base of the proximal phalanx of the thumb and first MCP radial sesamoid. The deep head of the FPB is innervated by the deep branch of the ulnar nerve, and the remainder of the thenar muscles is innervated by the recurrent branch of the median nerve. Although the adductor

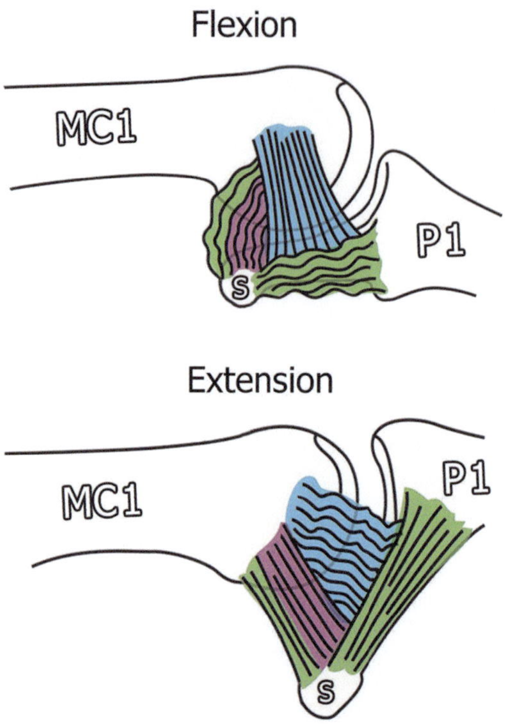

Fig. 10.18 *Ligaments of the first MCP joint*. The proper collateral ligaments (blue) traverse from the head of the first metacarpal (MC1) to the base of the first proximal phalanx (P1). The accessory collateral ligaments (purple) are more volar and extend from the metacarpal head to the volar plate and sesamoid bone (S). The metacarpal sesamoid and sesamoid phalangeal palmar ligaments are also shown in green. (Modified from Ref. [34])

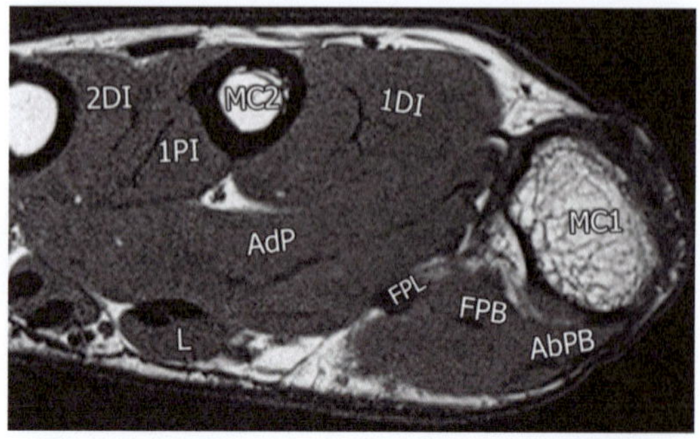

Fig. 10.19 *Thumb muscles*. Axial proton density-weighted MR image of the hand just proximal to the thumb MCP sesamoids demonstrates the thenar muscles: abductor pollicis brevis (AbPB) and flexor pollicis brevis (FPB) located palmar to the flexor pollicis longus (FPL) tendon; the opponens pollicis (not shown) inserts proximal to this level. Also shown are the adductor pollicis (AdP) muscle and central muscle group (lumbrical muscles (L), dorsal interosseous (DI), and palmar interosseous (PI)). The first (MC1) and second (MC2) metacarpal bones are indicated

pollicis (AdP) muscle does not belong to the proper thenar or the central muscle groups, it oftentimes grouped with a thenar musculature. The AdP has oblique and transverse heads that originate from the palmar aspect of the second and third metacarpal bones. AdP inserts onto the base of the first proximal phalanx, ulnar sesamoid, and adductor aponeurosis (see below) and receives innervation from the deep branch of the ulnar nerve.

The extrinsic flexor muscle group includes the FPL, AbPL, extensor pollicis brevis (EPB), and EPL muscles. The FPL muscle originates at the volar surface of the radius and the adjacent interosseous membrane. It has a long tendon that passes under the flexor retinaculum through the carpal tunnel, located dorsal and radial to the median nerve [30]. The FPL tendon passes between the thenar and AdP muscles. The distal tendon lies superficial to the volar plate between the two sesamoid bones at the MCP joint and inserts distal to the base of the distal phalanx of the thumb (Figs. 10.19 and 10.20). The FPL tendon flexes the IP joint and to a lesser degree the MCP joint. The FPL lacks a vinculum and adjacent lumbrical muscle that support the digital flexor tendons; therefore, the tendon has even less restriction and is more likely to retract if torn.

The first and third extensor tendon compartments have tendons that are important for thumb movement. In compartment one, the AbPL and EPB tendons are important for thumb abduction, extension, and rotation at the first CMC and MCP joints [30]. In the third extensor tendon compartment, the EPL tendon passes on the ulnar side of Lister's tubercle of the radius before extending distally and is responsible for extension of the interphalangeal joint.

The extensor mechanism is simpler in the thumb than in other digits [15]. The EPB tendon inserts to the dorsal base of the proximal phalanx and blends to the dorsal plate of the first MCP joint. The EPL tendon continues to the dorsal base of the distal phalanx. The EPB is variable

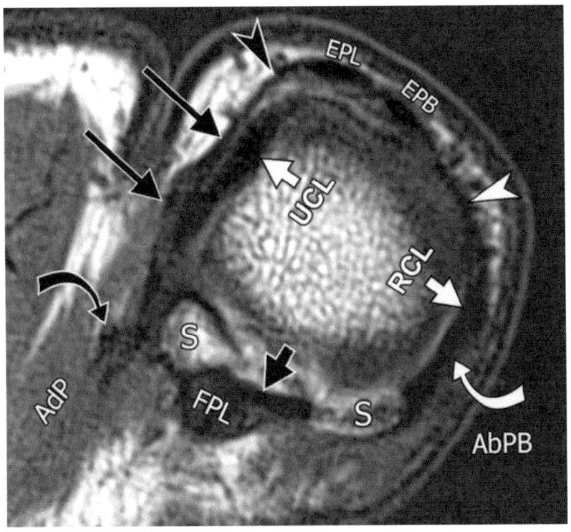

Fig. 10.20 *MRI anatomy of the first MCP joint.* Axial proton density-weighted image at the level of the first MCP joint. The adductor pollicis muscle (AdP) and its tendon (curved black arrow) attach to the ulnar sesamoid and adductor aponeurosis (long black arrows). The adductor aponeurosis overlies the UCL and is continuous with the sagittal band and extensor hood (black arrowhead) that attach to the extensor pollicis longus (EPL) tendon. The abductor pollicis brevis (AbPB) tendon is located on the radial aspect of the joint (curved white arrow). The abductor aponeurosis (white arrowhead) blends with the radial side of the sagittal band and extensor hood. The extensor pollicis brevis (EPB) tendon is located at the radial aspect of the EPL tendon and deep to the radial sagittal band and extensor hood. The AbPB tendon and RCL blend together and are difficult to separate. Volar plate (short black arrow). S sesamoids, FPL flexor pollicis longus, UCL ulnar collateral ligament, RCL radial collateral ligament

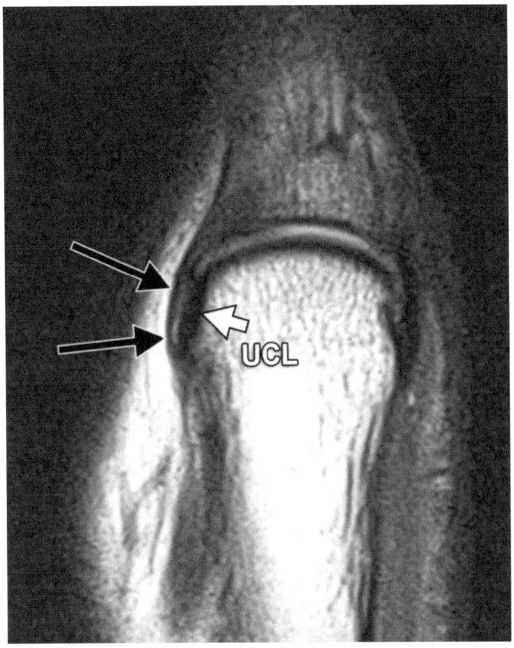

Fig. 10.21 *Ulnar collateral ligament (UCL) at the MCP joint.* Coronal PD-weighted image of the first MCP joint at the level of the proximal attachment of the UCL (white arrow). Note adductor aponeurosis (black arrows) depicted as a thin layer located superficially to the UCL

and can continue to attach to the distal phalanx along with the EPL tendon [35]. The dorsal plate does not have well-defined attachments to the metacarpal and proximal phalanx, and a synovial recess may be seen deep to the dorsal plate and EPB insertion, mimicking a dorsal plate injury [36]. The thumb extensor tendons do not branch into central and lateral slips as in the digits [30].

The extensor hood is the connective tissue that envelops the extensor tendons and consists of the sagittal band at the level of the MCP joint and the triangular expansion more distally. The sagittal band of the first MCP joint maintains the EPL tendon in the midline and is visible on MR imaging [30] (Fig. 10.20). The triangular expansion is the distal extension of the extensor hood beyond the sagittal band and envelops the EPL tendon as it extends to its insertion to the distal phalanx [30]. It is typically not visible on MR imaging. The AdP aponeurosis contributes fibers to the ulnar side of extensor hood (Fig. 10.20), whereas the AbPB and FPB tendons contribute fibers from the radial side [30]. The AdP aponeurosis overlies the UCL in a somewhat oblique plane and has an attachment to the EPL tendon (Figs. 10.20 and 10.21). The close relationship of the AdP aponeurosis and UCL predisposes to a stener lesion, where the AdP aponeurosis is interposed between a torn retracted UCL and prevents proper ligament healing. The AbPB tendon passes over the radial side of the joint to attach to the radial base of the proximal phalanx. The AbPB aponeurosis overlies the RCL and blends with radial side of the sagittal band and extensor hood (Figs. 10.17 and 10.20) [30]. The sagittal band blends with the collateral ligaments at the periphery at the MCP joint and is indirectly connected to the sesamoid bones and volar plate [30].

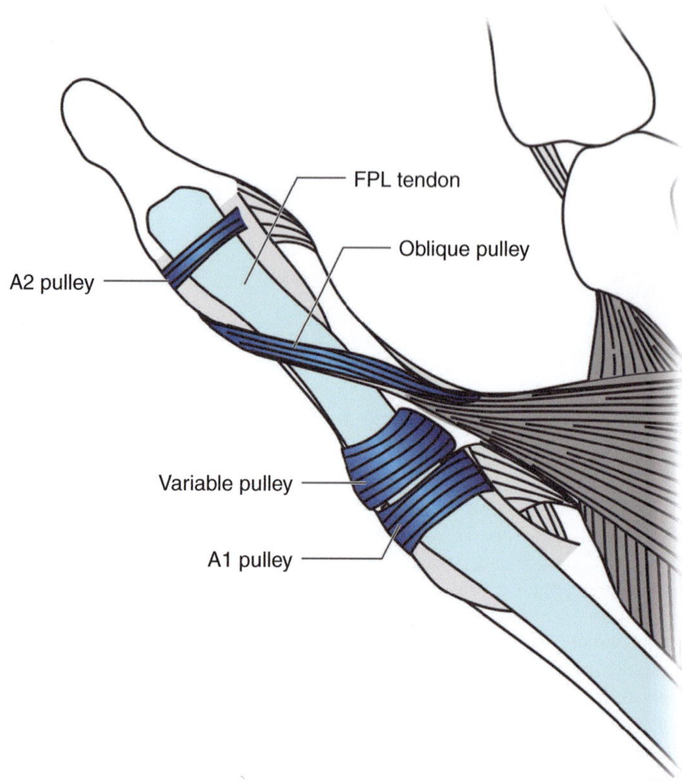

Fig. 10.22 *Pulleys of the thumb*. The A1 pulley is located at the level of the MCP, and the A2 pulley is at the level of the interphalangeal (IP) joint. The oblique pulley courses obliquely at the level of the mid-proximal phalanx and is associated proximally with the insertion of the adductor aponeurosis. The variable pulley is located between the A1 and the oblique pulley. FPL flexor pollicis longus tendon

Pulleys of the Thumb

The pulleys of the thumb function to keep the FPL tendon in close apposition to the phalanges and only consist of annular pulleys, unlike other fingers [30]. The first annular pulley (A1) is at the level of the MCP joint. It is a transverse retinacular structure that covers the MCP joint with the proximal two thirds of the volar plate [36]. It is intimately associated with the sesamoid bones [30]. It can be difficult to distinguish on MR imaging. The second annular pulley (A2) is a transverse retinacular structure at the level of the interphalangeal joint and is fused with the volar plate and the base of the distal phalanx [36] (Fig. 10.22).

The oblique annular pulley is located between the first and second annular pulleys at the level of the mid-proximal phalanx and courses obliquely from the ulnar side of the base of the proximal phalanx to the radial side of the base of the distal phalanx [36]. The proximal ulnar attachment of the oblique annular pulley is intimately associated with the attachment of the adductor aponeurosis [37]. The variable annular pulley is located between the first annular and the oblique annular pulley at the level of the proximal phalanx base. The radial limb is longer than the ulnar limb normally (Fig. 10.23) [30].

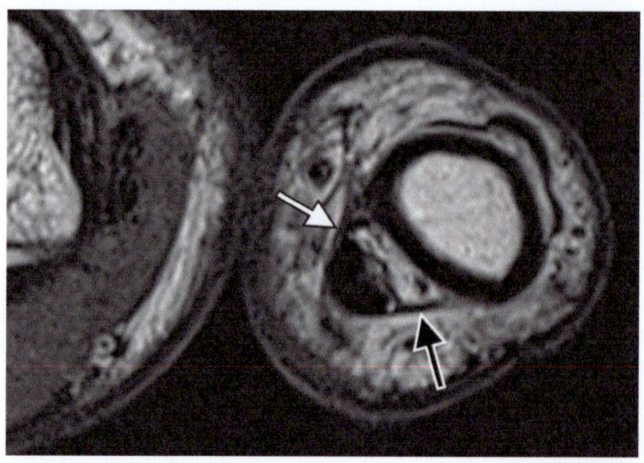

Fig. 10.23 *Normal MRI of pulley anatomy*. Variable pulley depicted on axial proton density-weighted image at the level of the first proximal phalangeal base, distal to the A1 pulley. The radial limb (black arrow) is normally longer than the ulnar limb (white arrow)

MRI Optimization

When imaging the hand, fingers, or thumb, MR imaging optimization strategies are focused on (1) proper patient and extremity positioning to ensure both patient's comfort and image quality, (2) selecting appropriate coverage with respect to the zonal anatomy to answer specific clinical questions, and (3) obtaining high-resolution images in planes prescribed to the region of interest.

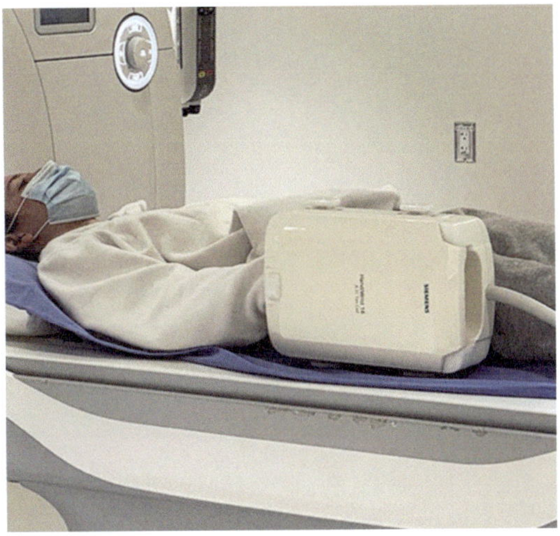

Fig. 10.24 *Optimizing patient positioning*. The arm is positioned at the side with the hand in the coil which maximizes patient comfort, reduces motion artifact, and allows for diagnostic images even though the area of interest is not centered in the magnet

For imaging of the fingers, the patient can be positioned supine or decubitus with the hand at the side of the patient (Fig. 10.24). This positioning may not always be achievable due to coil design and patient size. The image quality may also be negatively affected by field heterogeneity when the hand is located at the periphery of the bore of the MR imaging unit. A standard position of the hand in the magnet designed to place the hand close to the isocenter of the bore (the so called superman position, with the patient lying prone with the arm elevated above the head) is often poorly tolerated by patients. The discomfort can be alleviated by propping the patient's body with pillows to decrease the extension at the shoulder (Fig. 10.25). When bilateral hand MR imaging is requested, for example, for evaluation of inflammatory arthritis, both hands may be placed in the extremity coils and imaged simultaneously in the "prayer position" or "fetal-praying," allowing assessment of disease symmetry and minimizing the duration of the study (Fig. 10.26) [38, 39]. Padding and splint immobilization can increase comfort and minimize motion.

High-resolution imaging of the small structures in the fingers and thumb requires the use of a local coil. Although the coil should be as small as possible to provide a field of view (FOV) suitable for the area of interest to maximize the signal-to-noise (SNR) ratio, wrist or extremity coils can provide an extended FOV

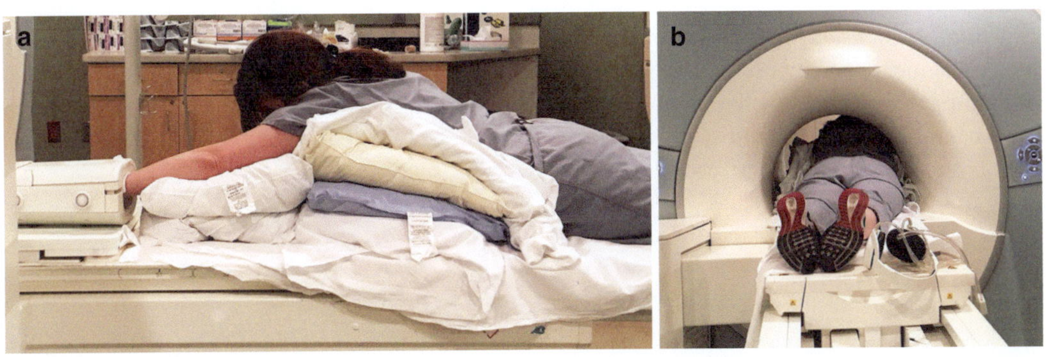

Fig. 10.25 *Optimizing patient positioning*. The so-called superman position is typically poorly tolerated by patients, in part due to hyperextension of the shoulder. The discomfort may be alleviated by propping the patient's body with pillows to decrease the angle of flexion at the shoulder joint. (Images courtesy of Dr. David A. Rubin, All Pro Orthopedic Imaging Consultants, ST Louis MO)

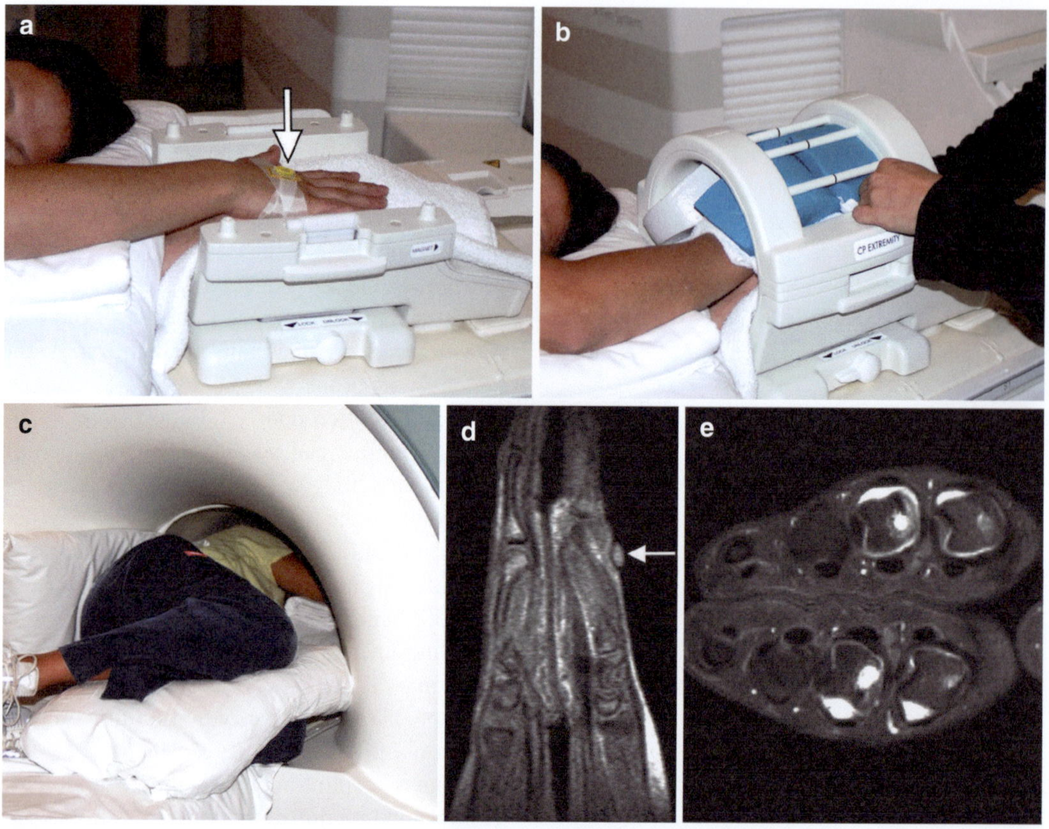

Fig. 10.26 *Optimizing patient positioning*. Decubitus positioning for simultaneous imaging of both hands and wrists. "Fetal-praying" position (**a**–**c**) with the patient lying on the side with the shoulders, elbows, hips, and knees flexed, the palms are placed in the extremity coil and positioned slightly cranial. Sufficient padding is utilized to ensure patient's comfort. Sagittal scout gradient echo recalled image (**d**) shows placement of the marker (arrow) to denote the right side. Axial T1-weighted contrast-enhanced fat-suppressed image of a patient with rheumatoid arthritis (**e**) allows simultaneous assessment of both hands with a single injection. (Images courtesy of Dr. David A. Rubin, All Pro Orthopedic Imaging Consultants, ST Louis MO)

which may be necessary to image the proximal extent of tendons, synovial sheath anatomy, tumor staging, or arthritis screening [40]. When evaluating flexor tendon injuries in particular, the imaging protocol should address both the site of the injury and the potential for significant retraction of the proximal tendon stump. Dependent on the degree of retraction, either extending or moving the FOV proximally may be necessary (Fig. 10.27).

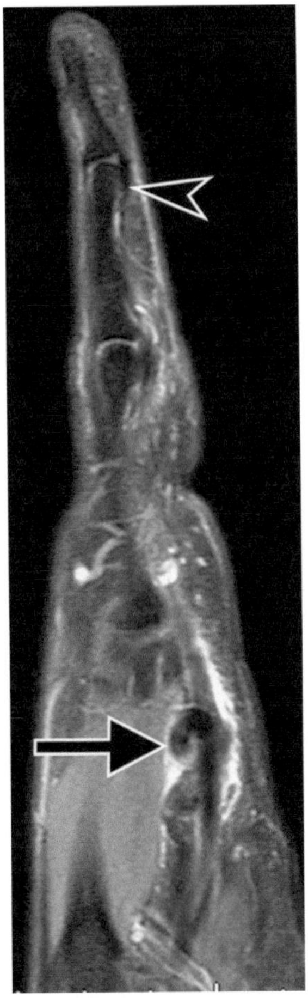

Fig. 10.27 *Optimizing coverage.* Sagittal proton density-weighted fat-suppressed image of the ring finger in a 46-year-old female with a tender mass at the palm of the hand and loss of fourth DIP flexion demonstrates full-thickness rupture of the fourth FDP (arrowhead) distally to Zone II with proximal tendon stump (arrow) retracted to Zone III

For dedicated imaging of the fingers and thumb, the FOV and slice thickness should be minimized in order to maximize spatial resolution with acceptable SNR. The FOV typically ranges from 6 to 12 centimeters, and slice thickness should be 2–3 millimeters in the sagittal and coronal planes and 3–4 mm in axial planes. The in-plane resolution should be less than 0.5 mm pixel size (FOV divided by the matrix size) [16, 40]. Higher resolution may be achieved with 3T MR imaging units and specially designed local coils. Increasing matrix size to achieve high resolution typically results in increased scanning time that can lead to patient discomfort and motion artifact. Parallel imaging and increase interslice gap may be used to mitigate this and decrease scanning time. Three-dimensional gradient echo sequences produce images of high SNR and spatial resolution and allow creating reformations in multiple planes.

The imaging planes must be prescribed with respect to a finger or a thumb rather than the hand or wrist. For internal comparison, the adjacent finger should be included in the FOV. In dedicated MR imaging of the thumb, the hand should be positioned so that the thumb is aligned parallel to the main magnetic field in a slightly abducted position. An axial image through the head of the first metacarpal and collateral ligaments may be used to prescribe true sagittal and coronal planes of the thumb (Fig. 10.28).

In order to minimize magic angle artifact, the fingers should be extended and aligned with their long axis parallel to the main magnetic field. The exception to this is imaging of an annular pulley injury, where the finger of interest can be imaged at 35–40 degrees of flexion to depict bowstringing of the tendon and provide a useful secondary sign of pulley injury [41, 42].

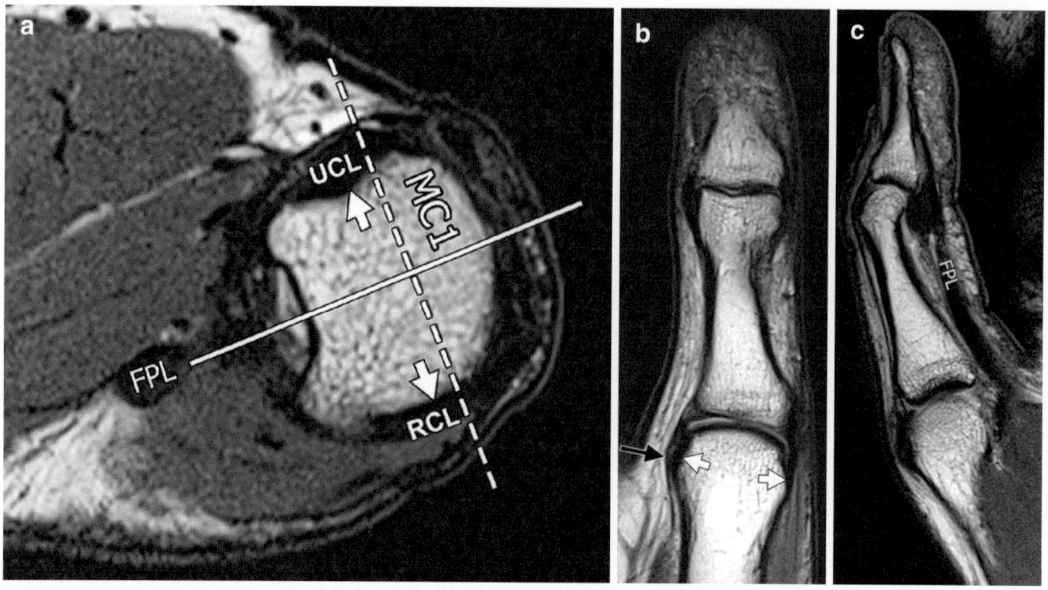

Fig. 10.28 *Optimizing imaging planes of the thumb.* Coronal and sagittal imaging planes are planned orthogonally on the axial image (**a**) at the level of the metacarpal (MC1) head. The coronal sections (dashed lines) should traverse parallel to the plane between the UCL and RCL (white arrows), producing a true coronal image at the MCP joint (**b**) depicting relationship between the UCL and adductor aponeurosis (black arrow, **b**). The sagittal images should be prescribed perpendicular to this plane and extend through the flexor pollicis longus tendon (FPL) producing a sagittal image (**c**) demonstrating the FPL tendon

References

1. Theumann NH, Pfirrmann CWA, Drapé JL, Trudell DJ, Resnick D. MR imaging of the metacarpophalangeal joints of the fingers. Part I. Conventional MR imaging and MR arthrographic findings in cadavers. Radiology. 2002;222(2):437–45. https://doi.org/10.1148/radiol.2222010181.
2. Chung CB, Steinbach LS. MRI of the upper extremity: shoulder, elbow, wrist and hand. Philadelphia: Wolters Kluwer Health/Lippincott Williams & Wilkins; 2010.
3. Clavero JA, Alomar X, Monill JM, et al. MR imaging of ligament and tendon injuries of the fingers. Radiographics. 2002;22:237–56.
4. El-Shennawy M, Nakamura K, Patterson RM, Viegas SF. Three-dimensional kinematic analysis of the second through fifth carpometacarpal joints. J Hand Surg Am. 2001;26(6):1030–5. https://doi.org/10.1053/jhsu.2001.28761.
5. De Maeseneer M, Van Roy P, Jacobson JA, Jamadar DA. Normal MR imaging findings of the midhand and fingers with anatomic correlation. Eur J Radiol. 2005;56(3):278–85. https://doi.org/10.1016/j.ejrad.2005.05.020.
6. Benjamin M, Kaiser E, Milz S. Structure-function relationships in tendons: a review. J Anat. 2008;212(3):211–28. https://doi.org/10.1111/j.1469-7580.2008.00864.x.
7. Garcia-Elias M, An KN, Berglund L, Linscheid RL, Cooney WP, Chao EYS. Extensor mechanism of the fingers. I. A quantitative geometric study. J Hand Surg Am. 1991;16(6):1130–6. https://doi.org/10.1016/S0363-5023(10)80079-6.
8. Alomar X, Monill JM, Esplugas M. Extensor mechanism of the fingers: MR imaging–anatomic correlation. Radiographics. 2003;23:593–611.
9. Petchprapa CN, Vaswani D. MRI of the fingers: an update. Am J Roentgenol. 2019;213(3):534–48. https://doi.org/10.2214/AJR.19.21217.
10. Von Schroeder HP, Botte MJ. Anatomy and functional significance of the long extensors to the fingers and thumb. Clin Orthop Relat Res. 2001;383:74–83. https://doi.org/10.1097/00003086-200102000-00010.
11. Kichouh M, Vanhoenacker F, Jager T, et al. Functional anatomy of the dorsal hood or the hand: correlation of ultrasound and MR findings with cadaveric dissection. Eur Radiol. 2009;19(8):1849–56. https://doi.org/10.1007/s00330-009-1383-9.
12. Jones FW. The principles of anatomy as seen in the hand. England J A Churchill, 1920;1920:222–33.
13. Lin GT, Amadio PC, An KN, Cooney WP. Functional anatomy of the human digital flexor pulley system. J Hand Surg Am. 1989;14(6):949–56. https://doi.org/10.1016/S0363-5023(89)80043-7.

14. Doyle JR. Anatomy of the finger flexor tendon sheath and pulley system. J Hand Surg Am. 1988;13(4):473–84. https://doi.org/10.1016/S0363-5023(88)80082-0.
15. Hauger O, Chung CB, Lektrakul N, et al. Pulley system in the fingers: normal anatomy and simulated lesions in cadavers at MR imaging, CT, and US with and without contrast material distention of the tendon sheath. Radiology. 2000;217(1):201–12. https://doi.org/10.1148/radiology.217.1.r00oc40201.
16. Gupta P, Lenchik L, Wuertzer SD, Pacholke DA. High-resolution 3-T MRI of the fingers: review of anatomy and common tendon and ligament injuries. Am J Roentgenol. 2015;204(3):W314–23. https://doi.org/10.2214/AJR.14.12776.
17. Scheldrup EW. Tendon sheath patterns in the hand; an anatomical study based on 367 hand dissections. Surg Gynecol Obstet. 1951;93(1):16–22.
18. Fussey JM, Chin KF, Gogi N, Gella S, Deshmukh SC. An anatomic study of flexor tendon sheaths: a cadaveric study. J Hand Surg Eur Vol. 2009;34(6):762–5. https://doi.org/10.1177/1753193409344529.
19. Gellman H, Botte MJ, Shankwiler J, Gelberman RH. Arterial patterns of the deep and superficial palmar arches. Clin Orthop Relat Res. 2001;383:41–6. https://doi.org/10.1097/00003086-200102000-00007.
20. Mitchell CH, Fayad LM, Ahlawat S. Magnetic resonance imaging of the digital nerves of the hand: anatomy and spectrum of pathology. Curr Probl Diagn Radiol. 2018;47(1):42–50. https://doi.org/10.1067/j.cpradiol.2017.02.009.
21. Ochiai N, Matsui T, Miyaji N, Merklin RJ, Hunter JM. Vascular anatomy of flexor tendons. I. Vincular system and blood supply of the profundus tendon in the digital sheath. J Hand Surg Am. 1979;4(4):321–30. https://doi.org/10.1016/S0363-5023(79)80068-4.
22. Tagliafico A, Cadoni A, Fisci E, et al. Nerves of the hand beyond the carpal tunnel. Semin Musculoskelet Radiol. 2012;16:129–36. https://doi.org/10.1055/s-0032-1311764.
23. Rhodes NG, Murthy NS, Lehman JS, Rubin DA. Pacinian corpuscles: an explanation for subcutaneous palmar nodules routinely encountered on MR examinations. Skeletal Radiol. 2018;47(11):1553–8. https://doi.org/10.1007/s00256-018-2934-4.
24. Rhodes NG, Murthy NS, Lachman N, Rubin DA. Normal Pacinian corpuscles in the hand: radiology–pathology correlation in a cadaver study. Skeletal Radiol. 2019;48(10):1591–7. https://doi.org/10.1007/s00256-019-03223-y.
25. Kleinert HE. Report of the committee on tendon injuries. J Hand Surg Am. 1989;14(2 Pt 2):3816. https://doi.org/10.1016/0363-5023(89)90118-4.
26. Melville DM, Taljanovic MS, Scalcione LR, et al. Imaging and management of thumb carpometacarpal joint osteoarthritis. Skeletal Radiol. 2015;44(2):165–77. https://doi.org/10.1007/s00256-014-1997-0.
27. Edmunds JO. Current concepts of the anatomy of the thumb trapeziometacarpal joint. J Hand Surg Am. 2011;36(1):170–82. https://doi.org/10.1016/j.jhsa.2010.10.029.
28. Ladd AL, Weiss APC, Crisco JJ, et al. The thumb carpometacarpal joint: anatomy, hormones, and biomechanics. Instr Course Lect. 2013;62:165–79.
29. Chiavaras MM, Harish S, Oomen G, Popowich T, Wainman B, Bain JR. Sonography of the anterior oblique ligament of the trapeziometacarpal joint: a study of cadavers and asymptomatic volunteers. Am J Roentgenol. 2010;195(6):428–34. https://doi.org/10.2214/AJR.10.4403.
30. Rawat U, Pierce JL, Evans S, Chhabra AB, Nacey NC. High-resolution MR imaging and US anatomy of the thumb. Radiographics. 2016;36(6):1701–16. https://doi.org/10.1148/rg.2016160015.
31. Kerr RM. The thumb carpometacarpal joint. Radsource MRI Web Clinic — July 2016. https://radsource.us/thumb-carpometacarpal-joint/. Published 2020. Accessed 28 Nov 2020.
32. Cardoso FN, Kim HJ, Albertotti F, Botte MJ, Resnick D, Chung CB. Imaging the ligaments of the trapeziometacarpal joint: MRI compared with MR arthrography in cadaveric specimens. Am J Roentgenol. 2009;192(1):13–9. https://doi.org/10.2214/AJR.07.4010.
33. Amar E, Rozenblat Y, Chechik O. Sesamoid and accessory bones of the hand-An epidemiologic survey in a Mediterranean population. Clin Anat. 2011;24(2):183–7. https://doi.org/10.1002/ca.21077.
34. Stener B. Displacement of the ruptured ulnar collateral ligament of the metacarpo-phalangeal joint of the thumb. J Bone Joint Surg Br. 1962;44-B(4):869–79. https://doi.org/10.1302/0301-620x.44b4.869.
35. Shigematsu S, Shimizu H, Beppu M, Hirata K. Anatomy of the extensor pollicis brevis associated with an extension mechanism of the thumb metacarpophalangeal joint. Hand Surg. 2014;19(2):171–9. https://doi.org/10.1142/S0218810414500166.
36. Hirschmann A, Sutter R, Schweizer A, Pfirrmann CWA. MRI of the thumb: anatomy and spectrum of findings in asymptomatic volunteers. Am J Roentgenol. 2014;202(4):819–27. https://doi.org/10.2214/AJR.13.11397.
37. Bayat A, Shaaban H, Giakas G, Lees VC. The pulley system of the thumb: anatomic and biomechanical study. J Hand Surg Am. 2002;27(4):628–35. https://doi.org/10.1053/jhsu.2002.34008.
38. Meier R, Thuermel K, Noël PB, et al. Synovitis in patients with early inflammatory arthritis monitored with quantitative analysis of dynamic contrast-enhanced optical imaging and MR imaging. Radiology. 2014;270(1):176–85. https://doi.org/10.1148/radiol.13130039.
39. Rubin DA. MRI and ultrasound of the hands and wrists in rheumatoid arthritis. I. Imaging findings. Skeletal Radiol. 2019;48(5):677–95. https://doi.org/10.1007/S00256-019-03179-Z.

40. American College of Radiology. ACR–SPR–SSR practice parameter for the performance and interpretation of magnetic resonance imaging (MRI) of the fingers and toes.
41. Parellada JA, Balkissoon AR, Hayes C, Conway WF. Bowstring injury of the flexor tendon pulley system: MR imaging. Am J Roentgenol. 1996;167(2):347–9. https://doi.org/10.2214/ajr.167.2.8686601.
42. Gabl M, Rangger C, Lutz M, Fink C, Rudisch A, Pechlaner S. Disruption of the finger flexor pulley system in elite rock climbers. Am J Sports Med. 1998;26(5):651–5. https://doi.org/10.1177/03635465980260050901.

11 Hand Pathology: Traumatic

Erin F. Alaia

Osseous Trauma

Metacarpal Fractures

Metacarpal fractures comprise approximately one-fifth of all hand fractures [1]. Metacarpal head fractures are considered rare injuries and, when encountered, are most commonly intra-articular and involve the second metacarpal head, due to the exposed border location and relative lack of second carpometacarpal joint mobility [2, 3]. Fractures with large articular surface defects are commonly treated surgically to restore congruence of the articular surface [3]. Metacarpal head fractures may be complicated by avascular necrosis [4].

Fractures of the metacarpal neck are commonly referred to as Boxer's fractures, observed when the metacarpophalangeal joint is clenched and strikes a solid object (i.e., a wall), most commonly observed at the fifth metacarpal neck [2]. Fractures of the metacarpal shaft may be transverse or oblique, with obliquely oriented fractures frequently commonly resulting in rotational deformity and shortening when displaced [1]. Surgical management may be considered for significant angular deformity, irreducibility, open fractures, and rotational malalignment [5].

Metacarpal base fractures should be closely examined for intra-articular involvement. The most common intra-articular fracture is seen at the base of the fifth metacarpal, mechanistically similar to fracture of the first metacarpal base, and occasionally referred to as "reverse Bennett" or "baby Bennett" fracture (Fig. 11.1). Optimal management of the "reverse Bennett" fracture is debated, although most recommend surgical management of displaced fractures to prevent premature osteoarthritis, weaker grip, and limitations in range of motion [4].

MRI is uncommonly indicated for the diagnosis of isolated metacarpal fracture but may be ordered to evaluate for radiographically occult fracture and intra-articular extension and to evaluate for injury of supporting structures or the regional soft tissues. T1-weighted images will display the fracture as discrete linear low T1 signal, with regional marrow edema on fluid-sensitive images (Fig. 11.2). Contusion will appear as marrow edema, but without a discrete fracture line.

E. F. Alaia (✉)
Department of Radiology, Musculoskeletal Division, NYU Langone Health/NYU Langone Orthopedic Hospital, New York, NY, USA
e-mail: Erin.Fitzgerald@nyulangone.org

B. U. Casagranda (ed.), *MRI of the Upper Extremity*, https://doi.org/10.1007/978-3-030-81612-4_11

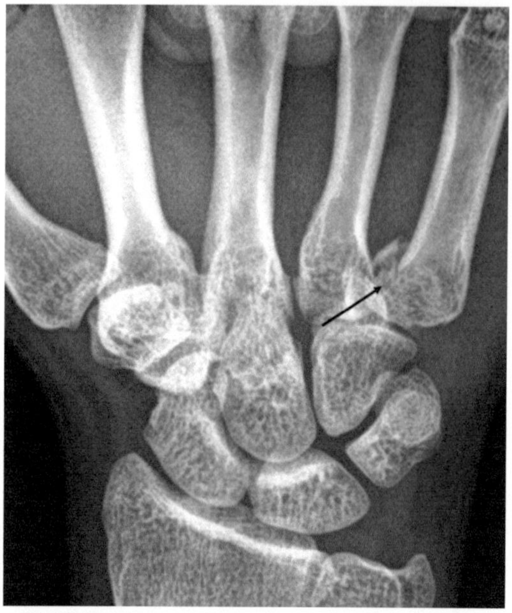

Fig. 11.1 *Reverse Bennett fracture in a 24-year-old female*. Frontal wrist radiograph demonstrates an obliquely oriented, mildly displaced intra-articular fracture along the radial base of the fifth metacarpal (arrow), also known as a reverse Bennett fracture

Phalangeal Fractures

Phalangeal fractures occur more commonly than fractures of the metacarpals. Over half of all phalangeal fractures involve the distal phalanx, followed by the proximal phalanx, and least commonly the middle phalanx. Fractures may involve the shaft, head, or base and should be classified as intra-articular or extra-articular. Avulsion fractures may occur at the flexor or extensor tendon, collateral ligament (Fig. 11.3), or capsular attachments. Pathologic fractures of the phalanges are rare and most commonly are seen in patients with enchondroma [1] (Fig. 11.4).

Distal phalanx fractures may include fracture of the tuft, shaft, or articular surface and inserting structures [6]. Distal phalanx tuft fractures may be accompanied by a subungual hematoma or injury to the nail plate [2]. Although tuft fractures may fail to achieve bony union, even months after the injury, they may instead achieve a stable fibrous union [6]. Fractures of the distal phalanx shaft may be transverse or longitudinal in

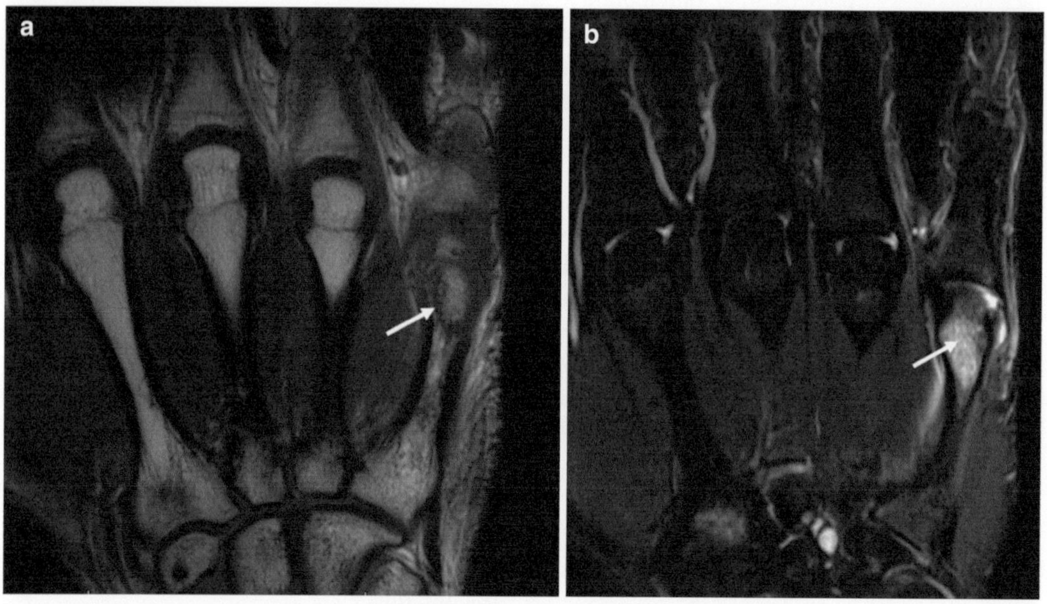

Fig. 11.2 *Fifth metacarpal fracture in a 22-year-old male*. Coronal T1 image (**a**) shows a nondisplaced hairline fracture (arrow) of the fifth metacarpal neck, with the coronal T2 fat-suppressed image (**b**) showing regional marrow edema (arrow)

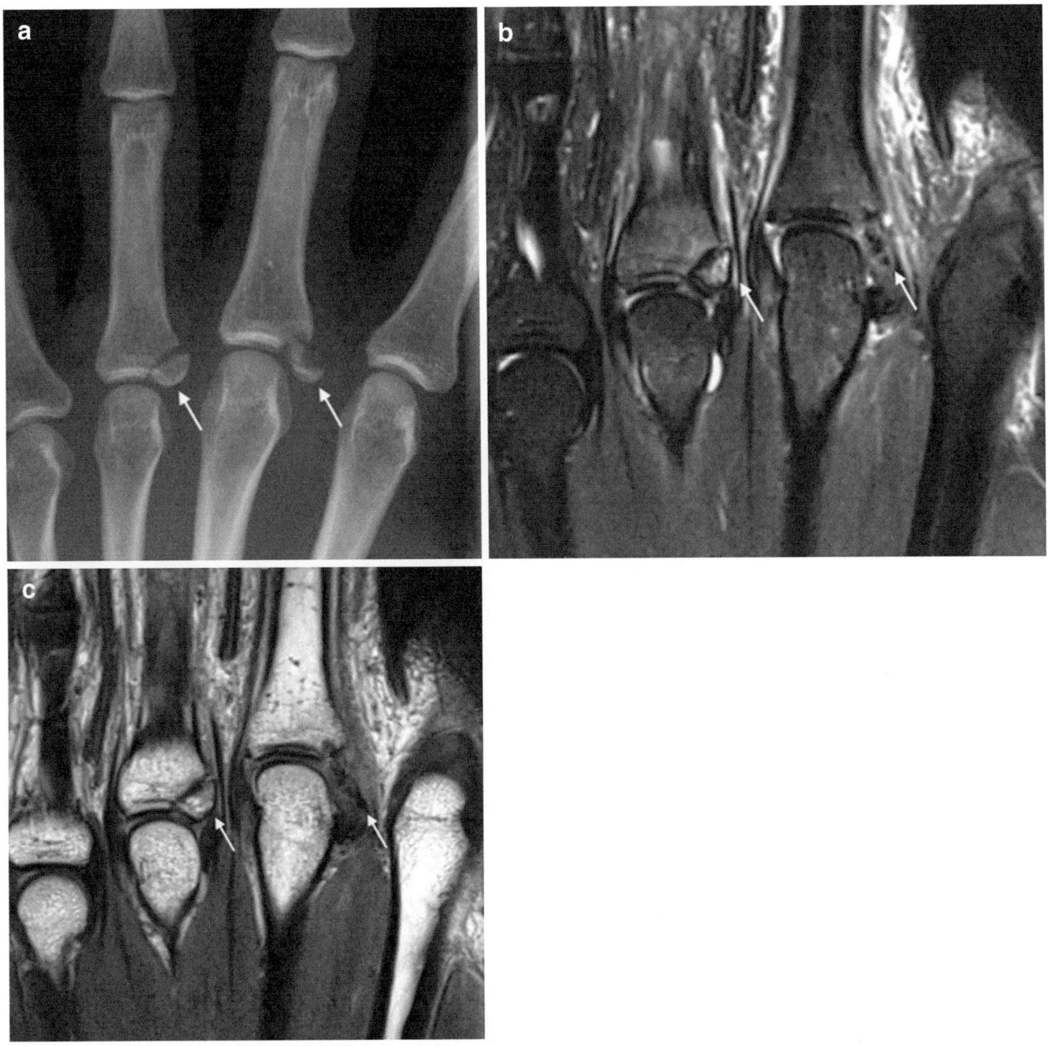

Fig. 11.3 *Displaced radial collateral ligament avulsion fractures in a 36-year-old female*. Frontal hand radiograph (**a**) demonstrates displaced avulsion fractures along the radial base of the third and fourth proximal phalanges (arrows), with rotation of the third phalangeal base fracture. Coronal T2 fat-suppressed (**b**) and proton density (**c**) images confirm bony avulsion of the third and fourth metacarpophalangeal radial collateral ligaments (arrows)

orientation. Nondisplaced shaft fractures, stabilized by the regional soft tissues, may heal with conservative measures alone, while displaced fractures may require percutaneous pinning [2].

Articular fractures of the distal phalanx, unlike fractures of the shaft and tuft, are more likely to occur due to closed injury. Articular fractures include fractures of the palmar base, the dorsal base, and, in the pediatric population, epiphyseal separation injuries. Palmar and dorsal base articular fractures will be discussed in detail under injury to the flexor and extensor tendons, respectively. Epiphyseal separation injuries include the pediatric Seymour fracture. Seymour fractures

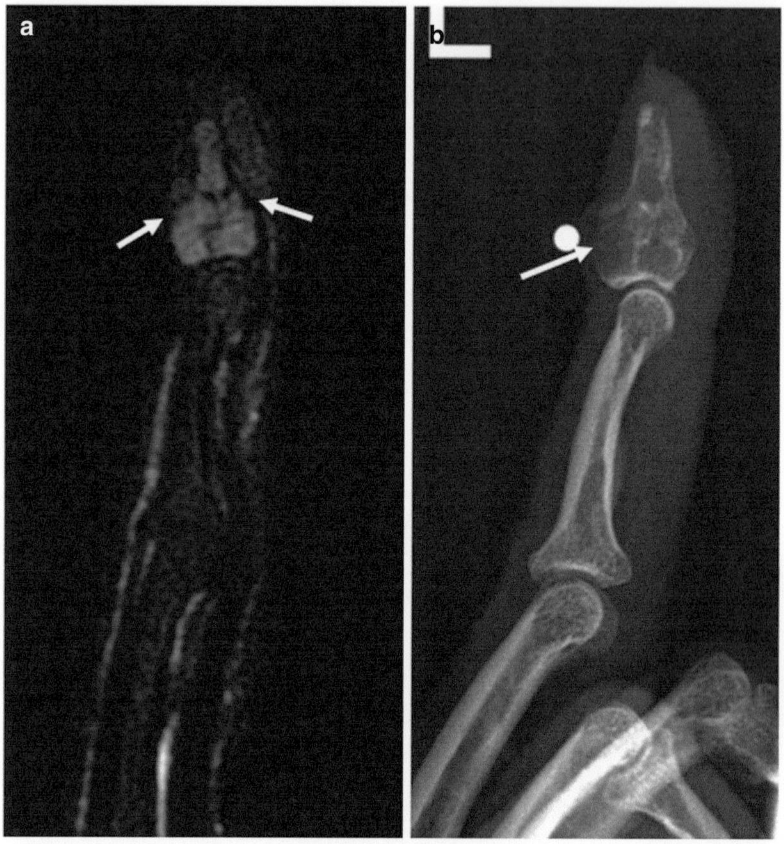

Fig. 11.4 *Pathologic fracture of a distal phalanx enchondroma in a 58-year-old female.* Sagittal T2 fat-suppressed MRI of the index finger (**a**) demonstrates near complete replacement of the distal phalanx by an expansile, lobular T2-hyperintense lesion with central mineralization, characteristic of an enchondroma (arrows). Dedicated lateral finger radiograph (**b**) better depicts a pathologic fracture along the dorsal base, with breakthrough of the cortex (arrow)

are displaced fractures of the distal phalanx which traverse the physis and have an associated nail bed laceration. Clinically, the distal phalanx may be dorsally angulated and may mimic a mallet finger injury, with the base of the nail lying superficial to the nail fold [7]. MRI may be indicated in Seymour fractures to evaluate for interposition of the nail germinal matrix between fracture fragments (Fig. 11.5). Failure to recognize and treat the Seymour fracture may result in physeal arrest, deformity of the nail plate, or chronic osteomyelitis [8].

The less common middle and proximal phalangeal fractures can be classified as articular or nonarticular. Nonarticular fractures include fractures of the neck, shaft, or phalanx base (Fig. 11.6). Articular fractures include condylar fractures (unicondylar or bicondylar) (Fig. 11.7), comminuted fractures, base fractures (involving the dorsal or volar lip or the lateral base), fracture dislocations, and finally intra-articular shaft fractures [2]. Open reduction and internal fixation may be indicated for significant displacement, instability, and malrotation or to restore congruency of the articular surface [2, 9]. Displaced unicondylar or bicondylar intra-articular fractures are considered unstable due to articular surface involvement and potential rotational instability and are usually indicated for surgery [5, 9].

MRI may be indicated for avulsion fractures at the collateral ligament (lateral base), volar plate (volar base lip), or extensor tendon central slip attachment (dorsal middle phalanx base). MRI will confirm involvement of the

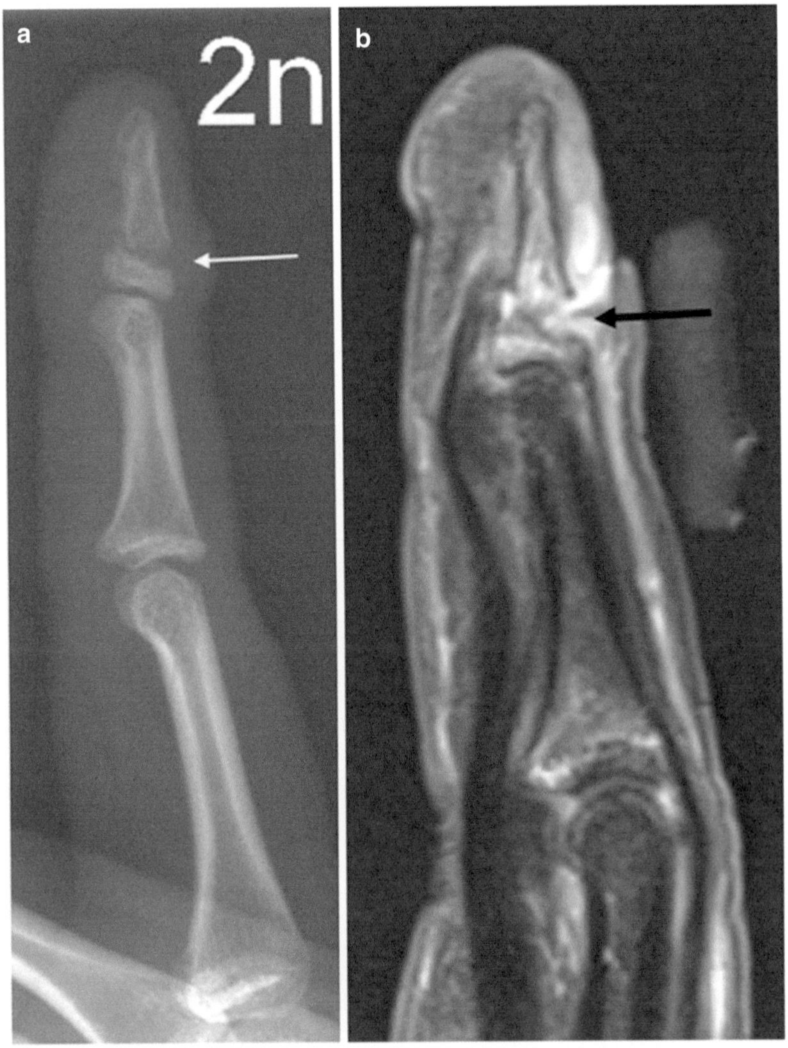

Fig. 11.5 *Fracture of the distal phalanx with interposed germinal matrix in a 13-year-old female*. Radiograph of the second digit (**a**) shows a fracture along the proximal metaphysis of the distal phalanx, with widening of the fracture gap along the dorsal margin (arrow). Sagittal T1 fat-suppressed post-contrast MRI (**b**) demonstrates enhancing soft tissue (arrow), confirmed at surgery to represent displaced germinal matrix, interposed along the dorsal fracture margin

capsuloligamentous or tendon attachment and the extent of soft tissue injury and will demonstrate any potential intra-articular displacement of the capsuloligamentous structures.

Ligamentous Pathology and Dislocations

Metacarpophalangeal and interphalangeal dislocations may be subcategorized as volar, dorsal, or lateral in direction and as simple or complex injuries. Dislocations are defined as simple when the joint is reduced by closed manipulation and complex when interposed soft tissue (i.e., collateral ligament, volar plate, joint capsule) prevents complete closed reduction. Subcategories are defined on the direction of the distal bone in relation to the proximal bone at the level of dislocation. Most dislocations are dorsal in direction. Lateral dislocations, or more commonly lateral subluxations, occur secondary to a rotatory mechanism and involve tears of one collateral ligament and at least partial tears of the volar

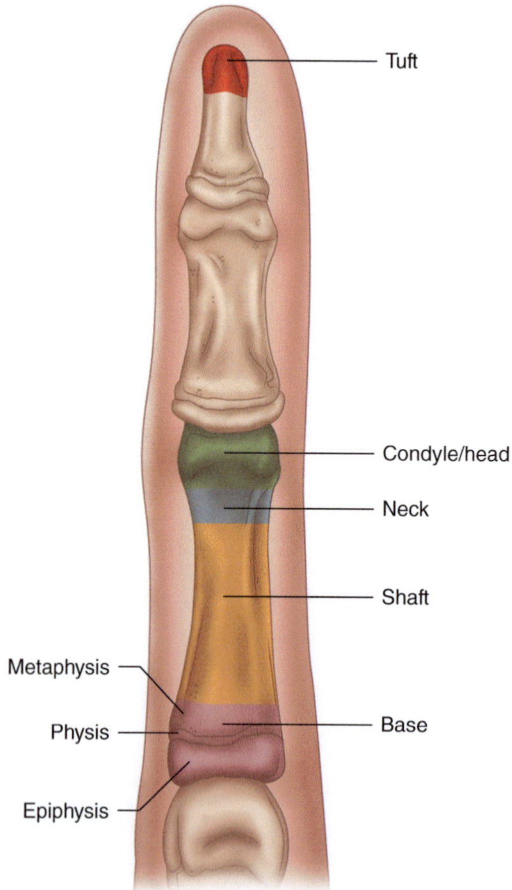

Fig. 11.6 *Phalanx anatomy.* Nonarticular fractures do not extend into the joint space and can involve the tuft (red) and neck (blue) of the phalanx. Articular fractures do extend into the joint space and can involve the condyles or head (green) of the phalanx. Base (pink) and shaft (orange) fractures may be articular or nonarticular depending on direction of force and extent of fracture line. In a skeletally immature patient, the base is comprised of the epiphysis, physis (growth plate), and metaphysis as annotated

plate. The rare volar dislocation is frequently irreducible due to soft tissue entrapment. The highly stable anatomic configuration of the finger interphalangeal joint resists dislocation, which will occur only if the structure is disrupted in at least two planes [2]. Most interphalangeal joint dislocations are dorsal and the result of hyperextension injury. Most interphalangeal dislocations are associated with a volar plate tear. If the volar plate tear has an associated fracture fragment, this may be the only imaging clue to severity of the injury if the joint is reduced at the time of radiographic imaging [1].

Most commonly, the collateral ligaments tear proximally, while the volar plate avulses distally at the phalanx base attachment [2]. Distal interphalangeal joint dislocations are less common than those of the proximal interphalangeal joint due to a shorter-level arm provided by the distal phalanx and stabilizing effects of the inserting flexor and extensor tendons [2].

Pilon injuries are occasionally seen and are the result of an axial load injury to the digit, typically fracturing the middle phalanx base, with involvement of both the volar and dorsal lip and with comminution and depression of the central articular surface [10] (Fig. 11.8).

Stability of interphalangeal fracture-dislocation injuries is evaluated by whether or not a well-aligned reduction is achieved [10]. The extent to which the fracture involves the articular surface is useful in predicting stability. Fractures involving less than 30% of the articular surface are typically stable, while those with more than 50% articular surface involvement are typically unstable, with stability harder to predict when 30–50% of the articular surface is involved [10]. Dedicated small field-of-view MRI of the injured finger can evaluate for incomplete reduction on sagittal images, which will appear as the "V" sign or a crescent-shaped gap along the dorsal or volar margin, indicative of instability [2, 11] (Fig. 11.9). MRI may also reveal intrasubstance or avulsive tears of the collateral ligaments, tears of the volar plate, contusion of the volar base of the middle phalanx and dorsal head of the proximal phalanx in dorsal dislocation, or contusion of one of the proximal phalanx head condyles if there is a rotatory component to the mechanism of injury [5] (Fig. 11.10).

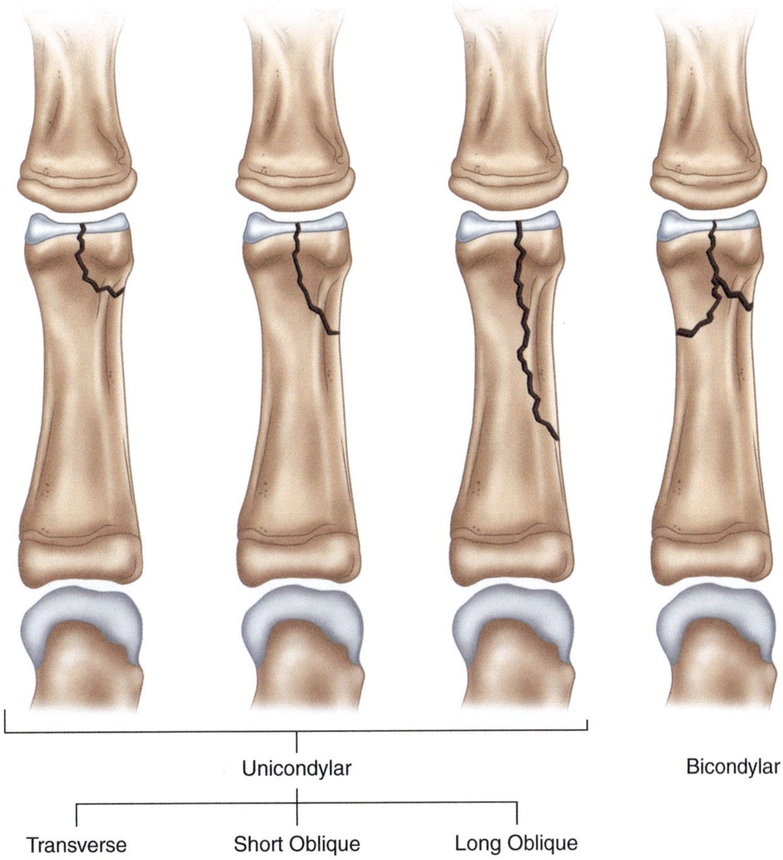

Fig. 11.7 *Condylar fracture types.* Unicondylar fractures involve one condyle of the phalanx head and are described as transverse, short oblique, or long oblique depending on fracture length and orientation. Bicondylar fractures involve both condyles of the phalanx head

Metacarpophalangeal joint dislocations occur less commonly than those of the interphalangeal joint and typically occur after fall on an outstretched hand, producing hyperextension and dorsal dislocation, most often involving the index finger. The hyperextension injury mechanism leading to dorsal dislocation causes avulsion of the volar plate from the metacarpal neck attachment, producing a simple injury when soft tissue is not interposed within the joint and closed reduction can be achieved and a complex injury when soft tissue (most often the volar plate) is interposed within the joint and closed reduction is not achieved. Occasionally, a rotational injury mechanism may lead to injury of the collateral ligaments [12].

MRI will evaluate the integrity of the volar plate and any displacement of the structure producing interposition within the metacarpophalangeal joint. Collateral ligaments should also be closely examined for sprain or tear, as well as occasional articular interposition, with isolated collateral ligament tears producing lateral deviation (Fig. 11.11).

Carpometacarpal dislocations of the second through fifth digits are uncommon. Of the carpometacarpal articulations, the fifth carpometacarpal joint is the most commonly injured, and in

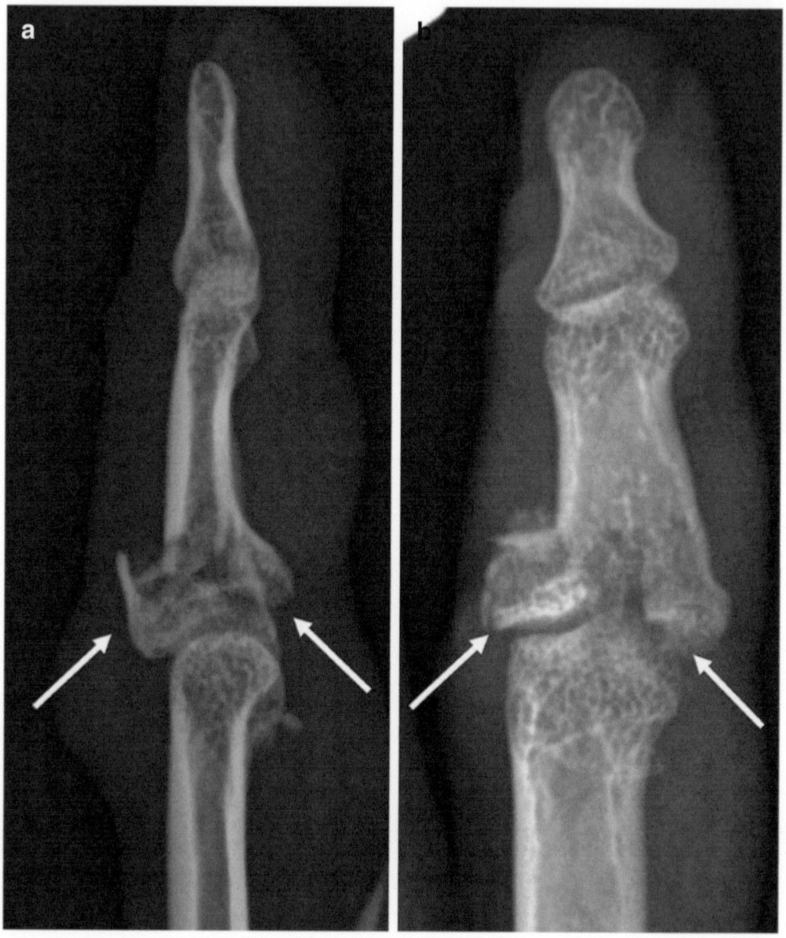

Fig. 11.8 *Pilon injury in a 21-year-old male.* Lateral (**a**) and oblique (**b**) radiographs show a pilon fracture of the middle phalanx base of the third digit (arrows) resulting from an axial load injury, with marked impaction and displacement of fracture fragments and offset along the articular surface

80% of injuries, fifth carpometacarpal joint dislocation occurs in combination with injury to another metacarpal [1]. Due to the extent and strength of regional supporting ligaments at the carpometacarpal joints, fracture dislocation and not pure dislocation injuries are more commonly observed [13]. Carpometacarpal dislocations are occasionally subtle and should be carefully scrutinized in patients with fractures of the metacarpal bases, as well as the dorsal and distal surfaces of the carpal bones, particularly the dorsal hamate. Dorsal hamate fractures associated with fifth carpometacarpal dislocations may demonstrate a range of appearances, ranging from simple dorsal avulsion fracture (Fig. 11.12), a comminuted dorsal compression fracture, or a split fracture in the coronal plane [1].

Soft Tissue Pathology

Extensor Tendon Injury

Finger extensor tendons are prone to injury due to the superficial location and thin, flat structure. Injuries are classified as either acute or chronic and open (i.e., laceration) or closed. Tears of the extensor tendons rarely demonstrate an appreciable gap, owing this to the complex intercommunicating extensor tendon network. Extensor tendons are reinforced at multiple levels and are extra-synovial in location, with the tendons covered by a paratenon instead of a discrete tendon sheath at the finger level. Thus, any retraction of a torn extensor tendon at the level of the finger is more likely due to disproportionate or unopposed

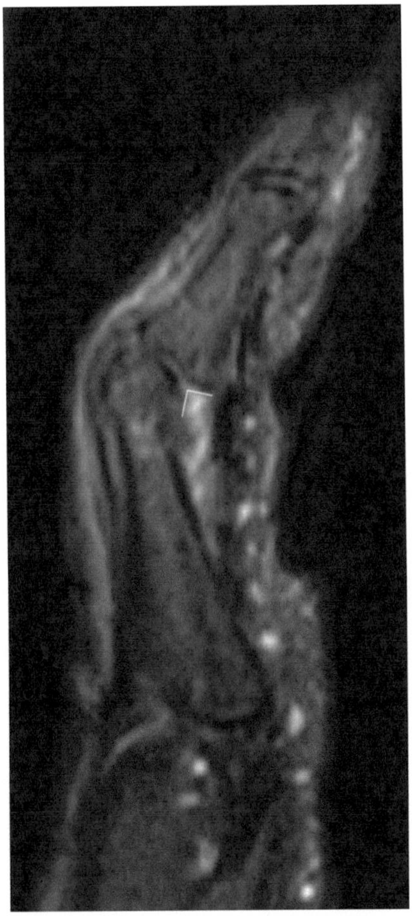

Fig. 11.9 *Volar subluxation producing the "V-sign" in a 75-year-old female*. Sagittal T2 fat-suppressed image demonstrates volar subluxation of the middle phalanx, producing abnormal V-shaped gapping along the volar joint, indicative of instability

flexor tendon pull [13]. Injuries to the complex extensor apparatus are best categorized by zone of injury. Chapter 10, Hand Anatomy, provides a detailed discussion of normal anatomic zones of the extensor tendons.

Zone 1

A classic injury to the finger extensor mechanism is the mallet finger injury, a zone 1 (distal interphalangeal joint) soft tissue or bony avulsion of the terminal extensor tendon [2] (Fig. 11.13). The injury pattern occurs when the actively extended distal interphalangeal joint is forced into sudden flexion [6]. The term mallet finger was employed due to the lateral view appearance of the injury, likened to a mallet, but due to the observation of this injury pattern in baseball players, the term baseball finger has also been used [1]. In approximately 5% of injuries, a swan-neck deformity will appear, with flexion of the distal interphalangeal joint and hyperextension of the proximal interphalangeal joint [1]. The secondary swan-neck deformity typically develops in patients with traumatic or congenital laxity of the proximal interphalangeal joint volar plate, with the central slip overcompensating at the proximal interphalangeal joint [2].

Doyle classified mallet finger injury pattern into four subtypes: closed injury with or without dorsal bony avulsion (type 1, most common), open injury with laceration (type 2), open injury with loss of tendon and soft tissue substance (type 3), and avulsion fractures (type 4) which are further subclassified into pediatric transepiphyseal plate fractures (type 4A), hyperflexion injury with fractures involving 20–50% of the articular surface (type 4B), and finally hyperextension injury, with fractures involving greater than 50% of the articular surface (type 4C) [2].

While there is some controversy over the treatment of mallet finger injuries, most agree that nondisplaced fractures may heal with splinting alone, while displaced fractures comprising more than one-third of the articular surface which do not reduce when the finger is splinted in extension are traditionally addressed with open reduction and internal fixation [6].

Zone 2

Zone 2 injuries involve tendon laceration at the level of the dorsal middle phalanx, with injury to one or both of the lateral bands, injury to the triangular ligament, or injury to both the lateral band(s) and the triangular ligament. Since only one lateral band is required to achieve full extension of the distal interphalangeal joint, single lateral band injuries can typically be managed with conservative measures alone, while more extensive injury will require surgical intervention [2, 14].

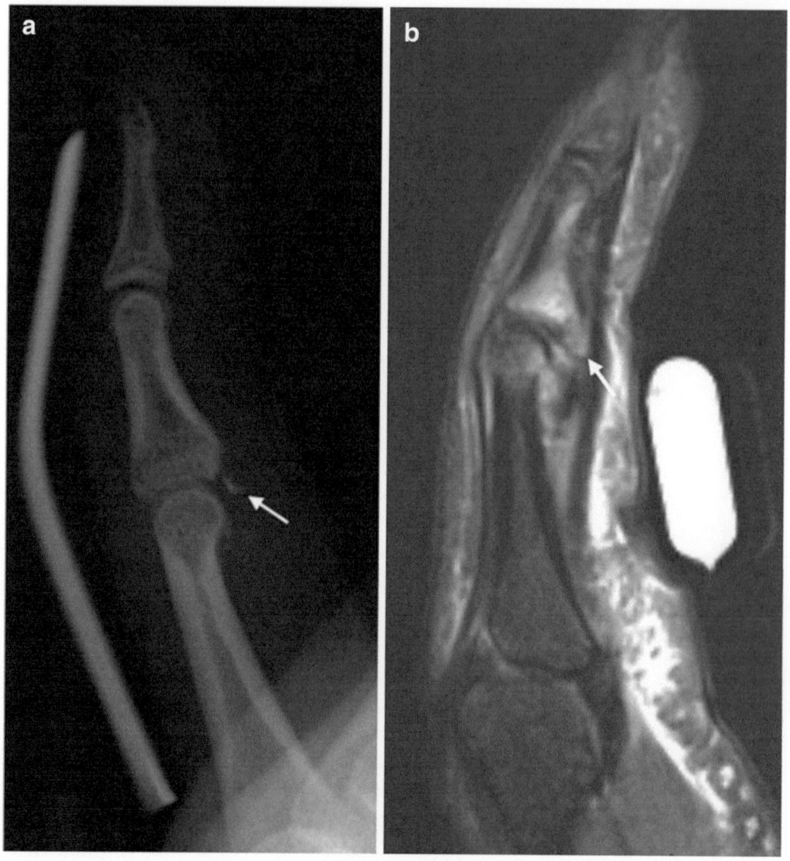

Fig. 11.10 *Volar plate avulsion fracture in a 21-year-old female.* Lateral radiograph of the index finger (**a**) and sagittal T2 fat-suppressed MR image (**b**) show a small distracted and rotated avulsion fracture at the middle phalanx base (arrows). MRI confirms involvement of the volar plate attachment, with contusion of the proximal phalanx head and middle phalanx base

Zone 3

At the proximal interphalangeal joint level, injury to the extensor apparatus may involve the lateral bands, the central slip, or both structures, producing the boutonnière deformity, with proximal interphalangeal joint extensor lag and distal interphalangeal joint hyperextension [2] (Fig. 11.14). Surgical management in central slip injuries is typically reserved for open injury, failed conservative management, displaced avulsion fractures, and proximal interphalangeal joint instability [14].

Zone 4

Zone 4 injuries are usually tendon lacerations at the level of the proximal phalanx. Close apposition of the extensor tendon to the convex bony contour of the proximal phalanx usually produces only partial tendon lacerations, and associated proximal phalanx fractures are occasionally seen. Lacerations greater than 50% tendon thickness and complete tears are traditionally treated surgically [2].

Zone 5

Zone 5 injuries to the extensor apparatus overlie the metacarpophalangeal joint and frequently occur when a clenched fist strikes someone in the mouth (fight bite), most often involving the middle finger. Extensor tendon injury frequently is only partial but has less clinical importance than the implications of inoculating the metacarpophalangeal joint with bacteria from the mouth, which may produce a septic joint [14].

Blunt injury to the extensor apparatus at the metacarpophalangeal joint level may cause laceration of the sagittal band. The middle finger,

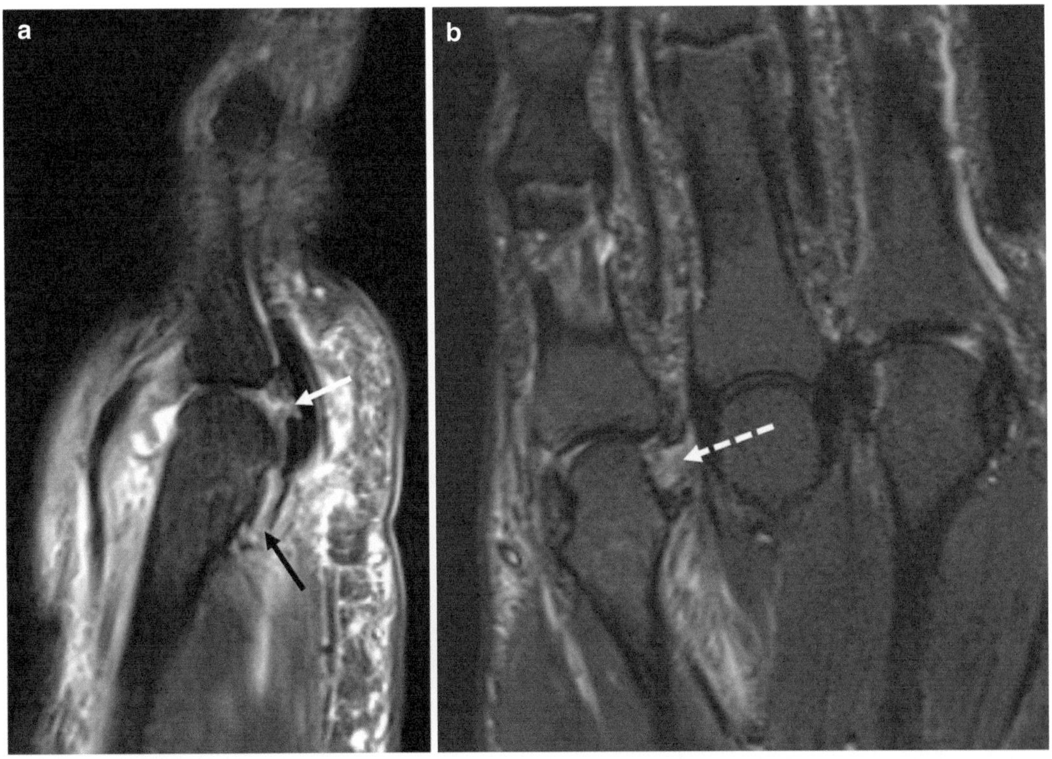

Fig. 11.11 *Fifth metacarpophalangeal joint volar plate and radial collateral ligament tear in a 68-year-old female.* Sagittal T2 fat-suppressed (**a**) and coronal STIR (**b**) MRI images show a complete tear of the volar plate (black arrow), at the level of the metacarpal neck attachment, as well as a tear more distally near the phalangeal base attachment (white arrow), while coronal image shows a complete intrasubstance tear of the radial collateral ligament (dashed arrow)

radial portion of the sagittal band, is the most common injury location, with resultant ulnar subluxation of the extensor tendon (Fig. 11.15). Three types of sagittal band injury have been described: *type 1* injury, in which the band is contused with mild injury, but no discrete tear; *type 2* injury, the sagittal band tears, with extensor tendon subluxation; and *type 3* injury, the band tears and the tendon completely dislocates [15].

Zone 6

Injury to the extensor tendon at the level of the metacarpal has a more favorable outcome, due to less common associated joint injury, decreased risk of adhesions, and lower probability of tendon imbalance [2].

MRI evaluation of the extensor apparatus should focus on integrity of the terminal tendon, lateral bands, and the central slip, best revealed in the sagittal and axial plane [16]. The tear should be characterized as low- (<50%) or high-grade (50% or greater) if partial thickness. Any associated avulsion fracture should be described in terms of size and extent of articular surface involvement [17, 18]. Sagittal band injuries can be evaluated for in the axial plane, which will show position of the extensor tendon relative to the metacarpal head, as well as sagittal band sprain/contusion, appearing as band thickening and increased T2 signal, but no discrete tear, versus partial or complete sagittal band tear. Adhesions, if present, will demonstrate blurring

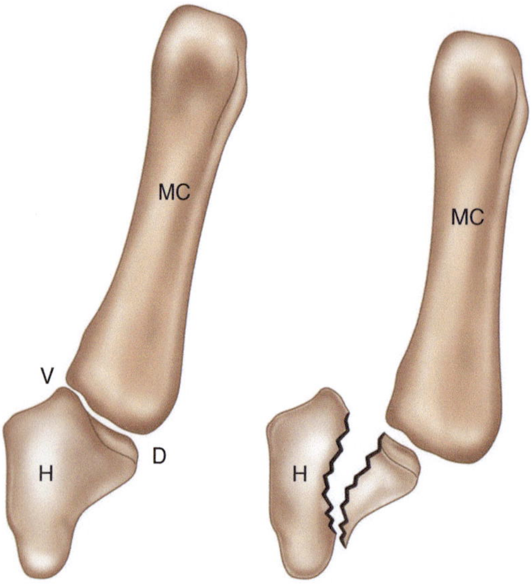

Fig. 11.12 *Carpometacarpal dislocation with dorsal hamate fracture.* Mechanism of injury for dorsal hamate fracture is illustrated in the setting of carpometacarpal dislocation. V Volar, D dorsal, H hamate, MC metacarpal

along the torn tendon margin and scarring of the regional subcutaneous fat, with the normal tendon anatomy distorted. Open wounds may show retained metallic foreign bodies appearing as susceptibility artifact [19].

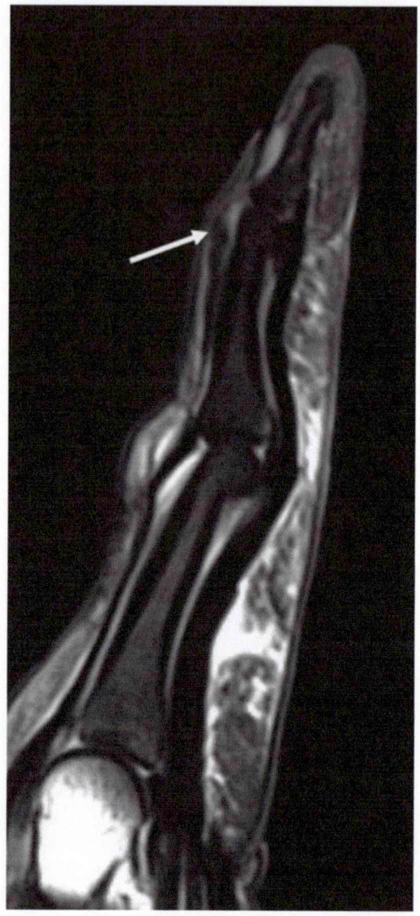

Fig. 11.13 *Soft tissue mallet finger injury in a 67-year-old male.* Sagittal T2 fat-suppressed image of the ring finger shows avulsion of the fourth digit terminal extensor tendon from the dorsal phalanx base attachment (arrow), with subtle flexion of the distal interphalangeal joint

Flexor Tendon Injury

Flexor tendon injuries should be classified as open or closed, with most avulsion injuries being closed injuries, and lacerations classified as open injuries. Flexor tendon injuries should be described according to one of the five anatomic zones of injury. Chapter 10, Hand Anatomy, provides a detailed discussion of normal anatomic zones of the flexor tendons.

Zone 1

Zone 1 injuries include laceration or avulsions of the flexor digitorum profundus distal to the flexor digitorum superficialis insertion [2]. Closed injury of the finger flexor tendon most commonly involves an avulsion of the flexor digitorum profundus attachment at the palmar base of the distal phalanx, referred to as the “jersey finger” (Fig. 11.16). This injury classically occurs when the actively flexed distal interphalangeal joint is forced into sudden hyperextension, as may occur when a player grabs a jersey and the opponent pulls away suddenly and forcefully. This injury pattern most commonly occurs in the ring finger, likely due to the weaker flexor tendon attachment of this digit [6].

Avulsions of the flexor digitorum profundus are categorized into three distinct injury pattern subtypes by Leddy and Packer: *Type 1* injuries include tendon avulsions retracted to the level of

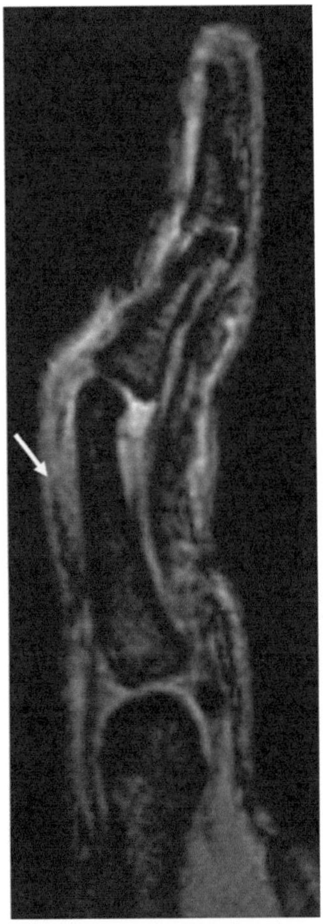

Fig. 11.14 *Central slip avulsion in a 27-year-old male.* Sagittal gradient echo image of the fifth digit demonstrates avulsion of the central slip of the fifth digit extensor tendon, with the stump proximally migrated and mildly redundant (arrow), with associated boutonniere deformity

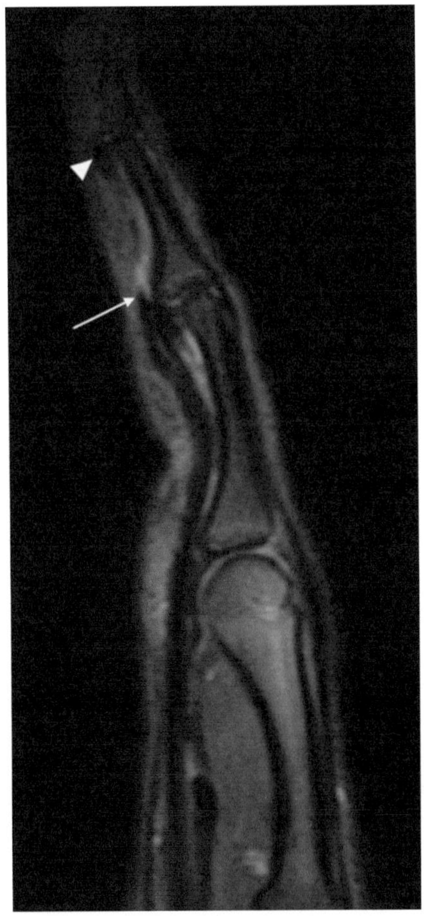

Fig. 11.16 *Flexor digitorum profundus avulsion in a 21-year old male.* Sagittal proton density fat-suppressed image of the middle finger shows a complete avulsion of the flexor digitorum profundus tendon from the volar distal phalanx base attachment with retraction (arrow). Note soft tissue along the volar distal interphalangeal joint represents an intact volar plate (arrowhead), and not the distal tendon stump

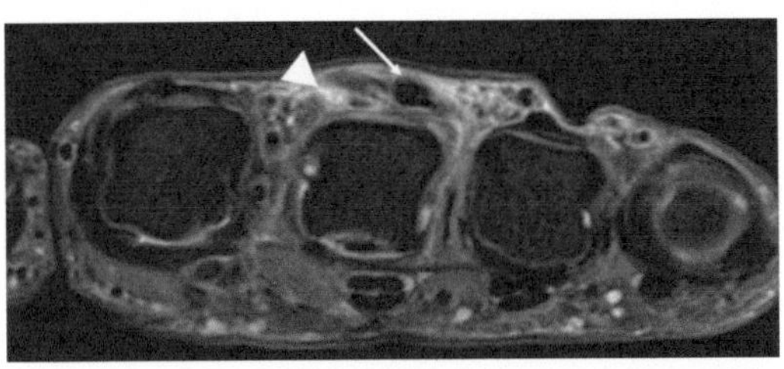

Fig. 11.15 *Sagittal band injury in a 73-year-old male.* Axial T2 fat-suppressed image of the hand shows a complete tear of the radial sagittal band of the third metacarpophalangeal joint (arrowhead), with resultant mild-ulnar subluxation of the third digit extensor tendon (arrow)

the palm with rupture of both the short and long vinculae which provide vascular supply to the phalangeal portion of the flexor tendon, thus requiring early surgical reattachment in order to avoid tendon necrosis and contraction. *Type 2* injuries include small bony avulsions which retract to the level of the proximal interphalangeal joint, with the long vinculum, and thus a portion of the tendon's blood supply, remaining intact. Surgical reattachment is advised for type 2

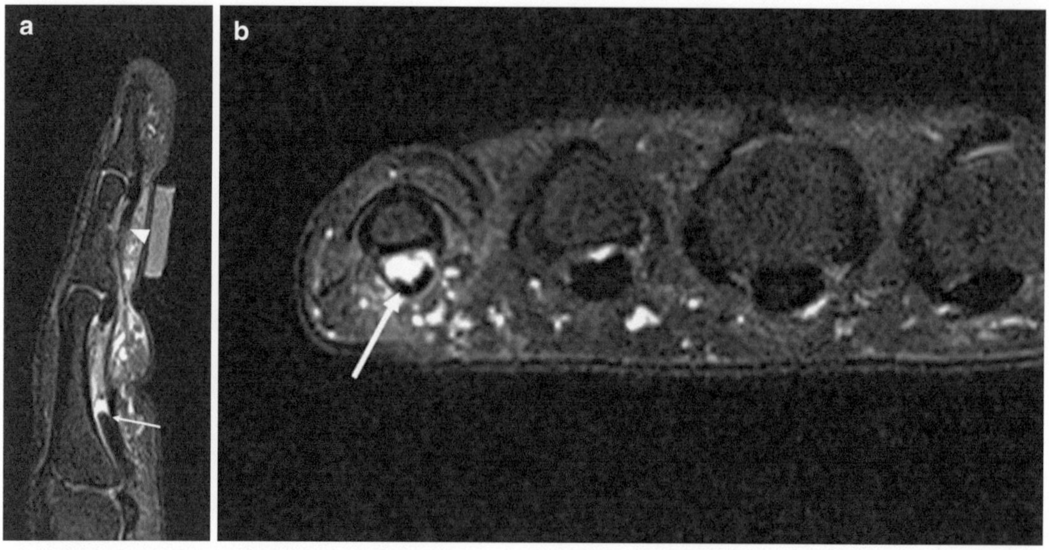

Fig. 11.17 *Zone 2 flexor tendon laceration in a 58-year-old female*. Sagittal T2 fat-suppressed image (**a**) reveals a zone 2 laceration of the fifth digit flexor digitorum profundus, with retracted proximal stump (arrow), distal stump fibers (arrowhead), and large intervening tendon gap. Axial T2 sat-suppressed image (**b**) shows the absence of the flexor digitorum profundus, with the flexor digitorum superficialis remaining intact (arrow)

injuries, although emergent intervention is not required, as in type 1 injuries, due to the remaining vascular supply. *Type 3* injuries have a large bony avulsion fragment which retracts just proximal to the distal interphalangeal joint, with the degree of retraction limited by the A4 pulley. Type 3 injuries are typically treated with open reduction and internal fixation [20].

Zone 2

Zone 2 injuries, the so-called no man's land, involve lacerations from the level of the A1 pulley to the level of the flexor digitorum superficialis attachment, often involving both the flexor digitorum and profundus tendons and carrying the worst prognosis [2, 21] (Fig. 11.17). The flexor digitorum superficialis tendon may be avulsed by closed injury mechanism but is rarely injured in isolation. A flexor digitorum superficialis avulsion will more commonly be seen in combination with a simultaneous flexor profundus injury [13].

Zones 3–5

Laceration of the flexor mechanism in zones 3–5 may involve injury to both the flexor digitorum superficialis and profundus tendon, as well as the neurovascular supply [2].

Timing of flexor tendon repair is dependent upon history and physical exam, with urgent repair indicated for compromised digital perfusion requiring microvascular repair or reconstruction [2].

High-resolution MRI tailored to the digit of concern will best demonstrate a fluid-filled defect at the site of flexor tendon tear, with the axial and sagittal plane most useful for flexor tendon pathology [16]. Larger avulsion fractures will show frank cortical disruption at the fracture site, with associated marrow edema. Smaller avulsion fractures, however, may only be appreciated on radiographs. Occasionally, flexor tendon tears will be accompanied by tenosynovitis, with the tendon sheath and involved pulleys thickening over time, mimicking a trigger finger on clinical exam [17].

Flexor Pulley Injuries

Pulley injuries are classically observed in rock climbers, most often affecting the ring finger,

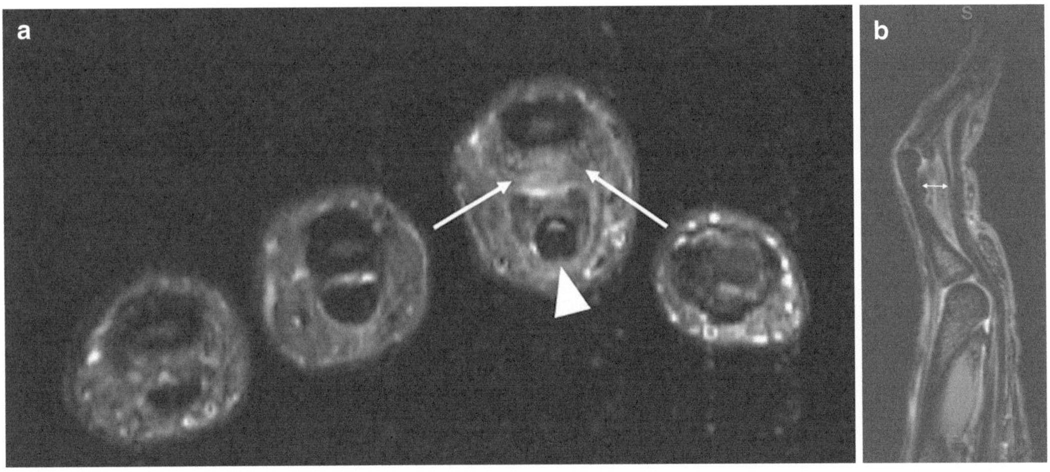

Fig. 11.18 *Pulley injury and bowstringing in a 41-year-old male*. Axial STIR (**a**) image shows complete tear of the third digit A2 pulley (arrows), with the flexor tendon (arrowhead) palmarly displaced, with marked gapping between the phalanx and the flexor tendon. Sagittal image (**b**) demonstrates bowstringing of the flexor tendon, due to sequential rupture of the A2 and A3 pulleys, with marked gapping between the flexor tendon and the proximal phalanx

with the A2 pulley the most commonly injured. Pulley rupture occurs when the finger is in the crimp position, wherein the PIP joint is in at least 90 degrees of flexion and the DIP joint is hyperextended, generating high tensile forces in the flexor digitorum profundus and superficialis, leading eventually to pulley rupture. Significant bowstringing of the flexor tendon will not occur unless sequential pulleys are ruptured, almost always including the A2 and A4 pulleys [22, 23].

On MRI, pulley tears demonstrate discrete discontinuity of pulley fibers, which will become more apparent with bowstringing, when the flexor tendon is displaced from the underlying phalanx (Fig. 11.18). Ancillary findings in pulley injury may include soft tissue edema surrounding the pulley and/or tenosynovitis [17].

References

1. Rogers LF. Radiology of skeletal trauma. 2nd ed. New York: NY Churchill Livingstone; 1992.
2. Green's operative hand surgery 2017. Philadelphia: Elsevier.
3. McElfresh EC, Dobyns J. Intra-articular metacarpal head fractures. J Hand Surg Am. 1983;8(4):383–93.
4. Diaz-Garcia R, Waljee J. Current management of metacarpal fractures. Hand Clin. 2013;29(4):507–18.
5. Wieschhoff GG, Sheehan SE, Wortman JR, Dyer GSM, Sodickson AD, Patel KI, Khurana B. Traumatic finger injuries: what the orthopedic surgeon wants to know. Radiographics. 2016;36(4):1106–28.
6. Schneider LH. Fractures of the distal phalanx. (0749-0712 (Print)).
7. Seymour N. Juxta-epiphysial fracture of the terminal phalanx of the finger. J Bone Joint Surg. 1966;48 B(2):347–9.
8. Abzug JM, Kozin SH. Seymour fractures. (1531-6564 (Electronic)).
9. Carpenter S, Rohde R. Treatment of phalangeal fractures. Hand Clin. 2013;29(4):519–34.
10. Elfar J, Mann T. Fracture-dislocations of the proximal interphalangeal joint. J Am Acad Orthop Surg. 2013;21(2):88–98.
11. Light TR. Buttress pinning techniques. Orthop Rev. 1981;10(5):49–55.
12. Dinh P, Franklin A, Hutchinson B, Schnall SB, Fassola I. Metacarpophalangeal joint dislocation. J Am Acad Orthop Surg. 2009;17(5):318–24.
13. Internal derangement of joints. 2nd ed. Vol. 1. Philadelphia: Saunders Elsevier; 2007.
14. Matzon JL, Bozentka D. Extensor tendon injuries. J Hand Surg Am. 2010;35(5):854–61.
15. Rayan GM, Murray D. Classification and treatment of closed sagittal band injuries. J Hand Surg Am. 1994;19A(4):590–4.
16. Ragheb D, Stanley A, Gentili A, et al. MR imaging of the finger tendons: normal anatomy and commonly encountered pathology. Eur J Radiol. 2005;56(3):296–306.
17. Gupta P, et al. High-resolution 3-T MRI of the fingers: review of anatomy and common tendon and ligament injuries. Am J Roentgenol. 2015;204:W314–23.

18. Clavero JA, Golanó P, Farinas O, et al. Extensor mechanism of the fingers: MR imaging-anatomic correlation. Radiographics. 2003;23(3):593–611.
19. Clavero JA, Alomar X, Monill JM, et al. MR imaging of ligament and tendon injuries of the fingers. Radiographics. 2002;22:237–56.
20. Leddy JP, Packer JW. Avulsion of the profundus tendon insertion in athletes. J Hand Surg Am. 1977;2(1):66–9.
21. Newmeyer WL, Manske P. No man's land revisited: the primary flexor tendon repair controversy. J Hand Surg Am. 2004;29(1):1–5.
22. Zafonte B, Rendulic D, Szabo RM. Flexor pulley system: anatomy, injury, and management. J Hand Surg Am. 2014;39(1531-6564 (Electronic)):2525–32.
23. Klauser A, et al. Finger pulley injuries in extreme rock climbers: depiction with dynamic US. (0033-8419 (Print)).

Thumb Pathology – Traumatic

12

Sarah I. Kamel and Suzanne S. Long

Carpometacarpal Joint

Stabilizers of the Carpometacarpal Joint

The first carpometacarpal joint, with a shallow articular surface, allows for wide range of motion of the thumb. While there have been numerous ligaments described at the level of the carpometacarpal joint in cadaveric specimens, many are below the resolution of imaging and may not be integral to joint stability. Essential ligamentous support of the carpometacarpal joint can be categorized by location: dorsal, intermetacarpal, volar, and ulnar (Fig. 12.1).

The dorsal support ligaments, the dorsal radial and posterior oblique ligaments, arise from the dorsal tubercle of the trapezium. At the dorsal aspect of the first metacarpal base, the dorsal radial ligament inserts radially and the posterior oblique ligament along the ulnar aspect. These structures act as the primary resistors to dorsoradial dislocation of the first metacarpal. The abductor pollicis longus and extensor pollicis brevis tendons lie immediately superficial to the dorsal radial and posterior oblique ligaments, respectively. These overlying tendons assist in stabilization of the joint and can aid in identification of the ligaments (Fig. 12.2). The two ligaments are usually not resolved individually on MRI and therefore can be identified as the dorsal ligament complex [1–3].

The intermetacarpal ligament, best seen on oblique coronal sequences at the base of the metacarpal, bridges the dorsoradial aspect of the second metacarpal to the volar-ulnar tubercle of the first metacarpal base (Fig. 12.3). It primarily resists radial translation of the thumb metacarpal.

Volarly, the anterior oblique ligament spans the trapezium and metacarpal base and is intimately associated with the joint capsule and overlying thenar muscles (Fig. 12.4). The anterior oblique ligament has also been described to have a superficial and a deep, intra-articular component, which may give it a striated appearance. Degeneration of the anterior oblique ligament is thought to be the primary contributor to osteoarthritis of the carpometacarpal joint, and repair of the anterior oblique ligament is the target of carpometacarpal joint reconstruction for its biomechanical significance [4].

S. I. Kamel (✉) · S. S. Long
Department of Musculoskeletal Radiology, Thomas Jefferson University Hospital, Philadelphia, PA, USA
e-mail: sarah.kamel@jefferson.edu

B. U. Casagranda (ed.), *MRI of the Upper Extremity*, https://doi.org/10.1007/978-3-030-81612-4_12

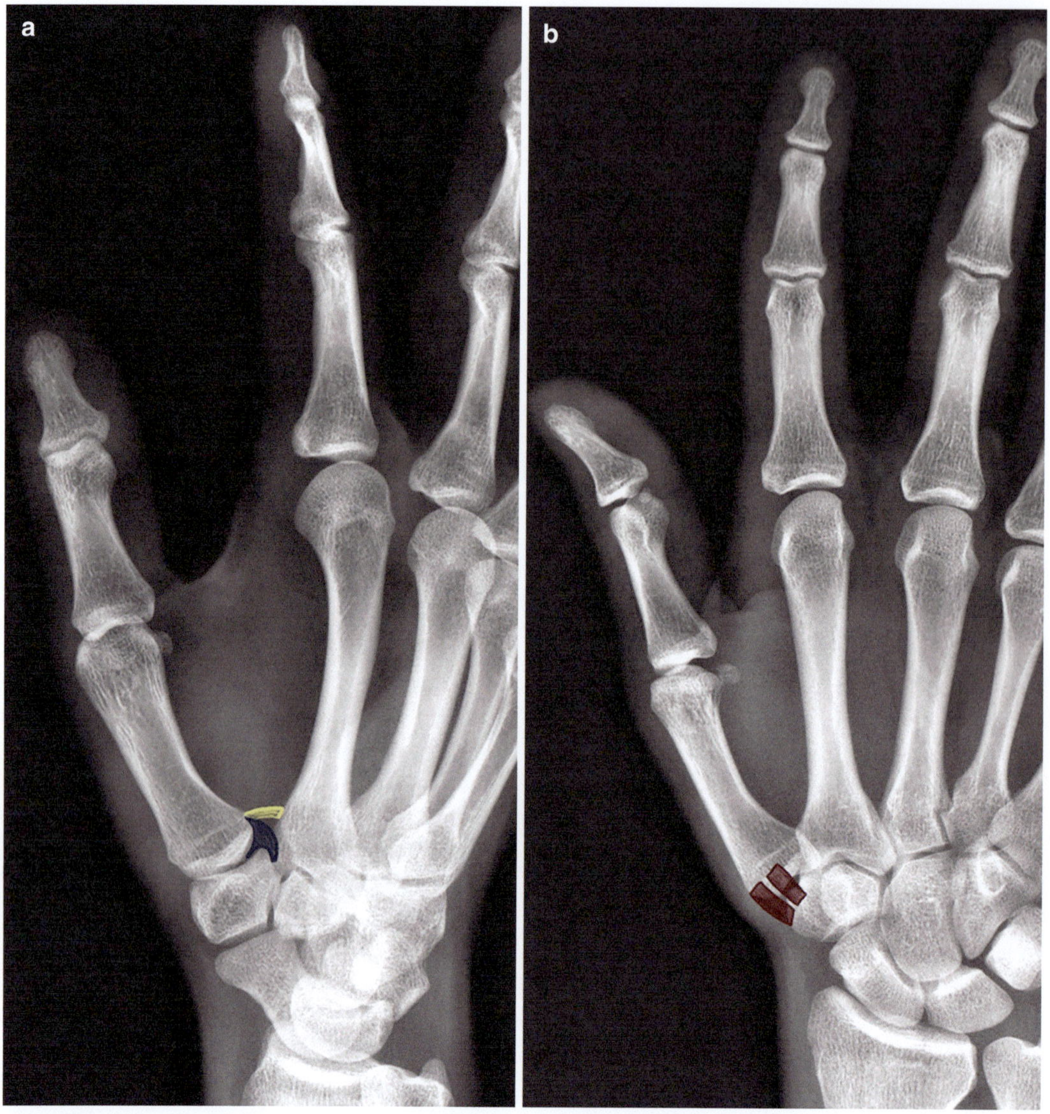

Fig. 12.1 Carpometacarpal ligamentous stabilizers. Posteroanterior (PA) oblique radiograph of the base of the thumb with the locations of the anterior oblique ligament (blue) and intermetacarpal ligament (yellow) highlighted (**a**). Note that the anterior oblique ligament has a superficial component and a deep, intra-articular component. PA radiographic view of the base of the thumb demonstrating the dorsal ligament complex (red) at the carpometacarpal joint (**b**). The dorsal radial ligament is located more radially, and the posterior oblique ligament is more ulnar, but identifying these structures as two separate ligaments typically is below the resolution of MRI

Finally, the ulnar collateral ligament spans the flexor retinaculum/trapezium and volar-ulnar base of the first metacarpal, providing additional support to the anterior oblique ligament. On MRI, it generally cannot be resolved as a separate structure from the anterior oblique ligament.

Osseous and Ligamentous Injury

The most common injury to the carpometacarpal joint, often elicited by punching an object with a clenched fist, is the Bennett fracture, an oblique intra-articular fracture of the metacarpal base.

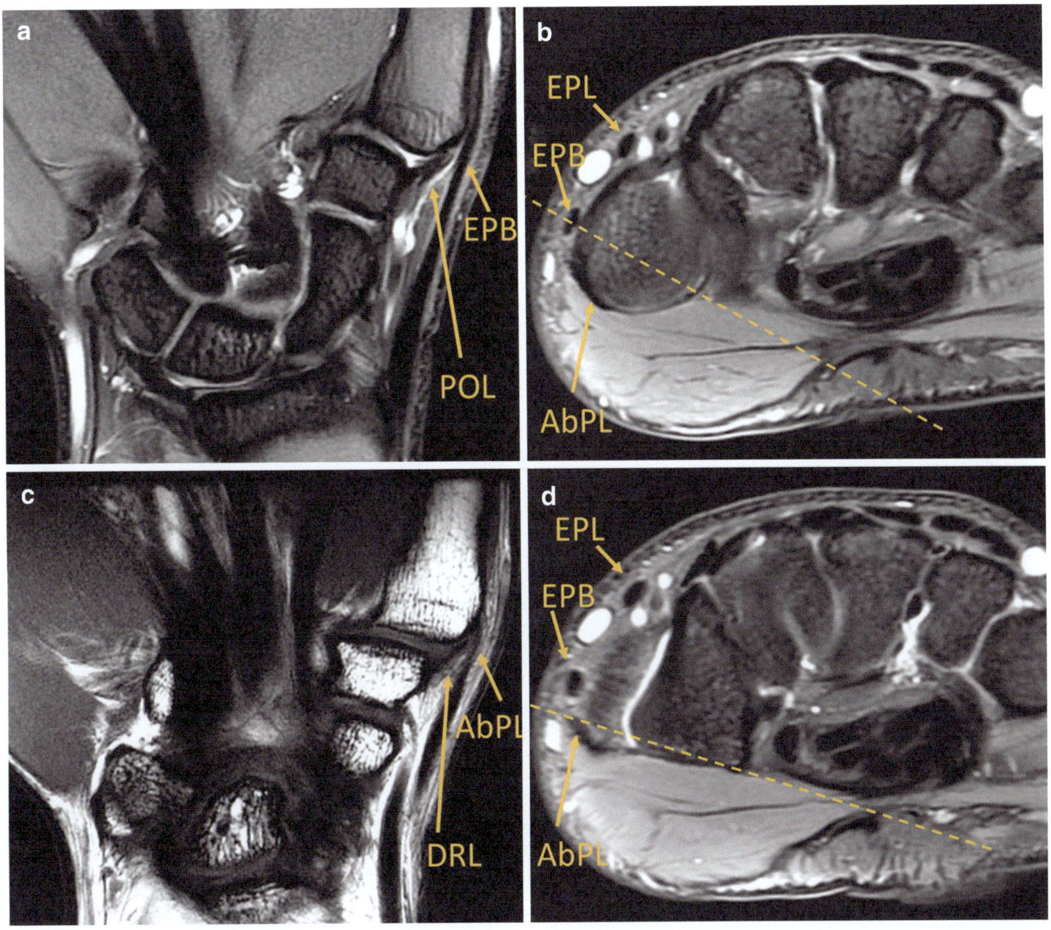

Fig. 12.2 Dorsal ligament complex. Coronal oblique (in the plane of the dotted line of Fig. 12.2b) T2 fat-saturated image (**a**) demonstrating the posterior oblique ligament (POL), which is the more ulnar component of the dorsal ligament complex and can be identified by the more superficial extensor pollicis brevis (EPB) tendon. T2 axial sequence through the base of the first metacarpal (**b**) demonstrating the locations of the EPB, abductor pollicis longus (AbPL), and extensor pollicis longus (EPL) tendons. Coronal oblique T1 sequence through the carpometacarpal joint (**c**), in the plane of the dotted line in Fig. 12.2d, demonstrating the dorsal radial ligament (DRL) which is radial to the POL and deep to the AbPL. T2 axial sequence (**d**) highlighting the position of the thumb extensors and AbPL

There is typically a volar avulsion fracture fragment which remains attached to the deep intra-articular band of the anterior oblique ligament. As a result, the fractured fragment maintains its articular surface attachment, and the remainder of the metacarpal is displaced radially by the abductor pollicis longus (Fig. 12.5). This often contributes to a wide articular diastasis. Treatment may include closed reduction with percutaneous pinning or open reduction with pinning. Long-term clinical outcomes are favorable if anatomic alignment is maintained postsurgically [5].

The Rolando fracture is a comminuted intra-articular fracture of the metacarpal base, with a "Y-" or "T"-shaped morphology. This typically appears as a transverse fracture through the metacarpal metadiaphysis and longitudinal intra-articular fracture dividing the articular surface into volar and dorsal fragments, with central depression of the articular surface (Fig. 12.6).

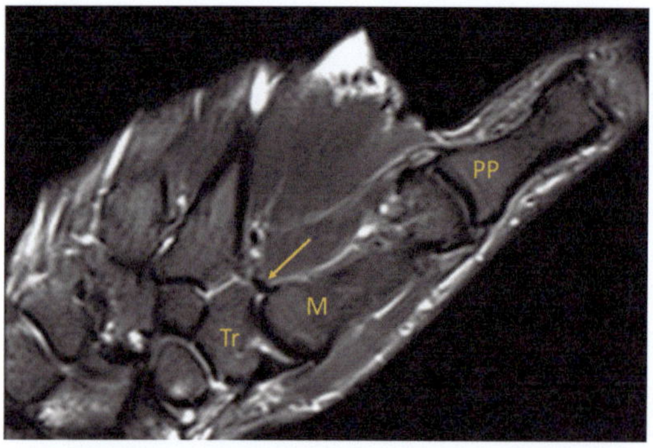

Fig. 12.3 Intermetacarpal ligament. T2 fat-saturated coronal sequence through the base of the carpometacarpal joint demonstrating the intermetacarpal ligament (arrow). Tr trapezium, M first metacarpal, PP first proximal phalanx

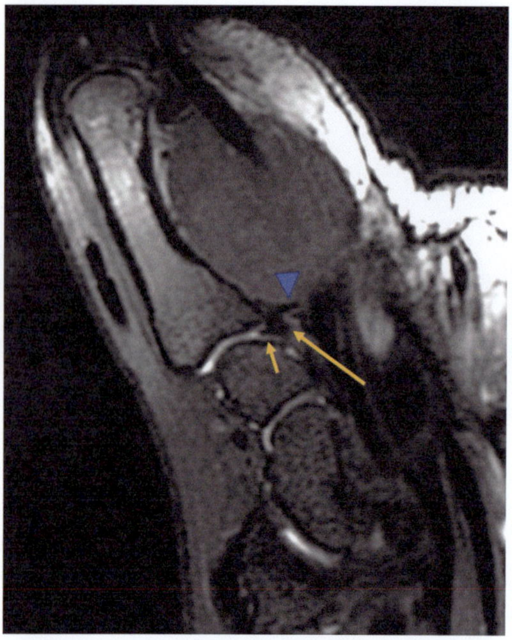

Fig. 12.4 Anterior oblique ligament. T2 coronal oblique through the carpometacarpal joint. The superficial, intra-articular (short arrow), and deep (long arrow) components of the anterior oblique ligaments are seen here. A portion of the intermetacarpal ligament (blue arrowhead) is also seen. (*Image courtesy of Ali B. Syed, MD from Stanford University Hospital*)

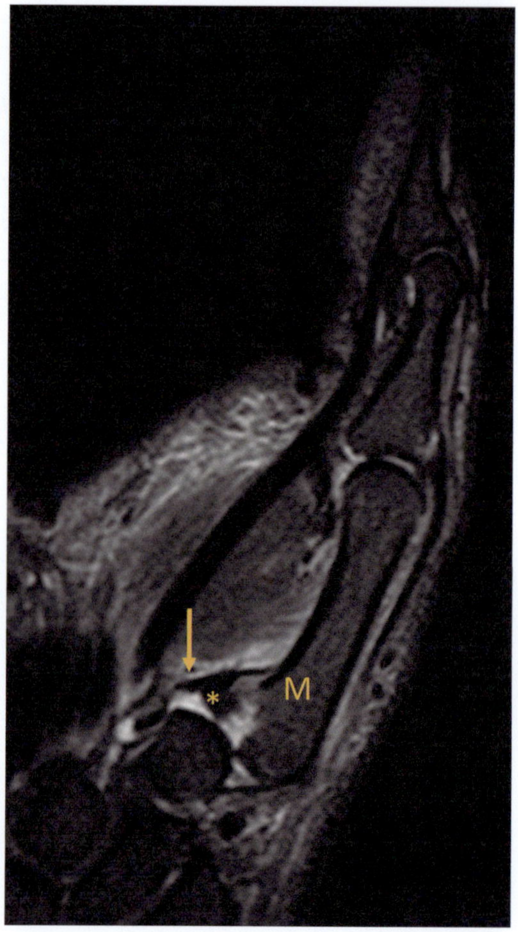

Fig. 12.5 Bennett fracture. A 23-year-old male following motor vehicle accident. T2 fat-saturated coronal oblique sequence through the carpometacarpal joint demonstrates an oblique, intra-articular fracture through the base of the thumb metacarpal, also known as a Bennett fracture. An avulsed fracture fragment (asterisk) remains attached to the anterior oblique ligament (arrow) with the remainder of the metacarpal (M) displaced radially by the abductor pollicis longus, contributing to articular diastasis

This injury is generally unstable, especially in the setting of displacement, necessitating surgical reduction and fixation. MRI is typically not performed in the setting of diagnostic radiographs as surgical fixation is the priority [6].

In the absence of fracture, the anterior oblique ligament is most commonly sprained (Fig. 12.7). Periligamentous edema, ligament discontinuity, or ligament avulsion can be seen with periosteal stripping from the metacarpal attachment. Injury to the dorsal ligaments will typically occur by a longitudinally directed force on the thumb in full

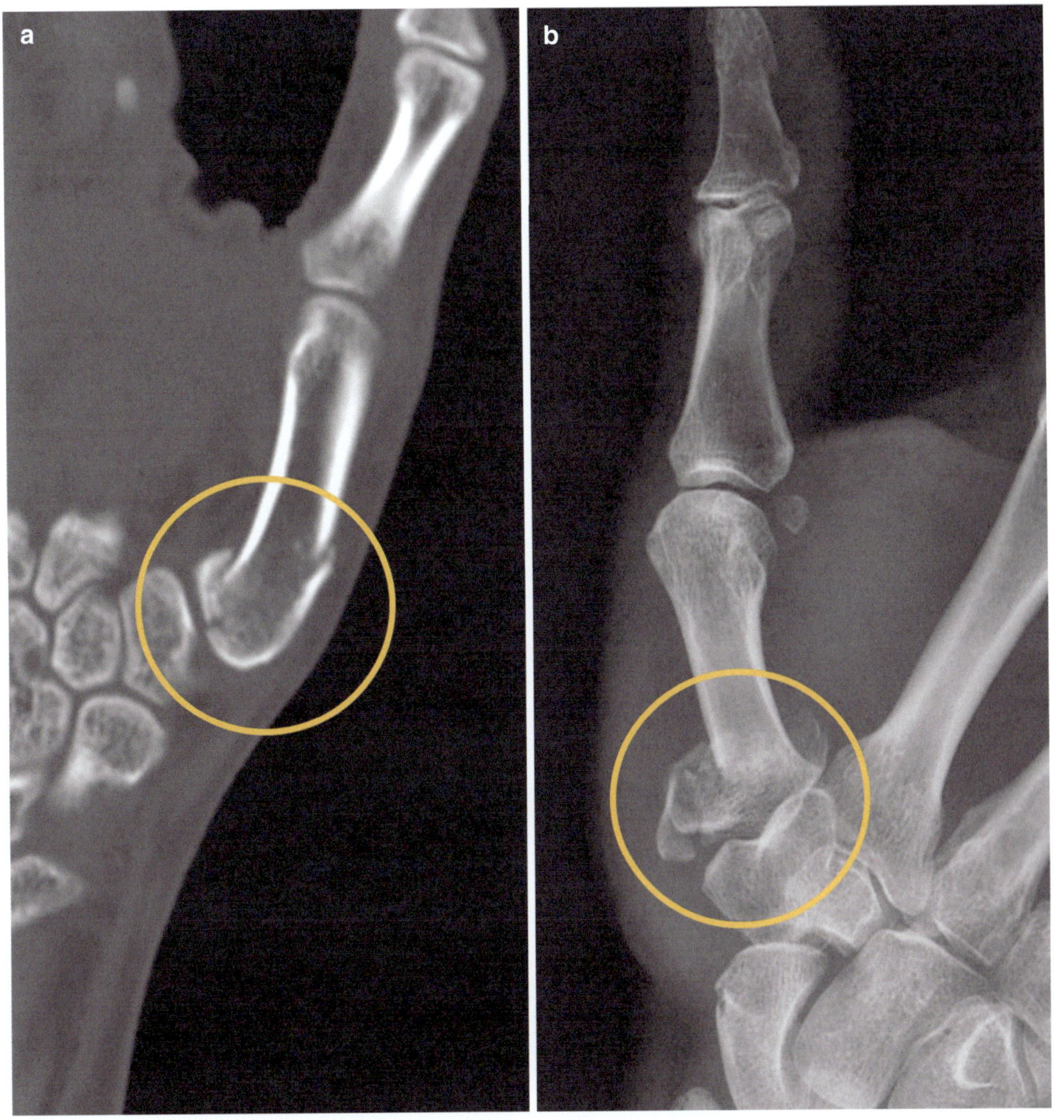

Fig. 12.6 Rolando fracture. Coronal section CT image through the base of the thumb (**a**) demonstrating the Y-shaped configuration of a Rolando fracture, an intra-articular fracture through the base of the first metacarpal. PA oblique radiograph of the thumb (**b**) shows a Rolando fracture in another patient, as a markedly comminuted and displaced intra-articular fracture

flexion or by a direct blow to the thumb web space, for example, when gripping a bike handlebar during impact. Secondary signs are helpful in identifying ligamentous injury, such as adjacent soft tissue edema, hematoma, or osseous contusion spanning the carpometacarpal joint. Ganglion cyst formation and ligament thickening suggest a chronic injury.

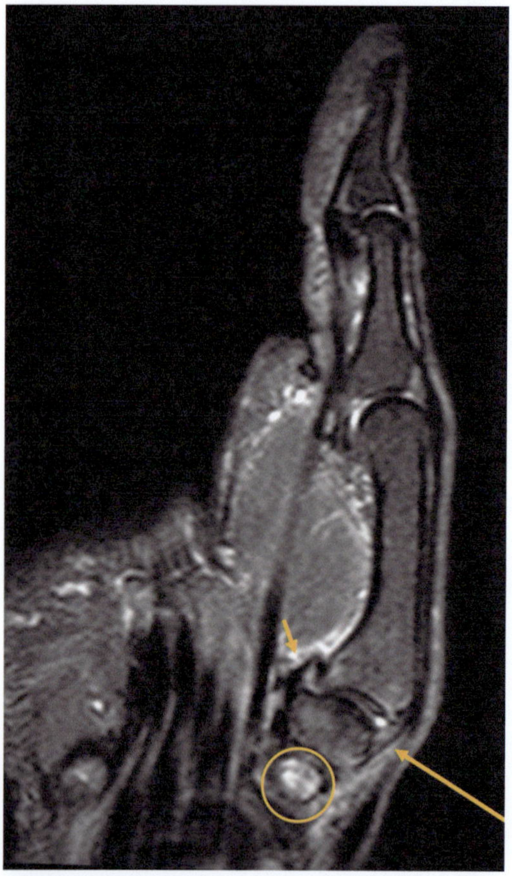

Fig. 12.7 Anterior oblique ligament sprain. T2 fat-saturated coronal oblique sequence through the carpometacarpal joint shows intrinsic and periligamentous edema of the dorsal ligament complex (long arrow) and anterior oblique ligament (short arrow), compatible with low-grade sprain. This patient suffered from a motor vehicle accident which also contributed to a nondisplaced fracture of the scaphoid (circle, partially imaged)

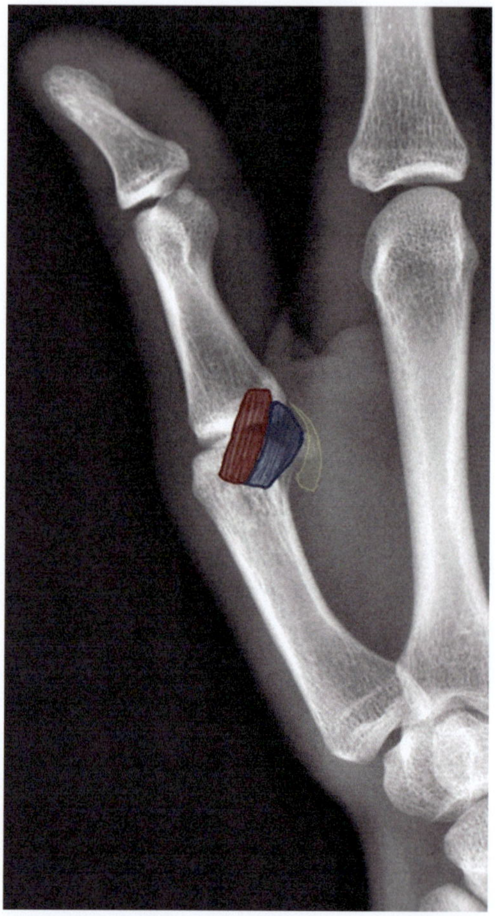

Fig. 12.8 Schematic of ulnar collateral ligaments of the thumb. Posteroanterior radiograph of the thumb with depiction of the ulnar collateral ligament. The ulnar collateral ligament is comprised of a proper component more dorsally (red) and a more volar accessory component (blue), both of which angle volarly. The accessory bundle inserts into the ulnar sesamoid and the volar plate (yellow) located between the sesamoids

Metacarpophalangeal Joint

Metacarpophalangeal Joint Anatomy

The primary static stabilizers of the thumb metacarpophalangeal (MCP) joint are the ulnar and radial collateral ligaments, which are each comprised of a proper and accessory bundle (Fig. 12.8). The proper ulnar collateral ligament originates from the medial tubercle of the metacarpal condyle and angles volarly to insert at the base of the proximal phalanx. Similarly, the proper radial collateral ligament arises from the lateral tubercle of the metacarpal condyle and courses in an oblique fashion volarly to insert at the tubercle of the proximal phalanx. The accessory ulnar and radial collateral ligaments are located volar to their proper counterparts and insert into the volar plate and respective ulnar and radial sesamoid. The ulnar collateral ligament is supported by the overlying aponeurosis of the adductor pollicis muscle, which is a dynamic stabilizer of the metacarpal joint, resisting valgus stress (Fig. 12.9). The MCP

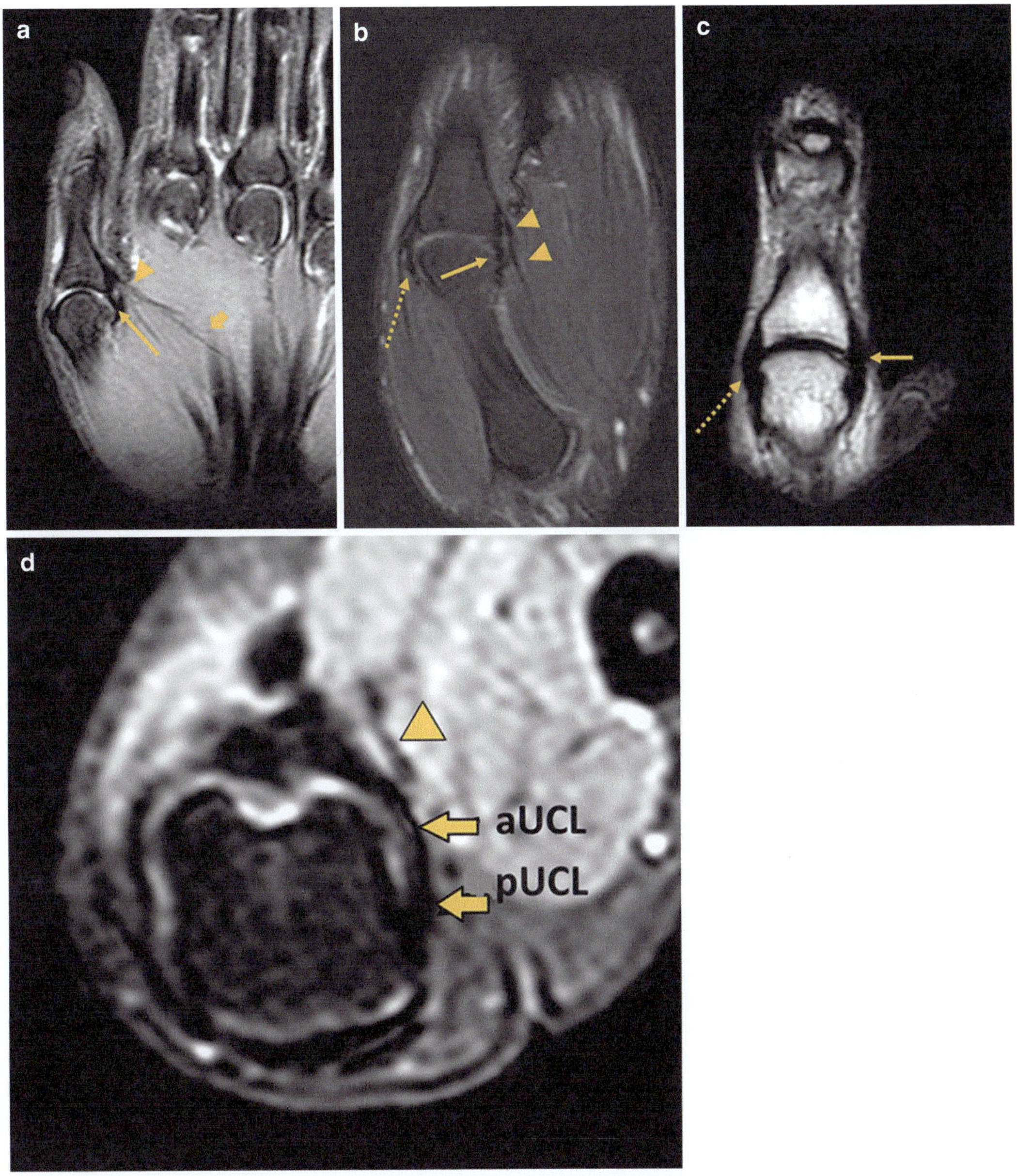

Fig. 12.9 Normal MRI appearance of the collateral ligaments. T2 fat-saturated sagittal sequence through the thumb metacarpophalangeal (MCP) joint (**a**). The ulnar collateral ligament (arrow) is seen deep to the aponeurosis of the adductor pollicis (arrowhead). There is partial visualization of the adductor pollicis muscle belly (short arrow) seen as it originates from the third metacarpal. Coronal STIR sequence of the thumb MCP joint (**b**) showing the ulnar collateral ligament (arrow) deep to the adductor pollicis aponeurosis (arrowheads). The radial collateral ligament (dotted arrow) is also seen on this slice. These intact ligaments are normally hypointense on T2/STIR sequences. Coronal T1-weighted sequence through the thumb MCP joint (**c**) showing the normal, hypointense, and continuous appearance of the ulnar (arrow) and radial (dotted arrow) collateral ligaments. Axial T2-weighted fat-saturated sequence through the MCP joint, above the level of the sesamoids (**d**). The proper (pUCL) and accessory (aUCL) collateral ligaments are seen with the adductor pollicis aponeurosis (arrowhead) just superficial to the ulnar collateral ligament

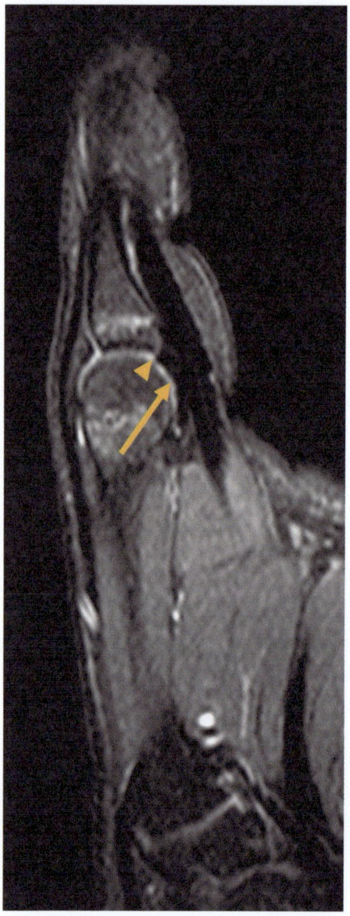

Fig. 12.10 Volar plate. T2 fat-saturated sequences in the midline sagittal plane of the thumb demonstrating the normal appearance of the volar plate (arrow) of the metacarpophalangeal joint in multiple patients. The volar plate bridges the sesamoid bones and attaches to the volar base of proximal phalanx, supporting the joint. There is a normal synovial recess deep to the volar plate (arrowhead)

joint is also stabilized by a triangularly shaped fibrocartilage volar plate which supports the joint capsule (Fig. 12.10). The volar plate extends between the sesamoid bones with attachments to the proximal phalanx and first metacarpal. Dorsally, the sagittal bands at the level of the metacarpophalangeal joint stabilize the extensor pollicis longus tendon as they are perpendicularly oriented to the tendon. A detailed axial view of these structures is later depicted in Fig. 12.11 [1–3].

Ulnar Collateral Ligament Injury

Injury to the ulnar collateral ligament of the metacarpal is the most common injury to the thumb. Ulnar collateral ligament tear may be secondary to chronic repetitive valgus stress on the thumb metacarpophalangeal joint or may be acutely injured during a valgus stress sustained during a fall on outstretched hand with the thumb abducted (typically while holding a ski pole – *Skier's thumb*). Accurate diagnosis of ulnar collateral ligament injury is necessary because if incorrectly treated, tears can lead to impaired thumb adduction function, such as pinching which is critical to activities of daily living, and may accelerate osteoarthritis at the metacarpophalangeal joint [7]. Clinical exam can be specific in making a diagnosis of ulnar collateral ligament injury; however, MRI is an excellent complement in diagnosis and treatment planning.

When evaluating the ulnar collateral ligament, axial and coronal sequences are most sensitive in identifying injury. Axial images should run perpendicular to the tubular bones and span the entire length of the thumb from the CMC joint through the distal phalanx. The proper coronal plane for assessing the collateral ligaments is prescribed from the axial plane with a line bisecting the sesamoid bones as described in Chap. 10.

Diagnosis of injury to the ulnar collateral ligament is based on multiple factors including abnormalities in size, contour, and signal of the ligament. The normal ulnar collateral ligament may have a striated appearance on fat-suppressed sequences but is typically hypointense on all sequences. Therefore, a partial tear should be diagnosed using a combination of intrinsic signal abnormality with focal ligament attenuation (Fig. 12.12). Complete ulnar collateral ligament tears are characterized on fluid-sensitive sequences with a fluid signal defect transecting the ligament, typically at the site of distal bony attachment, on the proximal phalanx. While less common, tears may also occur at the proximal bony attachment or midsubstance.

A common complication of complete ulnar collateral ligament tear is a Stener lesion, which

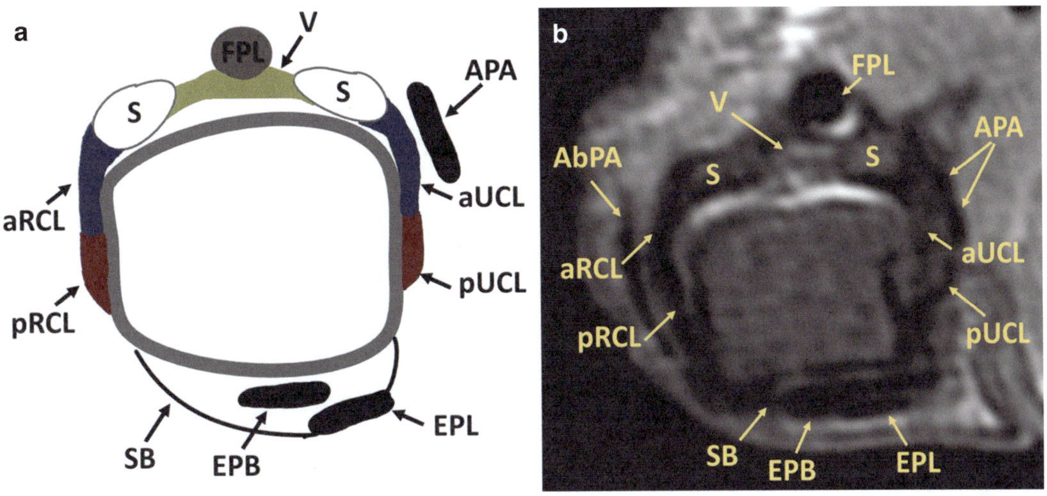

Fig. 12.11 Thumb MCP anatomy at the level of the sesamoids. Axial schematic (**a**) and T2 fat-saturated sequence (**b**) through the level of the sesamoids. The images are oriented with the volar thumb superiorly and the ulnar aspect on the right. APA adductor pollicis aponeurosis, AbPA abductor pollicis, aUCL accessory ulnar collateral ligament, aRCL accessory radial collateral ligament, EPB extensor pollicis longus, EPL extensor pollicis brevis, FPL flexor pollicis longus, pUCL proper ulnar collateral ligament, pRCL proper radial collateral ligament, S sesamoid, SB sagittal band, v volar plate

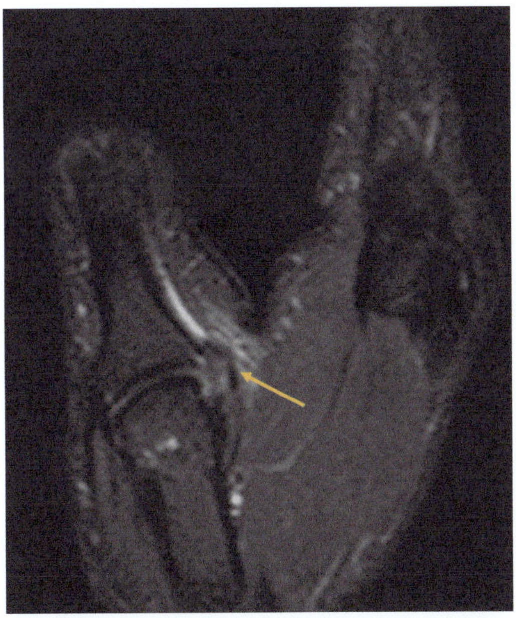

Fig. 12.12 Ulnar collateral ligament sprain. A 32-year-old male injured in a motor vehicle accident. Coronal T2 fat-saturated sequence through the metacarpophalangeal joint demonstrates thickening and edema of ulnar collateral ligament (arrow) with partial tearing of the deep fibers and periligamentous edema. Findings are compatible with a high-grade ulnar collateral ligament sprain

has been reported to occur in up to 88% of complete ulnar collateral ligament tears [8]. When the ulnar collateral ligament is torn from its distal attachment, the ligament retracts proximally toward the metacarpal origin, displaces beneath the proximal margin of the APA, and forms a ball superficial to the APA near or just proximal to the joint line. The APA then blocks the ligament from reapproximating the proximal phalangeal insertion, therefore preventing normal healing. This abnormality is best identified on coronal sequences (Fig. 12.13a, b). This has often been described as a "yo-yo on a string" sign. If there is difficulty in identifying the APA on coronal sequences in the setting of a Stener lesion, the axial sequences will highlight the APA surrounded with edema and without the normal underlying ulnar collateral ligament (Fig. 12.13b). Reporting the amount of ulnar collateral ligament displacement may guide clinicians in determining whether immobilization versus surgical intervention is adequate for healing. Surgical repair is often required for Stener lesions to maintain the function of the thumb metacarpophalangeal joint (Fig. 12.14) [7].

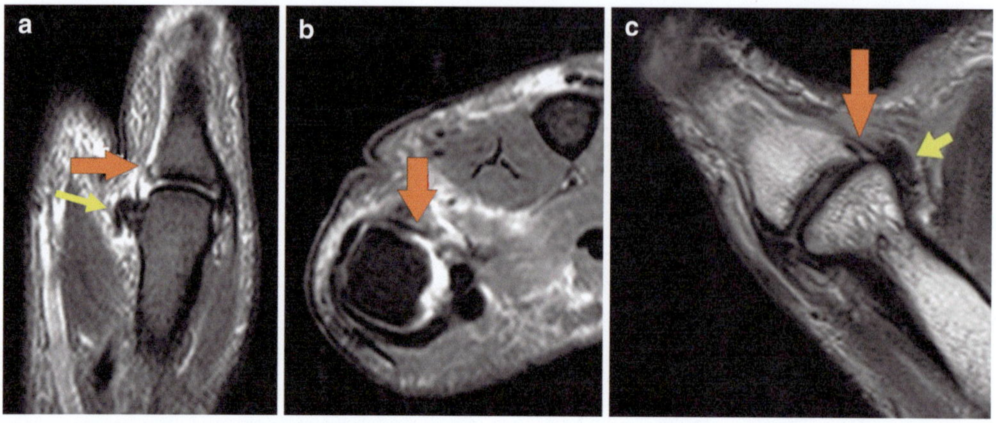

Fig. 12.13 Stener lesion. A 16-year-old male with thumb pain following ski injury. Coronal STIR sequence through the MCP joint demonstrates complete tear of the distal attachment of the ulnar collateral ligament. The ligament is retracted and balled up proximally (yellow arrow) with the adductor pollicis aponeurosis (orange arrow) interposed at the site of the former distal ligament insertion, forming the string of the yo-yo (**a**). The Stener lesion is confirmed on axial sequences where the adductor pollicis aponeurosis (orange arrow) is seen with the absence of the underlying ulnar collateral ligament and with surrounding edema (**b**). Another example of a Stener lesion in a 56-year-old female following slip and fall on ice. T1-weighted coronal sequence through the MCP joint (**c**) demonstrates the retracted ulnar collateral ligament (yellow arrow) and the interposed adductor pollicis aponeurosis (orange arrow)

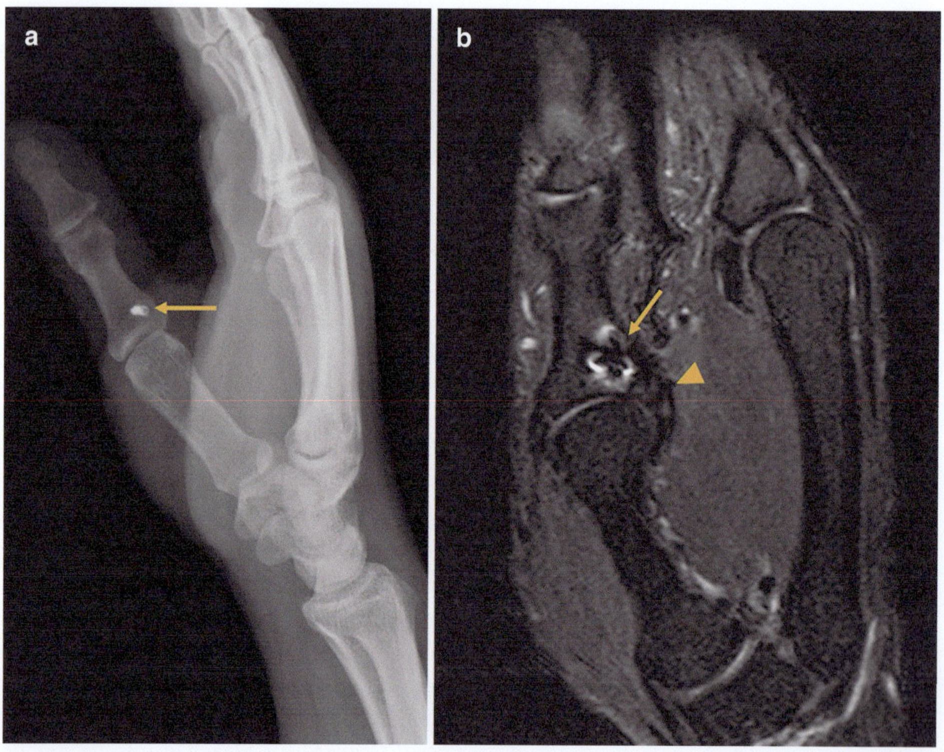

Fig. 12.14 Ulnar collateral ligament repair. A 23-year-old male following ulnar collateral repair. Lateral view of the wrist/hand (**a**) demonstrating a suture anchor at the ulnar base of the proximal phalanx (arrow) at the site of reattachment of the distal ligament. T2-weighted coronal sequence (**b**) shows susceptibility artifact at the site of the repair. The ulnar collateral ligament (arrowhead) appears thickened and scarred from prior injury, but without recurrent tear

Tears of the radial collateral ligament occur more often from the proximal attachment on the metacarpal, rather than the distal attachment on the phalanx (Fig. 12.15). Possible explanations for this may be related to the width of the distal ligament insertion which is broader than the origin, particularly when compared with the ulnar collateral ligament; alternatively, this may be

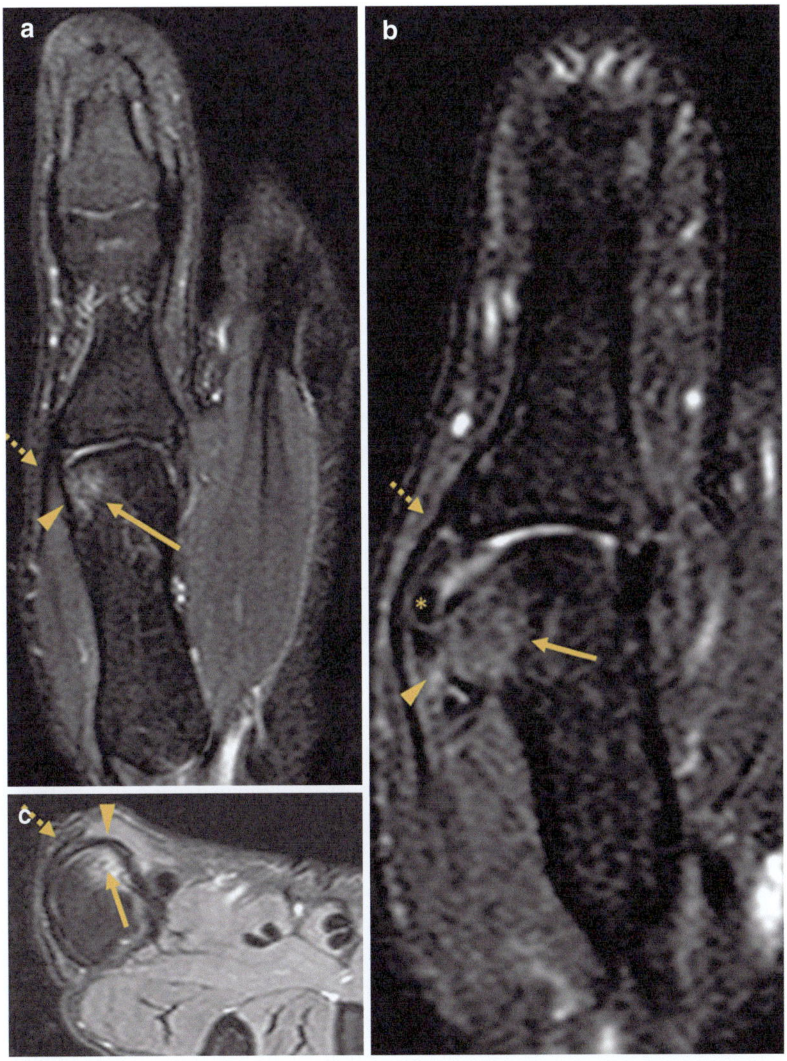

Fig. 12.15 Radial collateral ligament injuries. Coronal STIR sequence through the thumb (**a**) demonstrating avulsive osseous stress response (arrow) at the proximal attachment of the radial collateral ligament on the metacarpal. The ligament (arrowhead) does not appear discontinuous. Findings are compatible with low-grade radial collateral ligament injury. Also intact is the overlying abductor pollicis brevis aponeurosis (dotted arrow). Axial T2-weighted fat-suppressed sequence of the same patient through the level of the metacarpal head (**b**). Again seen is avulsive marrow edema (arrow) at the radial aspect of the metacarpal head. The overlying radial collateral ligament (arrowhead) and abductor pollicis brevis aponeurosis (dotted arrow) appear intact. Coronal STIR sequence in a different patient (**c**) who sustained a complete rupture of the radial collateral ligament with focal discontinuity of the ligament (arrowhead) at the proximal origin. There is partial retraction of the ligament (asterisk), periligamentous edema, and avulsive stress response in the metacarpal head (arrow). The overlying abductor pollicis brevis aponeurosis (dotted arrow) remains intact and in the expected position. Note ulnar subluxation of the proximal phalanx secondary to radial-sided injury with partially unopposed adductor pollicis

related to variation in mechanism of injury required to cause tear of the radial collateral ligament [9]. Injury to the radial collateral ligament is common in sports, caused by a fall with impact on the radial aspect of the thumb or direct impact trauma. A radial equivalent of the Stener lesion has been described with the overlying abductor pollicis longus tendon interposed between the proximal phalanx and a torn, proximally retracted radial collateral ligament. This is less commonly seen, however, because the abductor pollicis brevis aponeurosis is broader than its ulnar counterpart and, again, the ligament is more likely to tear proximally rather than distally.

Volar Plate Injuries

Trauma to the thumb MCP joint volar plate is produced by hyperextension injury or dislocation as seen in other digits. Volar plate injuries can be categorized into three types: I, avulsion of the distal plate; II, greater involvement of the surrounding collateral ligaments which may results in subluxation of the joint; and III, avulsion fracture and dislocation [10]. Avulsion fractures involving 40% of the articular surface will generally require surgery, as the collateral ligaments will likely be attached to the avulsed bone fragment and contribute to joint instability [11]. Careful consideration should be made to the presence of a normal synovial recess deep to the volar plate (Fig. 12.10). An acute volar plate injury will demonstrate a fluid signal gap in the expected location of the volar plate, with contour irregularity (Figs. 12.16 and 12.17).

Sagittal Band Injuries

Usually seen in conjunction with other MCP ligamentous injuries, sagittal band tears may result in subluxation and destabilization of the extensor pollicis longus tendon. Injury to the sagittal band is identified by deformity or discontinuity of the band with increased T2 signal intensity (Fig. 12.18). The extensor tendon typically subluxes away from the side of injury [12].

Interphalangeal Joint

Collateral ligament injuries, fractures, or dislocations of the thumb interphalangeal joint are relatively uncommon. Volar plate injuries may occur in instances of marked hyperextension, similar in appearance to those at the MCP joint. The interphalangeal joint volar plate inserts on the base of the distal phalanx, just proximal to the broad insertion of the flexor pollicis longus tendon. Sesamoid bones may be present in the volar plate, not to be mistaken for a volar plate avulsion fracture (Fig. 12.19).

Annular Pulley System

The pulley system of the thumb is a set of focally thickened transverse retinacular bands which stabilize and support mobility of the flexor pollicis longus tendon while preventing bowstringing of the tendon away from the underlying bone. There are no cruciform pulleys in the thumb as there are in other digits. While there may be some variability in number of annular pulleys detected in the thumb, most individuals have a first pulley at the level of the metacarpophalangeal joint (A1), a second at the level of the interphalangeal joint (A2), and an oblique annular pulley at the level of the proximal phalanx, between A1 and A2 (Fig. 12.20). The first annular pulley is closely associated with the sesamoid bones. Thumb flexion is primarily supported by the first annular pulley, which is reported to have a normal thickness of up to 0.5 mm [3].

Acute injury to the pulley is typically sustained by an episode of powerful flexion. Injury will demonstrate discontinuity of the pulley or increased intrasubstance signal intensity (Fig. 12.21). Bowstringing of the flexor pollicis longus tendon, or increased distance between the tendon and underlying bone, may be evident with a pulley tear.

Fig. 12.16 Thumb MCP volar plate injury. A 58-year-old female after fall. Sagittal T2-weighted fat-suppressed sequence (**a**) reveals a complete avulsion of the distal volar plate from the proximal phalanx. The retracted volar plate (arrow) has intrasubstance edema and irregularity distally. There is avulsive osseous stress response (arrowhead) along the volar aspect of the proximal phalanx. Traumatic stripping involves the dorsal and volar joint capsule (dotted arrows). There is mild volar subluxation of the proximal phalanx. There was concomitant ulnar collateral ligament injury (not pictured), which categorized this as a grade II injury. Sagittal T2-weighted fat-suppressed image (**b**) shows a normal volar plate (arrow) for comparison

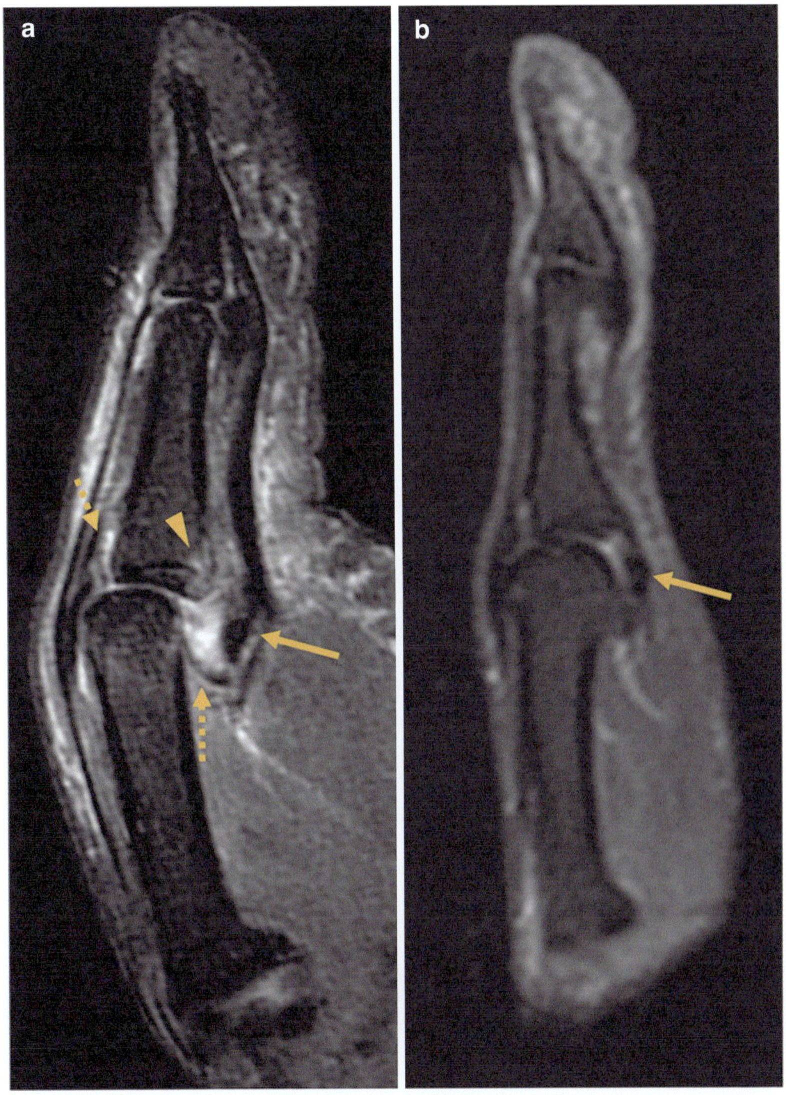

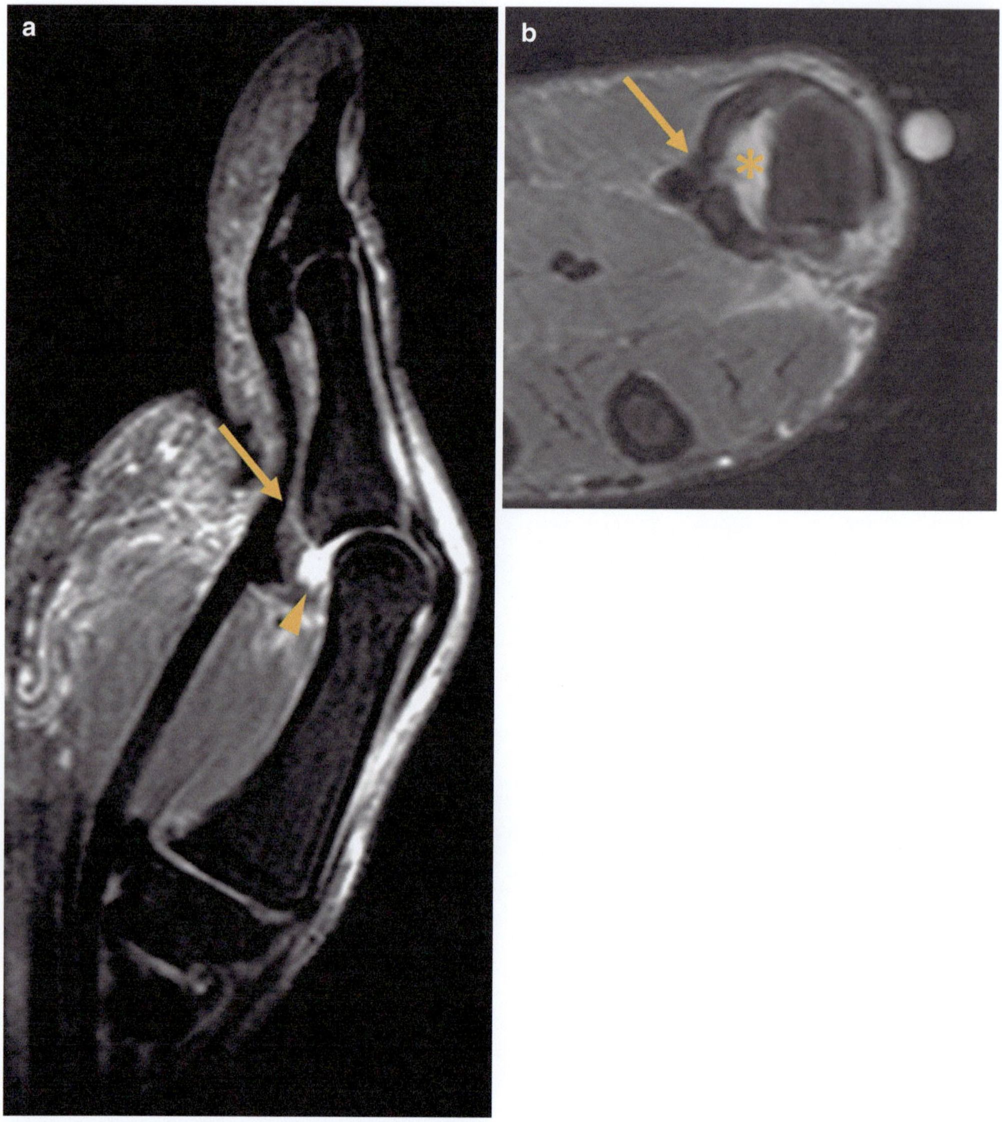

Fig. 12.17 Thumb MCP volar plate injury. A 28-year-old with volar plate avulsion following hyperextension injury playing sports. Sagittal T2-weighted fat-saturated sequence (**a**) shows complete discontinuity of the volar plate from the proximal phalanx (arrow) with marked posttraumatic joint fluid (arrowhead) displacing the plate volarly. This is compatible with a grade I volar plate injury. Findings are confirmed on T2-weighted fat-saturated axial sequence through the level of the sesamoids (**b**) which shows the sesamoids and flexor pollicis longus displaced volarly by the joint fluid (asterisk). There is edema within the volar plate (arrow), located between the sesamoids

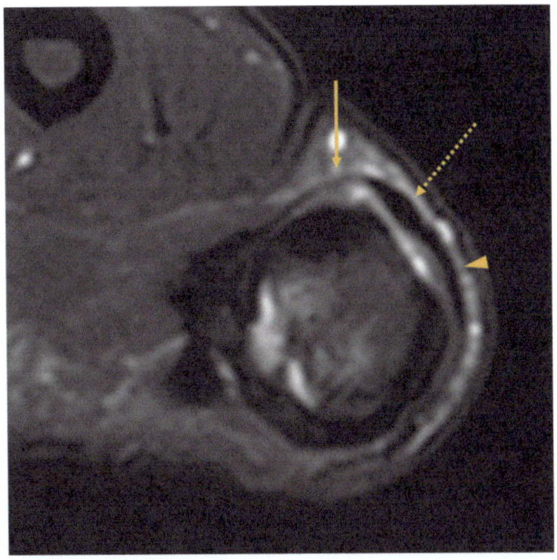

Fig. 12.18 Ulnar sagittal band sprain. At the level of the MCP joint, there is marked attenuation of the ulnar sagittal band (arrow), particularly relative to the radial sagittal band (arrowhead). Although there is no focal discontinuity of the band, there is moderate surrounding edema and attenuation. The extensor pollicis longus (dotted arrow) is in its normal eccentric position without subluxation. Findings support grade II sprain of the ulnar sagittal band

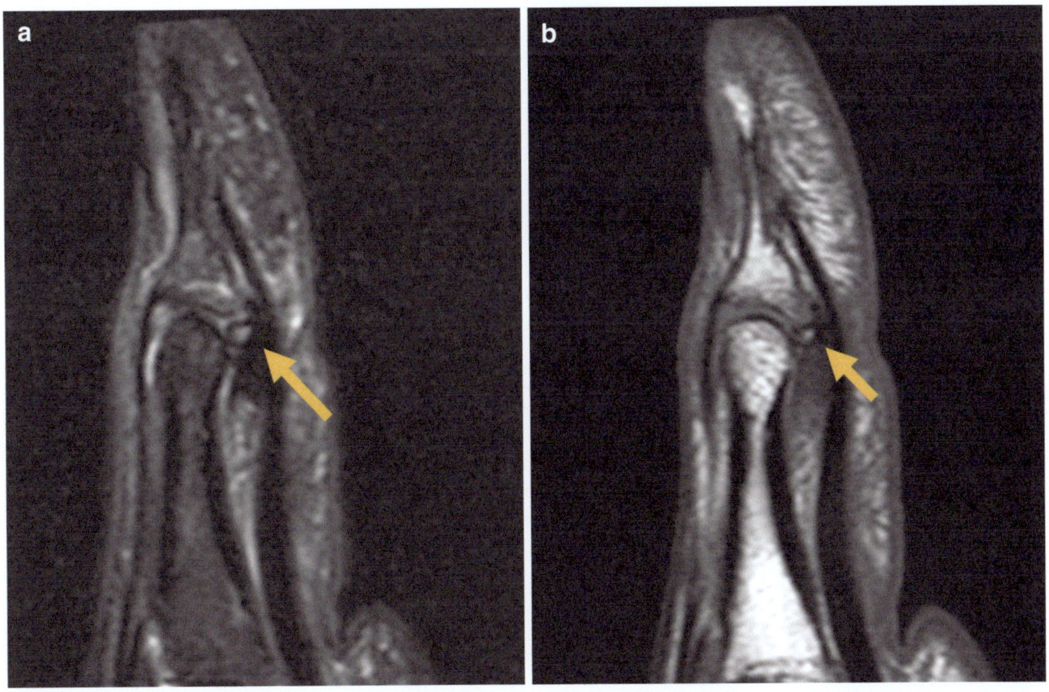

Fig. 12.19 Normal volar plate with sesamoid at the thumb interphalangeal joint. T2 fat-saturated sagittal sequence (**a**) and T1-weighted sagittal sequence (**b**) through the thumb interphalangeal joint demonstrating the normal volar plate, with the presence of a sesamoid (arrow), which is well corticated and not to be confused for an avulsive volar plate injury

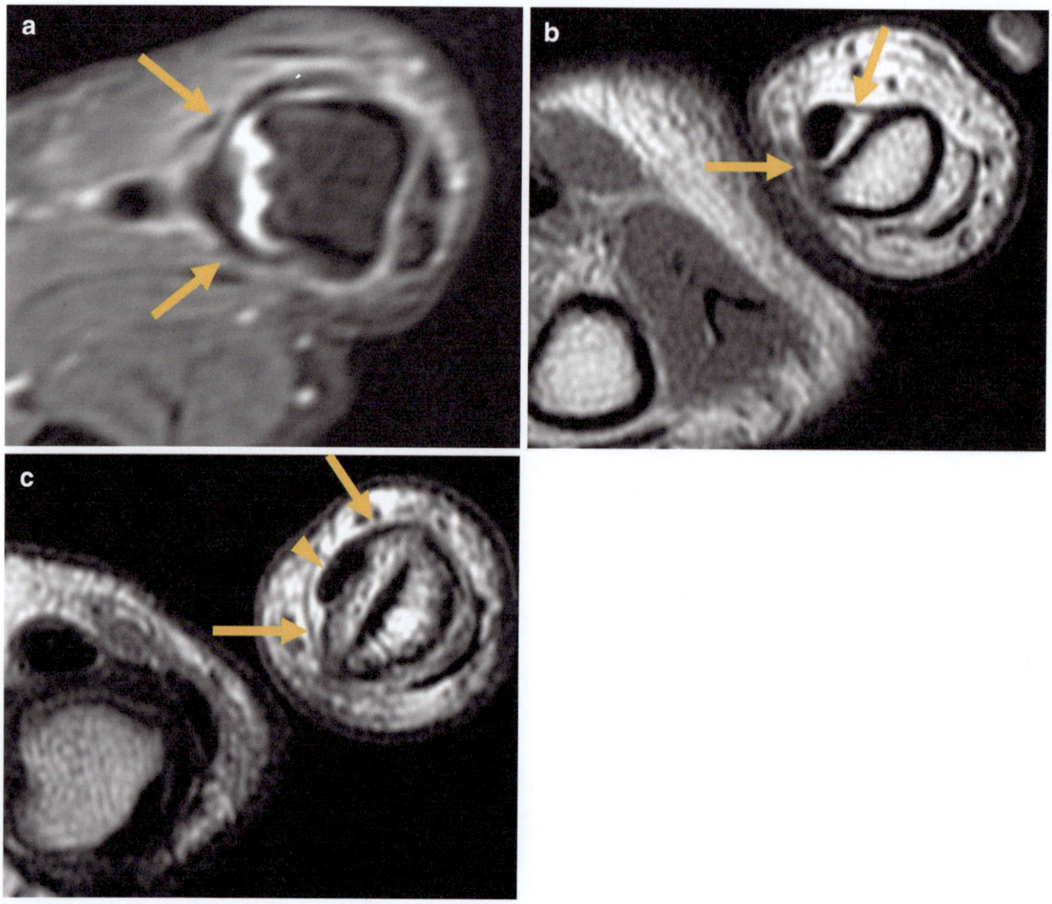

Fig. 12.20 Annular pulley system of the thumb. T2 fat-saturated axial sequence at the level of the MCP joint (**a**), just above the sesamoids, shows the A1 pulley (arrows) highlighted by the presence of a small joint effusion. T1 axial sequence at the mid-proximal phalanx (**b**) demonstrating the oblique pulley (arrows). T1 axial sequence at the level of the interphalangeal joint (**c**) showing the A2 pulley (arrows). At this level, the flexor pollicis longus (arrowhead) flattens out prior to inserting on the distal phalanx

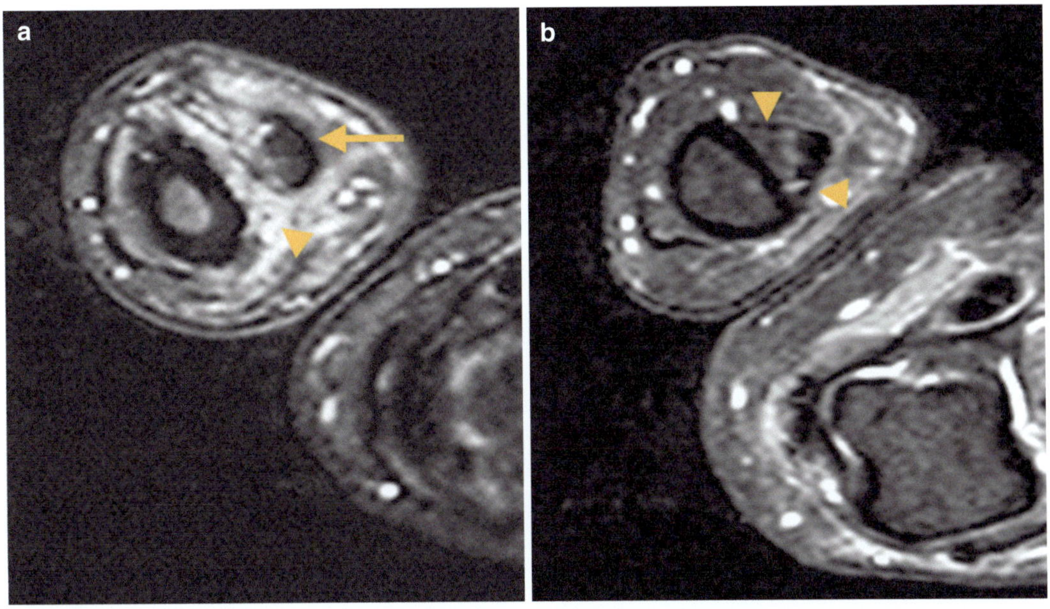

Fig. 12.21 Acute A2 pulley injury. T2-weighted axial sequence at the level of the mid-proximal phalanx demonstrating a completely torn A2 pulley (**a**). The fibers of the pulley are not clearly identified. There is bowstringing of the flexor pollicis longus tendon (arrow) with marked edema in the expected location of the pulley (arrowhead). Normal appearance of the oblique pulley (arrows) on a T2 fat-saturated axial sequence in a different patient (**b**). The fibers of the normal pulley should be dark and clearly delineated on T1 and T2 axial sequences

References

1. Rawat U, Pierce JL, Evans S, Chhabra AB, Nacey NC. High-resolution MR imaging and US anatomy of the thumb. Radiographics. 2016;36(6):1701–16. https://doi.org/10.1148/rg.2016160015.
2. Thumb CMC joint. Radsource, 1 July 2016. https://radsource.us/thumb-carpometacarpal-joint/. Accessed 18 Jun 2020.
3. Hirschmann A, Sutter R, Schweizer A, Pfirrmann CWA. MRI of the thumb: anatomy and spectrum of findings in asymptomatic volunteers. Am J Roentgenol. 2014;202(4):819–27. https://doi.org/10.2214/AJR.13.11397.
4. McCann MR, Rust PA, Wallace R. The stabilising effect of the anterior oblique ligament to prevent directional subluxation at the trapeziometacarpal joint of the thumb: a biomechanical cadaveric study. Arch Bone Jt Surg. 2018;6(2):105–11.
5. Carter KR, Nallamothu SV. Bennett fracture. In: StatPearls. Treasure Island (FL): StatPearls Publishing; 2021.
6. Feletti F, Varacallo M. Rolando Fractures. In: StatPearls. Treasure Island (FL): StatPearls Publishing; 2020.
7. Samora JB, Harris JD, Griesser MJ, Ruff ME, Awan HM. Outcomes after injury to the thumb ulnar collateral ligament--a systematic review. Clin J Sport Med Off J Can Acad Sport Med. 2013;23(4):247–54. https://doi.org/10.1097/JSM.0b013e318289c6ff.
8. Lark ME, Maroukis BL, Chung KC. The stener lesion: historical perspective and evolution of diagnostic criteria. Hand (N Y). 2017;12(3):283–9. https://doi.org/10.1177/1558944716661999.
9. Avery DM, Inkellis ER, Carlson MG. Thumb collateral ligament injuries in the athlete. Curr Rev Musculoskelet Med. 2017;10(1):28–37. https://doi.org/10.1007/s12178-017-9381-z.
10. Eaton RG, Malerich MM. Volar plate arthroplasty of the proximal interphalangeal joint: a review of ten years' experience. J Hand Surg Am. 1980;5(3):260–8. https://doi.org/10.1016/s0363-5023(80)80011-6.
11. Weintraub MD, et al. Avulsion injuries of the hand and wrist. Radiographics. 2020;40(1):163–80. https://doi.org/10.1148/rg.2020190085.
12. Jaibaji M, Rayan GM, Chung KW. Functional anatomy of the thumb sagittal band. J Hand Surg Am. 2008;33(6):879–84. https://doi.org/10.1016/j.jhsa.2008.01.039.

13 Hand Pathology: Nontraumatic

James Korf and M. K. Jesse

Arthritis

There are 27 bones and 27 joints in the hand. As with any synovial joint in the body, these joints are subject to osteoarthritis from the loss of articular cartilage and subsequent inflammatory response resulting in joint space narrowing, osteophytosis, and subchondral cystic change. While these findings are apparent and can be described with magnetic resonance (MR) imaging, radiography is typically the modality of choice to assess for the presence and degree of osteoarthritis. As such, MR imaging is more effectively utilized to identify and differentiate different forms of inflammatory arthritis, to guide treatment, and to prevent further secondary osteoarthritis.

Inflammatory Arthritis

Rheumatoid Arthritis

Rheumatoid arthritis is a common systemic inflammatory syndrome defined by polyarticular synovitis and autoantibodies [1]. It has an estimated prevalence of 1% of the adult population, with a steadily increasing incidence between the ages of 35 and 85 years old and is about twice as prevalent in women as in men [2]. Synovial inflammation from rheumatoid arthritis progresses with characteristic marginal osseous erosions and joint destruction; however, the rate of progression can vary widely. The diagnosis of rheumatoid arthritis is made by specific scoring criterion, which includes the number of joints involved, serologic factors, acute phase reactants, and chronicity of symptoms [3].

Given the clinical heterogeneity of the disease, imaging plays a role in establishing the diagnosis when the diagnosis is less certain, as well as characterizing the extent or progression of disease [4, 5]. As rheumatoid arthritis is primarily characterized by synovial inflammation, it follows that the hand is a prime location for the disease to manifest given its plethora of joints and synovial-lined tendon sheaths. Ultrasonography and radiography are widely available and affordable imaging modalities to establish and follow the degree of synovitis and osseous erosions, respectively. MR imaging serves as an excellent modality to obtain an overview of the carpus and fingers to assess for and qualitatively evaluate the presence of rheumatoid arthritis. MR imaging is also unique among other imaging modalities in that it can accurately assess for marrow edema within the subchondral bone, which is predictive of progression to osseous erosions [6].

J. Korf (✉) · M. K. Jesse
University of Colorado, Department of Radiology, Musculoskeletal Radiology and Intervention, Aurora, CO, USA
e-mail: James.Korf@cuanschutz.edu; Mary.Jesse@cuanschutz.edu

B. U. Casagranda (ed.), *MRI of the Upper Extremity*, https://doi.org/10.1007/978-3-030-81612-4_13

The hallmark for rheumatoid arthritis on MR imaging is the presence of synovitis. Synovitis will be most apparent on fat-saturated, fluid-sensitive, and post-gadolinium-enhanced images and appear as T2-isointense, enhancing frond-like material distending a synovial-lined space such as a joint or tendon sheath (Figs. 13.1 and 13.2) [7]. While these findings can manifest on non-contrast-enhanced sequences, intravenous gadolinium contrast administration improves the sensitivity and specificity for identifying synovitis and tenosynovitis [8]. Marrow edema and osseous erosive changes will occur and be more apparent in more advanced disease. These tend to occur at the margins of a joint where articular cartilage is the thinnest, and will be hyperintense on T2-weighted sequences, and may have peripheral or central enhancement depending on the size of erosion and presence of intervening tissue (Fig. 13.3). It is important to differentiate these pseudo-erosions such as intraosseous ganglia and synovial cysts [9]. Also, it is important to note the typical distribution of joints affected in the hand, which usually occurs proximal to distal, affecting the carpus and metacarpophalangeal joints prior to affecting the interphalangeal joints.

Psoriatic Arthritis and Peripheral Seronegative Spondyloarthropathy

Initially thought to be a subset of rheumatoid arthritis, Moll et al. first described the concept of seronegative spondyloarthropathy in the 1970s as a group of inflammatory arthritides including psoriatic arthritis, ankylosing spondylitis, reactive arthritis, and enteropathic spondylitis [10, 11]. The pathophysiology of these entities is not entirely understood, although there is a shared association with human leukocyte antigen B27 (HLA-B27) [12]. Contrary to the name, seronegative spondyloarthropathies can be subdivided into axial and peripheral subtypes depending on the location in the body primarily affected.

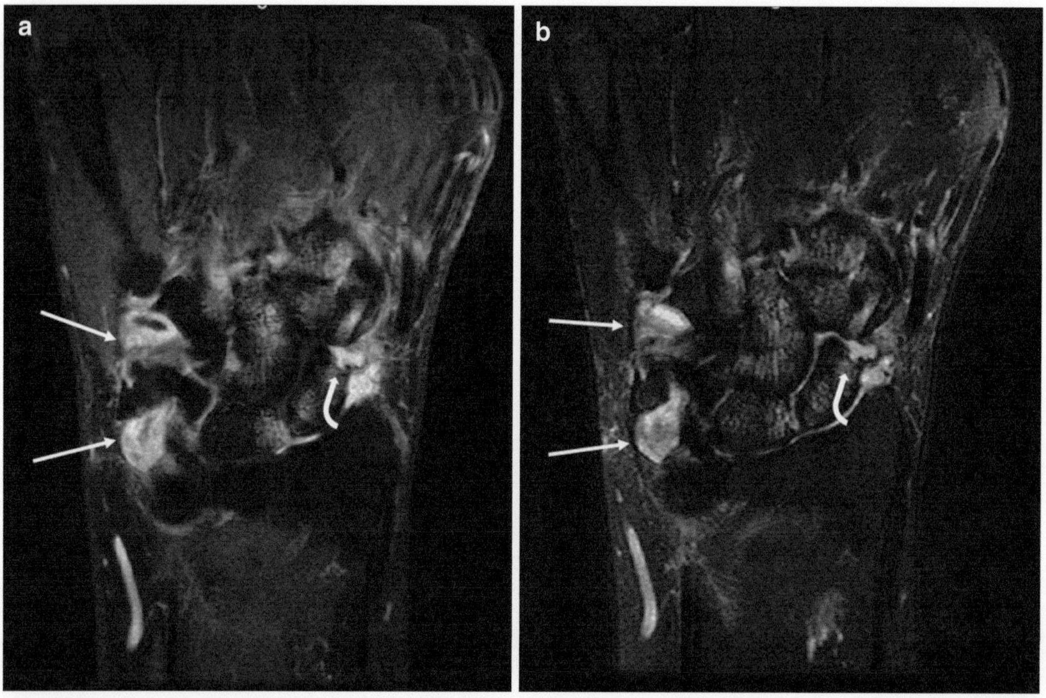

Fig. 13.1 Rheumatoid arthritis. Coronal T1 FS post-contrast (**a**) and coronal T2 STIR (**b**) MR images of the wrist in a patient with rheumatoid arthritis. Enhancing synovitis noted in the radiocarpal and midcarpal joints (arrows) with erosion in the distal scaphoid (arrowheads). Marrow edema and enhancement noted in the lunate and capitate bones

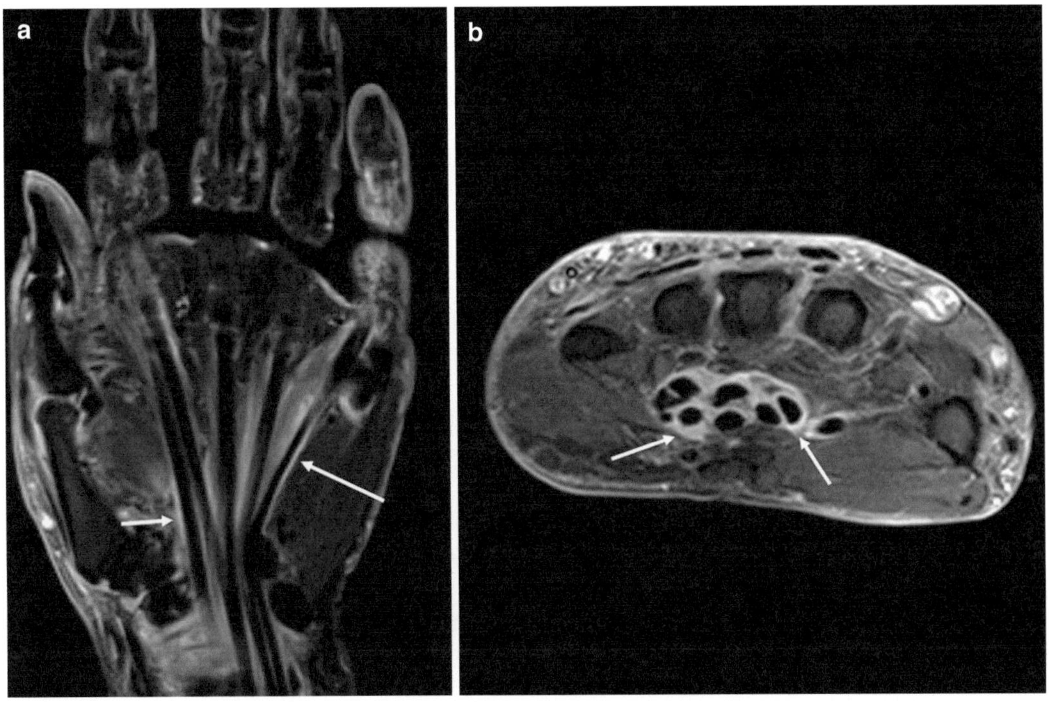

Fig. 13.2 Rheumatoid arthritis. Coronal (**a**) and axial (**b**) T1FS post-contrast images in a 68-year-old woman. Images reveal extensive tenosynovitis of the flexor tendons in the hand and wrist (arrows)

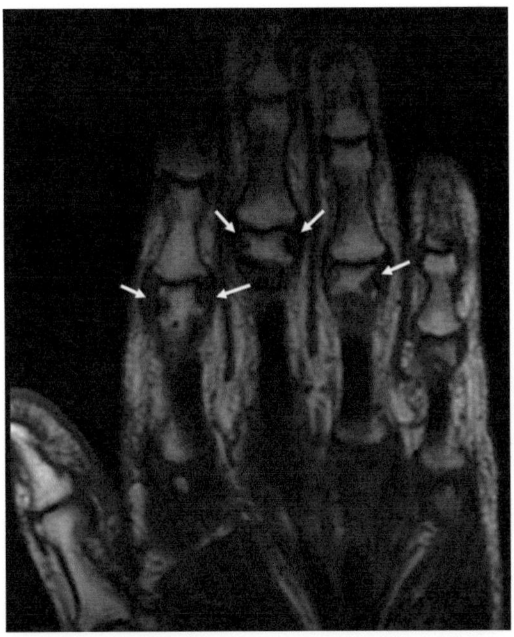

Fig. 13.3 Rheumatoid arthritis. Coronal T1-weighted MRI showing marginal erosions (arrows) of the proximal phalanges at the proximal interphalangeal joints in a patient with seropositive rheumatoid arthritis

Psoriatic arthritis is the most prevalent of the peripheral spondyloarthropathies, estimated between <0.1% and 0.4% [13]. Clinically the distinction of psoriatic arthritis from other peripheral seronegative spondyloarthropathies is made from the skin manifestations of psoriasis. The prevalence of psoriatic arthritis in patients with psoriasis is estimated at 13.8%, although some studies suggest there may be a higher subclinical prevalence [14, 15].

Understanding the entheseal region is critical to understanding the pattern of peripheral spondyloarthritis. The enthesis is the fibrocartilaginous transitional zone at the attachment site of ligament, tendon, or joint capsule to bone. Unlike rheumatoid arthritis, where inflammation is primarily a synovial-centered process, psoriatic arthritis pathology is centered on the enthesis. This pattern of inflammation informs the early imaging findings in psoriatic arthritis in the hand. MR imaging is particularly well suited to evaluate for and classify the findings in psoriatic arthritis as the findings may be subtle or occult radiographically early in the disease process [16].

The distribution of psoriatic arthritis tends to be monoarticular or oligoarticular early in the disease process, typically occurring in the smaller joints of the hands and fingers. MR imaging findings will demonstrate marrow edema and enhancement along the corner of a phalanx near a ligamentous or capsular attachment, reflecting the inflammation centered on the enthesis. There is often inflammation of the adjacent pericapsular and perienthetic soft tissues. Flexor tendon tenosynovitis and soft tissue edema throughout an entire digit can also occur resulting in dactylitis, a characteristic clinical finding (Fig. 13.4). Edema and enhancement can also extend along the adjacent periosteum resulting in a periostitis and eventually osseous proliferative change visible by radiography. It is also important to note any MR imaging findings of fingernail involvement, as the paronychia may help differentiate psoriatic arthritis from other spondyloarthropathies in patients with minor or occult skin manifestations of psoriasis [16].

In contradistinction from rheumatoid arthritis, marrow edema observed in joints affected by psoriatic arthritis does not necessarily progress into an osseous erosion. The osseous erosions seen in psoriatic arthritis tend to occur along the peripheral bare areas of a joint earlier in the disease process, although progression to the center of the joint space is commonly seen later in more advanced disease [17]. At later stages, there can also be ankylosis of the affected joint, dramatic subluxations, and classic pencil-in-cup deformities, which can be readily identified radiographically.

Crystalline Arthropathy and Crystal Deposition Disease

Gout

Gout is the most common inflammatory arthropathy in men and the most common crystalline arthropathy. Gout results from the supersaturation of uric acid and formation of monosodium urate crystals (MSU) in and around joints.

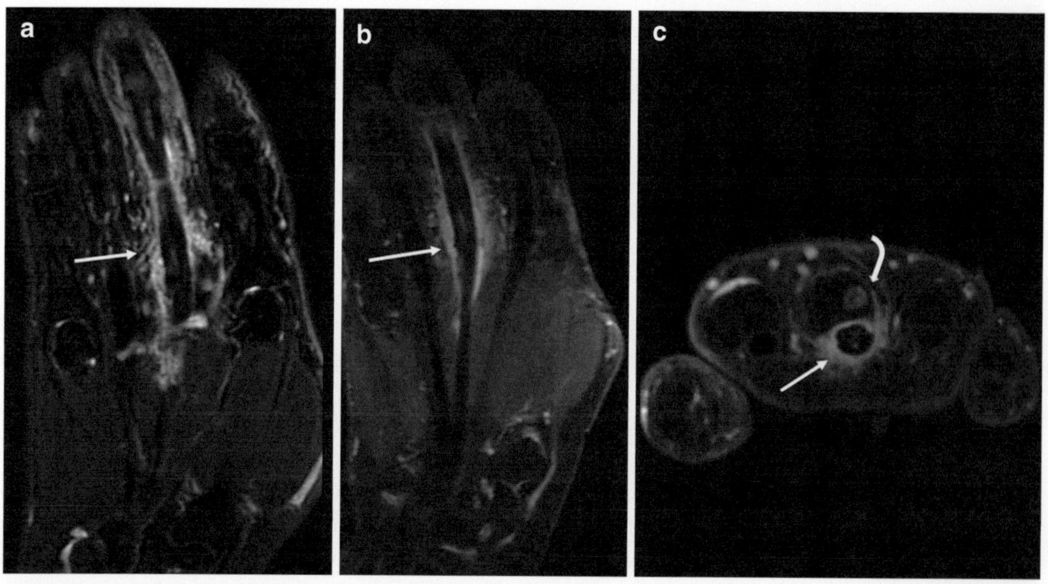

Fig. 13.4 Psoriatic arthritis. A 69-year-old woman presents with chronic hand pain and known history of psoriatic arthritis. Coronal T2FS (**a**), coronal T1FS post-contrast (**b**), and axial T1FS post-contrast (**c**) MR images demonstrating dactylitis with extensive peritendinous inflammation (arrows). Note the juxta-articular erosion in the proximal phalanx (curved arrow)

Epidemiologic studies have shown an increasing prevalence in recent history, increasing from 4.8/1000 in 1969 to ranging between 8.5 and 9.9/1000 since 1980 [18]. These studies have also established an understanding of the underlying etiologies predisposing for hyperuricemia including dietary factors, obesity, hypertension, renal dysfunction, and certain medications.

The diagnosis of gout is often made clinically with an acutely inflamed joint and elevated serum uric acid levels, subsequently confirmed with joint aspiration and identification of negatively birefringent needle-shaped crystals within synovial fluid with polarized microscopy. However, there are opportunities for false-negative results with this approach, as crystals may not be identifiable in approximately 25% of acute gout cases and serum uric acid may not be elevated in 42% of patients with acute gout attacks [19, 20]. Radiography has also been used often in the identification and characterization of gouty arthropathy, with characteristic juxta articular erosions and calcified tophi. But much like other arthropathies, the radiographic manifestations are often found late in the disease process [21]. As such, studies have suggested the overall quality of care for patients with gout is suboptimal [22]. Advanced imaging modalities such as dual-energy computed tomography (CT) and MR imaging have an increasing role in establishing the diagnosis earlier in the disease process.

MR imaging provides advantages in both soft tissue characterization and evaluation of deeper structures and joints which may be otherwise occult with radiography and ultrasound (US). The key finding in gout on MR imaging is the presence of tophi, which are the regions of concentrated MSU crystal deposition. Tophi can have a variable appearance on MR imaging. Most often tophi are intermediate signal intensity on T1-weighted sequences, with an intermediate or heterogeneously low signal on T2 and fluid-sensitive sequences. T2 signal characteristics have been described as more often variable as compared to T1, and the variance in low T1 and T2 signal is thought to be related to the degree of tophus calcification. Tophi can be homogeneously enhancing or show predominantly peripheral enhancement, which is attributed to the degree of surrounding and intervening inflammatory tissues (Fig. 13.5). There can be varying degrees of adjacent marrow and soft tissue edema and enhancement which reflects the amount of adjacent inflammation at the time of imaging [23].

Knowledge of the distribution patterns of gout in the hand and wrist can be useful in making the diagnosis by MR imaging. Traditional understanding of gout was focal concentric growth of a tophus, typically in a juxta-articular location, which would form the characteristic circumscribed erosion with overhanging edges. However, MSU crystal deposition can be multicompartmental with spread along adjacent tendon sheaths and fascial compartments, with diffuse soft tissue involvement described with advanced cases [23].

Calcium Pyrophosphate Deposition Disease

Calcium pyrophosphate deposition disease (CPPD) describes an array of disease processes related to the deposition of calcium pyrophosphate dihydrate crystals. The term "pseudogout syndrome" was first coined by Kohn et al. in 1962 after a series of cases aspirating synovial fluid from patient presenting with acute synovitis revealed rhomboid crystals with weakly positive birefringence in polarized microscopy, mimicking an acute gout flare [23]. These calcium pyrophosphate (CPP) crystals have since been recognized to contribute to a spectrum of disease ranging from asymptomatic deposition to a destructive arthropathy [24].

CPP crystals deposit in hyaline cartilage and fibrocartilaginous tissues of joints. In hyaline cartilage, these crystals form characteristic thin, fine calcifications, whereas when they deposit fibrocartilaginous structures such as the triangular fibrocartilage complex (TFCC) in the wrist, they can have a shaggy, irregular appearance. This calcification is termed chondrocalcinosis and is typically best seen radiographically or with CT. Asymptomatic presence of

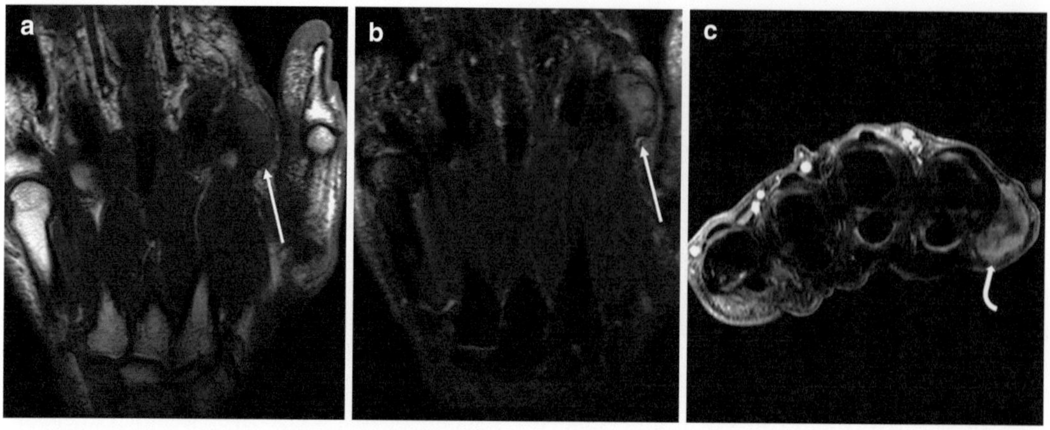

Fig. 13.5 Gout. A 70-year-old man presents with index finger pain. Coronal T1 (**a**), coronal T2FS (**b**), and axial T1FS post-contrast (**c**) MR images demonstrating a heterogeneous T1-isointense, mildly T2-hyperintense (arrows), and peripherally enhancing (curved arrow) tophus adjacent to the index finger metacarpophalangeal joint

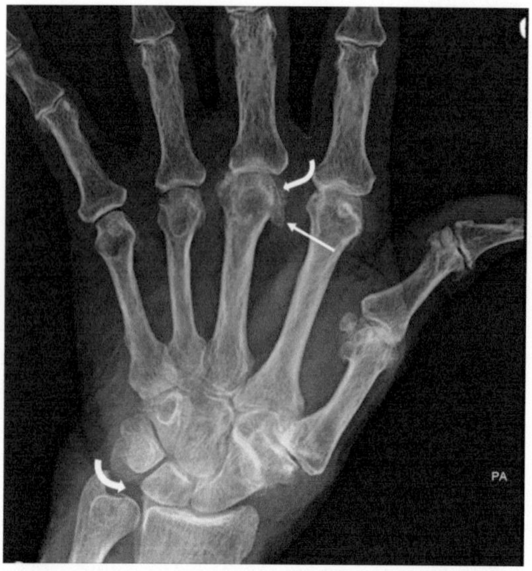

Fig. 13.6 CPPD arthropathy. Frontal radiograph of the hand demonstrating linear chondrocalcinosis of the triangular fibrocartilage and metacarpophalangeal joint capsule (curved arrows) with "hook osteophyte" formation from the long finger metacarpal head (arrow)

chondrocalcinosis is very common and increases with age [25]. Chondrocalcinosis as well as acute CPP arthritis has been associated with osteoarthritis, hyperparathyroidism, and use of loop diuretics [26].

Arthropathic changes related to CPPD mirror osteoarthritis but can be differentiated by their severe nature, with osseous destruction and characteristically large subchondral cyst formation, which are circumscribed and hyperintense on T2-weighted sequences. CPPD arthropathy has characteristic distribution and can affect weight-bearing and non-weight-bearing joints equally. In the hand, the metacarpophalangeal (MCP) joints are commonly affected with associated hooked osteophytes of the MCPs found to be a common radiographic finding (Fig. 13.6). In the wrist, CPP deposition has a predilection for the TFCC of the wrist, which can give it a heterogeneous signal on fluid-sensitive-weighted sequences. Studies have also shown a strong correlation between CPPD scapholunate advanced collapse (SLAC). CPPD of the hand is associated with and can be found in combination with arthropathy of hemochromatosis, although in these cases wrist manifestations are less frequently seen [27].

Hydroxyapatite (Basic Calcium Phosphate) Deposition Disease

Hydroxyapatite (HA) is the most common form of calcium phosphate in bone. The term basic calcium phosphate (BCP) refers to three types of calcium phosphate crystals, the most common of which is HA, although the terms are often used interchangeably. Hydroxyapatite deposition disease (HADD) was first described by McCarty et al. in 1966 as they described a series of patients with recurrent inflammatory syndromes within bursae, tendons, and joints with associated radiographically apparent "fluffy" calcifications, which they identified as HA crystals. The etiology for HA deposition is debated and not well understood. Prevailing theories suggest an underlying tendinous or capsular injury predisposing for mineral deposition [28, 29].

In the asymptomatic phase, this deposition forms large homogeneous and amorphous calcifications readily identified by radiography and differentiated from heterotopic ossification and sesamoid bone by their lack of cortication and trabecular bone pattern. While it is most often found in the shoulder, it can occur in any tendinous or joint capsular structure and frequently found in the wrist and hand. In the acute inflammatory setting, these deposits enter a resorptive phase where the calcification becomes less apparent radiographically and elicits a robust inflammatory calcific tendinitis or calcific periarthritis [28]. The symptoms can be severe in the acute setting, sometimes requiring hospitalization and mimicking an inflammatory or septic arthritis, and pose a diagnostic challenge given the less visible HA deposit radiographically. As with CPPD arthropathy, MR imaging is not the ideal modality for identifying subtle calcifications. However, given the acute presentation, it is not uncommon for an MR imaging to be obtained during the acute phase to evaluate for infection or other inflammatory conditions.

On MR imaging, the key findings will be focal low signal deposited along a joint capsule or tendon with surrounding inflammation. In the hand, this commonly occurs along the flexor carpi ulnaris tendon. HA deposits will have low signal on T1- and T2-weighted sequences, and the configuration will be amorphous or spiculated depending on the degree of resorption and configuration of the remaining HA deposit [27]. HA crystals can decompress into adjacent bursa or tendon sheaths and result in calcific bursitis or tendonitis. Occasionally these deposits can extend intraosseous or within the joint space and result in dramatic osseous erosions or a destructive arthritis; however, this has primarily been described in the shoulder [28].

Masses and Neoplastic Processes of the Hand

Soft Tissue Masses

Lumps and bumps of the hand and wrist are frequently encountered clinically, and the vast majority of them are benign. Primary soft tissue malignancies and metastases to the soft tissues are rare within the hand. In many cases, characteristic features with MR imaging can confirm a benign soft tissue mass diagnosis. However, given the nonspecific imaging findings of low-grade sarcomas, histopathologic correlation may be required with certain solid-enhancing masses.

Ganglia and Synovial Cysts

The distinction between synovial cysts and ganglion cysts is histologic. Ganglion cysts are pseudocysts, with a predominantly acellular fibrous wall containing few fibroblastic cells, whereas synovial cysts are true cysts with a synovial cellular lining. While the histologic distinction may imply a difference in etiology, their imaging and clinical manifestations are essentially identical, and the difference is mostly academic from a radiologic perspective. Ganglion and synovial cysts are common and together account for 60% of all hand masses [30]. They can occur at any age but are found most frequently between the ages of 20 and 40 years old, and there is an approximately 2–3:1 female predominance. The etiology of ganglia is not well understood. They mostly occur spontaneously; however, 15% of patients with ganglia report a prior injury [30, 31]. Because of these features, multiple theories of their etiology exist. Contrast injections of joint spaces and ganglion cysts have shown a one-way communication between the joint space and the ganglion cysts, suggesting a unidirectional valve mechanism. Others theorize an underlying capsular injury or degeneration with leakage of synovial fluid, with fibrous reaction of the adjacent tissues and subsequent ganglion formation [31].

US is often successful in the initial interrogation of a suspected ganglion secondary to the superficial location and cystic nature of the mass.

MR imaging can be subsequently utilized when the anechoic nature of a cyst is not demonstrated sonographically, typically with small cysts or with cysts with desiccated internal contents. MR imaging can also further characterize surrounding inflammatory change, mass effect on nearby neurovascular structures, intraosseous extension, as well as the deeper originating synovial or tenosynovial structure when it is not apparent sonographically. The imaging features of a cyst on MR include a well-circumscribed, T2-hyperintense cystic mass with a tail extending to the underlying joint or tendon sheath, with thin peripheral enhancement.

Ganglion and synovial cysts can arise from any articulation or tendon sheath. In the wrist, they are broadly divided into volar and dorsal ganglions, each with implications on potential interventions. Dorsal ganglia are more common, comprising of 57–70% of cysts within the hand and wrist, typically arising from the scapholunate interval and extending through the dorsal capsule. Volar cysts comprise of 13–20 of hand and wrist ganglions and are the second most common location. Volar cysts are more amenable to aspiration, whereas dorsal ganglion cysts are more likely to recur after aspiration and typically require surgical resection if treatment is necessary due to functional impairment or impingement on neurovascular structures. Mucous cysts refer to a specific ganglion or synovial cyst arising from the dorsal interphalangeal joint of the fingers. These tend to occur in older patients and can extend distally and result in deformity of the nail bed (Fig. 13.7). Like dorsal ganglion cysts, these are likely to recur with aspiration and typically require surgical resection when intervention is necessary [31].

Epidermal Inclusion Cysts

Epidermal inclusion cysts or epidermal cysts are epithelial-lined cystic structures centered within the dermis and subcutaneous tissues containing epidermal and keratin debris. They can arise from several mechanisms, including from displaced remnant ectodermal tissues, traumatic or surgical implantation of epidermal tissue, or occlusion of the pilosebaceous unit. Their

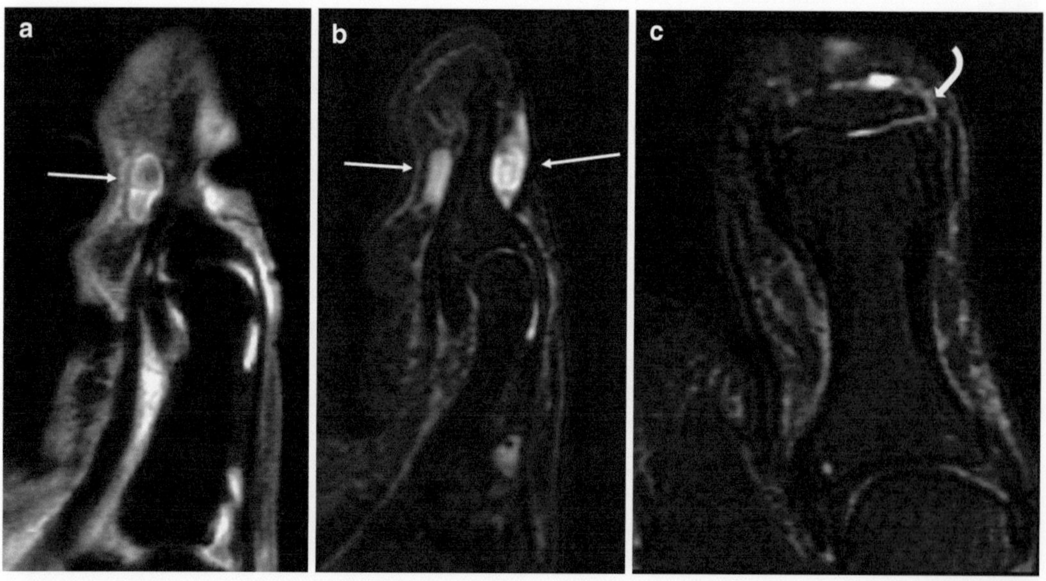

Fig. 13.7 Ganglion cyst. Sagittal T1FS post-contrast (**a**), sagittal T2FS (**b**), and coronal T2FS (**c**) MRI images of a mucous (ganglion) cyst arising from the thumb interphalangeal joint, with extension along the distal phalanx and subungual involvement (arrows). Note the thin T2 tail extending to the radial side of the thumb interphalangeal joint (curved arrow)

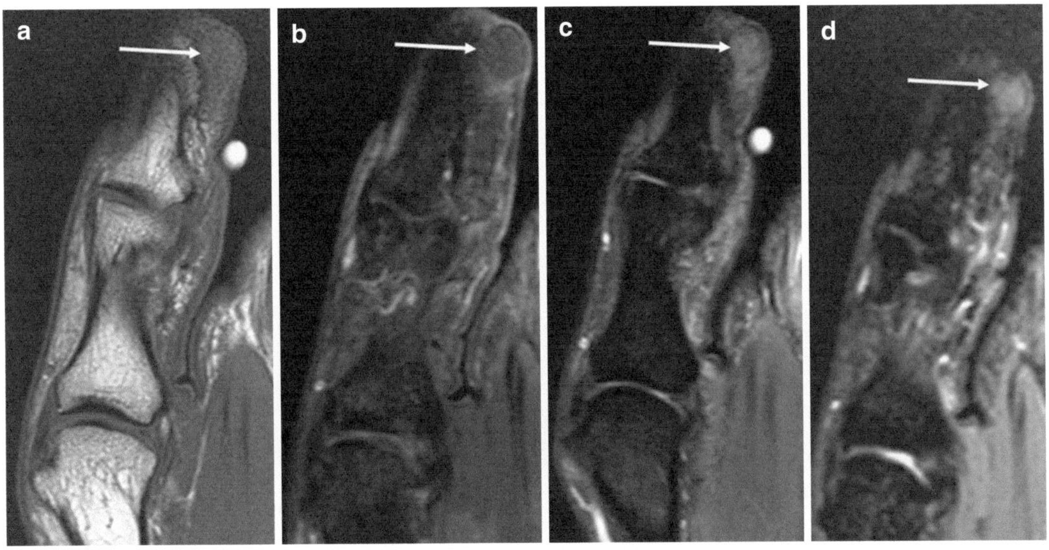

Fig. 13.8 Epidermal inclusion cyst. Sagittal T1 (**a**), T1FS post-contrast (**b**), T2FS (**c**), and GRE (**d**) sequences demonstrate a round, homogeneous mass with minimal thin peripheral enhancement

appearance on MR imaging can vary depending on whether the cyst has ruptured. When unruptured, they appear as a well-defined, peripherally enhancing round, or ovoid mass centered in the dermal tissues (Fig. 13.8). The internal signal characteristics depend on the nature of its internal contents. Typically epidermoid cysts have hyperintense internal signal on T2-weighted sequences, although there can be variable heterogeneously low T2 signal when the internal contents are dense or calcified. The internal signal on T1-weighted sequences can also vary from homogeneously hypointense to heterogeneously hyperintense, which is likely related to the degree of internal proteinaceous material. When the cyst ruptures in these, they can mimic a solid mass. The mural enhancement can become thick and shaggy, with enhancing internal septations. The internal intrinsic signal on T1- and T2-weighted sequences shows similar variation to their unruptured counterparts and depends on the nature of the internal contents [32]. Malignant degeneration to squamous cell carcinoma has been recorded in 2.2% of resected cysts, and this possibility should be considered with an irregular ruptured cyst or in the setting of cyst recurrence [33].

Fat-Containing Masses

Lipomatous masses are the most frequently encountered soft tissue masses clinically, and lipomas are the most common benign lipomatous mass [34]. While relatively less common compared to other locations in the body, lipomas are a common solid tumor of the hand [35]. They often occur between fifth and seventh decades and are divided into superficial or deep [34]. Superficial lipomas are located in the subcutaneous tissues, whereas deep lipomas may be intramuscular or along the deep investing fascia. MR imaging can localize relevant anatomy prior to resection. Lipomas are round or ovoid circumscribed masses which follow fat signal on all sequences (Figs. 13.9 and 13.10). They may contain a few thin internal and enhancing septa.

As with other malignancies, liposarcoma of the hand is exceedingly rare. Features concerning for malignancy in lipomatous lesions would mirror liposarcoma elsewhere in the body, with thickened enhancing septa or focal mass-like enhancing components within or adjacent to a lipomatous mass. If encountered, these areas should be the target for biopsy to avoid a false-negative result from sampling error.

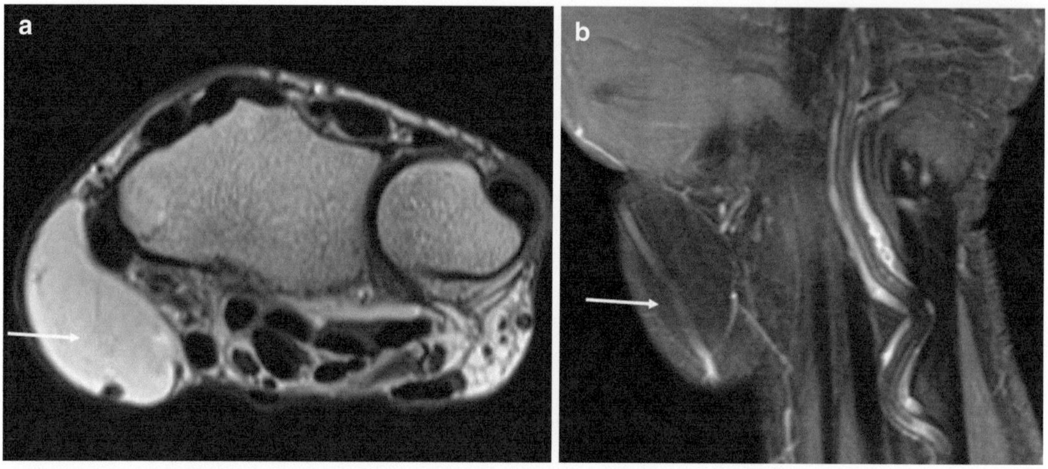

Fig. 13.9 Lipoma. Axial T1 (**a**) and coronal T1FS post-contrast (**b**) sequences show a lipoma (arrows) within the radial subcutaneous tissues of the hand, with minimal thin internal septations and following fat signal on all sequences

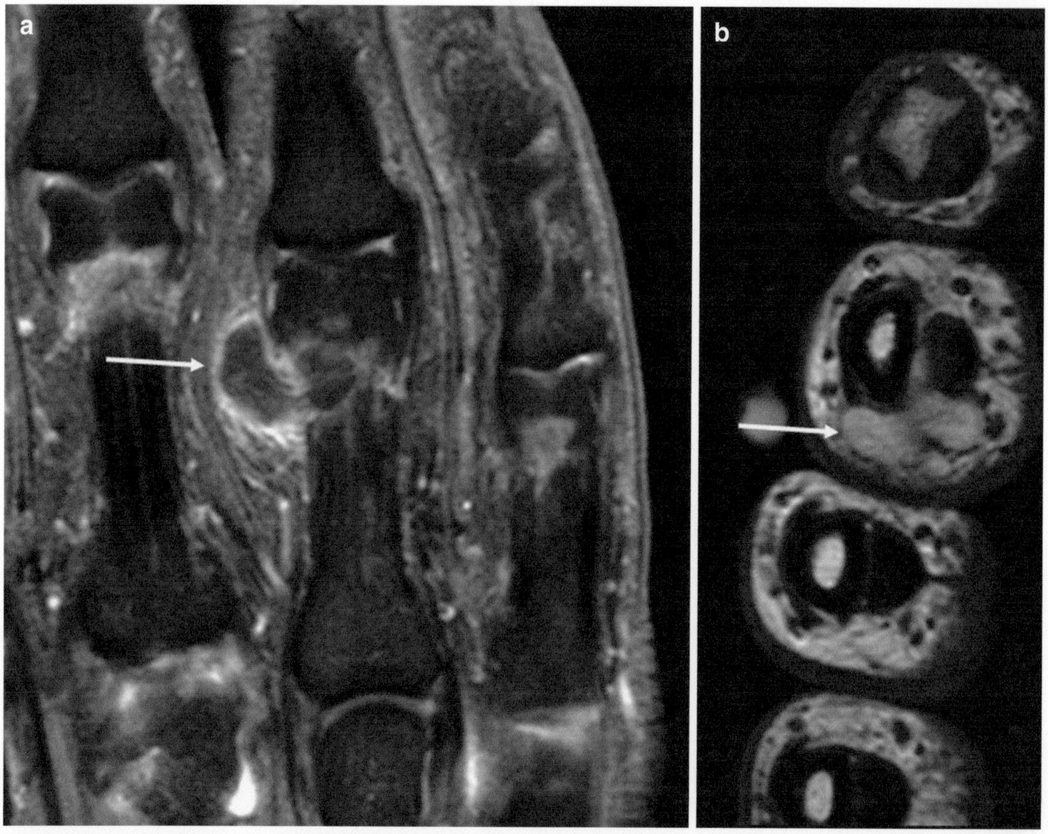

Fig. 13.10 Parosteal lipoma. Coronal T1FS post-contrast (**a**) and axial T1 (**b**) sequences reveal a parosteal lipoma within the subcutaneous tissues of the ring finger. Notice the thin enhancing peripheral capsule (arrow)

Hemangiomas and Vascular Malformations

Hemangiomas and vascular malformations include a heterogeneous grouping of benign vascular tumors and anomalies containing disorganized vascular elements with intermixed nonvascular mesenchymal elements. The International Society for the Studies of Vascular Anomalies now categorizes these lesions as "vascular tumors" for infantile hemangiomas, "low-flow vascular malformations" for venous and lymphatic malformations, and "high-flow vascular malformations" for arteriovenous malformations (AVMs) [36].

Low-flow vascular malformations are a relatively common soft tissue masses representing approximately 7% of all benign soft tissue masses [37]. Clinically these present as waxing and waning ill-defined palpable masses. On MR imaging, they are typically multilobulated with multiple internal T2-hypointense fibrous septa and can be found in subcutaneous or intramuscular locations. T1-weighted sequences reveal the signal to be generally low, with variable degrees of T1 hyperintensity. While these features are relatively nonspecific, some findings on MR imaging can help differentiate hemangiomas from malignant soft tissue neoplasms. Given their vascular nature, they contain increased water content from stagnant blood resulting in marked T2-hyperintense signal as well as avid post-contrast enhancement (Fig. 13.11). Phleboliths, which have a round hypointense appearance on T2-weighted and gradient echo sequences, are also associated with venous malformation [37]. Other case series have described atrophy of adjacent muscular and osseous structures in vascular malformations. The etiology for this is not delineated but may be related to altered perfusion of adjacent normal structures in the region [38, 39].

AVMs typically manifest clinically in late childhood or early adulthood. The key MR imaging finding is the presence of a serpentine nidus of feeding arteries and draining veins. These will typically appear as flow voids on gradient echo sequences and enhance on

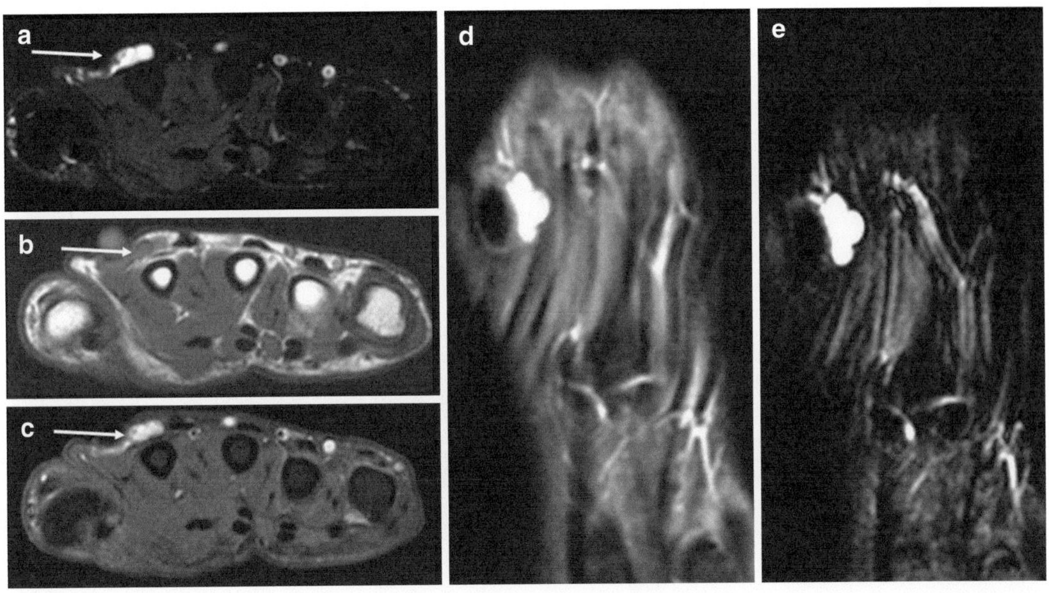

Fig. 13.11 Small soft tissue hemangioma. Axial T2FS (**a**), T1 pre-contrast (**b**) and T1FS post-contrast (**c**), and coronal T1FS post-contrast (**d**) and T2FS (**e**) sequences show a lobular markedly T2-hyperintense and avidly enhancing mass (arrows)

post-contrast sequences (Fig. 13.12). Contrast-enhanced and MR arteriography techniques can be used to delineate the involved arterial supply and venous drainage pathways before conventional angiographic imaging and therapies are performed [36]. Teo et al. also found that targetoid areas of central T2 hypointensity, which they theorized could be thrombosed vascular elements, were also found to be more common in hemangiomas [38].

Glomus Tumors

Glomus tumors are typically benign hamartomatous masses arising from the specialized neuromyo-arterial glomus body involved in thermoregulation. Seventy-five percent of glomus tumors occur in the hand, with 65% of those occurring in the fingertips, with a preponderance for the subungual space. Glomus tumors represent between 1% and 4.5% of all hand masses and typically occur between fourth and sixth decades. These clinically most often present with painful, temperature-sensitive masses in the fingers and can have discoloration of the nail bed. On radiographs, they often show scalloped erosion of the adjacent distal phalanx. MR imaging will reveal small round or oval masses with signal characteristics reflecting their vascular nature with homogeneous T1-hypointense and marked T2-hyperintense signal as well as avid homogeneous post-contrast enhancement (Fig. 13.13) [40].

Peripheral Nerve Sheath Tumors and Other Neural Masses

Benign peripheral nerve sheath tumors (PNST) include both schwannomas and neurofibromas. In the hand, they share similar imaging features, typically appearing as a fusiform mass growing along the distribution of a nerve. Although PNST signal characteristics are generally nonspecific, the following MR imaging findings can help distinguish PNST from other solid masses. On T2-weighted sequences, PNST can show a “target sign,” which is a central fibrous region with low T2 signal surrounded by a ring of myxoid T2-hyperintense material (Fig. 13.14). Identifying the presence of neural fascicles within or alongside the mass, also

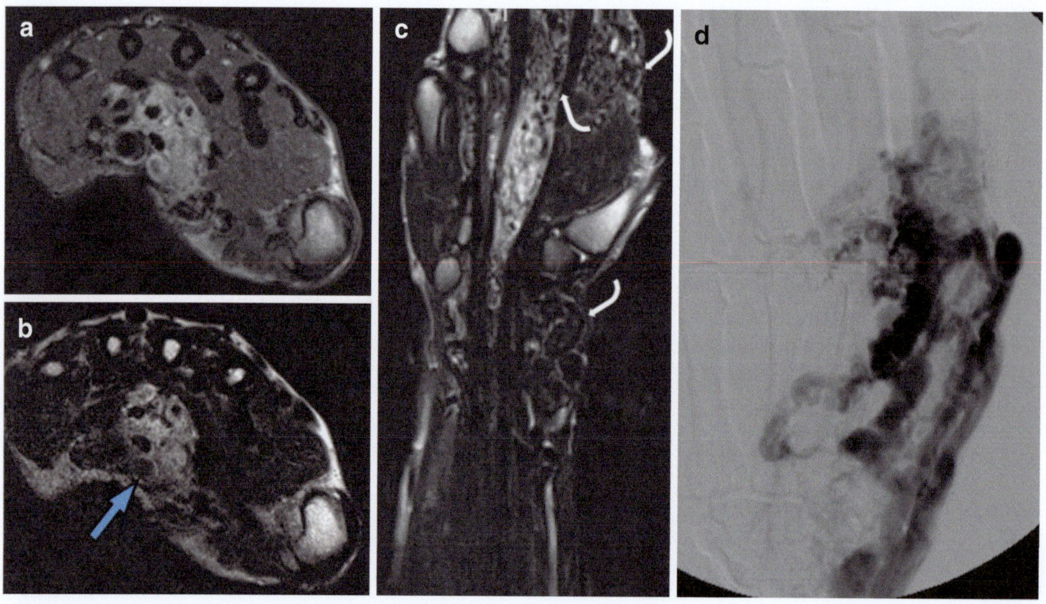

Fig. 13.12 Large arteriovenous malformation. Axial T1 post-contrast (**a**), axial T2 (**b**), coronal T2 (**c**), and digital subtraction angiography (**d**) showing arterial supply from the radial artery with a large nidus of tortuous vessels. Note the serpiginous flow voids on T2 sequences (curved arrows) and targetoid central T2 hypointensity (blue arrow)

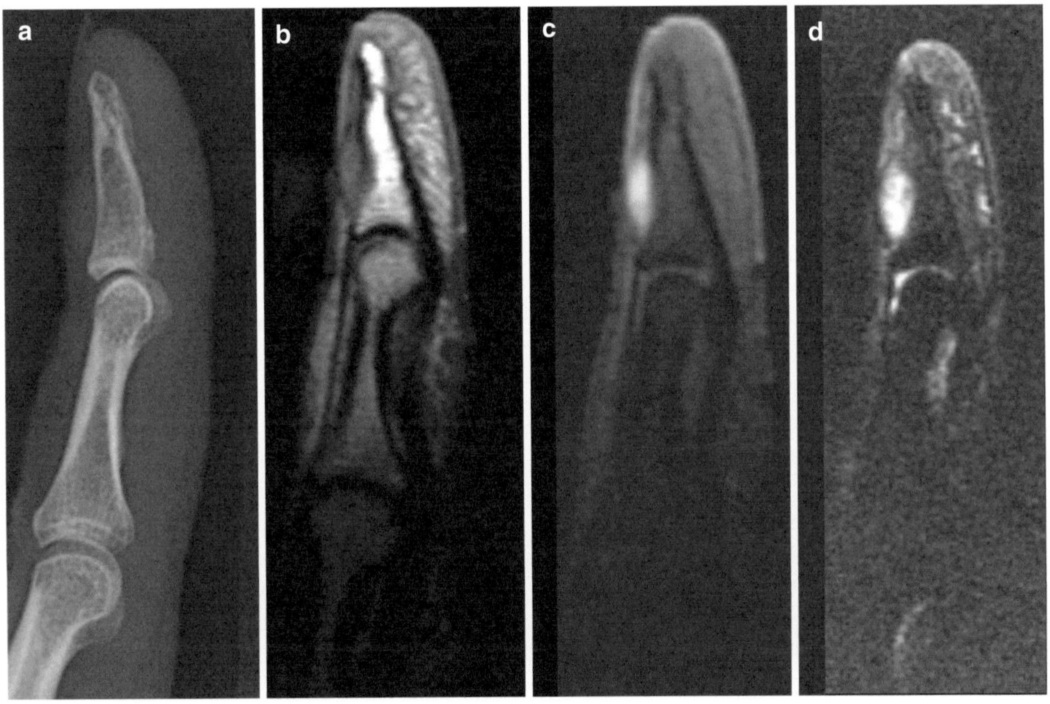

Fig. 13.13 Glomus tumor. Lateral radiograph (**a**), sagittal T1 (**b**), T1FS post-contrast (**c**), and T2FS (**d**) showing a subungual soft tissue mass of the distal phalanx. Glomus tumors demonstrate uniform T2 hyperintensity and enhancement

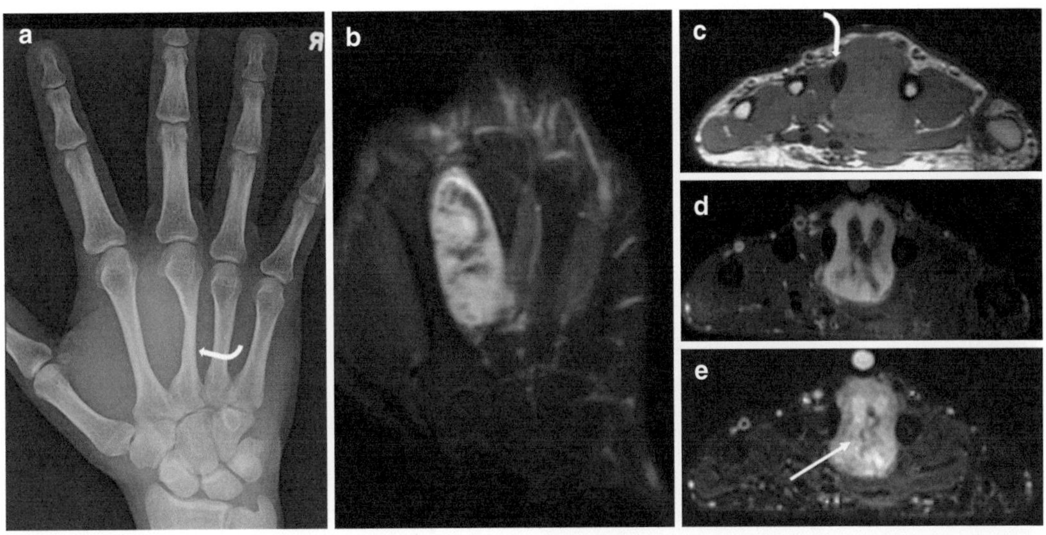

Fig. 13.14 Peripheral nerve sheath tumor. Frontal radiograph (**a**) and coronal T1FS post-contrast (**b**) sequence showing a fusiform mass extending along a distal branch of the radial nerve. Axial T1 (**c**), T1FS post-contrast (**d**), and T2FS (E) sequences along the central portion of the mass. Note the targetoid centrally T2-hypointense signal (arrow) on axial sequences and smooth remodeling of the adjacent metacarpal (curved arrows)

termed the "fascicular sign," can be an additional clue that a solid mass is a peripheral nerve sheath tumor. Also, the presence of peripheral fat, usually best identified on T1-weighted sequences, suggests the mass arises in an intermuscular space and is often seen with PNSTs arising along a neurovascular bundle. Malignant PNSTs are typically found more centrally in the body, although cases of malignant PNST in the hand have been reported. Malignant PNST share similar features to their benign counterparts but are often larger in size and show more irregular features such as prominent central necrosis and thickened, irregular margins extending proximally and distally along the affected nerve [41].

Pacinian corpuscles are neurologic mechanoreceptors and a normal anatomic structure to encounter in the hand. They are normally located in the subcutaneous tissues near the metacarpophalangeal joints. On MR imaging, they are small round or ovoid foci which demonstrate high signal on T2-weighted sequences (Fig. 13.15). Familiarity with their appearance on MR imaging is important as to not mistake them for a pathologic process [42].

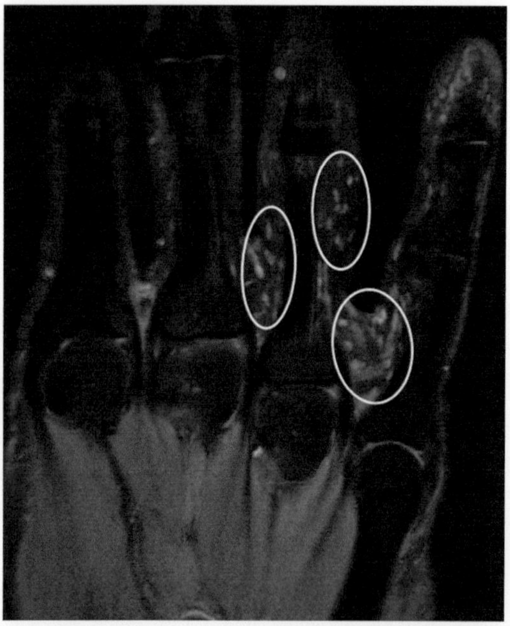

Fig. 13.15 Pacinian corpuscles. T2FS sequence showing numerous subcutaneous Pacinian corpuscles (circles), a normal anatomic structure

Fibroma of the Tendon Sheath and Palmar Fibromatosis

Fibromas of the tendon sheath in the hand are composed of tightly packed spindle cells surrounded by collagen. They are slow-growing, painless masses typically occurring between 20 and 50 years of age and occur approximately three times more commonly in men [43]. Fibromas are often found along the flexor tendons in the hand and are typically oval or round well-defined masses. MR imaging characteristics include homogeneously hypointense on T1- and T2-weighted sequences with little to no enhancement; however, enhancement and T2 signal can vary depending on degrees of internal cellularity and myxoid change histologically [43].

Palmar fibromatosis, also called Dupuytren's disease or Dupuytren's contractures, is a superficial fibromatosis that shares some imaging and histologic features with tendon sheath fibromas. However, palmar fibromatosis is a distinct clinical entity, found more commonly in men, with ill-defined fibrous proliferation occurring along the palmar aponeurosis, eventually forming chord-like extensions along the flexor tendons of the fingers and resulting in significant morbidity and loss of function. The signal characteristic with palmar fibromatosis also varies depending on the cellular content of the lesion, with increased intensity on both T1- and T2-weighted sequences noted with increasing cellularity (Fig. 13.16). It is also notable that recurrence of palmar fibromatosis after resection is higher in more cellular variants [44].

Tenosynovial Giant Cell Tumor

Also termed pigmented villonodular synovitis (PVNS) and tenosynovitis (PVNTS), synovial giant cell tumors are a benign neoplastic process of the synovium that can involve joints, bursa, or tendon sheaths. The intra-articular

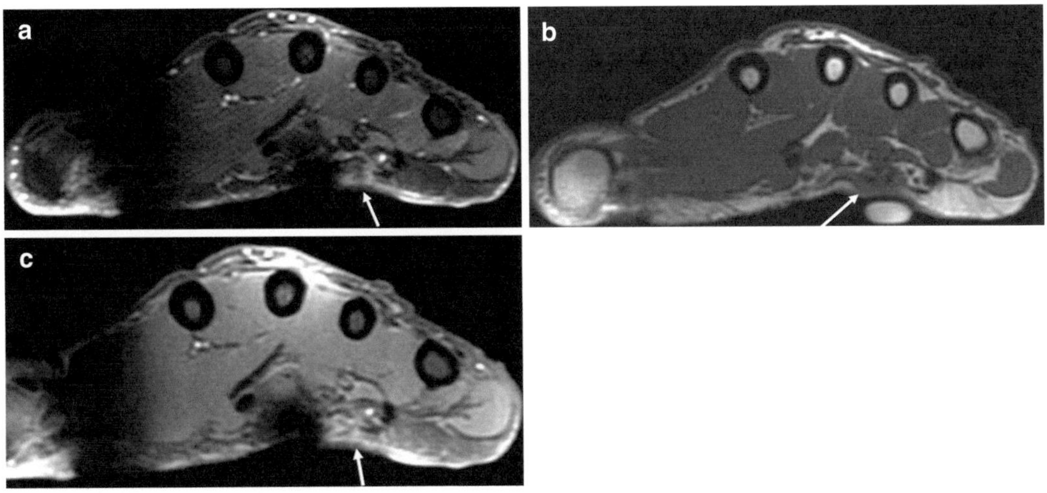

Fig. 13.16 Palmar fibromatosis (Dupuytren's disease). Axial T2 FS (**a**), T1 (**b**), and T1FS post-contrast (**c**) sequences of the hand showing a T1-hypointense, T2-hyperintense, and enhancing focus of fibromatosis (arrows) in a patient with clinically apparent Dupuytren's contractures

form has a predilection for large joints, and the tenosynovial form is much more frequently encountered in the hand. Approximately 65–89% of cases of tenosynovial giant cell tumor can be found within the hand and wrist. Histologically, there is villonodular synovial proliferation containing mononuclear histiocytoid cells, giant cells, and lipid-laden macrophages with associated hemosiderin deposition [45].

Tenosynovial giant cell tumors manifest as lobular mass lesions found along the tendon sheaths of the hand and can be described as localized when singular or diffuse when the extent is multifocal or extensive. They often have intermediate to low signal on T1- and T2-weighted sequences. There tends to be greater variability on T2-weighted sequences depending on the degree of hemosiderin deposition and relative presence of lipid-laden macrophages. Likewise, the degree of susceptibility and blooming artifact on GRE sequences varies based on the presence of hemosiderin deposition, which is typically more a feature of the intra-articular version. Associated erosions are characteristically smooth and saucer-like involving the adjacent osseous structures, which can be apparent radiographically (Fig. 13.17) [45].

Desmoid Fibromatosis (Desmoid Tumor)

Desmoid fibromatosis (DF) goes by several names, including desmoid tumor and aggressive fibromatosis. DF are rare locally aggressive fibroblastic neoplasms. Most of the masses are sporadic; however, they are associated with familial adenomatous polyposis (FAP), termed Gardner's syndrome when found in combination. DF does not metastasize, but its locally aggressive features and penchant for local recurrence after surgical resection can lead to significant morbidity in the extremities and hand [46].

MR imaging of DF typically reveals a round mass with a peripheral stellate appearance, which reflects the tendrils of invading tumor extending into local soft tissues [47]. Signal characteristics of DF vary reflecting the variable proportional composition of spindle cells and extracellular elements. In general, T1 signal tends to be isointense to the skeletal muscle, and T2 signal ranges from isointense to hyperintense relative to the skeletal muscle. A central nonenhancing, T2-hypointense band is present in 60–90% of DF formed of dense collagen and stromal bands (Fig. 13.18) [46].

There are wide varieties of treatment options for DF which are often used in combination. First-

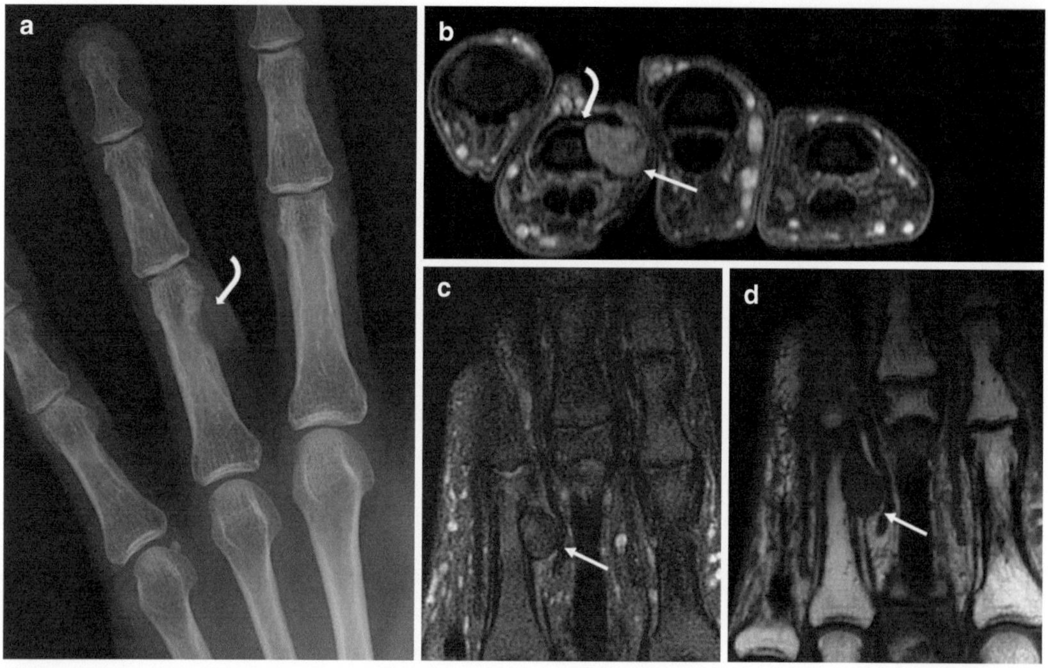

Fig. 13.17 Tenosynovial giant cell tumor. Frontal radiograph showing a typical saucer like erosion along the ring finger proximal phalanx (**a**). Corresponding MRI with axial T1FS post-contrast (**b**), coronal T2FS (**c**), and coronal T1 (**d**) sequences showing a round T1- and T2-hypointense mass with mild diffuse enhancement arising from the ring finger tendon sheath (arrows)

line treatment is typically a wide surgical excision; however, recurrence rate is high. Targeted chemotherapies and hormonal therapies can be employed to reduce the tumor burden prior to resection. Radiation therapy can also be used when surgical resection is otherwise prohibited. Localized therapy with percutaneous cryoablation is an emerging and promising therapy to achieve local control with minimal morbidity [48].

Nodular (Pseudosarcomatous) Fasciitis

Nodular fasciitis is an inflammatory pseudoneoplastic and self-limiting process that preferentially occurs in the upper extremities. Histologically, it appears similar to reparative tissues with proliferation of thin spindle cells demonstrating high mitotic activity, although lacking the cellular atypia found in sarcomatous neoplasms. The imaging features are nonspecific and can also mimic neoplasm with T1 signal isointense or hypointense to skeletal muscle, heterogeneous signal on T2 sequences, and typically diffuse but inhomogeneous enhancement [49]. Histopathologic correlation is necessary to establish the diagnosis. The self-limiting nature and lack of recurrence for nodular fasciitis are an important clinical feature. In patients with apparent recurrence of previously diagnosed nodular fasciitis, it is recommended the initial pathology be reviewed [50].

Primary Soft Tissue Sarcomas of the Hand

Primary soft tissue sarcomas of the hand are rare. The diagnosis is typically made histologically, often after excisional biopsy or when percutaneous core biopsy is pursued prior to resection. There are a few sarcoma subtypes which tend to occur in the distal extremities and can be found in the hand.

Acral myxoinflammatory fibroblastic sarcoma (AMFS) is a low-grade sarcoma typically found in the distal extremities. It typically presents as a slow-growing, painless mass. AMFS has been described to be an ovoid mass with well-defined borders and on MR imaging shows high signal on T2-weighted sequences, low

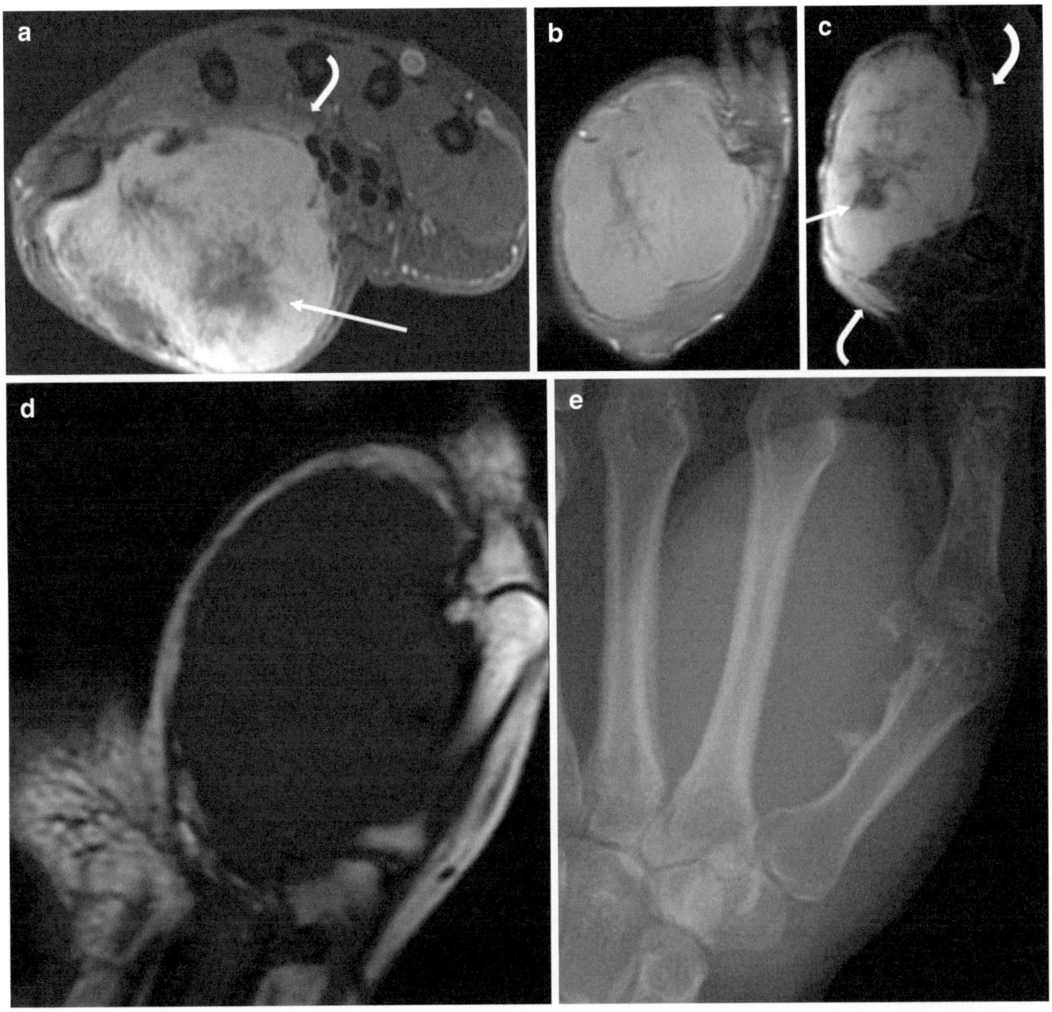

Fig. 13.18 Desmoid tumor. T1FS axial (**a**), sagittal PDFS (**b**), T1 FS post-contrast (**c**), and coronal T1 (**d**) sequences showing a recurrent desmoid tumor occupying the thenar soft tissues. Note the central nonenhancing band (arrows), peripheral tendril-like extensions (curved arrows), and involvement of the flexor tendons just distal to the carpal tunnel. Radiograph (**e**) shows reactive change to the adjacent thumb metacarpal

intrinsic signal on T1 sequences, and homogeneously enhances [51].

Epithelioid sarcoma is a primary soft tissue sarcoma found typically in young males between the ages of 16 and 35 years old. A small case series reviewing the imaging features of epithelioid sarcoma found a variable appearance on MR imaging, although most often showing an irregularly shaped soft tissue mass with predominately T1-hypointense signal with variably heterogeneous or homogeneous hyperintensity on T2-weighted sequences. This case series noted a predilection for regional lymphadenopathy, half of which were found to be metastatic [52].

Osseous Neoplasms

Most osseous neoplastic processes in the hand are benign and discovered incidentally. Radiographic features are often sufficient to make or strongly suggest the diagnosis. MR imaging is the modality of choice for characterizing lesions that are symptomatic, show aggressive radiographic features, or require surgical intervention.

Chondroid Lesions

Enchondromas are benign intramedullary lesions composed of hyaline cartilage and account for approximately 50% of all primary bone lesions in the hand and wrist. Radiographically they occur centrally in the distal metaphyseal region and are a circumscribed lucent lesion. Enchondromas of the hand often lack the ring-and-arc calcified chondroid matrix that is usually present in enchondromas found elsewhere in the body. Enchondromas can occur at any age but are most commonly found between the third and fifth decades. They tend to occur most commonly in the proximal phalanx, followed by the metacarpals and then middle phalanxes of fingers. MR characteristics include multilobular, T2-hyperintense intramedullary lesions with thin peripheral enhancement. Endosteal scalloping is a common feature in the hand, and although scalloping of greater than two-thirds of the cortex is considered an aggressive feature elsewhere in the body, this is commonly found in benign enchondromas of the hand. Chondrosarcoma of the hand is rare and typically manifests as malignant degeneration of multiple enchondromas such as Maffucci and Ollier's syndrome [53]. Maffucci's syndrome can be differentiated from Ollier's syndrome by the presence of multiple slow-flow vascular malformations (Fig. 13.19).

Surface enchondromas are a rare variant and arise from the periosteum rather than the medullary space. These occur in a similar demographic and distribution as intramedullary enchondromas. Other than the location, the MR imaging appearance is typical of enchondromas with lobar T2-hyperintense periosteal mass and scalloping the outer cortex [53].

Osteochondroma

Osteochondromas are benign osseous outgrowths of bone with characteristic cartilage cap and continuity to the intramedullary space (Fig. 13.20a). They can be pedunculated or sessile and typically grow away from the adjacent joint. Most commonly found in the second decade, they are often

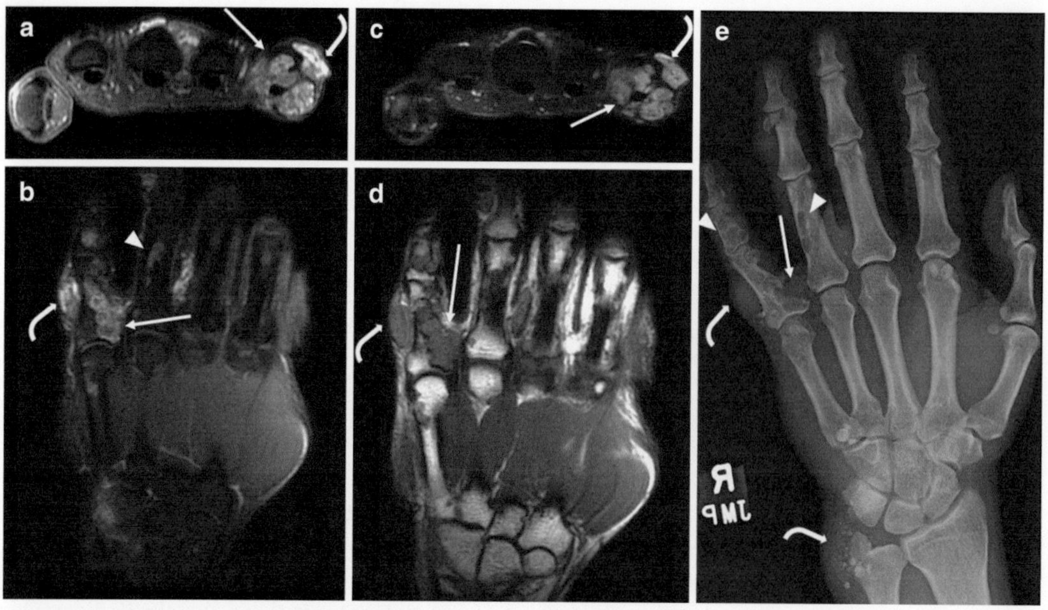

Fig. 13.19 Maffucci's syndrome. Axial (**a**) and coronal (**b**) T1 FS post-contrast, axial T2FS (**c**), and coronal T1 (**d**) sequences of a hand in a patient with history of Maffucci's syndrome. Note the aggressive chondroid lesion with extra-osseous extension along the adjacent flexor tendon (arrows). Corresponding radiograph (**e**) also demonstrates the presence of multiple venolymphatic malformations (curved arrows) and other chondroid lesions (arrow heads) and confirms the diagnosis of Maffucci's syndrome

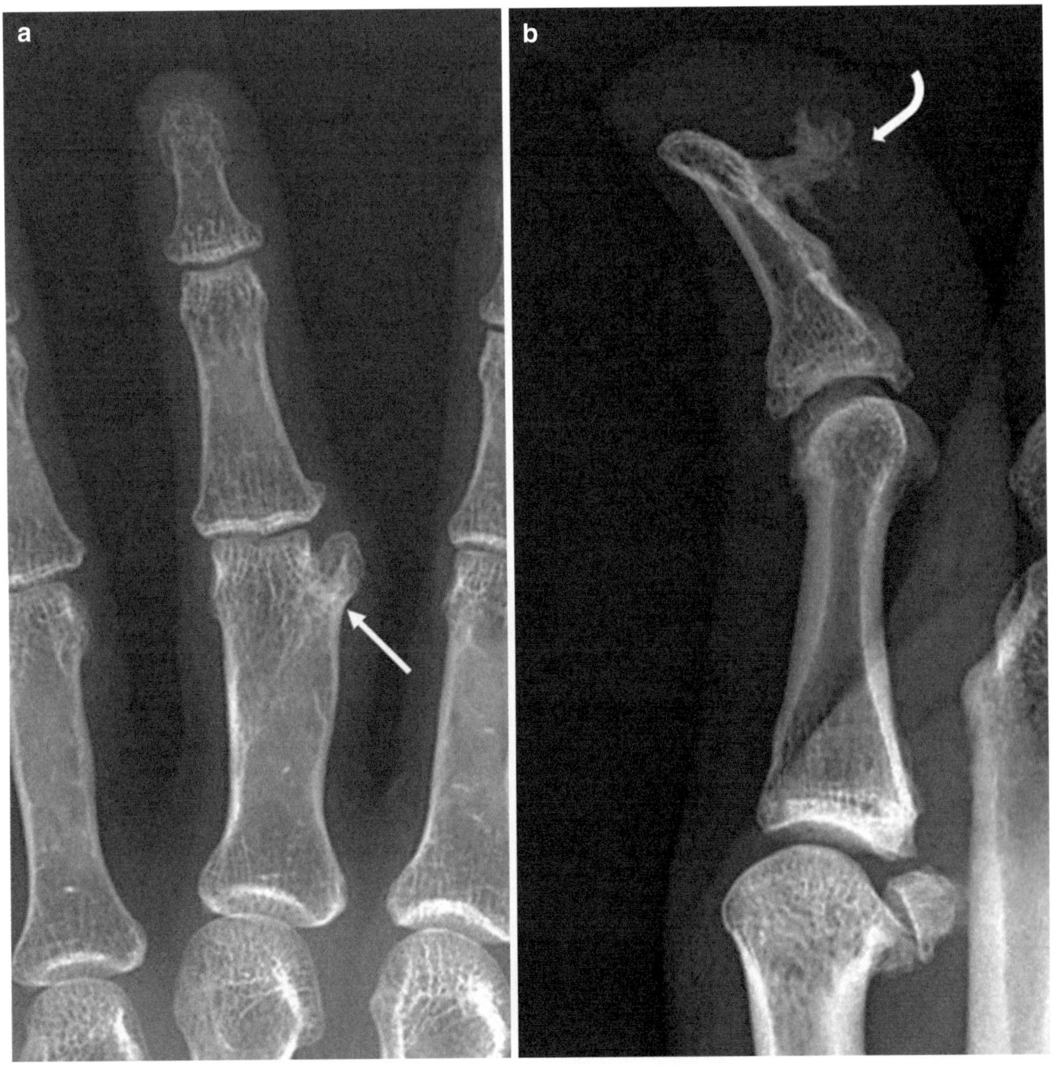

Fig. 13.20 Common benign osseous lesions of the hand. Osteochondroma (**a**) and BPOP (**b**) on radiograph. Note the medullary continuation of the osteochondroma (arrow) versus the absence of medullary continuation in BPOP (curved arrow)

asymptomatic. Osteochondromas have a potential for malignant degeneration to chondrosarcoma, which manifests initially by thickening of the cartilage cap. These lesions are usually painless, although new pain with these lesions should be investigated to rule out malignant degeneration. MR imaging is a useful modality to determine the cause of a newly painful osteochondroma, which can be sequela of malignant degeneration, fracture of the osseous stalk, or development of an adventitious bursitis from friction with the adjacent soft tissues [53].

Bizarre Parosteal Osteochondromatous Proliferation (Nora's Lesion)

Bizarre parosteal osteochondromatous proliferation (BPOP) is a benign entity characterized by the development of a surface-based osteochondral body along the phalanxes or metacarpals of the hand. Its etiology is not well understood, with neoplastic and posttraumatic origins proposed. BPOP is typically found in young patient between 20 and 30 years of age. These osteochondral bodies may be pedunculated or sessile; however, unlike osteochondromas, there is no continuity of the medullary space between the tubular bone and osteochondral body (Fig. 13.20b). MR imaging can be a useful modality to evaluate for this continuity and differentiate BPOP from an osteochondroma if the lesions are sufficient in size [53].

Osteoid Osteoma

Osteoid osteomas are small, cortically based, osteoblastic neoplasms that produce prostaglandins which result in an exquisite inflammatory response. Pain from osteoid osteomas is classically responsive to NSAIDs. On MR imaging, the inflammatory response manifests as marrow and periosteal edema with reactive thickening of the adjacent cortical bone. The diagnosis can be confirmed with MR imaging if the presence of a characteristic T2-hyperintense nidus is detected; however, if too small, CT may be necessary to confirm the diagnosis (Fig. 13.21). Radiofrequency ablation can be used to treat these lesions, although it is not the treatment of choice in the hand given the proximity of vital structures [53].

Aneurysmal Bone Cyst

Aneurysmal bone cysts (ABC) are benign lesions of bone, characterized by a "soap-bubble" appearance of an expansile lytic lesion, located eccentrically in the medullary space. In the hand, these typically occur in the metaphysis of tubular bones. Classically considered the sequela of a reparative process, genetic mutations suggest this lesion could be an immature osteoblastic neoplasm [53, 54]. MR imaging of ABCs reveal expansile, septated, cystic lesions with thin peripheral enhancement. The presence of internal fluid-fluid levels reflecting layering blood within the cyst is a characteristic finding. However, it should be noted that fluid-fluid levels are not unique to ABCs, as aggressive tumors such as giant cell tumor, osteoblastoma, and osteosarcoma can have an admixed ABC component with fluid-fluid levels. Post-contrast sequences should be obtained to confirm the presence or absence of a solid-enhancing component when evaluating a potential ABC.

Giant Cell Tumor of Bone

Giant cell tumor (GCT] of bone is a predominantly benign although locally aggressive osseous neoplasm, accounting for 5% of bone tumors of the hand. GCTs occur in young, skeletally mature patient with the mean age of 22 years old. Radiographically they are expansile lucent

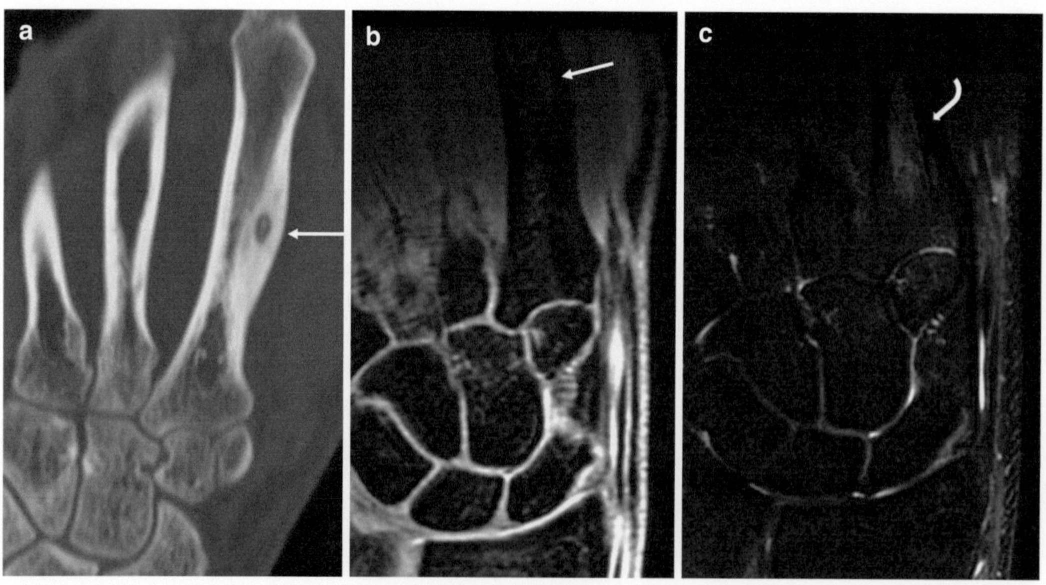

Fig. 13.21 Osteoid osteoma. CT of the index finger metacarpal with associated cortical thickening (**a**). Coronal 3D T2-weighted (**b**) and coronal T2 FS (**c**) MR sequences reveal the hyperintense nidus (arrow) as well as marrow edema of the proximal metacarpal (curved arrow)

lesions with a notable non-sclerotic narrow zone of transition. GCTs occur slightly more often in metacarpals as opposed to phalanxes. On MR imaging, they appear as a T1-hypointense, T2 iso-slight hyperintense, homogeneously enhancing mass (Fig. 13.22). Fluid-fluid levels may be present reflecting a coexisting ABC component. Their locally aggressive nature can be manifested by expansion and extension beyond the cortical bone into the adjacent soft tissues. They are often treated with curettage and cementing of the resection cavity. GCT has the propensity to form pulmonary metastases, and follow-up CT imaging of the chest is recommended [53].

Infectious Conditions of the Hand

The hands are a common site of penetrating trauma and prone to soft tissue infections. Given the superficial nature of the hand's complex communicating anatomy, infections of the hand are prone to spreading beyond the skin and subcutaneous tissues. Contrast-enhanced MR imaging has the ability to characterize soft tissues and delineate inflammatory changes, allowing it to be the ideal modality in assessing the extent of infection in the hand.

Superficial Infections

Cellulitis is an infection of the dermal and subcutaneous tissues and is characterized by the presence of skin thickening and edema which is high signal on T2-weighted, fat-saturated sequences. Edema from fluid overload or hypoalbuminemia can be differentiated from cellulitis with the presence of dermal and subcutaneous enhancement. Infections can progress and convalesce into abscesses, which are best seen as rim-enhancing fluid collections on T1 post-contrast fat-suppressed sequences.

Infections of the fingertips require special attention due to their ability to spread to deep structures. Paronychia is a specific soft tissue infection involving the nail bed. It is important to note the proximity of the nail bed to the distal interphalangeal joint and distal phalanx increases the propensity to advance to osteomyelitis and septic arthritis. Similarly, a "felon" is a term that describes an abscess of the volar pad of a fingertip, often as the result of penetrating trauma. This space is relatively confined with multiple septal divisions, and as pressure from an infection increases, it can spontaneously decompress, possibly deep into the distal phalanx or proximally along the flexor tendon sheath [55].

Deep Space Infections

More aggressive soft tissue infections can extend to the deep fascial tissues and result in a necrotizing soft tissue infection. The hallmark for these infections on imaging is perifascial soft tissue gas, which on MR imaging appears as a signal void on both fluid-sensitive and T1-weighted sequences (Fig. 13.23). MR imaging can be useful in detecting the extension of infection to the superficial and deep fascial structures but ultimately lacks specificity in distinguishing necrotizing fasciitis from other processes. There is a particular difficulty distinguishing necrotizing fasciitis from pyomyositis; however, a comparison of the two processes by Seok et al. determined thin smooth enhancement of the deep and superficial fascia, peripheral band like enhancement of the underlying muscle, and multicompartmental involvement are all findings favoring necrotizing fasciitis, whereas diffuse muscular enhancement, intramuscular abscess, and thick irregular enhancement of the deep and superficial fascial favor pyomyositis [56].

Pyogenic tenosynovitis occurs when bacteria seed and infection spread along the tendon sheaths. It occurs more commonly with flexor tendons rather than extensor tendons. Knowledge of anatomy is important when evaluating infection extent. For example, small finger flexor tendon sheath is contiguous with the flexor tendon sheath at the wrist, predisposing infectious spread from the hand to the wrist and vice versa. Infections of the thumb and small finger can also extend along the radial and ulnar bursa, respectively, and inoculate the flexor tendons at the level of the wrist through the potential space of

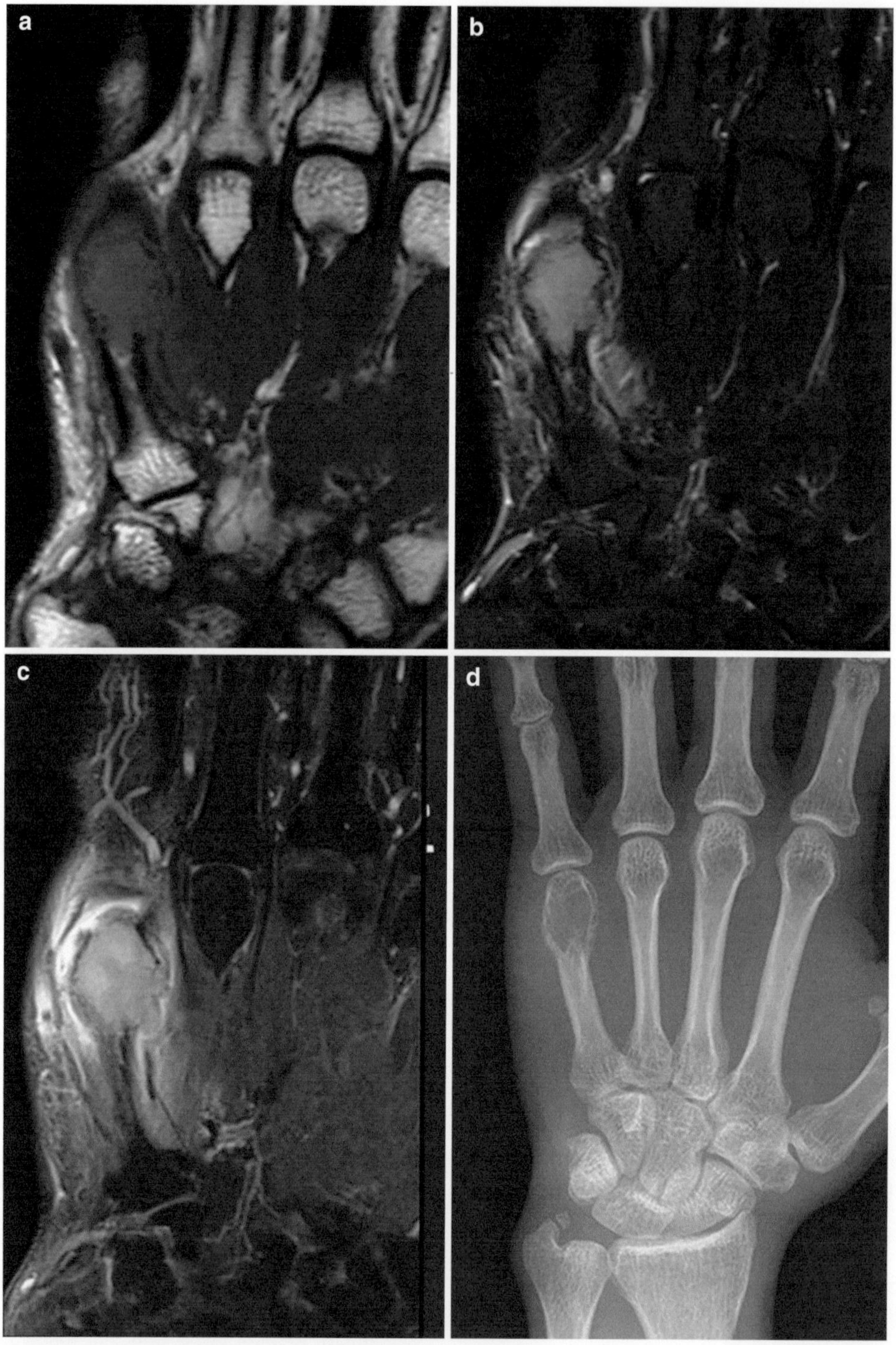

Fig. 13.22 Giant cell tumor of bone. T1 (**a**), T2FS (**b**), and T1FS post-contrast (**c**) coronal sequences showing an expansile, locally aggressive giant cell tumor of bone arising from the small finger metacarpal. Corresponding radiograph shows the typical thin circumscribed non-sclerotic margins (**d**)

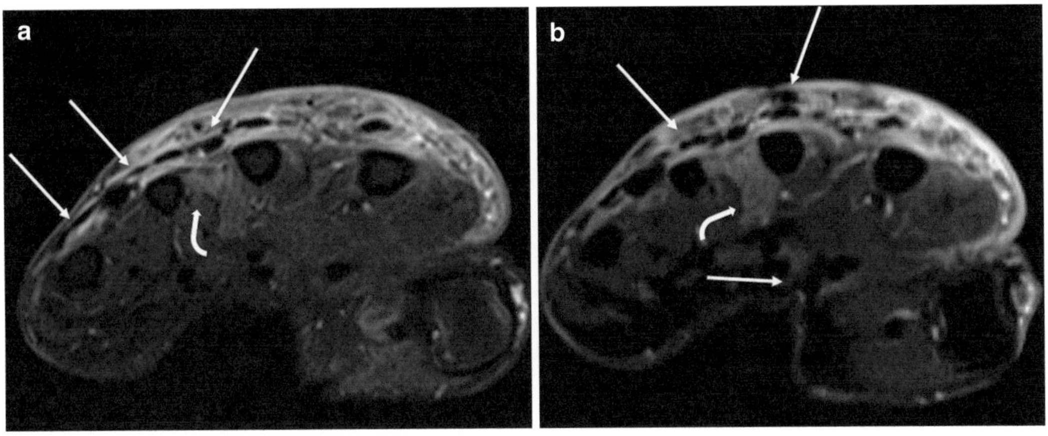

Fig. 13.23 Deep space infection. Axial T1FS post-contrast (**a**) and T2FS (**b**) sequences of the hand in a patient with a necrotizing soft tissue infection following a cat scratch. Note the low signal foci corresponding to soft tissue gas (arrows). Muscular edema and enhancement involve the adjacent lumbricals (curved arrows). Cultures grew polymicrobial organisms including *Pasteurella multocida*

Parona. This creates a classic "horseshoe" distribution of pyogenic tenosynovitis in the hand and wrist. Timely decompression and treatment of pyogenic tenosynovitis are critical as tendons can undergo pressure necrosis and subsequent rupture resulting in substantial functional deficit and morbidity [55].

Septic arthritis and osteomyelitis are not uncommon given the superficial nature of bones and joints comprising the hand. MR imaging findings of bone and joint infection mirror other locations in the body and can be characterized by the presence of joint effusions with marrow edema of the adjacent bone, progressing to cortical erosion and replacement of the normal T1-hyperintense yellow marrow signal.

Chronic Infections

Chronic infection can have a wide range of imaging presentations from soft tissue ulceration, abscesses, sinus tracts, and even mass-like lesions. Chronic osteomyelitis can be a destructive process, elicit sclerosis with reactive bone formation, or a complex combination thereof. This variety of possible presentations poses a diagnostic challenge from an imaging perspective, and the possibility of chronic infection should be considered in lesions without a clear diagnosis [55].

Atypical infectious organisms are frequently a causative agent in chronic infections, especially in immunocompromised patients. Mycobacteria, both tuberculosis and non-tuberculosis, are common pathogens in chronic infections of the hand. Mycobacterial infections of the hand have a predilection for synovium and can cause chronic septic arthritis or tenosynovitis. A characteristic finding of mycobacterial infection on imaging is the presence of "rice bodies," which are composed of fibrinous tissue formed around shed synovial fragments and named for their similar appearance to rice grains on gross examination. Specifically on MR imaging, rice bodies appear as T2-isointense oval foci within a synovial space (Fig. 13.24). While rice bodies can be seen in other inflammatory causes of synovitis, their presence should raise the possibility of mycobacterial infection [57].

Congenital Abnormalities

Numerous congenital abnormalities occur in the hand as manifestations of skeletal dysplasia, systemic syndromes, or in utero insults. Often these

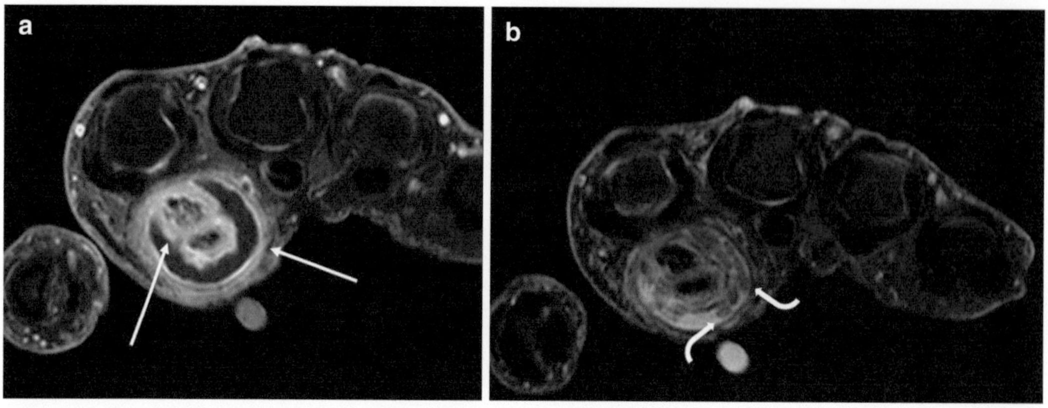

Fig. 13.24 Chronic infection. Axial T1FS post-contrast (**a**) and T2FS (**b**) sequences demonstrating a patient with chronic tenosynovitis from *Mycobacterium tuberculosis*. Note thick peritendinous and tenosynovial enhancement with irregularities of the flexor tendons (arrows) and distension of the tendon sheath with nonenhancing rice bodies (curved arrows)

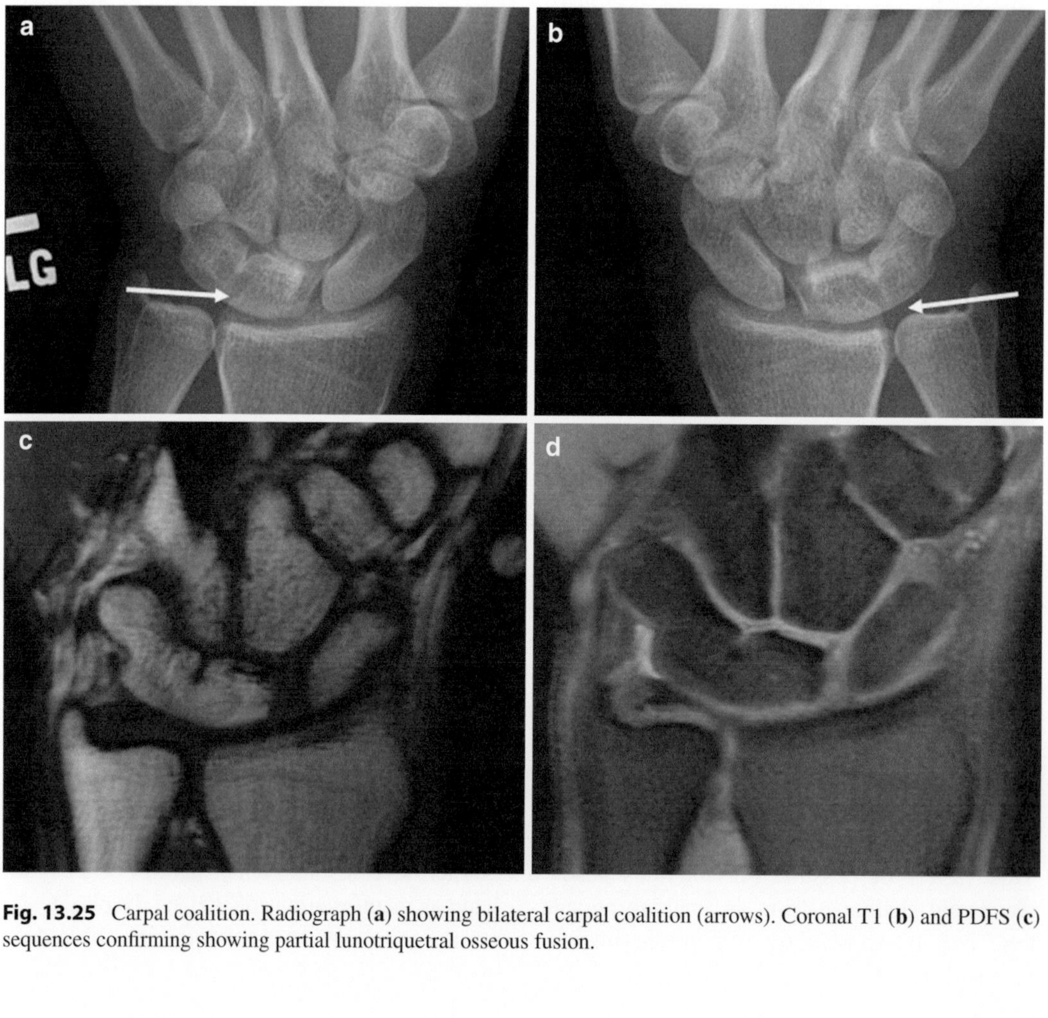

Fig. 13.25 Carpal coalition. Radiograph (**a**) showing bilateral carpal coalition (arrows). Coronal T1 (**b**) and PDFS (**c**) sequences confirming showing partial lunotriquetral osseous fusion.

abnormalities are clinically apparent early in life and characterized by radiography. However, other congenital abnormalities of the hand are less apparent clinically and can be noted incidentally or contributing to more indolent symptoms, presenting later in life.

Coalitions

Carpal coalition is one such example of an incidental or indolent abnormality. Carpal coalition occurs as a congenital or acquired synostosis of the carpal bones. It is estimated to be found in about 0.1% of the population and can be seen in isolation or as part of a syndrome with multiple congenital anomalies [58]. Congenital carpal coalition is thought to be a failure of differentiation during development. A.B. De Villiers Minnaar proposed a classification for lunotriquetral coalition, types 1–4: type 1, fibrocartilage coalition; type 2, partial osseous fusion (Fig. 13.25); type 3, complete osseous fusion; and type 4, complete osseous fusion with other carpal abnormalities present [59].

Carpal Boss

Carpal boss is a loosely defined term describing an osseous prominence dorsally along the capitate at the index and ring finger carpometacarpal joints, also referred to as the quadrangular joint. It is differentiated from an os styloideum by the presence of fusion or partial coalition to the adjacent capitate bone, analogous to the os trigonum and Stieda process of the talus. The exact etiology of carpal bossing is unknown, although a congenital process is a strong possibility given the nature of these lesions [60]. While carpal bossing can be diagnosed with radiography or CT, MR imaging is utilized to assess for bone marrow edema and inflammation or injury to the adjacent soft tissues. These findings allow the interpreter to establish the carpal boss's role in the presenting clinical syndrome (Fig. 13.26).

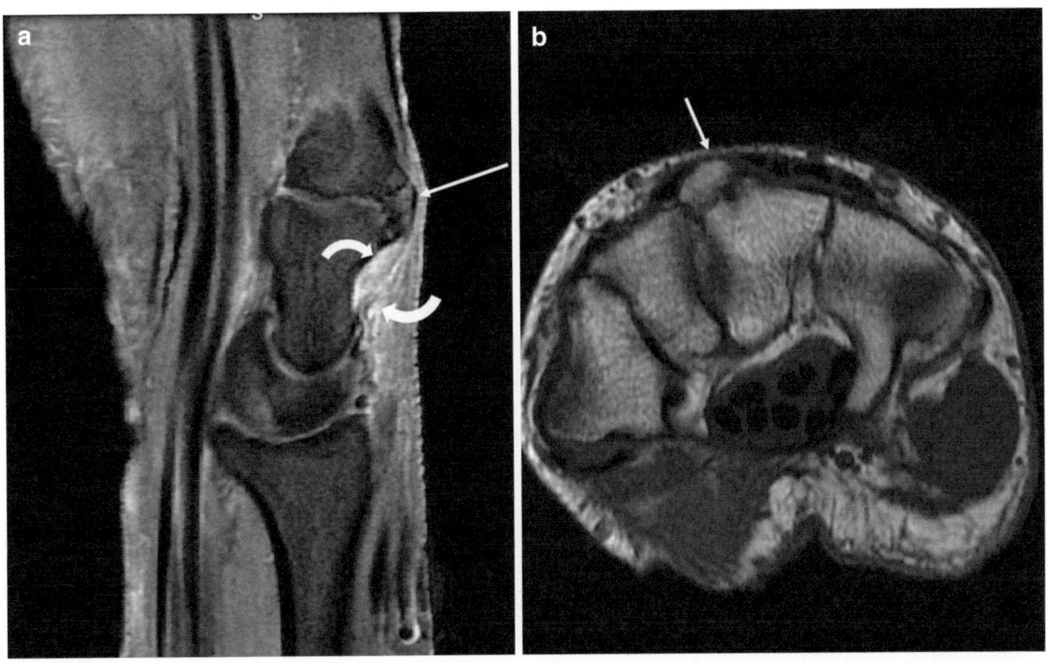

Fig. 13.26 Carpal boss. Sagittal PDFS (**a**) and axial T1 (**b**) MRI sequences of a patient with a symptomatic partially fused carpal boss (arrows). Note the mild adjacent soft tissue edema/inflammation (curved arrows)

References

1. Scott DL, Wolfe F, Huizinga TW. Rheumatoid arthritis. Lancet. 2010;376:1094–108.
2. Doran MF, Pond GR, Crowson CS, O'fallon WM, Gabriel SE. Trends in incidence and mortality in rheumatoid arthritis in Rochester, Minnesota, over a forty-year period. Arthritis Rheum. 2002;46:625–31.
3. Aletaha D, Neogi T, Silman AJ, et al. 2010 Rheumatoid arthritis classification criteria: an American College of Rheumatology/European League Against Rheumatism collaborative initiative. Arthritis Rheum. 2010;62:2569–81.
4. Colebatch AN, Edwards CJ, Østergaard M, et al. EULAR recommendations for the use of imaging of the joints in the clinical management of rheumatoid arthritis. Ann Rheum Dis. 2013;72:804–14.
5. Duer A, Ostergaard M, Horslev-Petersen K, Vallo J. Magnetic resonance imaging and bone scintigraphy in the differential diagnosis of unclassified arthritis. Ann Rheum Dis. 2008;67:48–51.
6. Bugatti S, Manzo A, Caporali R, Montecucco C. Inflammatory lesions in the bone marrow of rheumatoid arthritis patients: a morphological perspective. Arthritis Res Ther. 2012;14:229.
7. Rominger MB, Bernreuter WK, Kenney PJ, Morgan SL, Blackburn WD, Alarcon GS. MR imaging of the hands in early rheumatoid arthritis: preliminary results. Radiographics. 1993;13:37–46.
8. Stomp W, Krabben A, Heijde DVD, Huizinga TWJ, Bloem JL, Østergaard M, Van Der Helm-Van Mil AHM, Reijnierse M. Aiming for a simpler early arthritis MRI protocol: can Gd contrast administration be eliminated? Eur Radiol. 2015;25:1520–7.
9. Ejbjerg B, Narvestad E, Rostrup E, Szkudlarek M, Jacobsen S, Thomsen HS, Østergaard M. Magnetic resonance imaging of wrist and finger joints in healthy subjects occasionally shows changes resembling erosions and synovitis as seen in rheumatoid arthritis. Arthritis Rheum. 2004;50:1097–106.
10. Moll JMH, Haslock I, Macrae IF, Wright V. Associations between ankylosing spondylitis, psoriatic arthritis, Reiter's disease, the intestinal arthropathies, and Behcet's syndrome. Medicine. 1974;53:343–64.
11. Shiraishi M, Fukuda T, Igarashi T, Tokashiki T, Kayama R, Ojiri H. Differentiating rheumatoid and psoriatic arthritis of the hand: multimodality imaging characteristics. Radiographics. 2020;40:1339–54.
12. Drongelen VV, Holoshitz J. Human leukocyte antigen–disease associations in rheumatoid arthritis. Rheum Dis Clin N Am. 2017;43:363–76.
13. Stolwijk C, Boonen A, Tubergen AV, Reveille JD. Epidemiology of spondyloarthritis. Rheum Dis Clin N Am. 2012;38:441–76.
14. Ibrahim G, Waxman R, Helliwell PS. The prevalence of psoriatic arthritis in people with psoriasis. Arthritis Rheum. 2009;61:1373–8.
15. Gianluc AOAC. Subclinical joint involvement in psoriasis: magnetic resonance imaging and X-ray findings. Acta Derm Venereol. 1998;78:463–5.
16. Spira D, Kötter I, Henes J, Kümmerle-Deschner J, Schulze M, Boss A, Horger M. MRI findings in psoriatic arthritis of the hands. Am J Roentgenol. 2010;195:1187–93.
17. Cimmino MA, Parodi M, Zampogna G, Paparo F, Silvestri E, Garlaschi G, Scarpa R. Magnetic resonance imaging of the hand in psoriatic arthritis. J Rheumatol Suppl. 2009;83:39–41.
18. Roddy E, Choi HK. Epidemiology of gout. Rheum Dis Clin N Am. 2014;40:155–75.
19. Swan A. The value of synovial fluid assays in the diagnosis of joint disease: a literature survey. Ann Rheum Dis. 2002;61:493–8.
20. Schlesinger N, Norquist JM, Watson DJ. Serum urate during acute gout. J Rheumatol. 2009;36:1287–9.
21. Girish G, Glazebrook KN, Jacobson JA. Advanced imaging in gout. Am J Roentgenol. 2013;201:515–25.
22. Singh JA, Hodges JS, Toscano JP, Asch SM. Quality of care for gout in the US needs improvement. Arthritis Rheum. 2007;57:822–9.
23. Kohn NN. The significance of calcium phosphate crystals in the synovial fluid of arthritic patients: the "Pseudogout syndrome". Ann Intern Med. 1962;56:738.
24. Macmullan P, Mccarthy G. Treatment and management of pseudogout: insights for the clinician. Ther Adv Musculoskelet Dis. Sage Publishers. 2012;4(2):121–31. https://doi.org/10.1177/1759720X11432559. PMID: 22870500.
25. Ellman MH, Brown NL, Levin B. Prevalence of knee chondrocalcinosis in hospital and clinic patients aged 50 or older. J Am Geriatr Soc. 1981;29(4):189–92. https://doi.org/10.1111/j.1532-5415.1981.tb01764.x.
26. Abhishek A. Calcium pyrophosphate deposition disease. Curr Opin Rheumatol. 2016;28:133–9.
27. Omoumi P, Zufferey P, Malghem J, So A. Imaging in gout and other crystal-related arthropathies. Rheum Dis Clin N Am. 2016;42:621–44.
28. Mccarty DJ, Gatter RA. Recurrent acute inflammation associated with focal apatite crystal deposition. Arthritis Rheum. 1966;9:804–19.
29. Hayes CW, Conway WF. Calcium hydroxyapatite deposition disease. Radiographics. 1990;10:1031–48.
30. Freire V, Guérini H, Campagna R, Moutounet L, Dumontier C, Feydy A, Drapé J-L. Imaging of hand and wrist cysts: a clinical approach. Am J Roentgenol. 2012; https://doi.org/10.2214/ajr.11.8087y.
31. Thornburg LE. Ganglions of the hand and wrist. J Am Acad Orthop Surg. 1999;7:231–8.
32. Hong SH, Chung HW, Choi J-Y, Koh YH, Choi J-A, Kang HS. MRI findings of subcutaneous epidermal cysts: emphasis on the presence of rupture. Am J Roentgenol. 2006;186(4):961–6. https://doi.org/10.2214/ajr.05.0044.

33. Bauer BS, Lewis VL. Carcinoma arising in sebaceous and epidermoid cysts. Ann Plast Surg. 1980;5:222–4.
34. Gupta P, Potti TA, Wuertzer SD, Lenchik L, Pacholke DA. Spectrum of fat-containing soft-tissue masses at MR imaging: the common, the uncommon, the characteristic, and the sometimes confusing. Radiographics. 2016;36:753–66.
35. Calandruccio JH, Jobe MT. Tumors and tumorous conditions of the hand. In: Campbell's operative orthopaedics; 2013. https://doi.org/10.1016/b978-0-323-07243-4.00077-3.
36. Flors L, Leiva-Salinas C, Maged IM, et al. MR imaging of soft-tissue vascular malformations: diagnosis, classification, and therapy follow-up. Radiographics. 2011;31:1321–40.
37. Buetow PC, Kransdorf MJ, Moser RP, Jelinek JS, Berrey BH. Radiologic appearance of intramuscular hemangioma with emphasis on MR imaging. Am J Roentgenol. 1990;154:563–7.
38. Teo E-LHJ, Strouse PJ, Hernandez RJ. MR imaging differentiation of soft-tissue hemangiomas from malignant soft-tissue masses. Am J Roentgenol. 2000;174:1623–8.
39. Pourbagher A, Pourbagher MA, Karan B, Ozkoc G. MRI manifestations of soft-tissue haemangiomas and accompanying reactive bone changes. Br J Radiol. 2011;84:1100–8.
40. Baek HJ, Lee SJ, Cho KH, et al. Subungual tumors: clinicopathologic correlation with US and MR imaging findings. Radiographics. 2010;30:1621–36.
41. Murphey MD, Smith WS, Smith SE, Kransdorf MJ, Temple HT. From the archives of the AFIP. Radiographics. 1999;19:1253–80.
42. Rhodes NG, Murthy NS, Lachman N, Rubin DA. Normal Pacinian corpuscles in the hand: radiology–pathology correlation in a cadaver study. Skelet Radiol. 2019;48:1591–7.
43. Fox MG, Kransdorf MJ, Bancroft LW, Peterson JJ, Flemming DJ. MR imaging of fibroma of the tendon sheath. Am J Roentgenol. 2003;180:1449–53.
44. Murphey MD, Ruble CM, Tyszko SM, Zbojniewicz AM, Potter BK, Miettinen M. Musculoskeletal fibromatoses: radiologic-pathologic correlation. Radiographics. 2009;29:2143–83.
45. Murphey MD, Rhee JH, Lewis RB, Fanburg-Smith JC, Flemming DJ, Walker EA. Pigmented villonodular synovitis: radiologic-pathologic correlation. Radiographics. 2008;28:1493–518.
46. Braschi-Amirfarzan M, Keraliya AR, Krajewski KM, Tirumani SH, Shinagare AB, Hornick JL, Baldini EH, George S, Ramaiya NH, Jagannathan JP. Role of imaging in management of desmoid-type fibromatosis: a primer for radiologists. Radiographics. 2016;36:767–82.
47. Vandevenne JE, Schepper AMD, Beuckeleer LD, Marck EV, Aparisi F, Bloem JL, Erkorkmaz Z, Brijs S. New concepts in understanding evolution of desmoid tumors: MR imaging of 30 lesions. Eur Radiol. 1997;7:1013–9.
48. Tremblay KR, Lea WB, Neilson JC, King DM, Tutton SM. Percutaneous cryoablation for the treatment of extra-abdominal desmoid tumors. J Surg Oncol. 2019;120:366–75.
49. Coyle J, White LM, Dickson B, Ferguson P, Wunder J, Naraghi A. MRI characteristics of nodular fasciitis of the musculoskeletal system. Skelet Radiol. 2013;42:975–82.
50. Bernstein KE, Lattes R. Nodular (Pseudosarcomatous) fasciitis, a nonrecurrent lesion: Clinicopathologic study of 134 cases. Cancer. 1982;49:1668–78.
51. Narváez JA, Martinez S, Dodd LG, Brigman BE. Acral myxoinflammatory fibroblastic sarcomas: MRI findings in four cases. Am J Roentgenol. 2007;188:1302–5.
52. Hanna S, Kaste S, Jenkins J, Hewan-Lowe K, Spence J, Gupta M, Monson D, Fletcher B. Epithelioid sarcoma: clinical, MR imaging and pathologic findings. Skelet Radiol. 2002;31:400–12.
53. Ahmed O, Moore DD, Stacy GS. Imaging diagnosis of solitary tumors of the phalanges and metacarpals of the hand. Am J Roentgenol. 2015;205:106–15.
54. Oliveira AM, Chou MM. USP6-induced neoplasms: the biologic spectrum of aneurysmal bone cyst and nodular fasciitis. Hum Pathol. 2014;45(1):1–11. https://doi.org/10.1016/j.humpath.2013.03.005.
55. Patel DB, Emmanuel NB, Stevanovic MV, et al. Hand infections: anatomy, types and spread of infection, imaging findings, and treatment options. Radiographics. 2014;34(7):1968–86. https://doi.org/10.1148/rg.347130101.
56. Seok JH, Jee W-H, Chun K-A, Kim J-Y, Jung C-K, Kim YR, Eo W-K, Kim Y-S, Chung YG. Necrotizing fasciitis versus pyomyositis: discrimination with using MR imaging. Korean J Radiol. 2009;10:121.
57. Woon CY-L, Phoon E-S, Lee JY-L, Puhaindran ME, Peng Y-P, Teoh L-C. Rice bodies, millet seeds, and melon seeds in tuberculous tenosynovitis of the hand and wrist. Ann Plast Surg. 2011;66:610–7.
58. Spaans AJ, Beumer A. Carpal coalitions; failures of differentiation of the carpus: a description of cases. Open J Radiol. 2013;03:1–6.
59. Minnaar ABD. Congenital fusion of the lunate and triquetral bones in the south African bantu. J Bone Joint Surg. 1952;34-B:45–8.
60. Nevalainen MT, Roedl JB, Morrison WB, Zoga AC. MRI of a painful carpal boss: variations at the extensor carpi radialis brevis insertion and imaging findings in regional traumatic and overuse injuries. Skelet Radiol. 2019;48:1079–85.

Index

A
Accessory ossicles, 154, 155
Acral myxoinflammatory fibroblastic sarcoma (AMFS), 262
Aggressive osseous lesions
  giant cell tumor of the bone (GCTOB), 167, 168
  soft tissue sarcomas, 167
Alveolar rhabdomyosarcoma, 177
Aneurysmal bone cysts (ABC), 266
Annular pulley system, 240, 245
Anterior interosseous nerve (AIN) syndrome
  etiology and clinical presentation, 75
  imaging, 75, 76
  treatment, 75
Anterior oblique ligament sprain, 234

B
Benign neurogenic tumors, 172
Benign PNSTs
  MRI, 175, 176
  neurofibromas, 174
  radiography, 174
  schwannomas, 174
Bennett fracture, 232
Bicipitoradial bursitis, 100, 101
  etiology and clinical presentation, 76–77
  imaging, 77, 78
  treatment, 78
Bizarre parosteal osteochondromatous proliferation (BPOP), 265
Brachialis, 70–73

C
Calcium pyrophosphate dihydrate deposition disease (CPPD), 90, 163–164, 251, 252
Capitellum pseudodefect, 50, 52
Carpal boss, 271
Carpal coalitions, 271
  epidemiology, 151
  imaging features, 151
  lunotriquetral coalition, 152
  MRI, 152
  symptomatic scaphotrapezial coalition, 152
Carpal instability, 141, 142
Carpal tunnel syndrome (CTS), 142–144
  epidemiology, 155
  imaging features, 156
  MRI, 156, 157
Carpometacarpal dislocations, 219, 224
Cat-scratch disease, 101, 102
Chondrosarcoma, 97–99
Circle of Horii, 64
Congenital radial head dislocation, 103
Congenital radioulnar synostosis, 103, 104
Coronoid fractures
  etiology and clinical presentation, 43
  O'Driscoll classification system, 45, 46, 48
  Regan-Morrey classification, 43, 44, 46, 47
  treatment, 46
Cubital tunnel syndrome
  etiology and clinical presentation, 73–74
  imaging, 74
  treatment, 74

D
De Quervain tenosynovitis, 147, 148, 157, 158
Desmoid fibromatosis (DF), 261, 263
Diffuse giant cell tumor of tendon sheath (D-GCTTS), 171, 173
Diffuse idiopathic skeletal hyperostosis (DISH), 92, 93
Digital flexor tendon injuries, 145, 146
Displaced radial collateral ligament avulsion fractures, 215
Distal biceps tendon rupture
  classification/staging, 66
  complete tear, 65, 66
  etiology and clinical presentation, 65
  imaging, 65
  isolated short head biceps rupture, 68
  partial tear, 65–67
  tendinopathy, 67, 68
  treatment, 66
Distal interphalangeal joint dislocations, 218

B. U. Casagranda (ed.), *MRI of the Upper Extremity*, https://doi.org/10.1007/978-3-030-81612-4

Distal intersection syndrome, 158
Distal phalanx enchondroma, 216
Distal triceps tendon rupture
  etiology and clinical presentation, 68–69
  imaging, 69
  treatment, 69
Dorsal intercalated segment instability (DISI), 114
Dorsal intercarpal ligament (DICL) Injury, 141
Dupuytren's disease, 260

E
Elbow
  anatomy, 5
  annular ligament, 18, 19
  anterior compartment muscles, 6, 7
  anterior interosseous nerve, 12
  axis of rotation for flexion/extension, 2
  biceps brachii, 7–9
  brachial artery, 14, 15
  brachialis, 9–11
  brachioradialis, 11
  carrying angle, 2, 3
  common extensor tendon, 15, 16
  coronoid process, 1, 5
  distal humerus joint, 5
  dynamic (active) stabilizers, 1
  flexor carpi radialis, 19
  flexor carpi ulnaris, 19
  flexor digitorum profundus, 21
  flexor digitorum superficialis, 20
  flexor pollicis longus, 21
  Gantzer muscle, 22
  image optimization, 34
  lateral collateral ligaments, 1, 16, 17
  lateral compartment muscles & tendons, 15
  lateral ulnar collateral ligament, 17, 18
  ligaments, 58–64
  medial compartment muscles, 19, 20
  median nerve, 11, 12
  MRI optimization
    axial non-fat saturated imaging, 28
    COR image, 28
    for coronal acquisition, 28
    coronal plane imaging, 29
    MR arthrography, 29, 31, 32
    pre-contrast fat saturated TI-weighted imaging, 29
    routine elbow MRI protocol, 29
    for sagittal imaging, 28, 29
    technical parameters, 30, 31
  musculocutaneous nerve, 14
  osseous and soft tissue structures, 1
  osseous articulations, 5
  osseous stabilizers, 6
  palmaris longus, 21
  posterior compartment muscles
    anconeus, 24–26
    cubital tunnel, 26, 27
    olecranon bursa, 27
    olecranon process, 27
    triceps muscle, 24, 25
    ulnar nerve (C8-T1), 26
  posterior interosseous nerve, 14
  pronator teres, 19, 21
  PRUJ, 1
  radial collateral ligament, 17
  radial nerve, 12, 13
  radiocapitellar joint, 1, 5, 6
  radioulnar joints, 5
  "ring" concept, 1
  ulna joint, 5
  UCL, 1, 22, 23
    anterior bundle, 22–24
    posterior bundle, 22, 24
    transverse/oblique ligament, 23, 24
  ulnohumeral joint, 1, 5
Elbow synovial fold syndrome, 53
Enchondromas, 94, 166
Epithelioid sarcoma, 263
Essex-Lopresti fractures, 37
Ewing sarcoma, 97, 98
Extensor carpi ulnaris (ECU) tendon, 148
Extensor tendon injury
  zone 1, 221
  zone 2, 221
  zone 3, 222
  zone 4, 222
  zone 5, 222
  zone 6, 223
Extra-skeletal chondroma, 177

F
Fall on an outstretched hand (FOOSH) injury, 134
Fibromas of tendon sheath, 260
Fibrous dysplasia, 93–95
Flexor carpi radialis (FCR) tenosynovitis, 146, 147
Flexor carpi ulnaris (FCU) tendinopathy, 146
Flexor digitorum profundus (FDP), 119
Flexor pulley injuries, 226–227
Flexor tendon injuries
  zone 1, 224, 226
  zone 2, 226
  zone 3-5, 226

G
Giant cell tumor (GCT), 266
Giant cell tumor of the bone (GCTOB), 167, 168
Glomus tumors, 258, 259
Gout, 250–252
Gout arthropathy, 88, 89, 163

H
Hamate fractures, 138, 139
Hand
  biomechanics, 183–185
  capsular anatomy, 189, 190
  Carpal boss, 271

Carpal coalition, 271
cellulitis, 267
chronic infection, 269, 270
CPPD, 251, 252
curvatures of radius and ulna, 185
deep space infections, 267, 269
definition, 183
desmoid fibromatosis, 261, 263
digits of, 184
directional grip maneuver, 186
epidermal inclusion cysts, 254, 255
fat containing masses, 255, 256
fibromas of tendon sheath, 260
finger
capsuloligamentous anatomy, 191
extensor and flexor zones, 199, 200
extensor apparatus, 190, 192, 193
flexor apparatus, 194–197
MR imaging optimization, 207–210
vascular and digital nerve anatomy, 196–198
ganglia and synovial cysts, 253, 254
glomus tumors, 258, 259
gout, 250–252
hemangiomas and vascular malformations, 257–258
hook grip maneuver, 186
hydroxyapatite (basic calcium phosphate) deposition disease, 252–253
intrinsic muscles, 190, 192
key pinch maneuver, 186
nodular fasciitis, 262
oppositional pinch maneuver, 186
osseous neoplasms, 263–267
pacinian corpuscles, 199
palmar fibromatosis, 260, 261
pigmented villonodular synovitis (PVNS) and tenosynovitis (PVNTS), 260
PNST, 258–260
power grasp maneuver, 187
precision pinch maneuver, 186
primary soft tissue sarcomas, 262, 263
psoriatic arthritis, 250
rheumatoid arthritis, 247–249
seronegative spondyloarthropathy, 248
soft tissue masses, 253
span grasp maneuver, 187
thumb
CMC joint, 200–202
extensor and flexor zones, 199, 200
IP joint, 203
MCP joint, 201, 203, 204
MR imaging optimization, 207–210
muscle and tendon anatomy, 203–205
pulleys of, 206
vascular and digital nerve anatomy of finger, 199
Hemophilia, 91, 92, 164, 165
Hydroxyapatite (basic calcium phosphate) deposition disease, 252–253
Hydroxyapatite crystal deposition disease (HADD), 90–92

I
Infectious tenosynovitis, 159, 160
Interphalangeal fracture-dislocation injuries, 218
Intersection syndrome, 147, 148
Intra-articular bodies
classification/staging, 55, 56
etiology and clinical presentation, 54
imaging, 54, 55
treatment, 56
Intra-articular tenosynovial giant cell tumor (ITGCT), 95–97
Intraosseous ganglion cysts, 165, 166

K
Kienböck's disease, 116, 137, 138

L
Lateral epicondylitis, 62
Lateral epicondylosis
classification, 71
etiology and clinical presentation, 70–71
imaging, 71
treatment, 72
Lateral ulnar collateral ligament (LUCL)
etiology and clinical presentation, 62–63
imaging, 63, 64
treatment, 63, 64
Lipomas, 169–171
Little League elbow
etiology and clinical presentation, 56
imaging, 57, 58
treatment, 57
Localized giant cell tumor of the tendon sheath (L-GCTTS), 171, 172
Lunate morphologies, 153
Lunotriquetral ligament (LTL), 140

M
Madelung's deformity, 154–156
Maffucci's syndrome, 264
Medial epicondylosis (Common flexor tendinopathy)
etiology and clinical presentation, 72
imaging, 72, 73
treatment, 73
Median nerve schwannoma, 176
Metacarpal fractures, 213
Metacarpophalangeal and interphalangeal dislocations, 217, 219

N
Negative ulnar variance, 116
Neural fibrolipoma, 173–174
Neuropathic arthropathy, 86
Nodular fasciitis, 262

Non traumatic elbow pathologies
bicipitoradial bursitis, 100, 101
cat-scratch disease, 101, 102
chondrosarcoma, 97–99
congenital radial head dislocation, 103
congenital radioulnar synostosis, 103, 104
CPPD, 90
DISH, 92, 93
enchondroma, 94
Ewing sarcoma, 97, 98
fibrous dysplasia, 93–95
gout arthropathy, 88, 89
HADD, 90–92
hemophilia, 91, 92
ITGCT, 95–97
neuropathic arthropathy, 86
olecranon bursitis, 99, 100
osteoarthrosis, 85–86
osteochondroma, 93, 94
osteosarcoma, 96, 97
psoriatic arthritis, 88
rheumatoid arthritis, 86–88
septic arthritis, 101, 102
supracondylar spur, 104, 105
synovial cell sarcoma, 99
synovial chondromatosis, 95, 96

O
Olecranon bursitis, 99, 100
etiology and clinical presentation, 78–79
imaging, 79
treatment, 79
Olecranon fractures
AO classification, 40, 43
Colton classification, 40–42
etiology and clinical presentation, 39–40
Mayo classification, 40, 44
Schatzker classification system, 41, 42, 45
treatment, 42, 43, 45
Oligoarticular psoriatic arthritis, 162
Osborne-Cotterill lesion, 62
Osseous neoplasms
ABC, 266
chondroid lesions, 264
GCT, 266
Nora's Lesion, 265
osteochondromas, 264
osteoid osteomas, 266
Osseous trauma
metacarpal fractures, 213
phalangeal fractures, 214, 216, 218, 219
Osteoarthrosis, 85–86
Osteochondral fractures
coronal shear fractures, 49
diagnosis, 50
long term complications, 50
Osborne-Cotterill lesion, 49–51
physical examination, 50
type 2 (Kocher-Lorenz) coronal shear fracture, 50
Osteochondral lesions
etiology and clinical presentation, 46–47
imaging, 48–50
treatment, 53
Osteochondritis dissecans (OCDs), 46, 47
Osteochondromas, 93, 94, 264
Osteoid osteomas, 166–167, 266
Osteomyelitis, 269
Osteosarcoma, 96, 97

P
Palmar fibromatosis, 260, 261
Panner's disease, 46
etiology and clinical presentation, 56
imaging, 56, 57
treatment, 56
Panner's disease, 46
Peripheral nerve sheath tumors (PNST), 258–260
Phalangeal fractures, 214, 216, 218, 219
Pigmented villonodular synovitis (PVNS), 171–173
Pilon injuries, 218
Positive ulnar variance, 116
Posterior interosseous nerve (PIN) syndrome
etiology and clinical presentation, 75–76
imaging, 76
treatment, 76
Posterolateral rotatory Instability, 63
Primary soft tissue sarcomas, 262, 263
Pronator syndrome
etiology and clinical presentation, 74–75
imaging, 75
treatment, 75
Psoriatic arthritis, 88, 162–163, 250
Pyogenic tenosynovitis, 267

R
Radial collateral ligament injuries, 239
Radial head/neck fractures
etiology and clinical presentation, 37
imaging/classification, 37, 38
Mason classification, 38
treatment, 38, 39
Reverse Bennett fracture, 214
"Reverse Popeye" sign, 65
Rheumatoid arthritis (RA), 86, 88, 161–162, 247–249
Rolando fracture, 233

S
Sagittal band injuries, 240
Scaphoid fractures, 134
Scaphoid non-union, 135–137
Scaphoid nonunion advanced collapse (SNAC), 135
Scapholunate ligament injury, 139, 140
Septic arthritis, 101, 102, 159–161, 269
Seronegative spondyloarthropathy, 248
Sporotrichosis tenosynovitis, 160
Stable scaphoid fracture, 134

Stener lesion, 238
Supracondylar spur, 104, 105
Synovial cell sarcoma, 99
Synovial chondromatosis, 95, 96
Synovial cysts
  clinical course, 168
  epidemiology, 168
  imaging, 169
  MRI, 169, 170
Synovial fringe
  etiology and clinical presentation, 53
  imaging, 53, 54
  treatment, 53, 54
Synovial sarcoma, 177–178

T
Tennis elbow, 62
Thenar motor branch (TMB), 119
Thumb
  annular pulley system, 240, 245
  carpometacarpal Joint, 229–232
  interphalangeal joint, 240, 243
  metacarpophalangeal joint anatomy, 234–237
  osseous and ligamentous injury, 230, 233
  sagittal band injuries, 240
  ulnar collateral ligament injury, 236–240
  volar plate injuries, 240, 242
Traumatic neuromas, 172
Triangular fibrocartilage complex (TFCC), 142, 143
Triquetrum fractures, 139
Trochlear pseudodefect, 52

U
Ulnar collateral ligament (UCL)
  etiology and clinical presentation, 59
  imaging, 59–61
  injury, 236, 238, 239
  repair, 238
  treatment, 61, 62
Ulnar impaction syndrome, 116
Ulnar styloid fractures, 138
Ulnar tunnel syndrome (UTS), 144, 145
Ulnocarpal abutment syndrome, 137
Unstable scaphoid fracture, 135

V
Volar intercalated segment instability (VISI), 114, 140–141
Volar plate avulsion fracture, 222
Volar plate injuries, 240, 242
Volar subluxation, 221

W
Wartenberg syndrome, 145
Wrist
  biomechanics, 109–110
  carpal tunnel, 118–120
  dart throwing motion, 110
  De Quervain tenosynovitis, 147
  digital flexor tendon injuries, 145, 146
  ECU tendon, 148
  extensor retinaculum, 120–123
  extensor tendons, 120
  extrinsic ligaments, 109, 123–125
    dorsal and volar radioulnar ligaments, 127
    ECU subsheath, 129
    meniscal homologue, 128, 129
    radiocarpal ligaments, 124, 127
    TFCC, 127–129
    triangular fibrocartilage disc, 127
    triangular ligament, 127, 128
    ulnar collateral ligament, 129
    volar ulnocarpal ligaments, 129
  FCR tenosynovitis, 146, 147
  FCU tendinopathy, 146
  Guyon's canal, 116–118
  imaging protocols, 129
  intersection syndrome, 147, 148
  intrinsic ligaments, 109, 123–125
    distal interosseous ligaments, 124
    dorsal intercarpal ligaments, 124
    palmar midcarpal ligaments, 124
    proximal interosseous ligaments, 123
  ligament injuries
    capsular ligaments, 141
    carpal instability, 141, 142
    intrinsic/interosseous ligaments, 139
    lunotriquetral ligament, 140
    scapholunate ligament injury, 139, 140
    TFCC, 142, 143
  MR imaging, 133
  movements of freedom, 109
  nerve injuries
    carpal tunnel syndrome, 142–144
    ulnar tunnel syndrome, 144, 145
    Wartenberg syndrome, 145
  osseous anatomy, 113, 114, 116
  osseous injuries
    hamate fractures, 138, 139
    Kienböck's disease, 137, 138
    scaphoid fractures, 133–135
    scaphoid non-union, 135–137
    triquetrum fractures, 139
    ulnar styloid fractures, 138
  radial and ulnar deviation, 110
  range of motion, 110
  T2-weighted images, 133
  three-dimensional rotational movements, 133
  3T system, 133

MIX
Papier aus verantwortungsvollen Quellen
Paper from responsible sources
FSC® C105338

If you have any concerns about our products,
you can contact us on
ProductSafety@springernature.com

In case Publisher is established outside the EU,
the EU authorized representative is:
Springer Nature Customer Service Center GmbH
Europaplatz 3, 69115 Heidelberg, Germany

Printed by Libri Plureos GmbH
in Hamburg, Germany